RADIOLOGY

CASE REVIEW SERIES | **Musculoskeletal Imaging**

Notice

Medicine is an ever-changing science. As new research and clinical experience broaden our knowledge, changes in treatment and drug therapy are required. The authors and the publisher of this work have checked with sources believed to be reliable in their efforts to provide information that is complete and generally in accord with the standards accepted at the time of publication. However, in view of the possibility of human error or changes in medical sciences, neither the authors nor the publisher nor any other party who has been involved in the preparation or publication of this work warrants that the information contained herein is in every respect accurate or complete, and they disclaim all responsibility for any errors or omissions or for the results obtained from use of the information contained in this work. Readers are encouraged to confirm the information contained herein with other sources. For example and in particular, readers are advised to check the product information sheet included in the package of each drug they plan to administer to be certain that the information contained in this work is accurate and that changes have not been made in the recommended dose or in the contraindications for administration. This recommendation is of particular importance in connection with new or infrequently used drugs.

RADIOLOGY

CASE REVIEW SERIES | Musculoskeletal Imaging

Sayed Ali, MD
Associate Professor of Clinical Radiology
Musculoskeletal Radiology Fellowship Program Director
Temple University School of Medicine
Philadelphia, Pennsylvania
USA

Sanjay Patel, MBBS, MRCS, FRCR
Consultant Musculoskeletal Radiologist
Department of Imaging
Royal Derby Hospital
Derby
United Kingdom

Dhiren Shah, MA(Cantab), MRCS, FRCR
Consultant Musculoskeletal Radiologist
North West London Hospitals NHS Trust
London
United Kingdom

SERIES EDITOR

Roland Talanow, MD, PhD
President
Department of Radiology Education
Radiolopolis, a subdivision of InnoMed, LLC
Stateline, Nevada

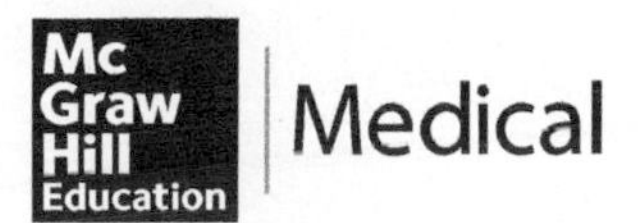

New York Chicago San Francisco Athens London
Madrid Mexico City Milan New Delhi Singapore
Sydney Toronto

Radiology Case Review Series: Musculoskeletal Imaging

7 LKV 23

ISBN 978-0-07-178703-1
MHID 0-07-178703-8

This book was set in Times LT Std. by Thomson Digital.
The editors were Michael Weitz and Regina Y. Brown.
The production supervisor was Richard Ruzycka.
Project management was provided by Shaminder Pal Singh, Thomson Digital.
The cover designer was Anthony Landi.
LSC Communications was the printer and binder.

This book is printed on acid-free paper.

Catalog-in-Publication Data is on file for this title at the Library of Congress.

To my parents and siblings, for their unwavering support.
To my wife Chandra, for her incomparable work ethic.
To my sons Rayhan and Kian, you make it all worthwhile.

—SA

Dedicated to my wife Sonia, and my little stars Kaushal and Anusha.
Without their endless support and encouragement, this dream
would not have been possible. I would also like to thank
my parents Raman and Seeta for their
continuous blessings.

—SP

Dedicated to Maya, Tiana, and Rishaan. Without your patience
and support over the last two years, this ambitious
project would never have come to fruition.

—DS

Contents

Series Preface ix
Preface xi

Easy Cases 1

Moderately Difficult Cases 153

Most Difficult Cases 355

Subject Index 409
Difficulty Level Index 411
Author Index 412
Acknowledgement Index 413

Series Preface

Maybe I have an obsession for cases, but when I was a radiology resident I loved to learn especially from cases, not only because they are short, exciting, and fun—similar to a detective story in which the aim is to get to "the bottom" of the case—but also because, in the end, that's what radiologists are faced with during their daily work. Since medical school, I have been fascinated with learning, not only for my own benefit but also for the sake of teaching others, and I have enjoyed combining my IT skills with my growing knowledge to develop programs that help others in their learning process. Later, during my radiology residency, my passion for case-based learning grew to a level where the idea was born to create a case-based journal: integrating new concepts and technologies that aid in the traditional learning process. Only a few years later, the *Journal of Radiology Case Reports* became an internationally popular and PubMed indexed radiology journal—popular not only because of the interactive features but also because of the case-based approach. This led me to the next step: why not tackle something that I especially admired during my residency but that could be improved—creating a new interactive case-based review series. I imagined a book series that would take into account new developments in teaching and technology and changes in the examination process.

As did most other radiology residents, I loved the traditional case review books, especially for preparation for the boards. These books are quick and fun to read and focus in a condensed way on material that will be examined in the final boards. However, nothing is perfect and these traditional case review books had their own intrinsic flaws. The authors and I have tried to learn from our experience by putting the good things into this new book series but omitting the bad parts and exchanging them with innovative features.

What are the features that distinguish this series from traditional series of review books?

To save space, traditional review books provide two cases on one page. This requires the reader to turn the page to read the answer for the first case but could lead to unintentional "cheating" by seeing also the answer of the second case. Doesn't this defeat the purpose of a review book? From my own authoring experience on the *USMLE Help* book series, it was well appreciated that we avoided such accidental cheating by separating one case from the other. Taking the positive experience from that book series, we decided that each case in this series should consist of two pages: page 1 with images and questions and page 2 with the answers and explanations. This approach avoids unintentional peeking at the answers before deciding on the correct answers yourself. We keep it strict: one case per page! This way it remains up to your own knowledge to figure out the right answer.

Another example that residents (including me) did miss in traditional case review books is that these books did not highlight the pertinent findings on the images: sometimes, even looking at the images as a group of residents, we could not find the abnormality. This is not only frustrating but also time consuming. When you prepare for the boards, you want to use your time as efficiently as possible. Why not show annotated images? We tackled that challenge by providing, on the second page of each case, the same images with annotations or additional images that highlight the findings.

When you are preparing for the boards and managing your clinical duties, time is a luxury that becomes even more precious. Does the resident preparing for the boards truly need lengthy discussions as in a typical textbook? Or does the resident rather want a "rapid fire" mode in which he or she can "fly" through as many cases as possible in the shortest possible time? This is the reality when you start your work after the boards! Part of our concept with the new series is providing short "pearls" instead of lengthy discussions. The reader can easily read and memorize these "pearls."

Another challenge in traditional books is that questions are asked on the first page and no direct answer is provided, only a lengthy block of discussion. Again, this might become time consuming to find the right spot where the answer is located if you have doubts about one of several answer choices. Remember: time is money—and life! Therefore, we decided to provide explanations to *each* individual question, so that the reader knows exactly where to find the right answer to the right question. Questions are phrased in an intuitive way so that they fit not only the print version but also the multiple-choice questions for that particular case in our online version. This system enables you to move back and forth between the print version and the online version.

In addition, we have provided up to 3 references for each case. This case review is not intended to replace traditional textbooks. Instead, it is intended to reiterate and strengthen your already existing knowledge (from your training) and to fill potential gaps in your knowledge.

However, in a collaborative effort with the *Journal of Radiology Case Reports* and the international radiology community Radiolopolis, we have developed an online repository with more comprehensive information for each case, such as demographics, discussions, more image examples, interactive image stacks with scroll, a window/level feature, and other interactive features that almost resemble a workstation. In addition, we are planning ahead toward the new Radiology Boards format and are providing rapid fire online sessions and mock examinations that use the cases in the print version. Each case in the print version is crosslinked to the online version using a case ID. The case ID number appears to the right of the diagnosis heading at the top of the second page of each case. Each case can be accessed using the case ID number at the following web site: www.radiologycasereviews.com/case/ID, in which "ID" represents the case ID number. If you have any questions regarding this web site, please e-mail the series editor directly at roland@talanow.info.

I am particularly proud of such a symbiotic endeavor of print and interactive online education and I am grateful to McGraw-Hill for giving me and the authors the opportunity to provide such a unique and innovative method of radiology education, which, in my opinion, may be a trendsetter.

The primary audience of this book series is the radiology resident, particularly the resident in the final year who is preparing for the radiology boards. However, each book in this series is structured on difficulty levels so that the series also becomes useful to an audience with limited experience in radiology (nonradiologist physicians or medical students) up to subspecialty-trained radiologists who are preparing for their CAQs or who just want to refresh their knowledge and use this series as a reference.

I am delighted to have such an excellent team of US and international educators as authors on this innovative book series. These authors have been thoroughly evaluated and selected based on their excellent contributions to the *Journal of Radiology Case Reports*, the Radiolopolis community, and other academic and scientific accomplishments.

It brings especially personal satisfaction to me that this project has enabled each author to be involved in the overall decision-making process and improvements regarding the print and online content. This makes each participant not only an author but also part of a great radiology product that will appeal to many readers.

Finally, I hope you will experience this case review book as it is intended to be: a quick, pertinent, "get to the point" radiology case review that provides essential information for the radiology boards in the shortest time available, which, in the end, is crucial for preparation for the boards.

Roland Talanow, MD, PhD

Preface

The whole purpose of education is to turn mirrors into windows.
—Sydney J. Harris

Musculoskeletal radiology has inspired great joy and fear amongst radiology trainees, who are excited by the varied pathology inherent in this discipline, but also somewhat apprehensive of its complexity.

We are fortunate to have the current imaging armamentarium at our disposal, but could you imagine the musculoskeletal radiologist of a past generation, making diagnoses solely on plain films? They were the real detectives, hunting for the most subtle of findings that would probably elude most of us currently in practice! We therefore owe them tremendous respect, because they have taught us that we should follow a stepwise approach to our specialty, and that often times a careful review of the radiograph is all that is needed.

The goal of this book is to provide quick and simple explanations of increasingly complex cases, and to slowly change that apprehension into a quiet understanding that somehow, somewhere there is an answer, or at the least, a logical explanation.

This book is for all radiology trainees, and their lifelong quest for knowledge.

SA, SP, DS

Ankle and leg pain following trauma

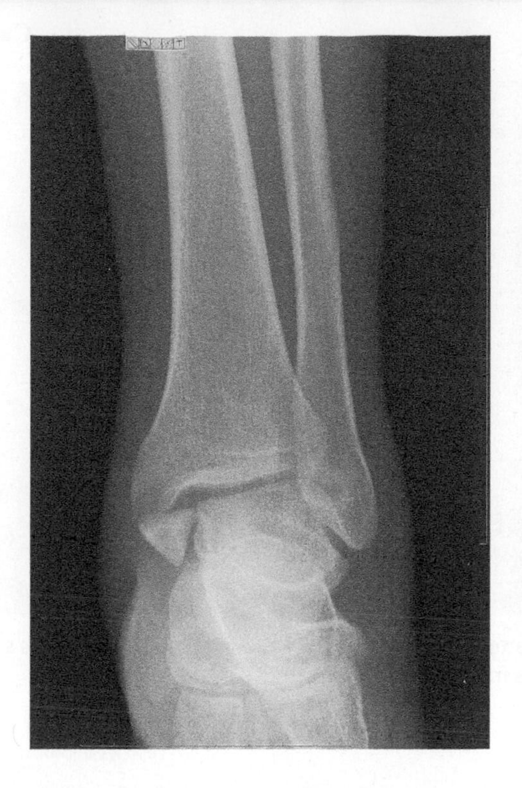

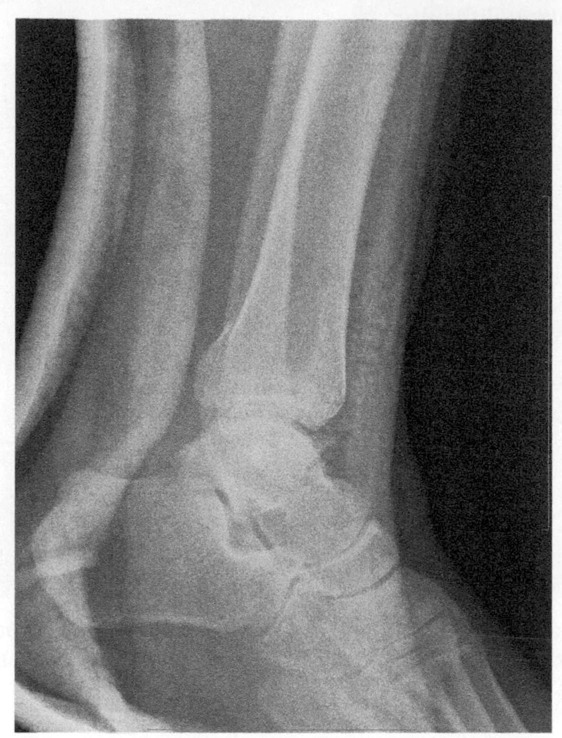

1. What are the findings?

2. What is the next most appropriate study?

3. What is the proposed mechanism of injury, using the Lauge Hansen classification?

4. What is the best method of assessing the stability of this injury?

5. What is the treatment?

Maisonneuve fracture 1362

Case ranking/difficulty: 

Category: Trauma

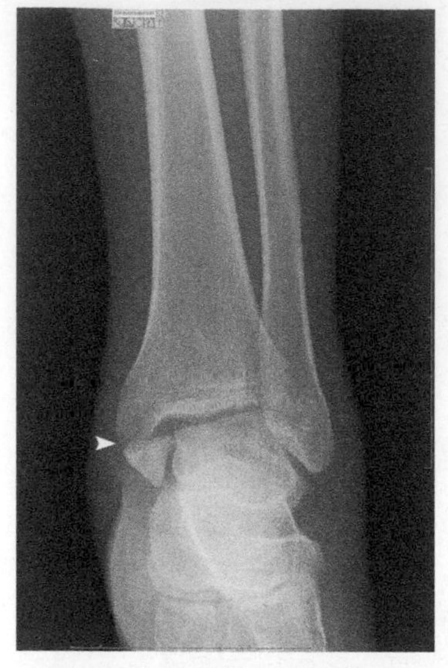

Transverse displaced medial malleolus fracture.

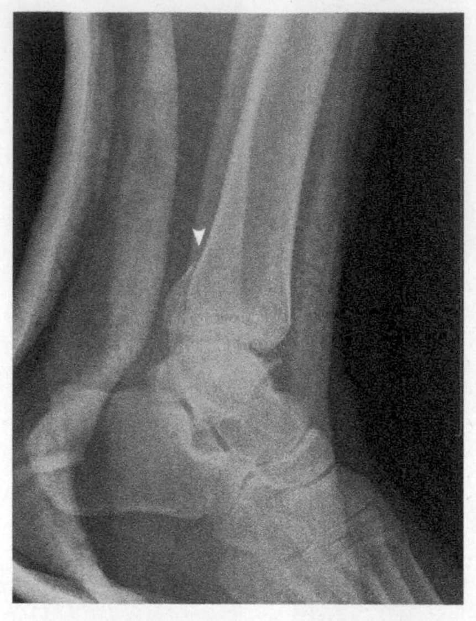

Postsplinting image better demonstrates the posterior malleolus fracture.

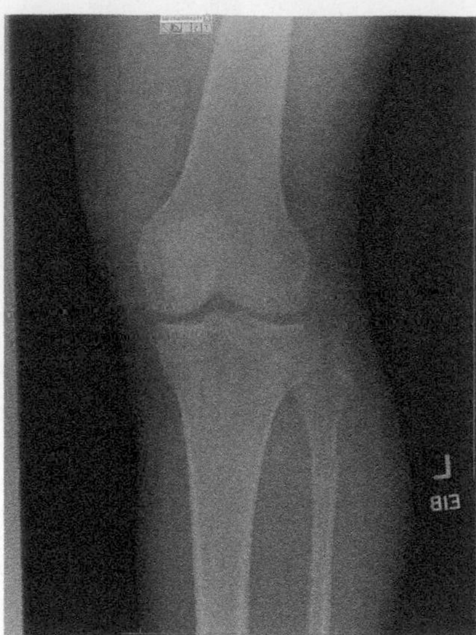

High fibula fracture is seen.

Answers

1. There is a displaced medial malleolus fracture, and a minimally displaced posterior malleolus fracture. The syndesmotic space does not appear widened.
2. A tibia-fibula film is needed to exclude a Maisonneuve fracture. Stress views may also be useful, but examination under anesthesia to assess stability is usually indicated.
3. Pronation-external rotation is the usual mechanism of injury.
4. Examination under anesthesia is the best way to assess for stability.
5. A long leg cast is suitable for stable Maisonneuve injuries, and open reduction and internal fixation (ORIF) with syndesmotic screws for unstable injuries. The proximal fibula fracture is not usually fixed.

Pearls

- The distal tibia, fibula, and talus along with the collateral and syndesmotic ligaments form a fibro-osseous ring.
- Disruption of one portion of the ring warrants exclusion of a fracture on the other side of the ring. In a Maisonneuve fracture, that fracture is a high fibula fracture.
- The interosseous membrane is injured as the forces are transmitted up to the proximal fibula.
- Instability is caused by the interosseous membrane rupture.
- The mechanism of this injury is pronation-external rotation.
- Management depends on the stability of the injury. The fibula fracture is not surgically corrected, but the interosseous membrane rupture may need to be.

Suggested Readings

Hanson JA, Fotoohi M, Wilson AJ. Maisonneuve fracture of the fibula: implications for imaging ankle injury. *AJR Am J Roentgenol.* 1999;173(3):702.

Wilson FC. Fractures of the ankle: pathogenesis and treatment. *J South Orthop Assoc.* 2000;9(2):105-115.

Pain and clicking in the shoulder after recurrent dislocation

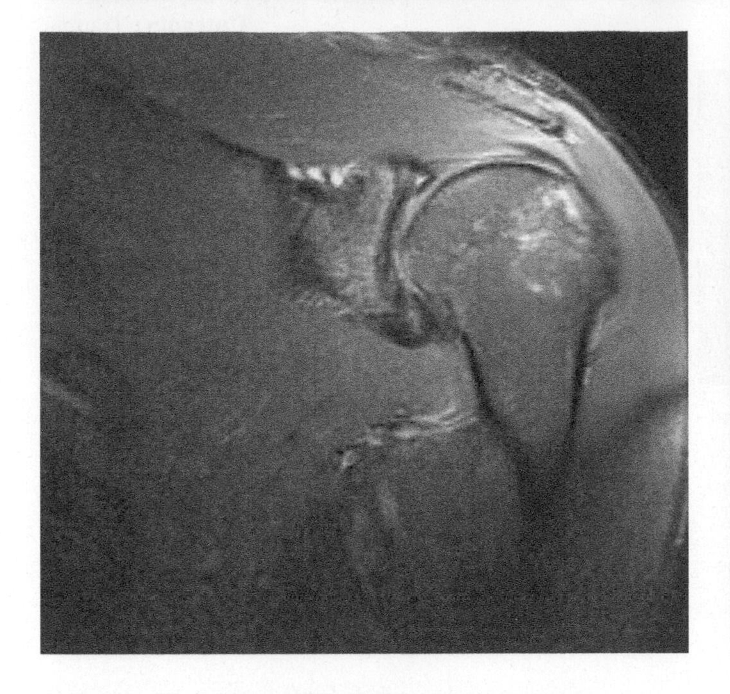

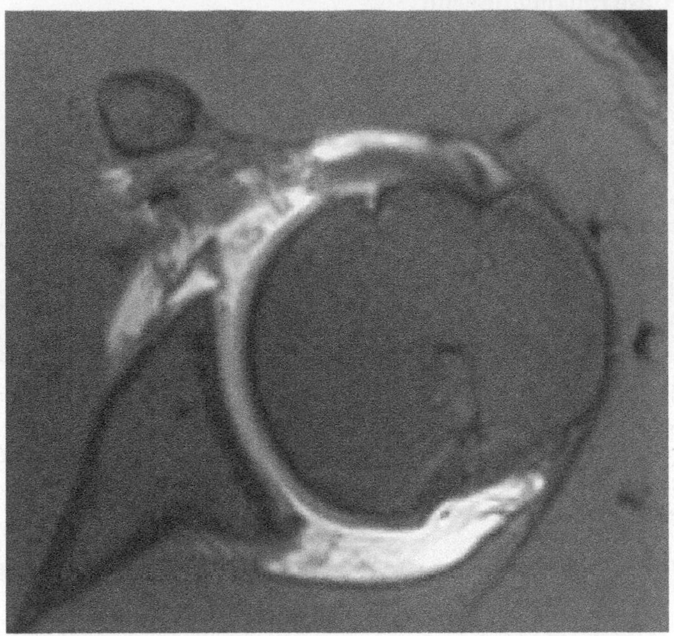

1. What are the characteristic MRI features of this entity?
2. What structures should be evaluated on MRI if this diagnosis is suspected?
3. What percentage of cases of this entity occurs in the direction that this injury was sustained?
4. What is a SLAP lesion?
5. What structures are at risk of damage in the acute presentation?

Hill-sachs defect (anterior dislocation of the shoulder) 526

Case ranking/difficulty: **Category:** Trauma

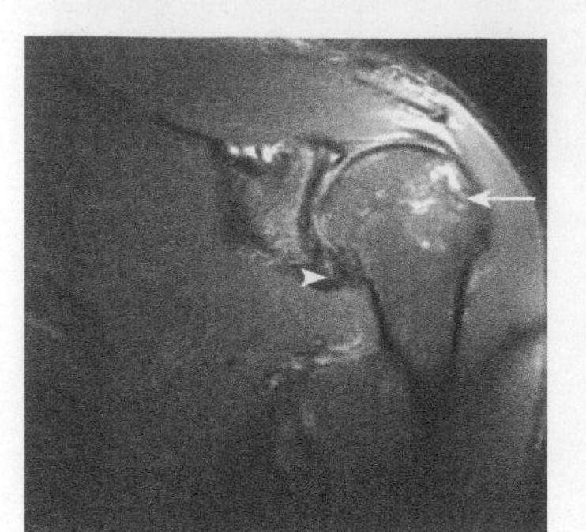

Hill-Sachs defect in posterolateral humeral head (*arrow*). Cleft in inferior labrum is seen consistent with a Bankart lesion (*arrowhead*).

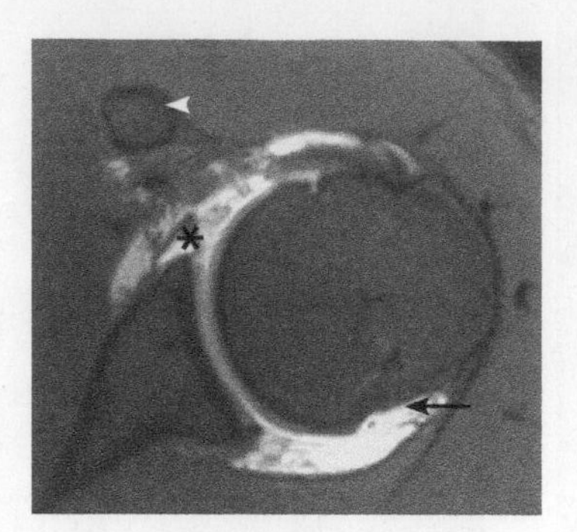

Contour abnormality of humeral head is best appreciated on axial images (*arrow*). This must be high (at or above the level of the coracoid—*arrowhead*). There is extensive tearing of the anterior labrum, from the level of the inferior Bankart lesion, extending more superiorly as shown here (*asterisk*).

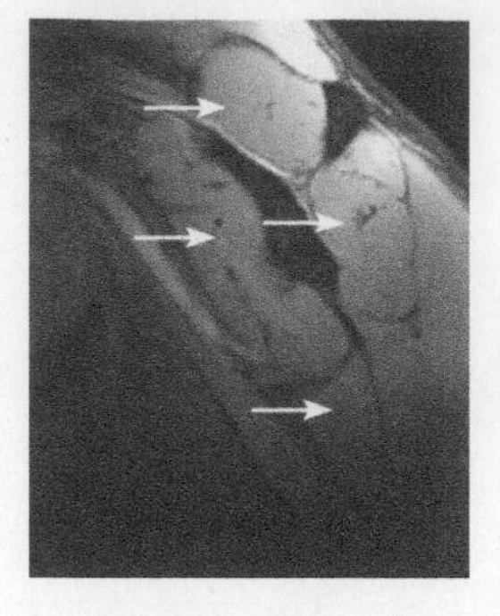

Sagittal images confirm integrity of rotator cuff muscle bulk with no denervation edema or fatty atrophy.

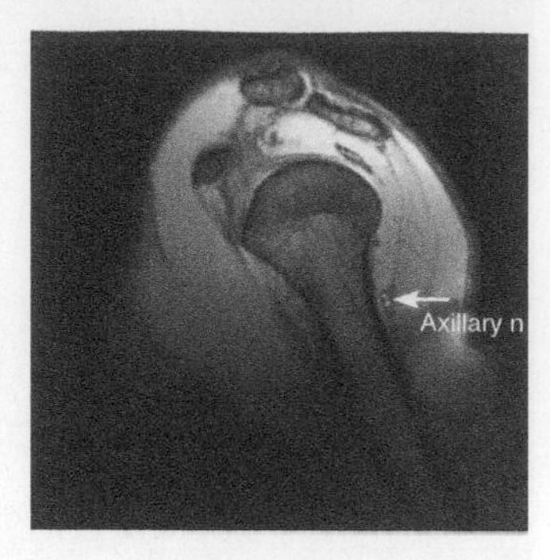

The coracoacromial arch, AC joint, and axillary neurovascular bundle are not damaged. The latter, in particular, is at risk of injury acutely with anterior dislocations.

Answers

1. Bankart lesions are highly specific and sensitive findings for previous anterior dislocation. A Hill-Sachs lesion is an impaction fracture of the posterolateral humeral head. A reverse Hill-Sachs lesion is a feature of posterior dislocation. Greater tuberosity fractures are also associated with anterior dislocation.
2. Careful inspection of the glenoid labrum is important to assess for Bankart lesions, in addition to bony Bankart fractures. The axillary nerve is particularly vulnerable from anterior inferior dislocation, and rotator cuff atrophy may be seen in late (missed) presentations as a result of nerve damage.
3. The vast majority of shoulder dislocations are anteroinferior (95%).

   Only 5% are posterior.
4. A SLAP lesion is a superior labral tear (anterior to posterior), which often is related to overhead throwing movements, for example, in athletics/baseball. It can also be seen in the context of a large anteroinferior tear (Bankart), which extends superiorly to the level of the biceps anchor.
5. The axillary neurovascular bundle is at direct risk from anterior dislocation, and its integrity must be confirmed clinically prior to reduction.

Pearls

- Anterior dislocations are very common, making up 95% of all glenohumeral dislocations.
- Hill-Sachs defects and Bankart lesions should be routinely evaluated in shoulder examinations, as they are highly specific for previous anterior dislocation.
- Routine imaging evaluation post dislocation should include assessment of the rotator cuff integrity, presence of a bony Bankart fracture, and evidence of labroligamentous injury.
- MR or CT arthrography are the investigations of choice post dislocation. MR has the advantage of assessing associated soft-tissue structures, for example, rotator cuff tendons and muscles.
- Specific imaging features of interest to the surgeon are (a) size of Hill-Sachs defect, (b) presence and size of a bony Bankart fracture in terms of percent of glenoid diameter fractured, (c) status of entire labrum, (d) integrity of rotator cuff, and (e) presence of intra-articular "loose" bodies.
- Presence of both Hill-Sachs plus reverse Hill-Sachs lesions and corresponding Bankart plus reverse Bankart lesions is suggestive of multidirectional instability.

Suggested Readings

Farin PU, Kaukanen E, Jaroma H, Harju A, Väätäinen U. Hill-Sachs lesion: sonographic detection. *Skeletal Radiol.* 1996;25(6):559-562.

Hendey GW, Kinlaw K. Clinically significant abnormalities in postreduction radiographs after anterior shoulder dislocation. *Ann Emerg Med.* 1996;28(4):399-402.

Imhoff AB, Hodler J. Correlation of MR imaging, CT arthrography, and arthroscopy of the shoulder. *Bull Hosp Jt Dis.* 1996;54(3):146-152.

Fall from a bridge

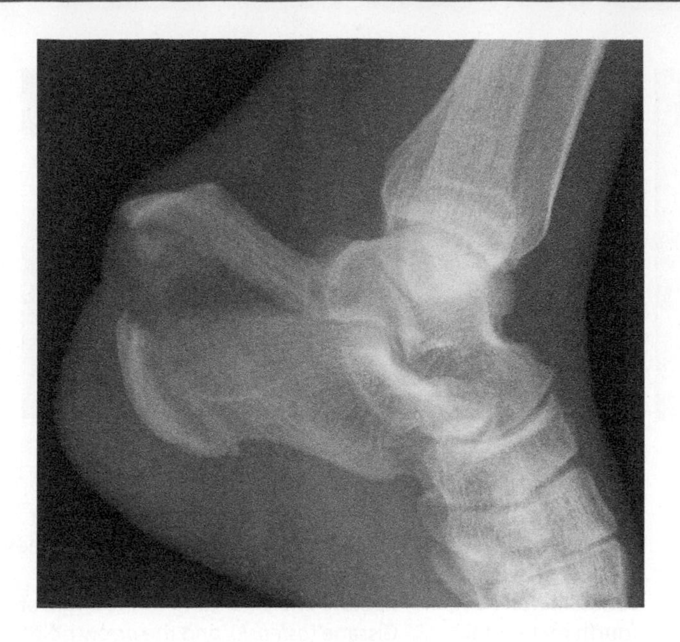

1. What type of calcaneal fracture is demonstrated?

2. What is the mechanism of injury?

3. How often are these fractures bilateral?

4. What is the change in Böhler angle in depressed calcaneal fractures?

5. What are the associated findings in this injury?

Calcaneus fracture: tongue type 2328

Case ranking/difficulty: 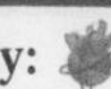 **Category:** Trauma

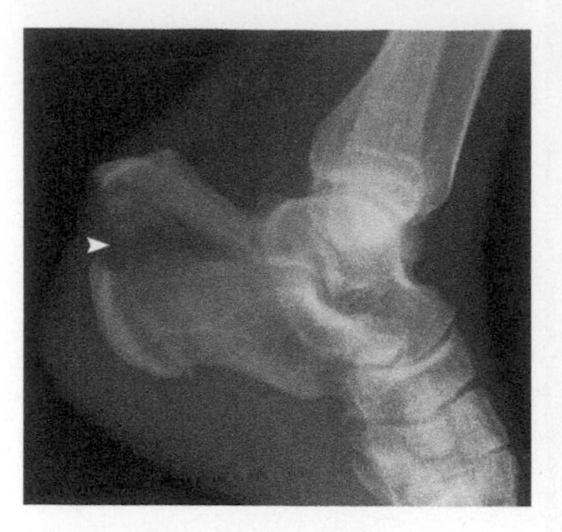

Intra-articular "tongue"-type calcaneus fracture. The secondary fracture line (*arrowhead*) is well depicted here, but the primary fracture line was only seen on CT.

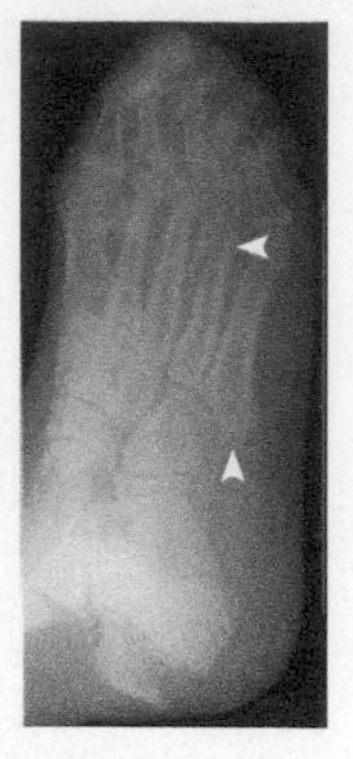

Different patient. Other tarsal fractures are common; in this case, a fifth metatarsal avulsion (pseudo-Jones fracture) and fourth metatarsal shaft fracture.

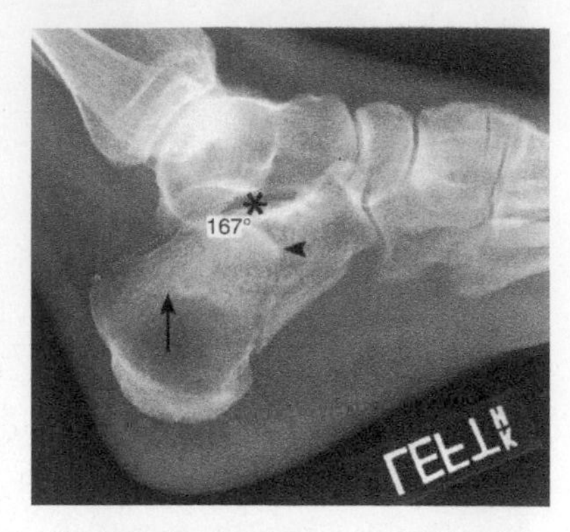

Different patient. Comminuted joint depression intra-articular calcaneus fracture, with flattening of the Böhler angle, which now measures 13 degrees. *Arrowhead* points to the primary fracture line extending to the angle of Gissane (*asterisk*), and the *arrow* points to the secondary fracture line.

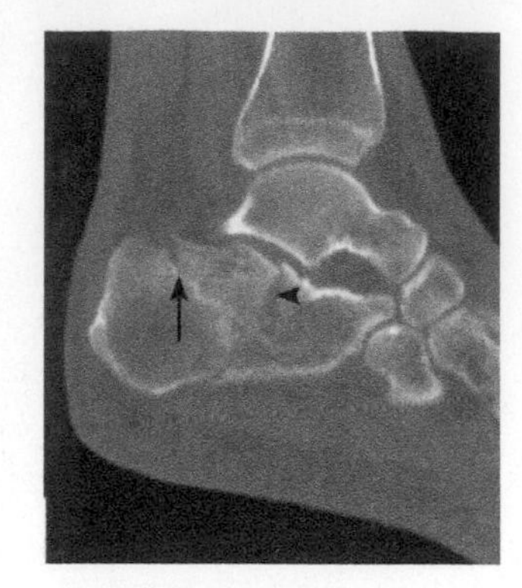

Joint depression type of fracture. *Arrowhead* points to the primary fracture line extending to the angle of Gissane, and the *arrow* points to the secondary fracture line.

Answers

1. There is a markedly displaced horizontal fracture of the calcaneus, known as a "tongue" fracture.
   These fractures, and the more common joint depression type, are intra-articular fractures.
2. Intra-articular calcaneal fractures, both the tongue and joint depression types, are a result of high-velocity axial loading, including from parachuting and falls from a height (usually greater than 6 feet).
3. Intra-articular calcaneal fractures are bilateral in 5% to 10% of injuries.
4. The Böhler angle is measured from the anterior calcaneal process to the peak of the articular facet, and from there to the peak of the posterior tuberosity. The normal angle is 20 to 40 degrees; in depressed calcaneal fractures, that angle is less than 20 degrees.
5. The high axial loading forces can result in thoracic or lumbar compression fractures, and bilateral fractures in 10% of injuries. Pilon fractures and other tarsal fractures may occur. Soft-tissue injuries include peroneal tendon dislocation, neurovascular injuries, and flexor hallucis tendon entrapment. A compartment syndrome may occur in up to 10% of injuries.

Pearls

- Calcaneal fractures are the most common tarsal bone fractures.
- Of all adult fractures, 2% are of the calcaneus. Of these, 10% are bilateral.
- The typical mechanism is axial loading.
- Seventy-five percent of fractures are intra-articular, the majority of which are joint depression type and, less commonly, the tongue type.
- The primary fracture line starts at the angle of Gissane and exits posteromedially.
- The secondary fracture line determines the type of fracture: in the tongue type, it exits posteriorly and produces a split in the calcaneus, often displaced by the traction of the Achilles tendon.
- In the joint depression type, the secondary fracture line starts posteriorly then exits dorsally just posterior to the posterior articular facet. Radiographically, the Böhler angle is reduced from the normal 20- to 40-degree angle in a joint depression type.
- The Sanders classification is used on CT scanning to further define the anatomy.
- A "beak" fracture is a calcaneal tuberosity avulsion fracture that will cause pressure erosion of the skin and conversion to an open fracture.
- Extra-articular fractures are much less common, and most commonly involve the calcaneal body, followed by the anterior calcaneal process. The latter fracture is the only calcaneus fracture that is more common in women.

Suggested Readings

Badillo K, Pacheco JA, Padua SO, Gomez AA, Colon E, Vidal JA. Multidetector CT evaluation of calcaneal fractures. *Radiographics.* 2011;31(1):81-92.

Daftary A, Haims AH, Baumgaertner MR. Fractures of the calcaneus: a review with emphasis on CT. *Radiographics.* 2005;25(5):1215-1226.

25-year-old runner presenting with severe left hip pain

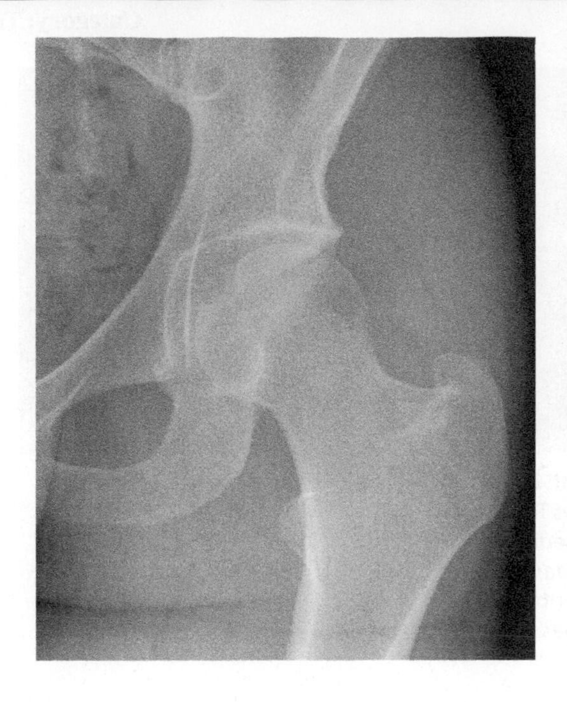

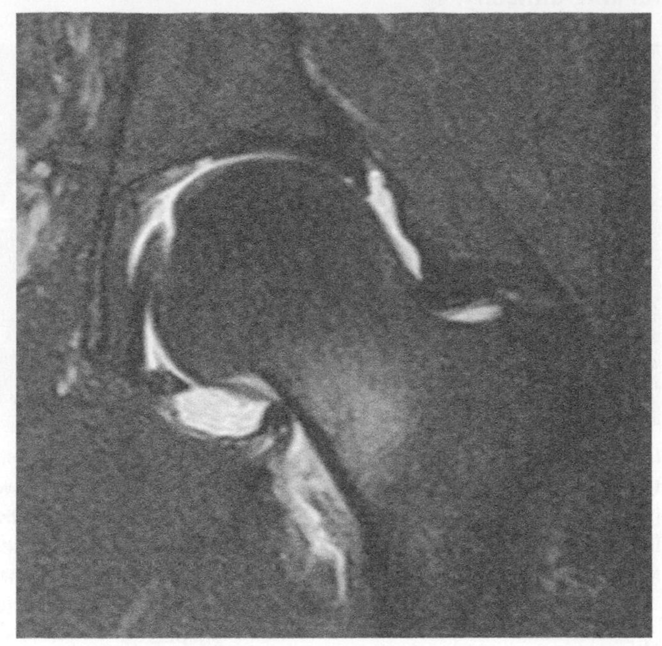

1. What are the radiographic findings?
2. What is the next most appropriate study?
3. What is the differential, and the most likely diagnosis?
4. What are the types of this condition, and which has the best prognosis?
5. What is the management for this condition?

Femoral neck stress fracture 1384

Case ranking/difficulty:

Category: Trauma

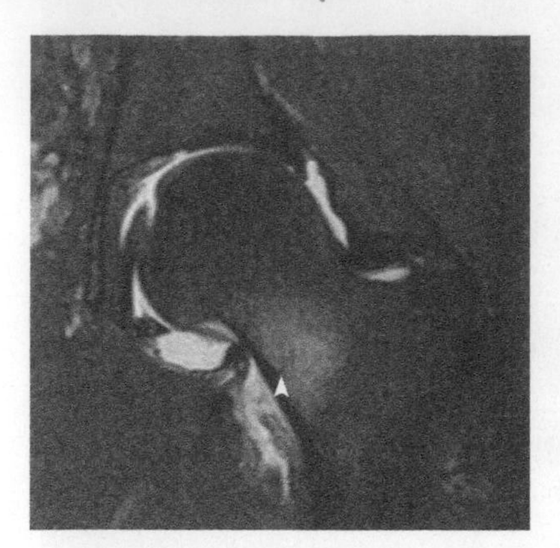

Intense bone marrow edema in the medial femoral neck with an incomplete T2 hypointense fracture line abutting the medial cortex (*arrowhead*).

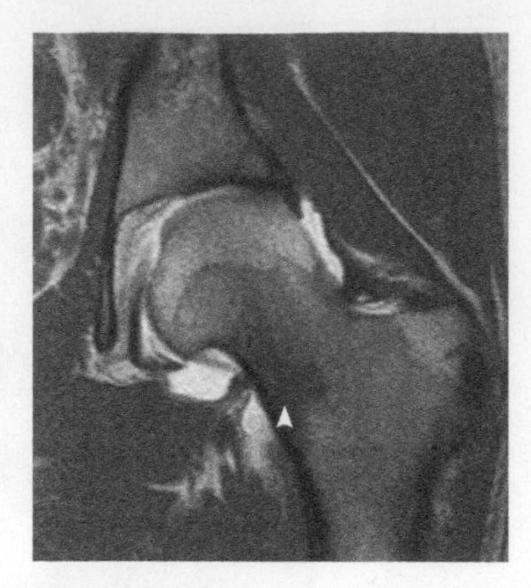

T1-weighted image with intra-articular contrast shows T1 hypointensity in the medial femoral neck (*arrowhead*). An MR arthrogram was performed because a labral tear was initially suspected.

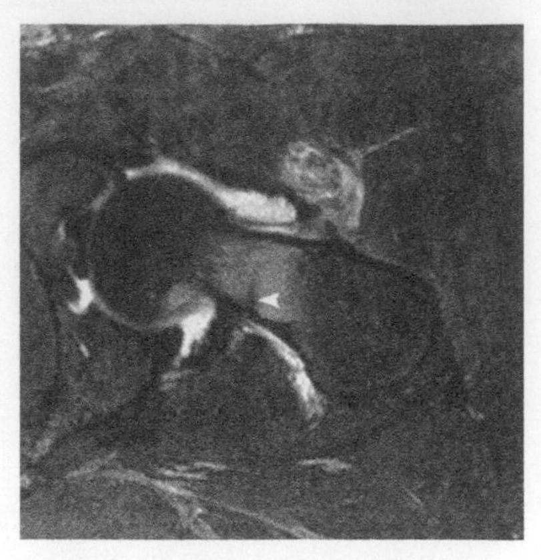

The fracture line is well appreciated.

Answers

1. The radiograph is normal.
2. An MRI would be the most sensitive and specific test to exclude a stress fracture.
3. Early septic arthritis, osteomyelitis, avascular necrosis, and stress fracture can have normal radiographs. The MRI shows centering in the medial femoral neck suggesting either stress fracture or osteoid osteoma. The absence of a nidus, and a clear fracture line, confirms a femoral neck stress fracture as the diagnosis.
4. There are 2 types of femoral neck stress fractures: the medial compressive type and the lateral tensile type.
5. Rest with gradual mobilization is the management for compressive femoral neck stress fracture. Tensile types may have to be percutaneously pinned, to avoid progression to a complete fracture.

Pearls

- Femoral neck stress fracture are either compressive or tensile types.
- The compressive type are located in the medial cortex and occurs in young active patients.
- The tensile types occur in the lateral femoral neck, in older more osteoporotic patients.
- The risks are progression to complete fractures, or avascular necrosis. These are greatest with the tensile-type stress fracture.
- Radiographs are often initially negative. When positive, there is a lucent fracture line that abuts the cortex and is perpendicular to the cortex, with surrounding sclerosis.
- MRI shows bone marrow edema and an incomplete fracture line.

Suggested Readings

Dorne HL, Lander PH. Spontaneous stress fractures of the femoral neck. *AJR Am J Roentgenol.* 1985;144(2): 343-347.

Meaney JE, Carty H. Femoral stress fractures in children. *Skeletal Radiol.* 1992;21(3):173-176.

Lower back pain with radicular symptoms in the legs

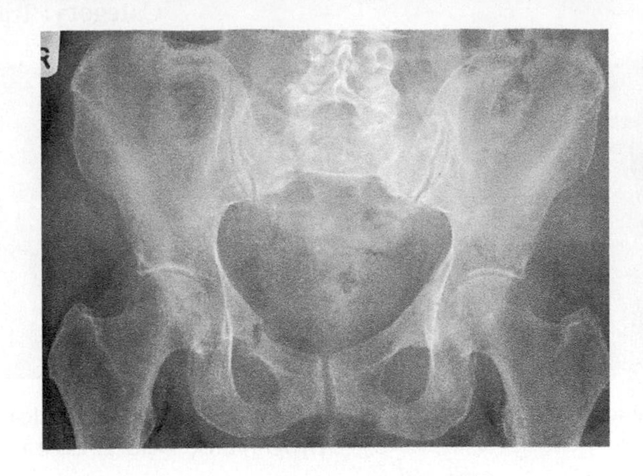

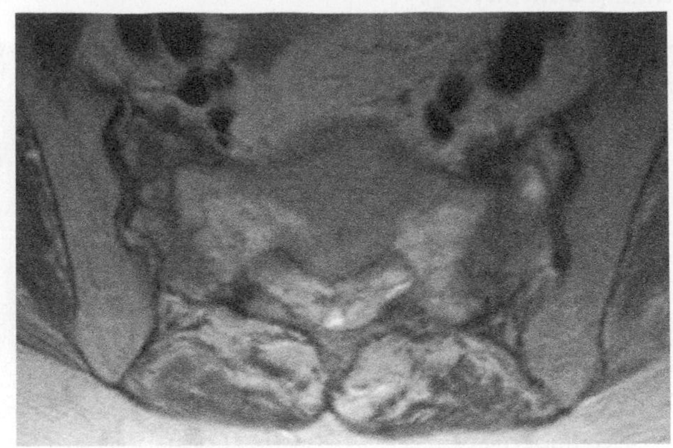

1. What are the radiographic findings?
2. What are the 2 main types of stress fractures?
3. What are the expected bone scan findings?
4. What are risk factors for this abnormality?
5. Which zone is most commonly involved?

Sacral insufficiency fracture 1537

Case ranking/difficulty: 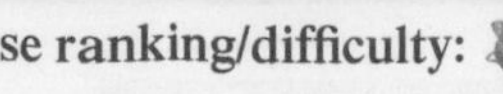 **Category:** Trauma

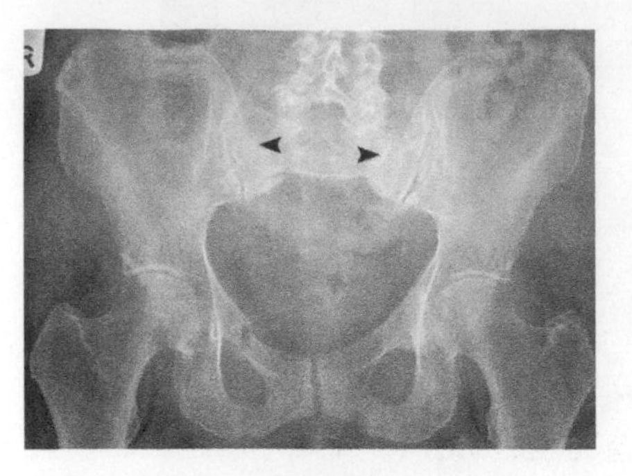

Bilateral sacral insufficiency fractures with compressed trabeculae.

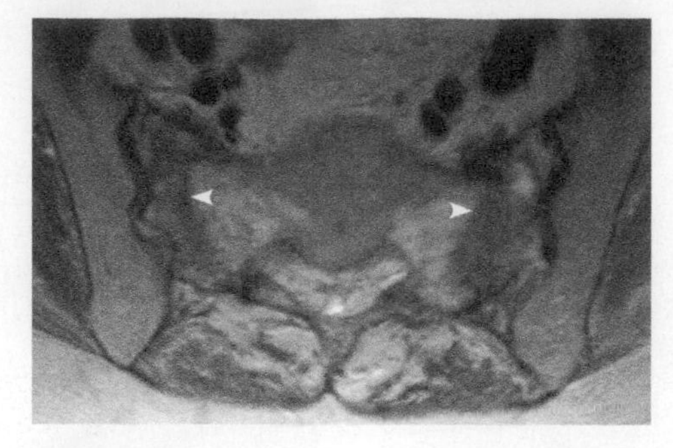

Bilateral sacral insufficiency fractures with low T1 signal fracture lines.

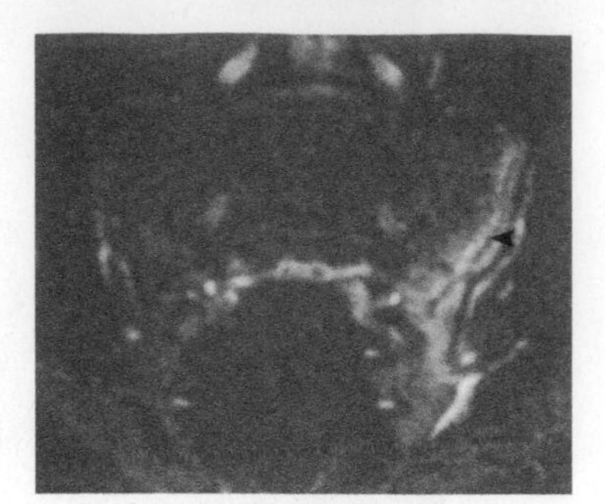

Another patient with a vertical T2 hyperintense sacral stress fracture.

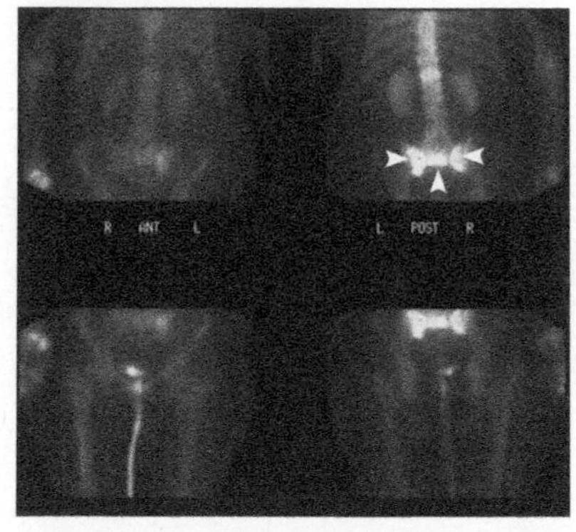

Bone scan in another patient showing the classic "H" or "Honda" sign of bilateral sacral insufficiency fractures.

Answers

1. Bilateral compressed trabeculae consistent with sacral insufficiency fractures.
2. Fatigue fractures are a result of abnormal stresses on normal bone, such as March fractures.
   Insufficiency fractures are a result of normal stresses on abnormal bone.
3. Although the bone scan is nonspecific, it may show a Honda or butterfly sign, with a horizontal and 2 vertical areas of increased uptake. Depending on the acuity, the bone scan may be positive on all 3 phases.
4. Osteoporosis is a major cause of sacral insufficiency fractures. Other causes include Paget disease, steroid use, sequelae of hip arthroplasties, and pregnancy/breastfeeding (the latter can induce a temporary osteoporotic state).
5. Denis classified sacral insufficiency fractures into 3 zones:
   - Zone I: Fractures in the sacral ala which are lateral to the neural foramina.
   - Zone II: Fracture through the neural foramina.
   - Zone III: Fracture through the body of the sacrum.

   Zone I fractures are the most common.

Pearls

- There are 2 types of stress fractures: fatigue fractures (normal bones with abnormal stresses), and insufficiency fractures (abnormal bones with normal stresses).
- Sacral insufficiency fractures are usually bilateral in the postmenopausal female.
- Risk factors include osteoporosis, rheumatoid arthritis, and Paget disease.
- Radiographs can show a sclerotic line, but this could be difficult to see because of bowel gas shadows and iliac vessel calcification. There is only a 12% accuracy of radiographs.
- Bone scan will show a Honda sign or butterfly sign, which is a horizontal fracture line with bilateral vertical sacral fractures.
- MRI will show low T1 fracture line and high STIR signal intensity marrow edema with or without fluid in the fracture line.
- CT can show an insufficiency fracture line clearly and can also show other associated fractures.
- Treatment is usually bed rest, pain killers, and immobilization. Sacral kyphoplasty and sacroplasty are now being introduced for some cases.

Suggested Readings

Blake SP, Connors AM. Sacral insufficiency fracture. *Br J Radiol.* 2004;77(922):891-896.

Brahme SK, Cervilla V, Vint V, Cooper K, Kortman K, Resnick D. Magnetic resonance appearance of sacral insufficiency fractures. *Skeletal Radiol.* 1990;19(7):489-493.

Hip pain for a few months, now progressing to limping

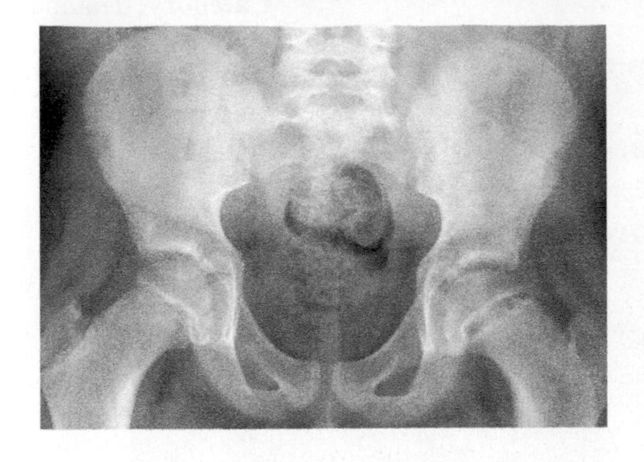

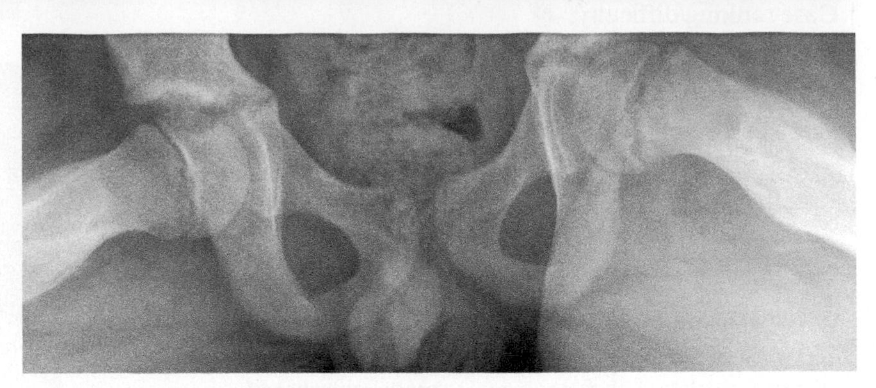

1. What are the radiographic findings?

2. How often is the disease bilateral?

3. What are the risk factors?

4. What are the treatment options?

5. What are the complications of this entity?

Slipped capital femoral epiphysis (SCFE) 1445

Case ranking/difficulty: 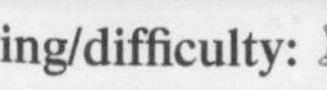 **Category:** Trauma

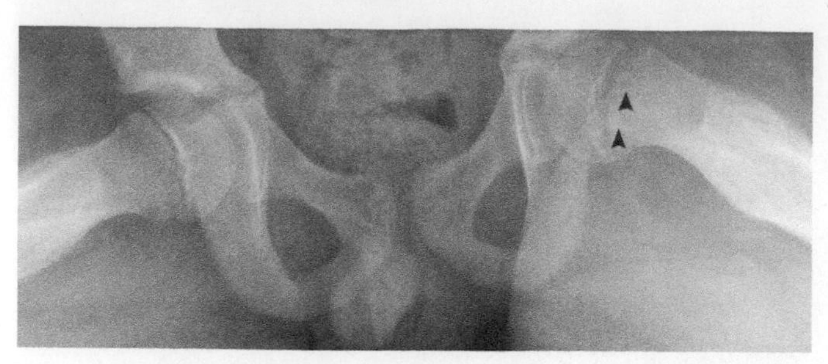

Frog lateral view of the left hip showing irregularity and widening of the growth plate, with metaphyseal sclerosis (*arrowheads*).

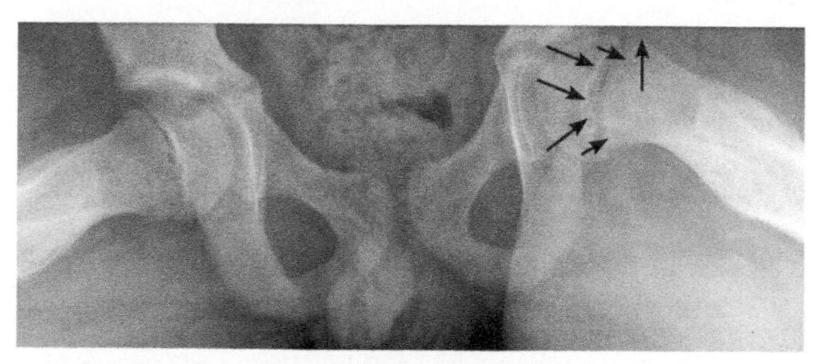

Frog lateral view with *long arrows* demonstrating widened and irregular epiphyseal growth plate of the left femur, and metaphyseal sclerosis (*short arrows*).

Answers

1. There is a blurring and irregularity of the physeal plate, posteromedial slip of the epiphysis, metaphyseal sclerosis, and abnormality of the line of Klein, which does not intersect the epiphysis. Slippage of the epiphysis gives the appearance of a reduction in height of the epiphysis because of foreshortening.
2. SCFE is bilateral in 20% of patients.
3. Obesity, rapid growth spurt, rickets, growth hormone therapy, and trauma are all predisposing factors, along with Afro-Caribbean origin.
4. Conservative treatment with analgesics and crutches in mild cases.

   Surgical pinning, corrective osteotomies, hip replacement, and contralateral prophylactic pinning are the main treatment options. Pinning should be performed without correction of the slippage, as there is an increased risk of avascular necrosis if correction is attempted.
5. Avascular necrosis, chondrolysis, limb length discrepancy, pistol grip deformity, and degenerative changes are recognized complications.

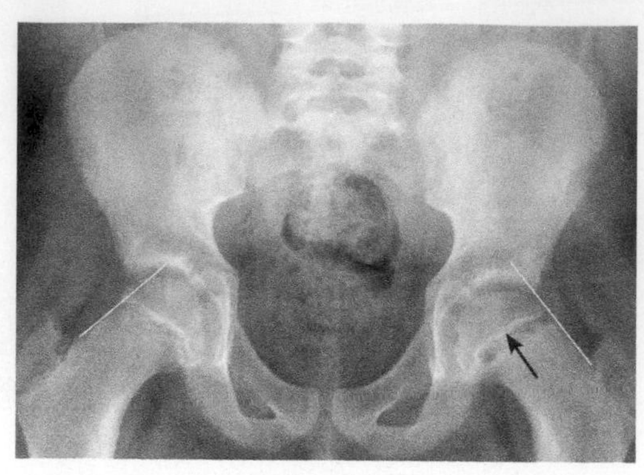

Widening of the left epiphyseal plate with irregularity of the growth plate suggesting a chronic stage of slip (*arrow*). Line of Klein is abnormal on the left, with no intersection of the epiphysis.

Pearls

- SCFE affects boys ages 10 to 17 years and girls ages 8 to 15 years. There is a 3:1 ratio of boys to girls.
- The early stage is a preslip phase in which there is a widening of the growth plate, irregularity and blurring of the physeal plate. The metaphysis is demineralized.
- In an acute slip, a line along the superior edge of the femoral neck fails to intersect the femoral epiphysis (line of Klein). There is posteromedial slippage of the epiphysis. This is best demonstrated on the crosstable lateral view, as positioning for a frog lateral can cause more displacement.
- In a chronic slip, there is a sclerosis and irregularity of the widened physis. There is also increased sclerosis of the metaphysis because of overlap, which is called the *metaphyseal blanche of Steel*.
- MRI shows early marrow edema on T2-weighted images, and sometimes the slippage is seen. It is important to check the opposite site as the disease can be bilateral. Associated mild effusion is also described, but nonspecific.
- Limb-length discrepancy is caused by early closure of the epiphysis.

Suggested Readings

Boles CA, El-Khoury GY. Slipped capital femoral epiphysis. *Radiographics*. 1997;17(4):809-823.

Dawes B, Jaremko JL, Balakumar J. Radiographic assessment of bone remodelling in slipped upper femoral epiphyses using Klein's line and the α angle of femoral-acetabular impingement: a retrospective review. *J Pediatr Orthop*. 2011;31(2):153-158.

Fall on outstretched hand with wrist pain

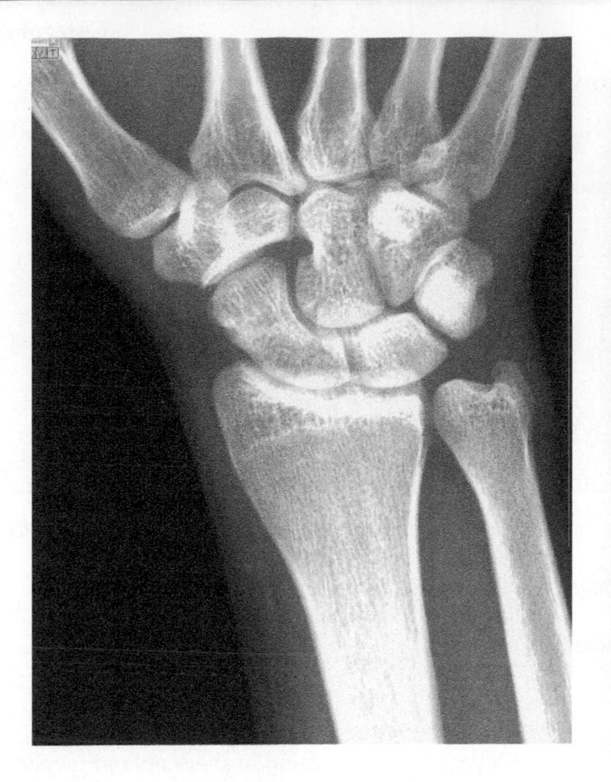

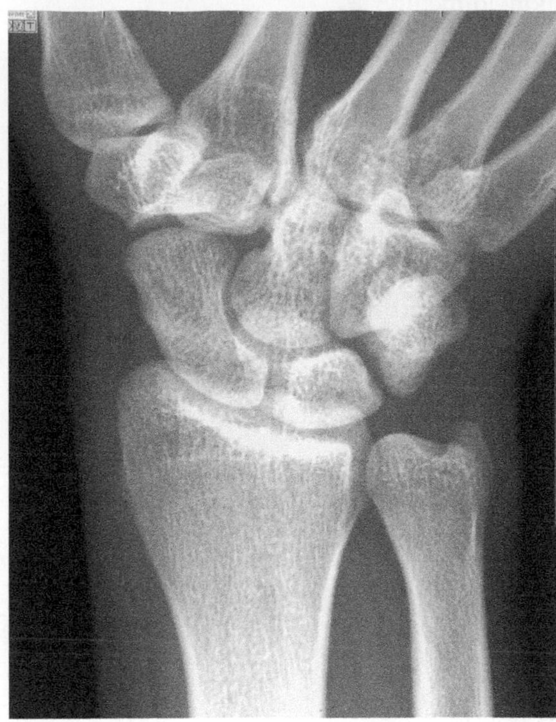

1. What are the radiographic findings?

2. What is a finding on the radiographs that may be helpful?

3. What scaphoid fractures are most common in children?

4. What scaphoid fractures are most prone to avascular necrosis?

5. What parameters are used to assess whether the fracture is considered displaced?

Occult scaphoid fracture 1387

Case ranking/difficulty:

Category: Trauma

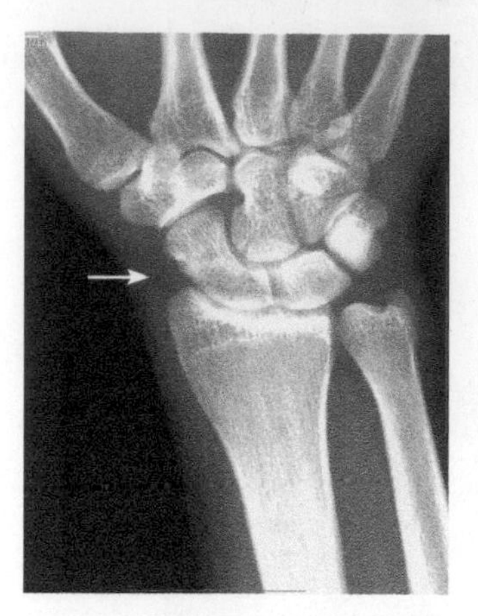

The scaphoid appears normal. The scaphoid fat pad (*arrow*) appears preserved.

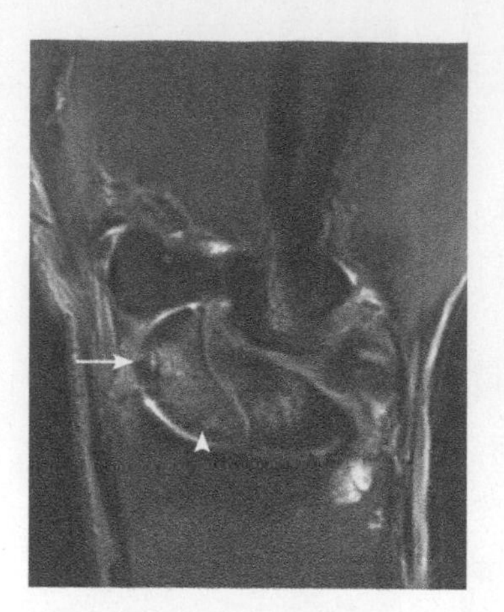

Nondisplaced fractures of the proximal scaphoid pole (*arrowhead*), and tubercle (*arrow*) are seen, with bone marrow edema. Lunate contusion is noted.

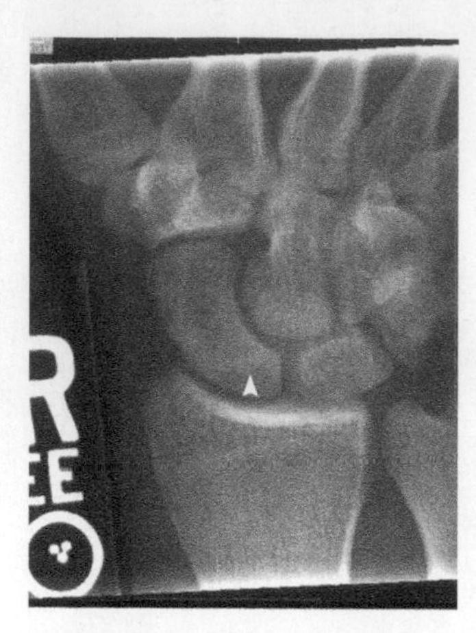

Repeat film 3 months later shows healed proximal pole fracture (*arrowhead*), with no evidence of avascular necrosis.

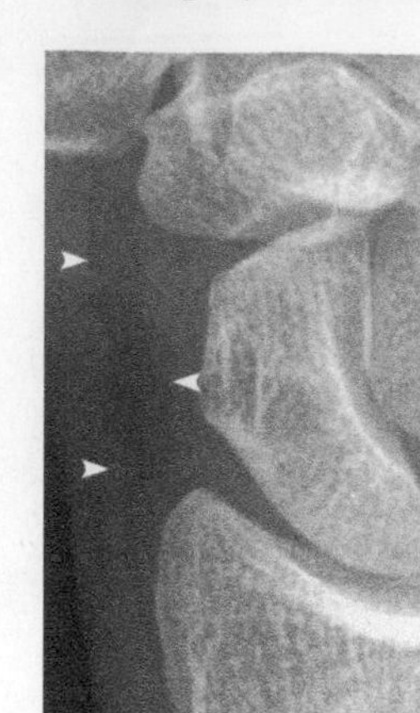

A normal scaphoid fat pad.

Answers

1. The radiographic appearances are normal. The scaphoid fat pad is preserved.
2. If a scaphoid fracture is suspected, elevation or displacement of the scaphoid fat pad may be seen. It is however not sensitive or specific. Pronator fat pad elevation occurs in distal radius fractures.
3. Tubercle fractures are most common in children. Waist fractures are most common in adults.
4. The scaphoid blood supply is from the dorsal branch of the radial artery and branches of the volar interosseous artery, and enters the scaphoid mainly through the dorsal ridge. Therefore, proximal pole fractures are the most prone to avascular necrosis because of the relatively poor perfusion.
5. Scaphoid fractures are considered to be displaced when there is a separation of 1 mm or angulation of 15 degrees.

Pearls

- Scaphoid fractures are a result of a fall on the outstretched hand.
- Ten percent to 20% of fractures are missed on radiographs.
- Elevation and distortion of the scaphoid fat pad can be helpful in detecting scaphoid fractures. It is, however, neither sensitive nor specific for such fractures.
- Seventy percent of fractures are at the waist, 10% to 20% at the distal pole, and 5% to 10% at the proximal pole.
- Proximal pole fractures have the greatest risk of avascular necrosis, and proximal pole fractures also have the greatest risk of delayed or nonunion.
- MRI is the most useful modality for the early detection of scaphoid occult fractures. Radionuclide bone scan may also be useful. However, many non-displaced scaphoid fractures can be treated with conservative splinting or casting, and advanced imaging is often not required.

Suggested Readings

Pierre-Jerome C, Moncayo V, Albastaki U, Terk MR. Multiple occult wrist bone injuries and joint effusions: prevalence and distribution on MRI. *Emerg Radiol.* 2010;17(3):179-184.

Stevenson JD, Morley D, Srivastava S, Willard C, Bhoora IG. Early CT for suspected occult scaphoid fractures. *J Hand Surg Eur Vol.* 2012;37(5):447-451.

Fall on the outstretched hand

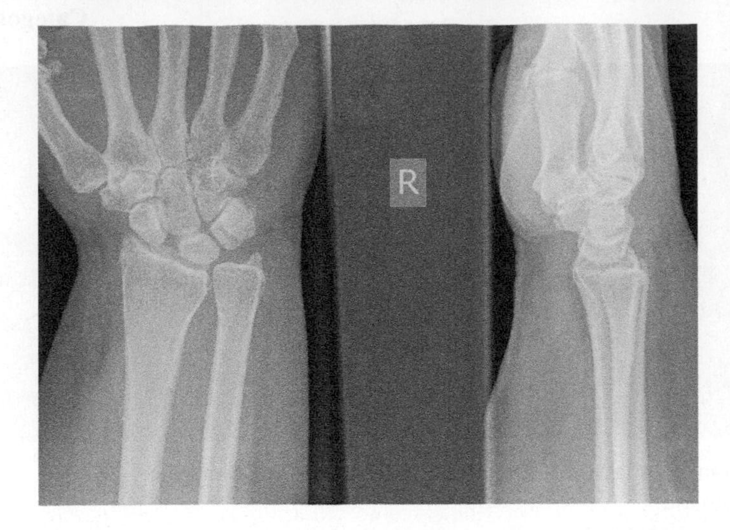

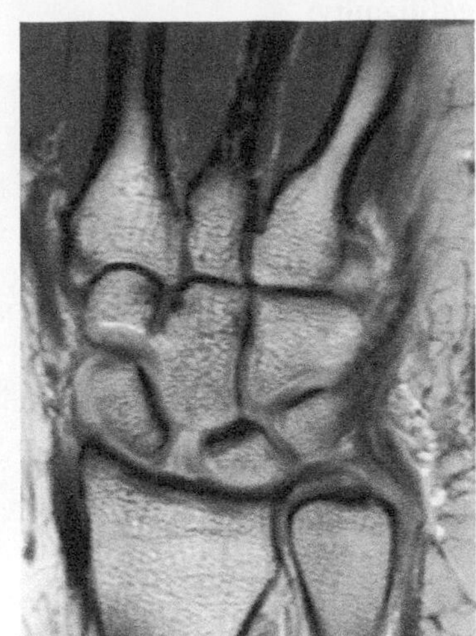

1. What is the main abnormality on the radiographs of the wrist?
2. What is the normal scapholunate distance on a PA radiograph?
3. What are the most useful tests to confirm scapholunate ligament injury?
4. What are the associated complications of this injury?
5. How can scapholunate dissociation be treated?

Scapholunate dissociation 1538

Case ranking/difficulty:

Category: Trauma

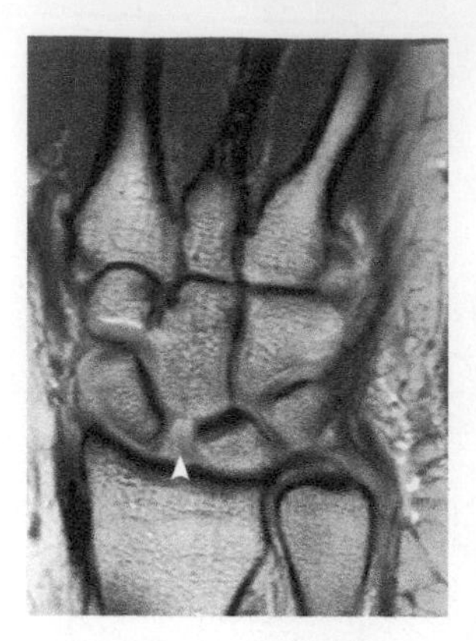

Increased scapholunate (SL) distance, with torn SL ligament.

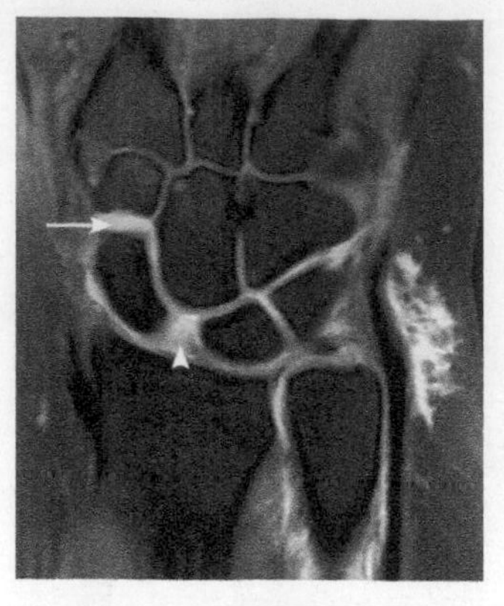

MR arthrogram. Contrast migrates from the radioscaphoid joint to the midcarpal joint (*arrow*) through a torn scapholunate ligament (*arrowhead*).

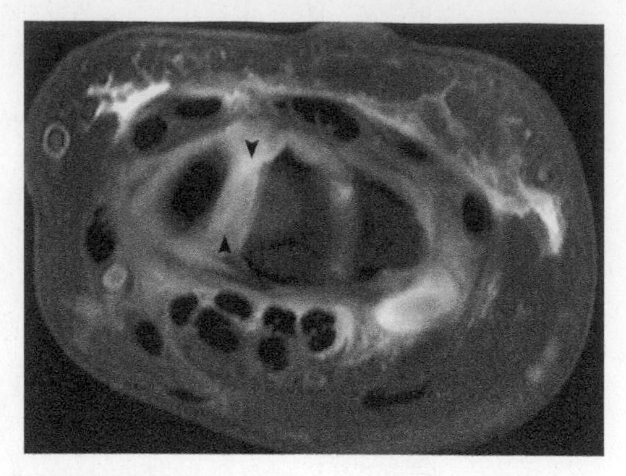

Disrupted SL ligament.

Answers

1. There is an increased gap between scaphoid and lunate, which suggests scapholunate dissociation. The scaphoid adopts a "signet-ring" appearance, and both the scapholunate and capitolunate angles are increased.
2. Normal is 1 to 3 mm. Abnormal scapholunate (SL) distance is more than 3 mm.
3. Although CT and MR arthrograms are both very useful, CT arthrography has higher accuracy, especially for partial nonsurgical tears of the scapholunate and lunotriquetral ligaments. In many cases, nonarthrographic CT or MRI is adequate.
4. SLAC (scapholunate advanced collapse), radioscaphoid osteoarthritis, and DISI (dorsal intercalated segmental instability) are recognized complications of scapholunate dissociation.
5. Depending upon the presentation, an acute SL tear is repaired with SL ligament repair or dorsal capsulodesis. The subacute and chronic tears without arthritis are treated with SL ligament or bone-ligament-bone repair, or tenodesis. Triscaphoid arthrodesis is performed in advanced cases.

Pearls

- SL dissociation is one of the most common patterns of carpal instability. It is the first injury in that spectrum.
- On AP radiographs, the SL distance is more than 3 mm, and the widened gap is known as the Terry-Thomas sign. This is well demonstrated on the clenched fist views, and PA views with ulnar deviation.
- The SL angle is more than 60 degrees, suggesting DISI. The capitolunate angle is also increased, usually more than 30 degrees.
- Other signs are a triangular-shaped lunate, and possible disruption of the carpal arcs of Gilula. As a consequence of the rotatory subluxation of the scaphoid, the scaphoid may demonstrate a "signet-ring" appearance.
- The SL ligament has 3 bands; the volar, central membranous, and dorsal bands. The dorsal band is structurally the most important, unlike the lunotriquetral ligament where the volar band is most important.
- MRI demonstrates the disrupted SL ligament. On MR arthrography, the contrast migrates from the radioscaphoid compartment into the midcarpal compartment.
- CT arthrography has higher accuracy than MR arthrography for the detection of SL and lunotriquetral ligament tears, especially partial nonsurgical tears.
- Complications include SLAC wrist, DISI, and degenerative changes of the radiocarpal joint.

Suggested Readings

Rominger MB, Bernreuter WK, Kenney PJ, Lee DH. MR imaging of anatomy and tears of wrist ligaments. *Radiographics.* 1993;13(6):1233-1246.

Timins ME, Jahnke JP, Krah SF, Erickson SJ, Carrera GF. MR imaging of the major carpal stabilizing ligaments: normal anatomy and clinical examples. *Radiographics.* 1995;15(3):575-587.

Fell down the stairs

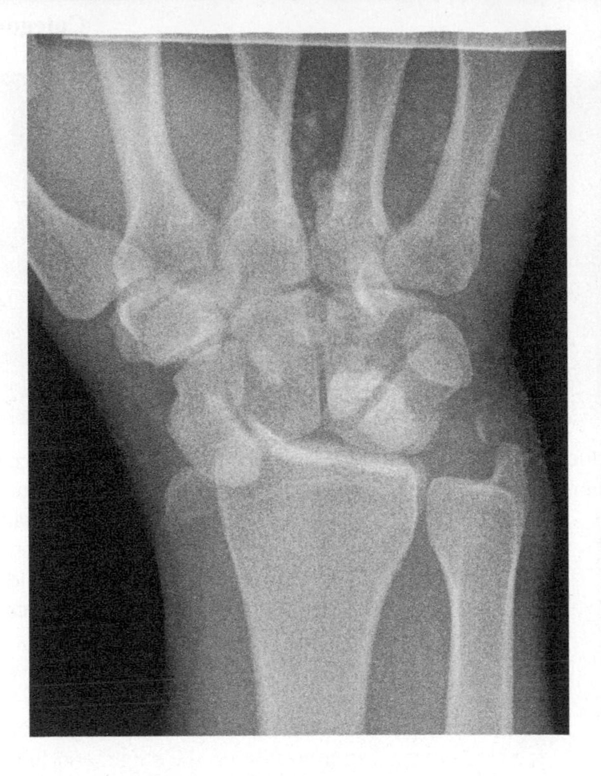

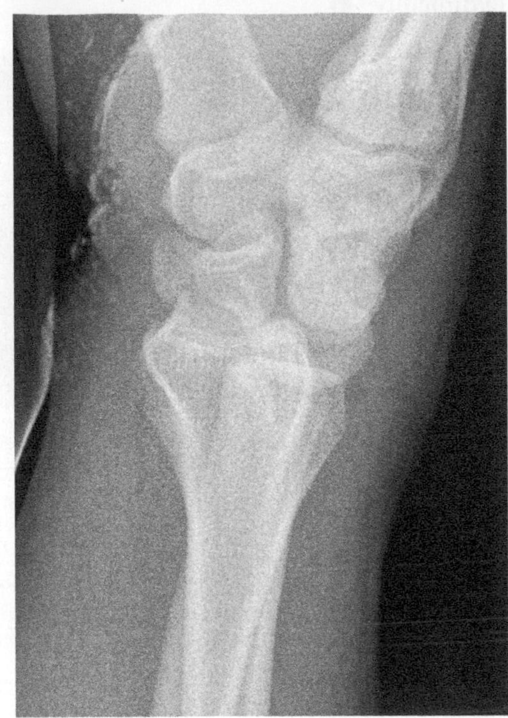

1. What are the radiographic findings?

2. What is the mechanism of injury?

3. What is the most severe injury in the spectrum of traumatic carpal instability?

4. What is the Terry Thomas sign?

5. What is the space of Poirier?

Perilunate dislocation **1394**

Case ranking/difficulty:

Category: Trauma

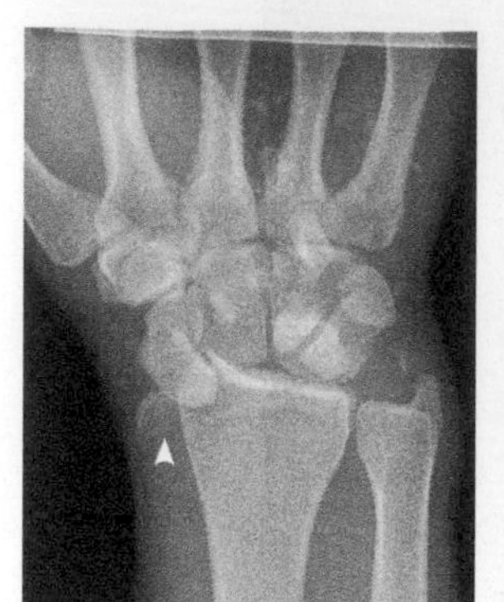

Marked disruption of the carpal arcs, with a displaced radial styloid fracture (*arrowhead*) and ulnar styloid process fracture. Numerous glass foreign bodies are also seen.

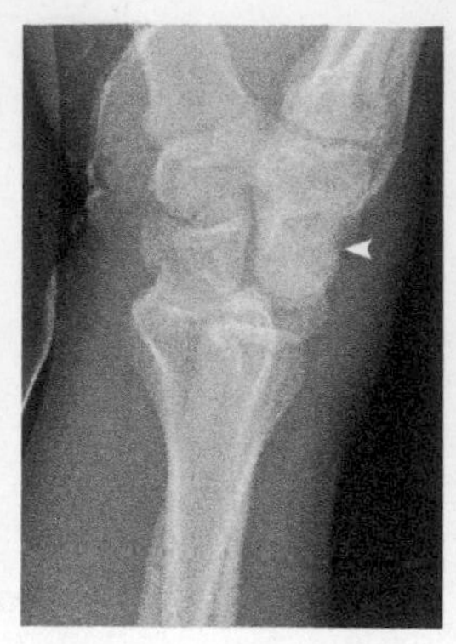

Perilunate dislocation. Lunate remains articulating with the radius, and the capitate dislocates posteriorly (*arrowhead*).

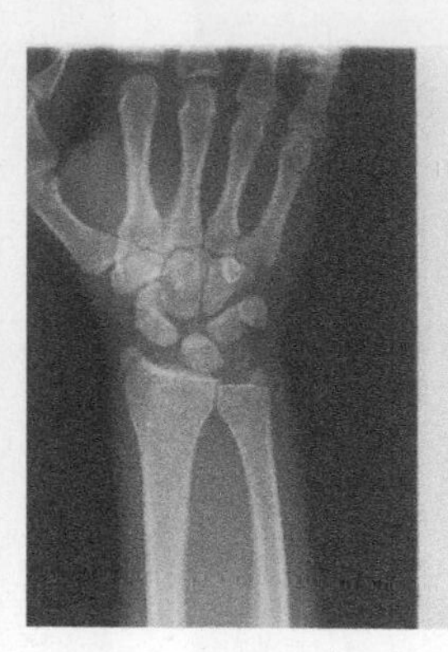

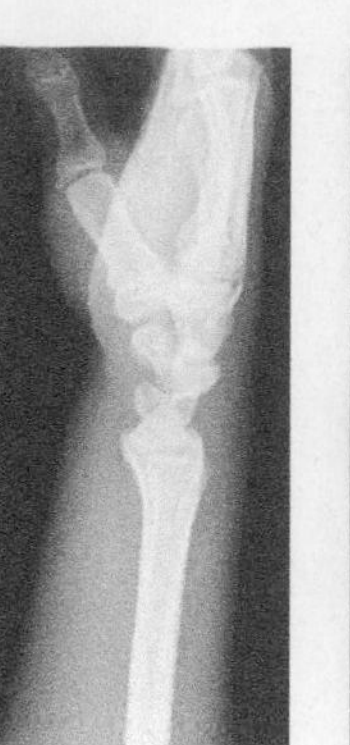

Postreduction radiographs show improved alignment. Some disruption of the carpal arcs persists.

Post second reduction, radial and ulnar styloid fractures are seen, with mild widening of the scapholunate space.

Answers

1. There is a radial styloid fracture with interrupted carpal arcs, perilunate dislocation, and multiple foreign bodies.
2. The mechanism is a fall on the outstretched hand held in hyperextension and ulnar deviation.
3. The spectrum is rotary subluxation of the scaphoid, perilunate dislocation, midcarpal dislocation, and finally lunate dislocation. The most severe injury is lunate dislocation.
4. This is a widened scapholunate space from scapholunate ligament tear.
5. The space between the radioscaphocapitate and palmar radiolunate ligament is known as the space of Poirier, and is a weak spot through which the lunate can dislocate into the carpal tunnel.

Pearls

- Lesser arc carpal injuries are purely ligamentous.
- Greater arc injuries have an associated fracture, most commonly of the scaphoid.
- Other fractures included the radial styloid, and less commonly the capitate and triquetrum.
- Four stages have been described, with the sequence being: rotary subluxation of the scaphoid, perilunate dislocation, midcarpal dislocation, and, finally, lunate dislocation.
- The severity increases with the stage, and lunate dislocation is the most serious.
- In perilunate dislocation, the carpal arcs are interrupted and the lunate often has a triangular configuration on an AP radiograph. The carpal arcs are usually disrupted.
- Post-traumatic arthrosis is the major complication.

Suggested Readings

Linscheid RL, Dobyns JH, Beabout JW, Bryan RS. Traumatic instability of the wrist: diagnosis, classification, and pathomechanics. *J Bone Joint Surg Am.* 2002; 84-A(1):142.

Schreibman KL, Freeland A, Gilula LA, Yin Y. Imaging of the hand and wrist. *Orthop Clin North Am.* 1997;28(4): 537-582.

Motor vehicle accident

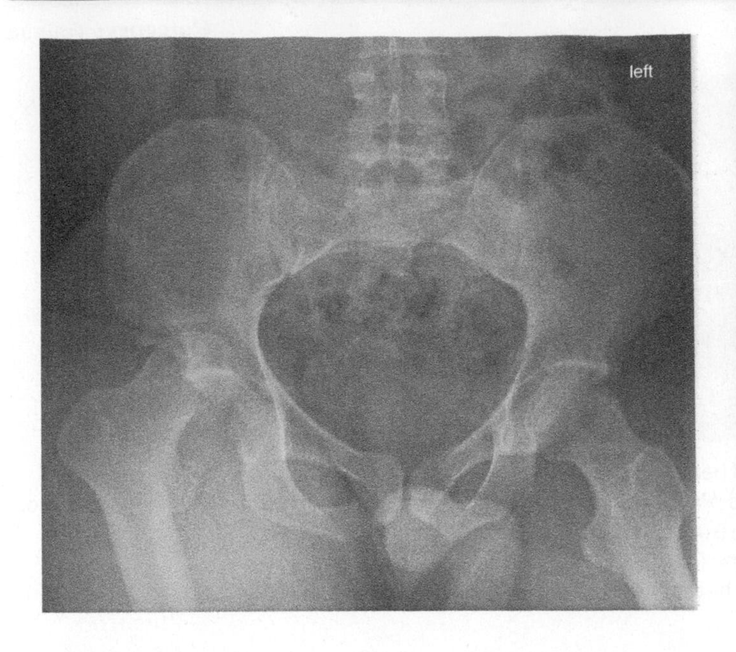

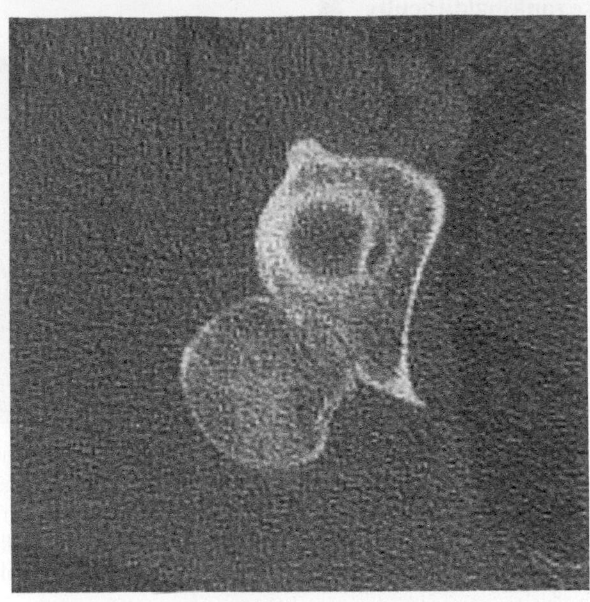

1. What is the most common direction of hip dislocation?

2. What are complications of hip fracture–dislocation?

3. What is the Pipkin classification?

4. Hip dislocations are usually isolated injuries. True or False?

5. What is the most common etiology for posterior hip dislocations?

Posterior hip dislocation 1471

Case ranking/difficulty: 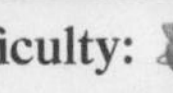

Category: Trauma

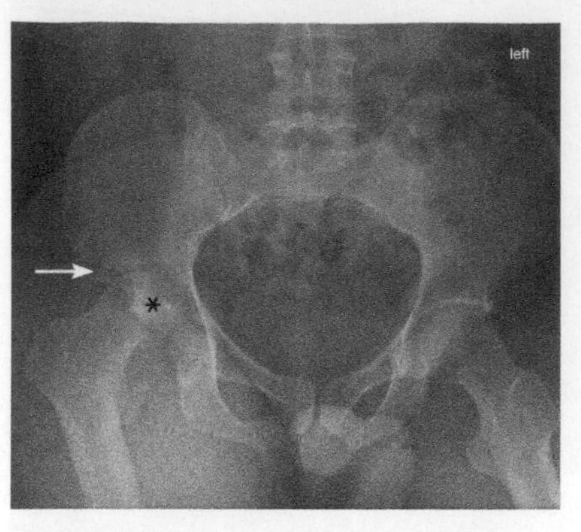

Dislocation of the right femoral head (*asterisk*) is demonstrated. A fracture fragment (*arrow*) is visible adjacent to the femoral head. The left femoral head is anatomically located.

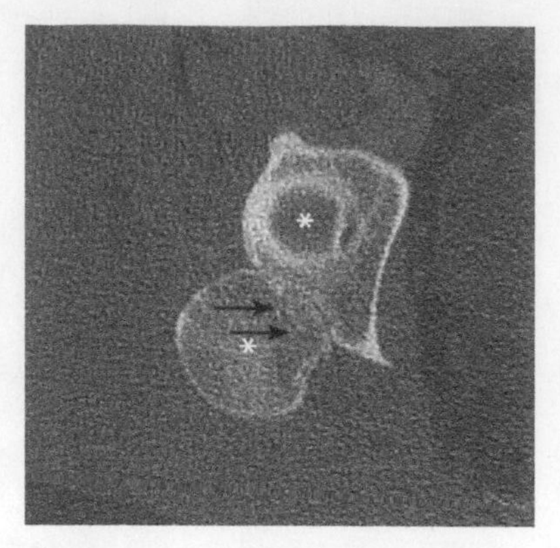

The femoral head (*inferior asterisk*) is dislocated posteriorly from the acetabulum (*superior asterisk*). A fracture line (*arrows*) is visible in the femoral head.

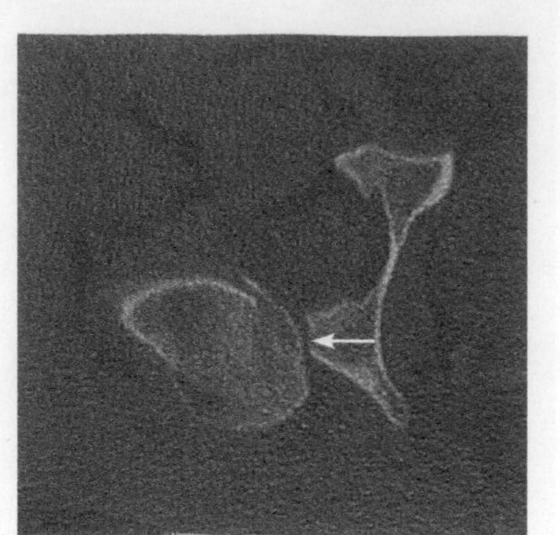

Fracture of the posterior wall of the acetabulum (*arrow*) is also demonstrated.

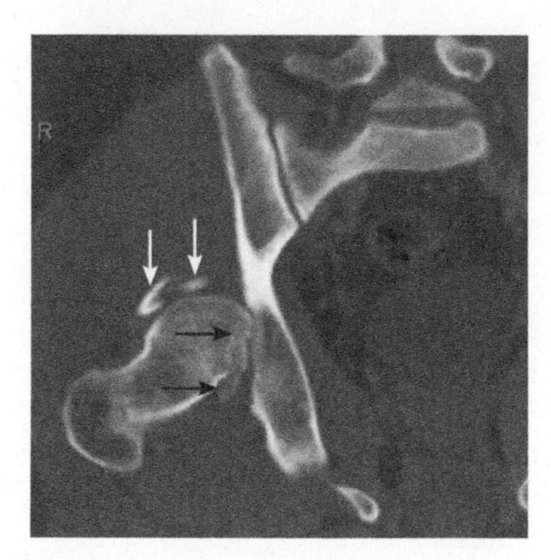

Fracture fragments arising from the posterior wall of the acetabulum are demonstrated (*white arrows*). Fracture of the femoral head is demonstrated (*black arrows*).

Answers

1. Of traumatic hip dislocations, 90% are posterior and 10% are anterior.
2. Complications of hip fracture–dislocation include osteonecrosis of the femoral head, post-traumatic osteoarthritis, hip instability, and heterotopic ossification.
3. The Pipkin classification is a classification system of hip dislocations with associated femoral head fractures.
4. Associated injuries are common, and 95% of patients with hip dislocations also sustain injury elsewhere in the body.
5. Motor vehicle accidents account for the majority of posterior hip dislocations. Other common causes of hip dislocations include athletic injuries and falls from a height.

Pearls

- Traumatic hip dislocations and fracture–dislocations are orthopedic emergencies.
- Of traumatic hip dislocations, 90% are posterior.
- Motor vehicle accidents account for the majority of posterior hip dislocations, and lack of seat belt use is common.
- Other common causes include athletic injuries and falls from height.
- The right hip is more commonly affected than the left hip by a ratio of 3:1.
- Associated femoral head shear fractures, and acetabular posterior wall/column fractures often occur.
- On radiographs, the hip is adducted and the femoral head is usually displaced posteriorly, laterally, and superiorly. In anterior dislocations, the hip is usually abducted, and displaced anteriorly, medially, and inferiorly.
- Of patients with hip dislocations, 95% also sustain injury elsewhere in the body.
- Complications of hip fracture–dislocation include osteonecrosis of the femoral head, post-traumatic osteoarthritis of the hip, instability, and heterotopic ossification.

Suggested Readings

Lang-Stevenson A, Getty CJ. The Pipkin fracture-dislocation of the hip. *Injury.* 1987;18(4):264-269.

Sahin V, Karakaş ES, Aksu S, Atlihan D, Turk CY, Halici M. Traumatic dislocation and fracture-dislocation of the hip: a long-term follow-up study. *J Trauma.* 2003;54(3):520-529.

Pain and inability to move shoulder after injury

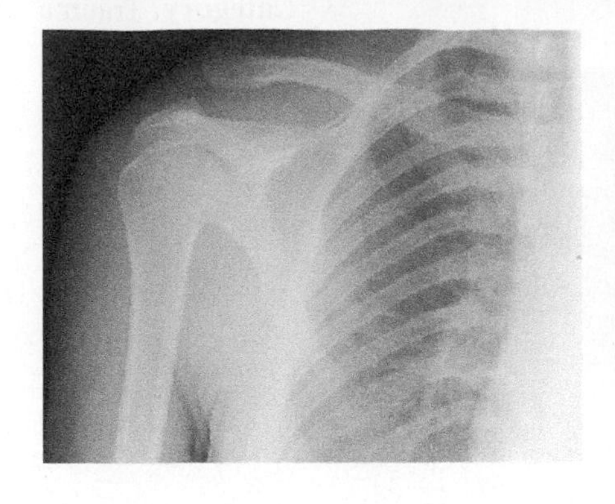

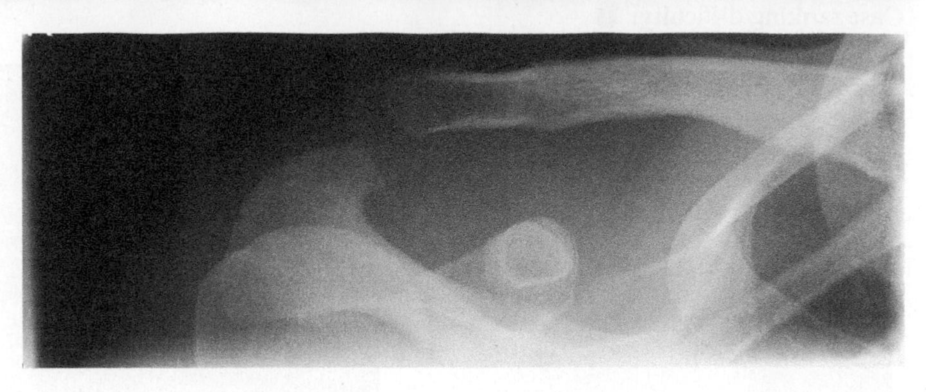

1. What ligaments are at risk of rupture with injuries to this joint?
2. What is the recommended treatment for grade 2 injuries of this structure?
3. What activities are risk factors for this injury?
4. What imaging modalities are appropriate for imaging this structure?
5. What is the treatment of choice for grade 3 injuries of this structure?

Acromioclavicular joint subluxation 480

Case ranking/difficulty: 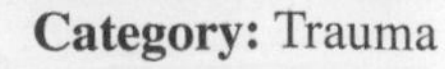 **Category:** Trauma

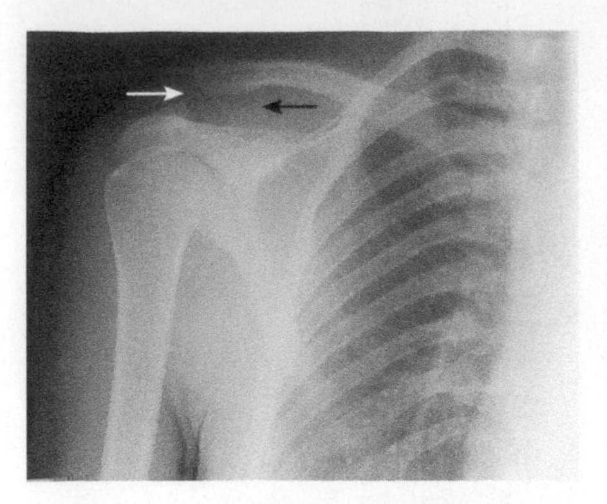

AC and CC ligament rupture consistent with a grade 3 injury.

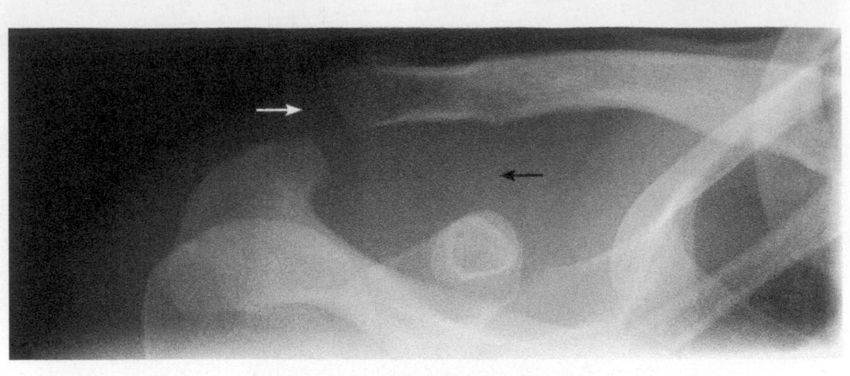

AC and CC ligament rupture on dedicated coned view of AC joint.

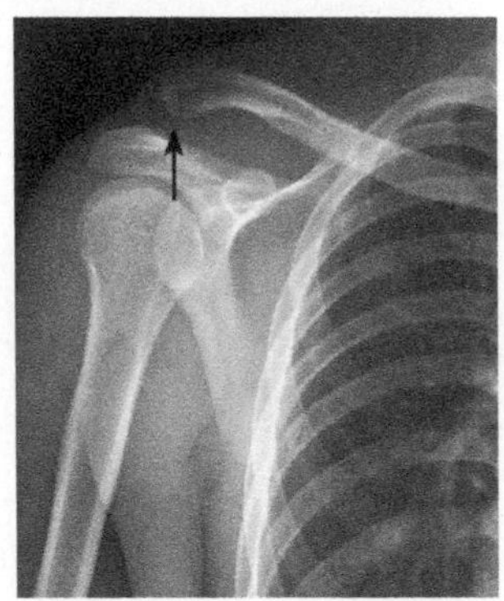

A further stepoff between the acromioclavicular articular margins and a posteriorly driven clavicle is a feature of grade 4 injuries.

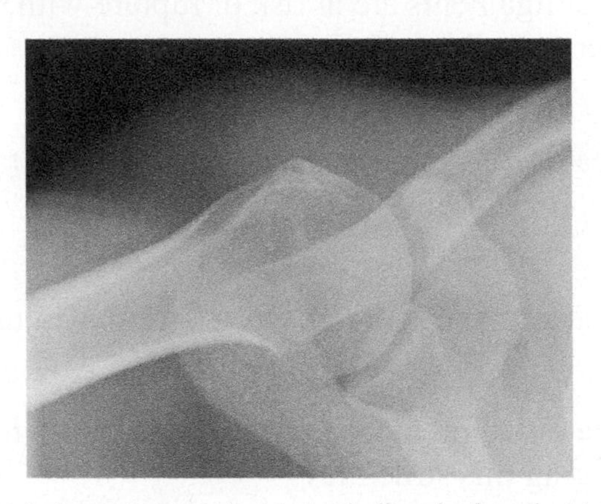

A posteriorly positioned clavicle is a hallmark of grade 4 injuries.

Answers

1. The acromioclavicular and coracoclavicular ligaments are at risk of rupture and may need surgical stabilization.
2. Grades 1 to 2 AC joint injuries generally have an excellent prognosis when managed conservatively. Grades 3 to 6 may require surgical repair.
3. High-energy direct trauma can lead to AC joint injury. Sports such as rugby and hockey are, therefore, high-risk activities for AC joint injury.
4. Plain film and CT are useful for demonstrating the bony injuries around the AC joint best. Ultrasound is useful for assessing the integrity of the acromioclavicular joint and coracoclavicular ligament. MRI can provide the same information, although does not allow dynamic assessment.
5. AC joint dislocations with disruption of the coracoclavicular ligament (grade 3 and above) are likely to lead to permanent disability and pain unless surgically repaired. An operation that is currently favored is the Nottingham repair, which involves passing synthetic ligament substitute material from the clavicle to the coracoid by looping it under tension around the coracoid to bring the bones closer together.

Pearls

- Superior subluxation of the distal clavicle is consistent with AC ligament and capsular injury of at least grade 2 by the Rockwood classification.
- The coracoclavicular distance should be evaluated to determine whether the CC ligament is ruptured (normal = 13 mm or less). Obtain an axillary view to determine posterior displacement of the clavicle into the trapezius muscle that is grade 4 injury, which usually requires operative repair.
- Approximately 6% of cases result in the complication of post-traumatic osteolysis.
- The Nottingham repair is a commonly used operation for AC joint stabilization.

Suggested Readings

Melenevsky Y, Yablon CM, Ramappa A, Hochman MG. Clavicle and acromioclavicular joint injuries: a review of imaging, treatment, and complications. *Skeletal Radiol.* 2011;40(7):831-842.

Reuter RM, Hiller WD, Ainge GR, et al. Ironman triathletes: MRI assessment of the shoulder. *Skeletal Radiol.* 2008;37(8):737-741.

History of MVA and left-sided chest pain

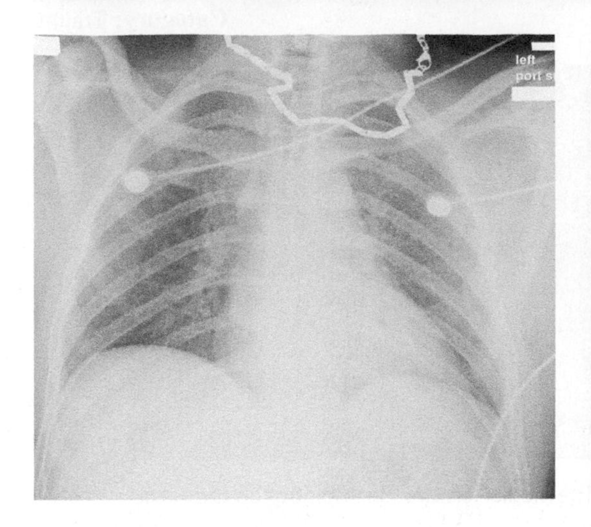

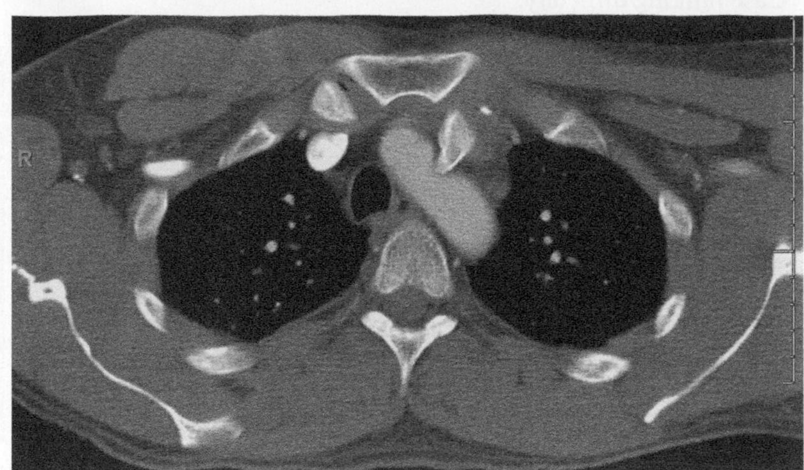

1. What is the finding on the chest X-ray?

2. What is the next most appropriate study?

3. What is the most common form of this injury?

4. What is the main risk of this injury?

5. What is the most appropriate management?

Posterior sternoclavicular joint dislocation 1364

Case ranking/difficulty:

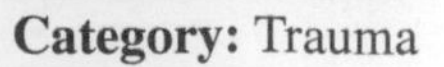

Category: Trauma

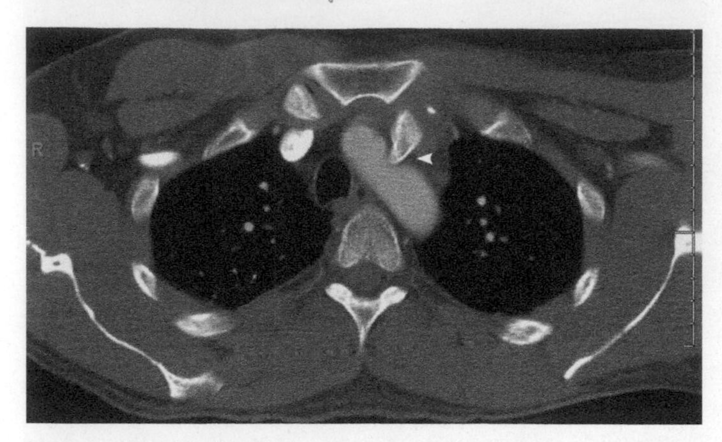

Posterior dislocation of the medial left clavicle with impingement on the aorta.

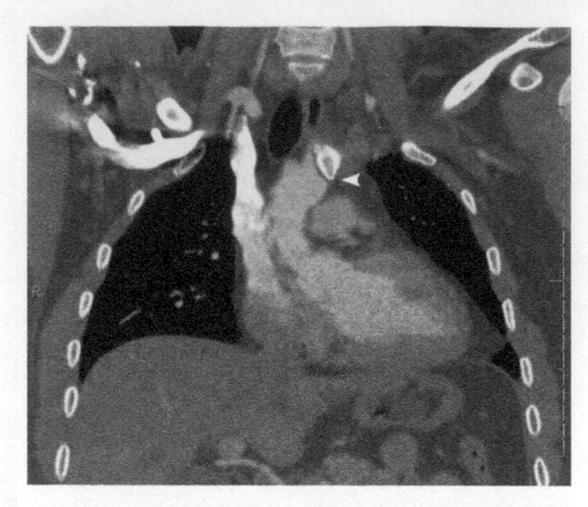

The medial left clavicle impinges on the aorta.

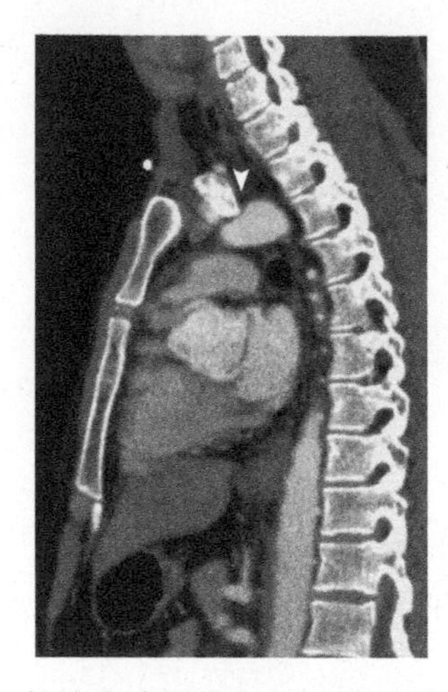

The medial left clavicle impinges on the aorta.

Answers

1. There is no abnormality on the chest X-ray.
2. If a sternoclavicular separation is suspected, then a CT scan is the next most appropriate study. A "serendipity" view is an AP film with 40-degree cranial angulation, used to evaluate the sternoclavicular joints.
3. This is a sternoclavicular dislocation, and the anterior form is nine times more common than the posterior form.
4. The main risk of a posterior sternoclavicular dislocation is mediastinal injury, including tracheal rupture and vascular injury.
5. Posterior sternoclavicular dislocations require closed reduction under anesthesia, or if this fails or the injury is life threatening, then open reduction.

Pearls

- Anterior sternoclavicular dislocations are 9 times more common than posterior.
- Posterior dislocations have a much higher morbidity.
- The mechanism for anterior dislocations is usually hyperabduction, and for posterior dislocations it is usually high-impact direct trauma as in an MVA.
- Mediastinal injury including great vessel and tracheal injuries can be devastating in this injury.
- AP chest may be normal. The posteriorly dislocated clavicle may be slightly inferior to the normal location. Anteriorly dislocated clavicle may be slightly superior.
- Findings are accentuated with a "serendipity" radiograph.

Suggested Readings

McCulloch P, Henley BM, Linnau KF. Radiographic clues for high-energy trauma: three cases of sternoclavicular dislocation. *AJR Am J Roentgenol.* 2001;176(6):1534.

Patten RM, Dobbins J, Gunberg SR. Gas in the sternoclavicular joints of patients with blunt chest trauma: significance and frequency of CT findings. *AJR Am J Roentgenol.* 1999;172(6):1633-1635.

Tsai DW, Swiontkowski MF, Kottra CL. A case of sternoclavicular dislocation with scapulothoracic dissociation. *AJR Am J Roentgenol.* 1996;167(2):332.

Road traffic accident

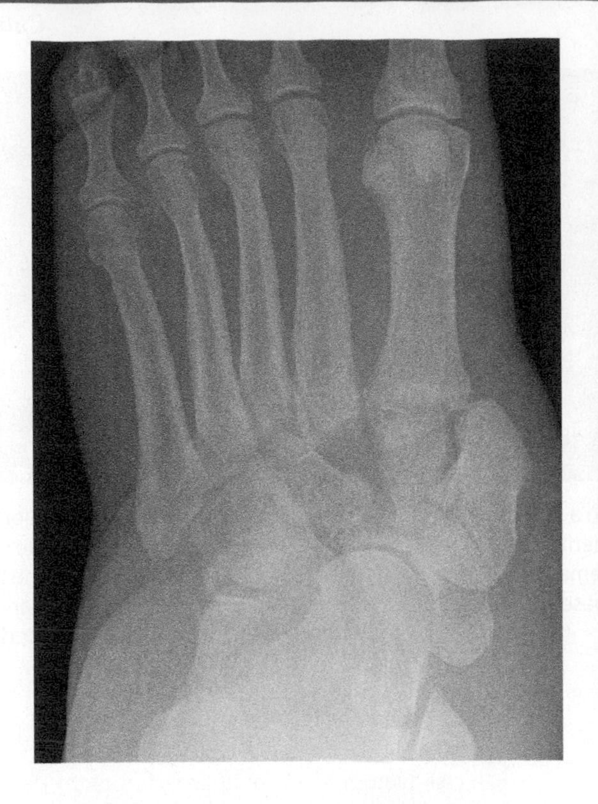

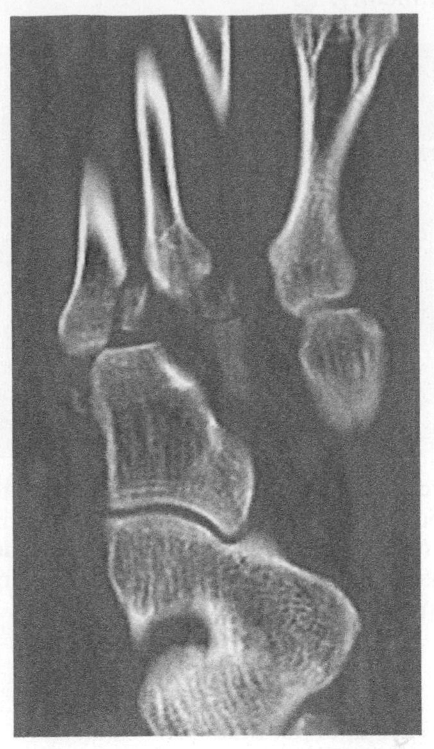

1. What are the imaging findings?
2. What are the different types of this entity?
3. What is the usual mechanism of injury?
4. What are the components of the Lisfranc ligament?
5. What imaging modality is best for evaluation of the major ligamentous structure involved in this entity?

Lisfranc fracture dislocation 1539

Case ranking/difficulty:  **Category:** Trauma

Fracture of the third (*arrowhead*) and fourth (*arrow*) metatarsal bases, with malalignment. Lateral cuboid fracture is also seen (*asterisk*).

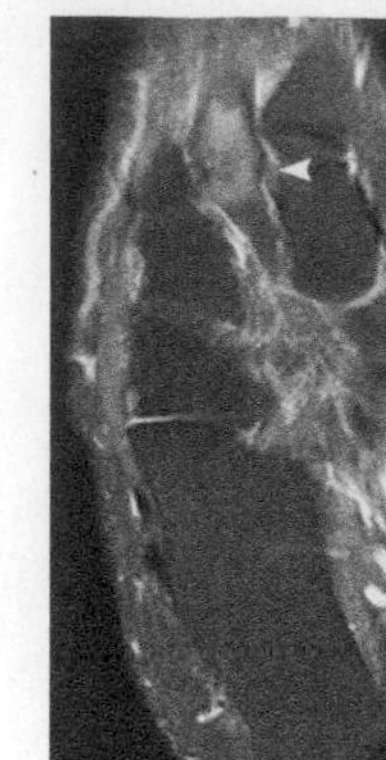

Another patient with a sprain of the Lisfranc ligament (*arrowhead*) and edema in the second metatarsal base.

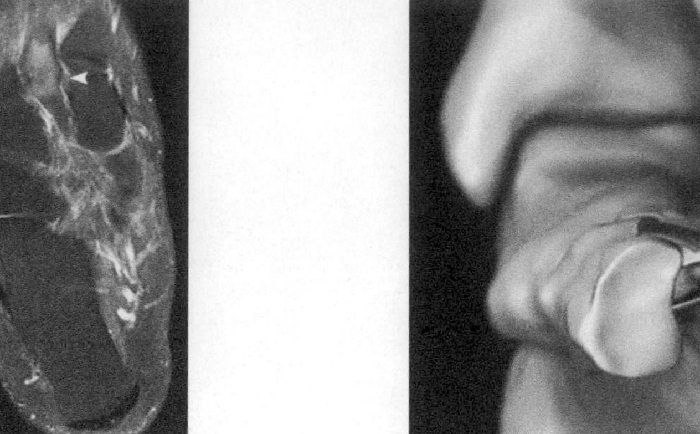

Illustration demonstrating the major components of the Lisfranc ligamentous complex. *Black band* is the weak dorsal band, *thick grey* the interosseous band, and *thin white* the plantar band. (Reproduced with permission from Radsource and Dr. Michael Stadnick.)

Answers

1. The plain radiograph demonstrates a homolateral Lisfranc fracture dislocation and fracture of the base of the second metatarsal with malalignment of the intercuneiform articulations.
2. Homolateral, divergent, isolated, and first ray separation are the described types of Lisfranc injury.
3. Road traffic accident, fall from height, Charcot joint, and forced plantar flexion are typical mechanisms.
4. The Lisfranc ligament connects the first cuneiform with the base of the second metatarsal. It has 3 main components: the plantar, central interosseous and dorsal bands. The ligament fails sequentially from dorsal to plantar. The dorsal capsule of the Lisfranc joint lacks sufficient reinforcement and is weak, hence dorsal subluxation is a primary feature.
5. Although the diagnosis of a Lisfranc fracture is usually made on CT, MRI best evaluates Lisfranc ligament, especially in partial tears and sprains. Of particular importance is the plantar component of the ligament: if there is a high-grade sprain or it is torn, it implies an unstable midfoot. CT and MRI also detects additional injuries not detectable on plain film.

Pearls

- The Lisfranc joint is a tarsometatarsal joint ligamentous complex, which is made up of the intermetatarsal, intertarsal, and tarsometatarsal joints and ligaments of the foot.
- High impact sports, falls, and MVAs are important risk factors. Charcot neuroarthropathy can also disrupt the joint.
- There are several types of injury:
  - Homolateral: All 5 metatarsals are displaced laterally. This may be associated with a cuboid fracture.
  - Divergent: Medial displacement of the first metatarsal and lateral displacement of the others.
  - Isolated: The second to fifth metatarsals are displaced laterally, the first is normally located.
  - First ray separation: The second to fifth metatarsals are normally located, the first metatarsal displaces medially.
- Plain film is the mainstay of diagnosis, although 20% of injuries are missed on radiographs. This injury could be associated with other fractures such as base of second metatarsal fracture, cuboid, navicular, and fractures of the shaft of the metatarsals.

Suggested Readings

Goiney RC, Connell DG, Nichols DM. CT evaluation of tarsometatarsal fracture-dislocation injuries. *AJR Am J Roentgenol.* 1985;144(5):985-990.

Kalia V, Fishman EK, Carrino JA, Fayad LM. Epidemiology, imaging, and treatment of Lisfranc fracture-dislocations revisited. *Skeletal Radiol.* 2012;41(2):129-136.

Macmahon PJ, Dheer S, Raikin SM, et al. MRI of injuries to the first interosseous cuneometatarsal (Lisfranc) ligament. *Skeletal Radiol.* 2009;38(3):255-260.

Twisting injury to knee, sensation of "giving way"

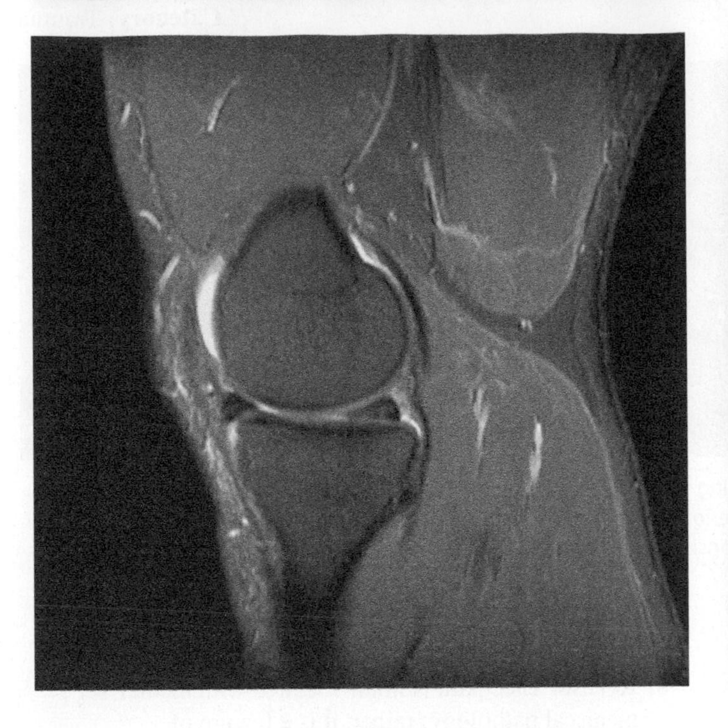

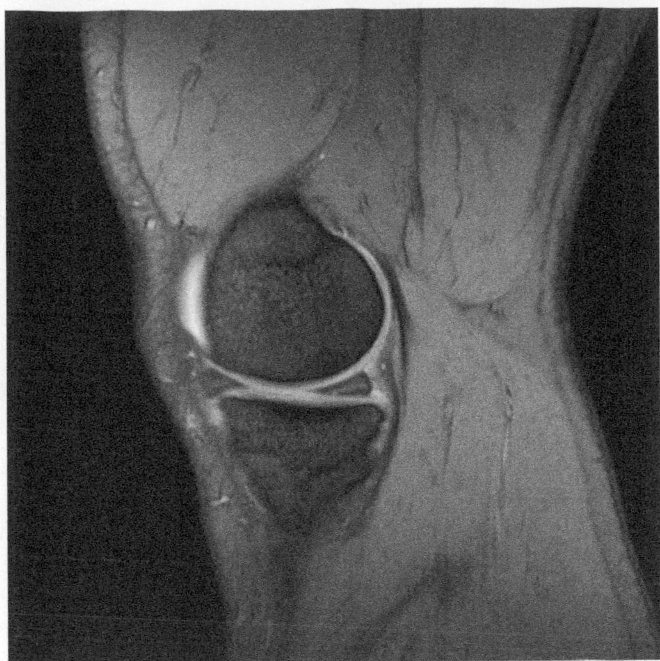

1. What are the imaging features of this entity?

2. Which associated ligamentous injuries may occur with injuries of this structure?

3. When making a decision regarding meniscal repair versus partial meniscectomy, which factor is least important?

4. Which are the recognized types of meniscal tear?

5. What are the symptoms of this condition?

Case ranking/difficulty:

Category: Trauma

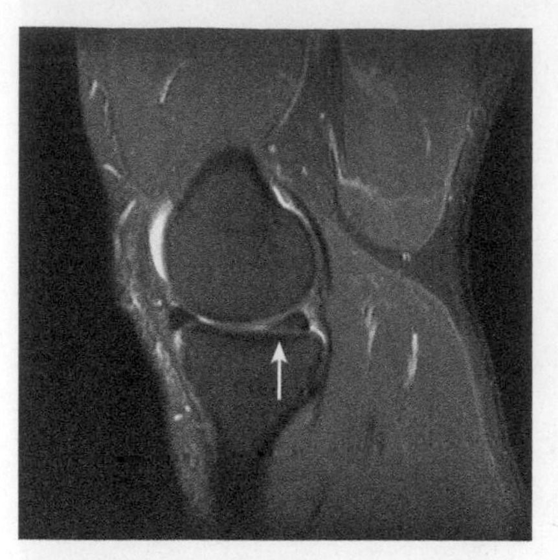

High signal extending to the inferior surface of the posterior horn of the medial meniscus consistent with a tear.

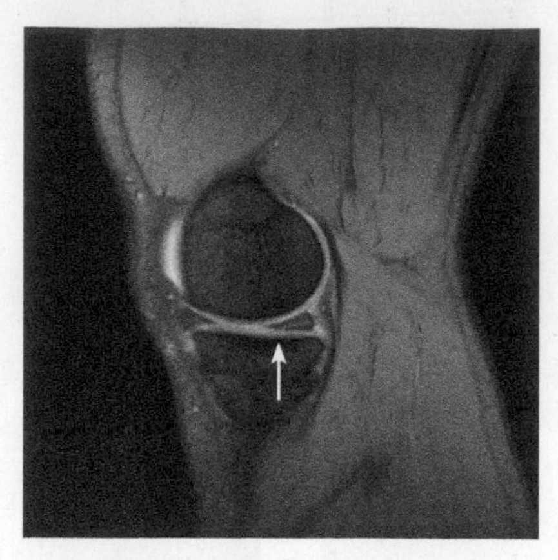

High signal extending to the inferior surface of the posterior horn of the medial meniscus consistent with a tear.

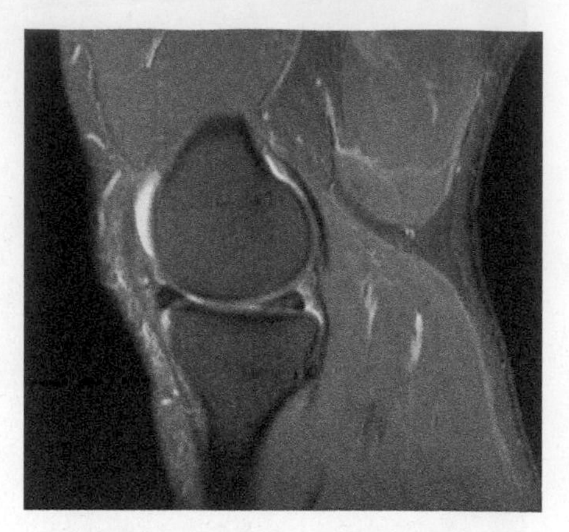

The lack of marrow edema and effusion is consistent with a chronic degenerative tear.

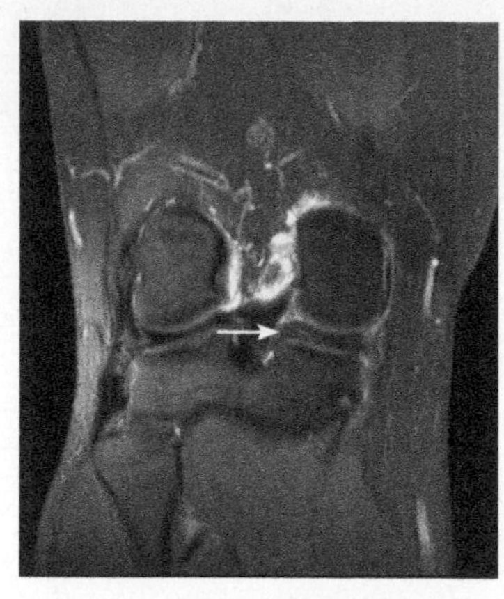

Horizontal configuration of degenerative tear is well appreciated on coronal images.

Answers

1. The clear definition of a meniscal tear is high signal within a meniscus extending to the articular surface. High signal per se is not diagnostic of a tear, and may reflect myxoid degeneration or artefact.
2. A medial meniscus injury is associated with ACL, PCL, capsular, and collateral ligament injuries. However, in this instance, the cause of the meniscal tear is more likely to be degeneration rather than a pivot-shift mechanism, hence other injuries are not present.
3. Severe tears on imaging appearances are often completely asymptomatic. Treatment should be geared to the patient's symptoms rather than to imaging appearances alone.
4. Known classifications of meniscal tears include radial, longitudinal, horizontal, flap, bucket-handle, and complex (which are a combination of 2 or more types). Flap and bucket-handle tears are particularly easy to miss, often lying in anatomically "hidden" sites, for example, the intercondylar notch.
5. Anterior knee pain is not associated with medial meniscal pathology; rather, it is a feature of patellofemoral dysplasia and osteoarthritis.

   The symptoms arising from meniscal pathology range from virtually no symptoms other than mild joint line tenderness to instability, locking, and giving way.

Pearls

- High signal on fluid-sensitive sequences extending to the articular surface is diagnostic of a meniscal tear.
- It is of paramount importance to look for meniscal fragments (loose bodies) that may be missed at arthroscopy.
- When diagnosing a medial meniscal tear, always evaluate other ligaments, for example, the ACL, carefully.
- Consideration of the site of tear is crucial when determining the likelihood of spontaneous healing and success of surgical repair; peripheral "red-zone" tears have the best prognosis.

Suggested Readings

Galea A, Giuffre B, Dimmick S, Coolican MR, Parker DA. The accuracy of magnetic resonance imaging scanning and its influence on management decisions in knee surgery. *Arthroscopy.* 2009;25(5):473-480.

Poulsen MR, Johnson DL. Meniscal injuries in the young, athletically active patient. *Phys Sportsmed.* 2011;39(1):123-130.

Pain on medial aspect of knee after being kicked from the side

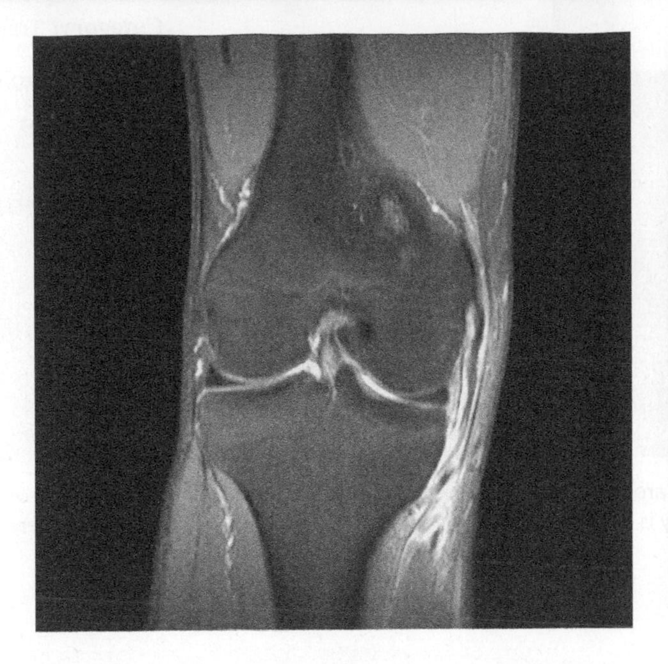

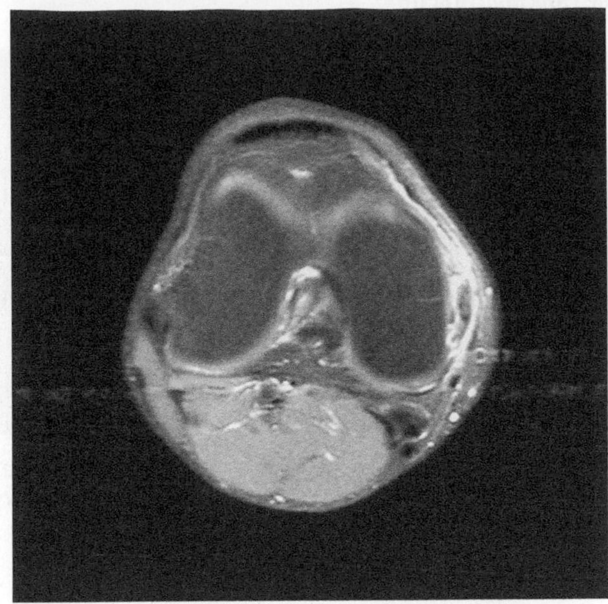

1. What is the structure injured in this patient?

2. What is the likely mechanism of injury?

3. What other injuries are associated with this mechanism of impact?

4. What statements are true regarding treatment for grade 1 injuries of the structure shown?

5. What is the expected recovery time for grade 2 injuries of the above structure?

Isolated MCL sprain of knee 1703

Case ranking/difficulty: **Category:** Trauma

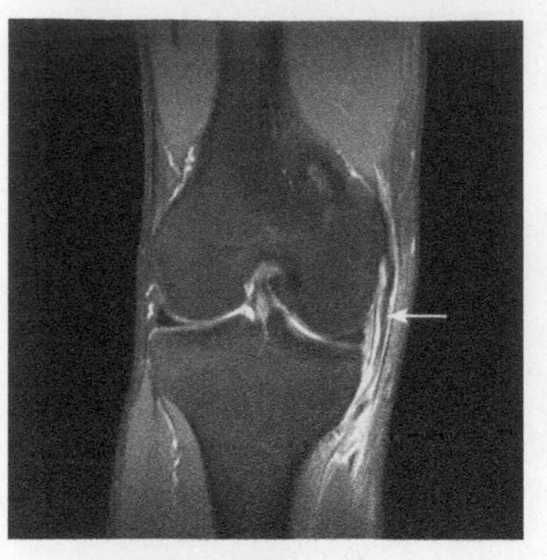

High signal around a thickened but intact MCL consistent with a grade 2 sprain.

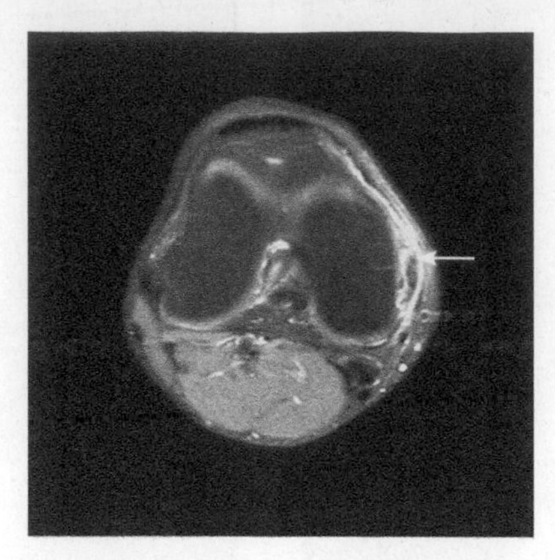

Extensive edema around MCL, but no other major injury is present.

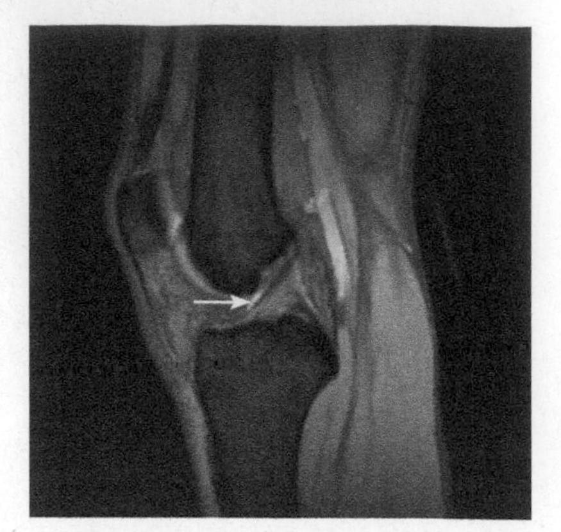

There is edema within the fibers of the ACL consistent with a sprain. There is no tear however.

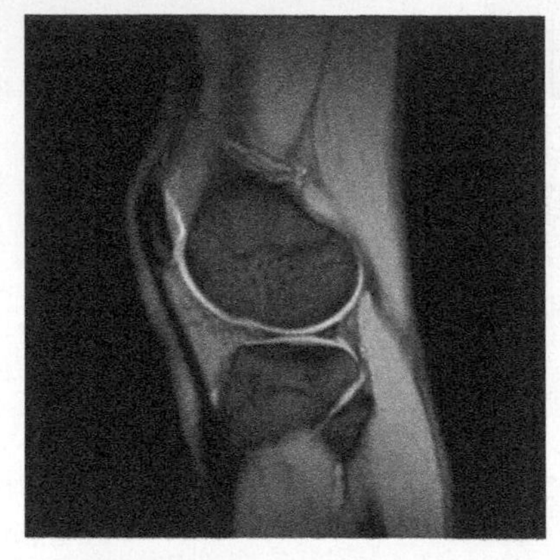

There is no other evidence of internal derangement. The menisci are normal and there is no effusion.

Answers

1. Edema is seen tracking around the MCL consistent with a grade 2 sprain.
2. Valgus strain affects the medial structures of the knee. No rotational force is present in cases of isolated MCL sprain.
3. A valgus-strain injury is an example of a flexion-distraction injury. The lateral structures are subjected to a flexion force, resulting in bone contusions and fractures of the lateral femoral condyle and lateral tibial plateau, and tears of the lateral meniscus.

   The medial structures are subjected to a distraction force, resulting in MCL injury and avulsion fractures of the medial compartment.
4. Grade 1 sprains do not require surgery. Early immobilization may be advisable, for example, lightweight cast/hinged-brace, although a rehabilitation program with a physical therapist is important for the best outcomes.
5. Most grade 2 MCL sprains should be healed in 10 to 12 weeks, assuming appropriate rest, rehabilitation, and avoidance of sports during the recovery period.

Pearls

- MRI is the investigative modality of choice for all cases of internal derangement.
- Isolated MCL sprains are associated with a valgus strain injury.
- Accurate grading is important for prognostic purposes, as it determines the period of rehabilitation required to enable athletes to return to their sport.
- MCL injuries are commonly classified into grades 1 to 3.
  - Grade 1: Intact ligament. High signal is seen superficial to ligament only. Return to normal function in 1 to 2 weeks.
  - Grade 2: Intact ligament. High signal is seen superficial and deep to the fibers of the ligaments. Return to normal function (eg, competitive sport) is approximately 8 to 12 weeks.
  - Grade 3: Complete tear, which is frequently in association with other injuries, for example, ACL. Return to normal function depends on associated injuries, for example ACL rupture, and consequently surgical correction and recovery time.

Suggested Readings

Edson CJ. Conservative and postoperative rehabilitation of isolated and combined injuries of the medial collateral ligament. *Sports Med Arthrosc.* 2006;14(2):105-110.

Järvinen M, Kannus P, Johnson RJ. How to treat knee ligament injuries? *Ann Chir Gynaecol.* 1991;80(2):134-140.

Reider B. Medial collateral ligament injuries in athletes. *Sports Med.* 1996;21(2):147-156.

Twisting injury of the knee

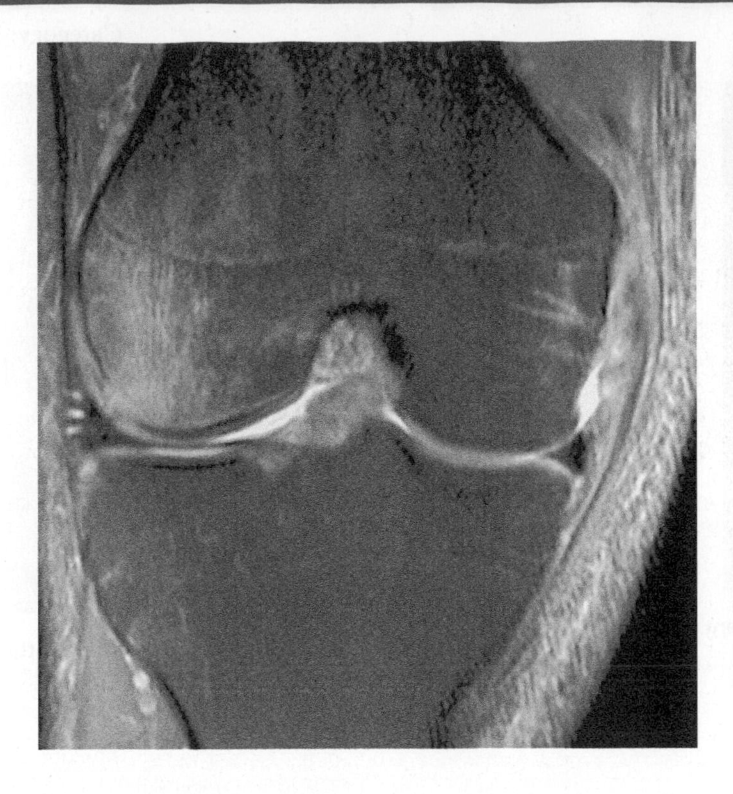

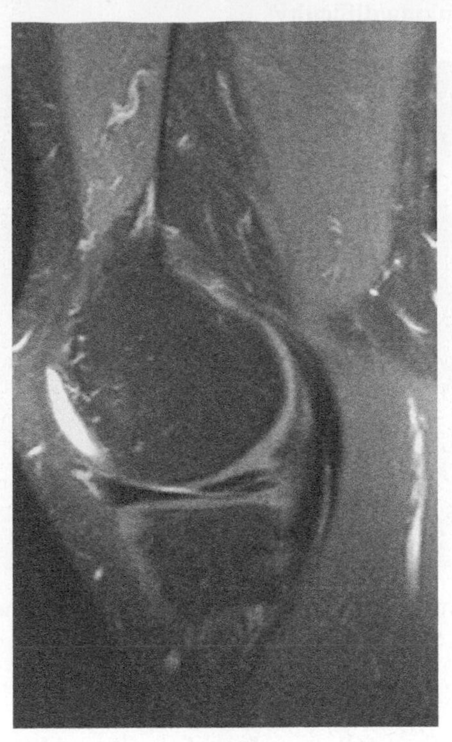

1. What are the imaging findings?

2. What is the O'Donoghue triad?

3. What is a Wrisberg rip tear?

4. What are the arthroscopic zones of the meniscus?

5. What are the medial supporting layers of the knee?

O'Donoghue triad 1541

Case ranking/difficulty: 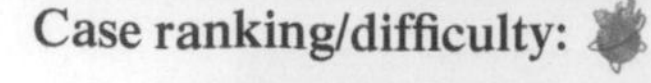

Category: Trauma

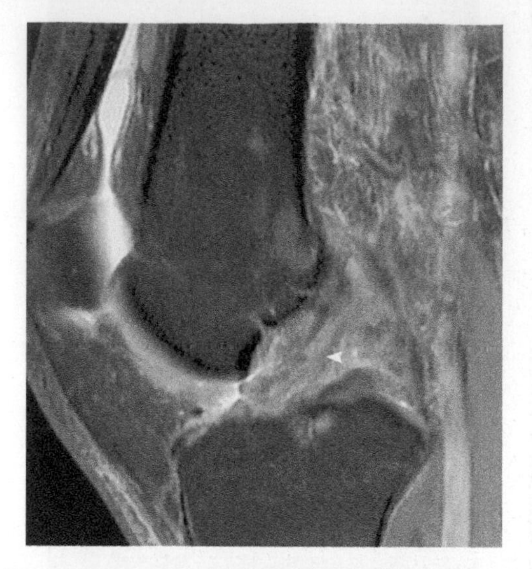

Complete rupture of the anterior cruciate ligament.

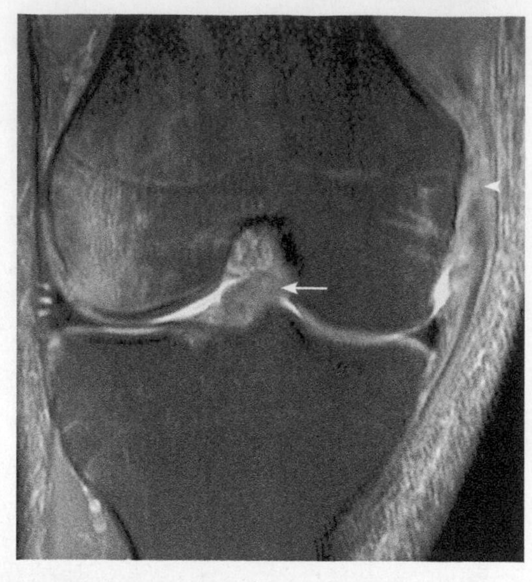

Grade III medial collateral ligament tear at its femoral attachment (*arrowhead*). Complete ACL tear (*arrow*).

Answers

1. There is an ACL rupture, medial collateral ligament injury, and associated horizontal medial meniscal tear.
2. ACL, MCL, and medial meniscal injury, although lateral meniscal tears are in fact more common.
3. A Wrisberg rip tear is a longitudinal tear of the posterior horn of the lateral meniscus, postulated as a sequela of an ACL tear.
4. The meniscus is divided into a red-on-red peripheral zone, an intermediate white-on-red zone, and the innermost white-on-white zone. Tears in the red zones are likely to heal and are repaired, and white zone tears are debrided.
5. There are 3 medial supporting layers. The outermost layer is the crural fascia, which also envelopes the sartorius posteriorly. The second layer is the superficial MCL, and the third layer is the deep MCL. Layers 1 and 2 are fused anteriorly, layers 2 and 3 are fused posteriorly.

Pearls

- The O'Donoghue triad is made up of a combination of injuries: medial collateral ligament rupture, ACL rupture, and meniscal tears. It is also called the *unhappy triad.*
- It was first described by O'Donoghue in 1950, and he reported injuries to the ACL, MCL, with a medial meniscal tear. It is now known that the meniscal injury could be either a medial or lateral meniscal tear, and that lateral meniscal tears are more common.
- Plain film may show an avulsion fracture of the medial femoral condyle (Stieda fracture), and genu valgus position of the knee.
- MRI is the investigative modality of choice. It shows all the direct and indirect signs of an anterior cruciate ligament injury, as well as the meniscal and MCL tears.
- Medial collateral injury:
  - Type 1: Increased T2 signal of the MCL, and edema external to the MCL.
  - Type 2: Stretching of the MCL with increased signal and thickening. Usually edema superficial and deep to the MCL.
  - Type 3: Rupture and discontinuity with high signal, sometimes associated with an avulsion fracture (Stieda fracture).

Suggested Readings

Shelbourne KD, Nitz PA. The O'Donoghue triad revisited. Combined knee injuries involving anterior cruciate and medial collateral ligament tears. *Am J Sports Med.* 1994;19(5):474-477.

Staron RB, Haramati N, Feldman F, et al. O'Donoghue's triad: magnetic resonance imaging evidence. *Skeletal Radiol.* 1994;23(8):633-636.

Twisted knee with swelling

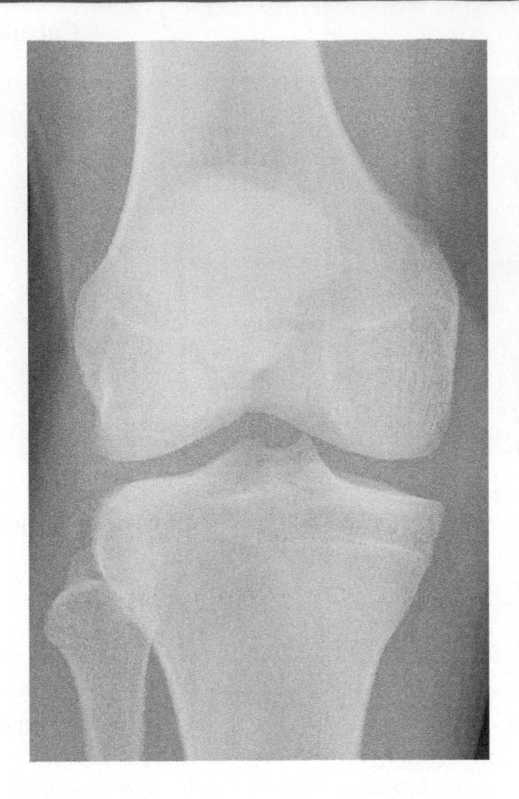

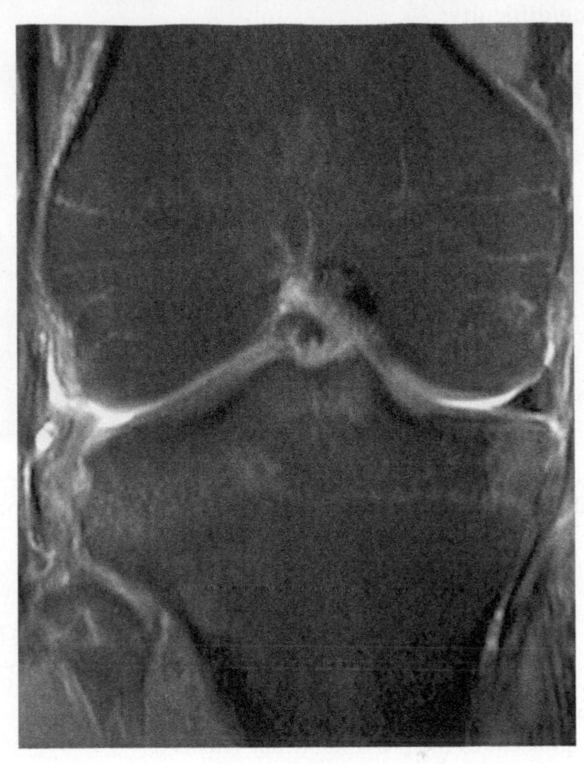

1. What are the radiographic findings?
2. What are the MRI findings?
3. What are the other associated injuries with this abnormality?
4. What is the mechanism of injury for this fracture?
5. A reverse Segond fracture occurs at the posteromedial tibia. What are the associated injuries of this fracture?

Segond fracture 1540

Case ranking/difficulty:

Category: Trauma

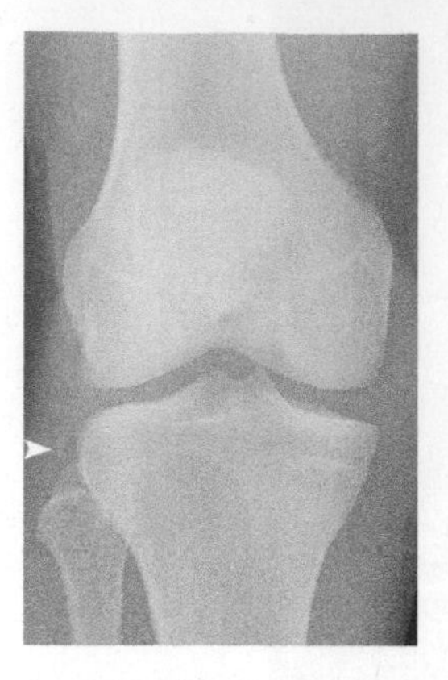

Avulsion fracture at the anterolateral tibia.

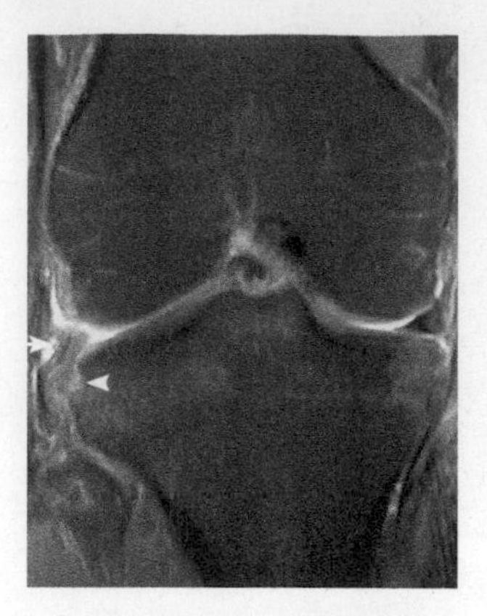

Complete rupture of fibular collateral ligament (*arrow*), and there is a fracture donor site with edema in the anterolateral tibia (*arrowhead*).

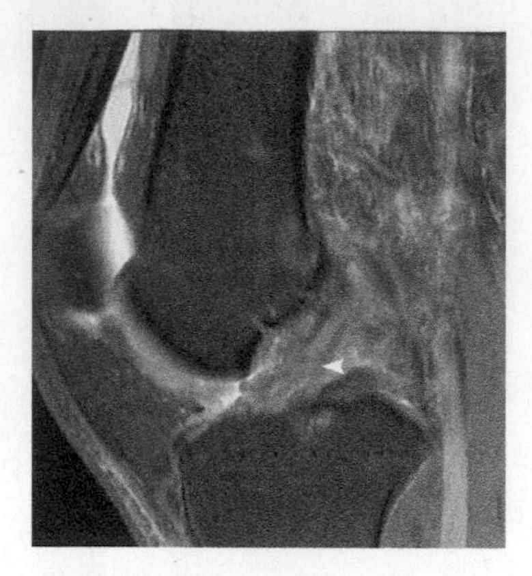

Complete ACL rupture in the same patient.

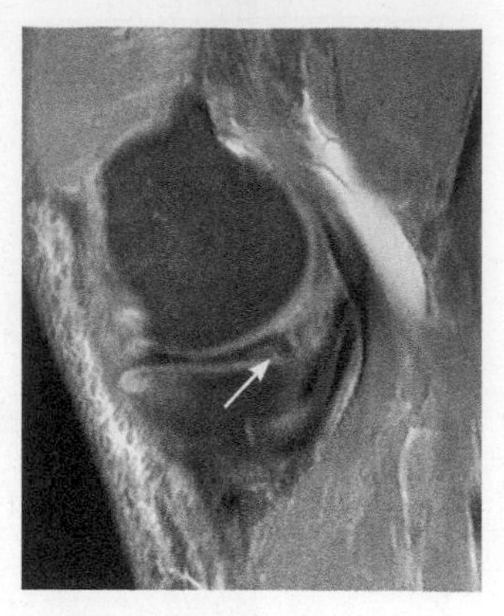

Medial meniscal tear is seen, an associated injury.

Answers

1. There is a bony fragment on the lateral aspect of the knee just adjacent to the proximal tibia. This is a Segond fracture.
2. The MRI shows high-grade rupture of the fibular collateral ligament, complete ACL rupture and bone bruising with subchondral edema at the lateral tibial plateau, the donor site for the Segond fracture.
3. The associated injuries with a Segond fracture are ACL or PCL rupture, medial meniscal tear, biceps femoris avulsion fracture and arcuate fracture.
4. Internal rotation and varus strain are the main mechanisms of injury in a Segond fracture, as compared to valgus stress in the majority of ACL tears.
5. PCL and medial meniscal tears are associations with a reverse Segond fracture.

Pearls

- A Segond fracture is a cortical avulsion fracture of the tibial insertion of the middle third of the lateral capsular ligament, but also may involve an avulsion of the posterior fibers of the iliotibial band.
- The mechanism is internal rotation and varus rotation, as opposed to the classic valgus strain for the majority of ACL ruptures.
- These fractures are associated with ACL tears, medial meniscal tears, MCL sprains, and biceps femoris and fibular collateral ligament avulsions (posterolateral corner injuries).
- They may also be associated with ACL footprint avulsions.
- Reverse Segond fracture is at the posteromedial tibia and is seen in association with PCL tears.

Suggested Readings

Campos JC, Chung CB, Lektrakul N, et al. Pathogenesis of the Segond fracture: anatomic and MR imaging evidence of an iliotibial tract or anterior oblique band avulsion. *Radiology.* 2001;219(2):381-386.

Escobedo EM, Mills WJ, Hunter JC. The "reverse Segond" fracture: association with a tear of the posterior cruciate ligament and medial meniscus. *AJR Am J Roentgenol.* 2002;178(4):979-983.

Gottsegen CJ, Eyer BA, White EA, Learch TJ, Forrester D. Avulsion fractures of the knee: imaging findings and clinical significance. *Radiographics.* 2008;28(6): 1755-1770.

Pain and locking of knee following twisting injury after playing soccer

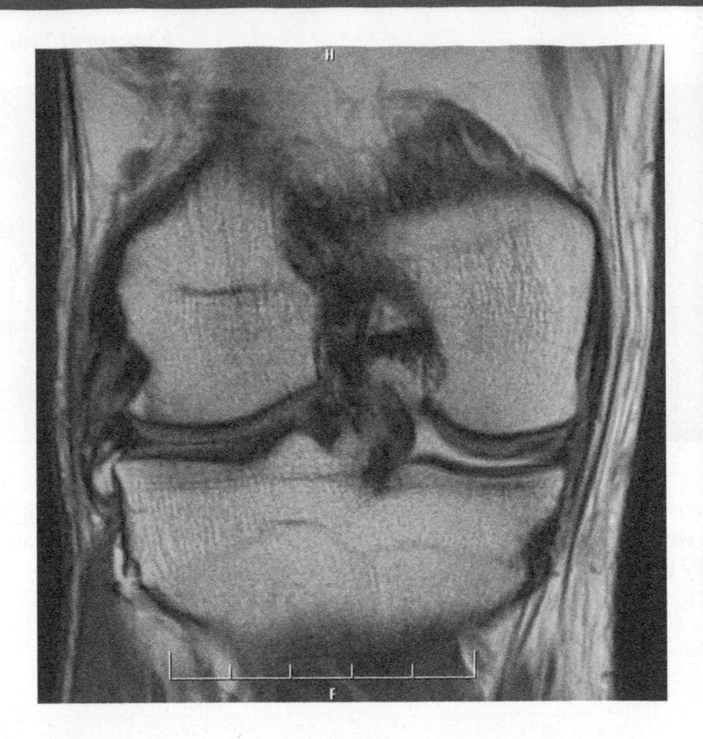

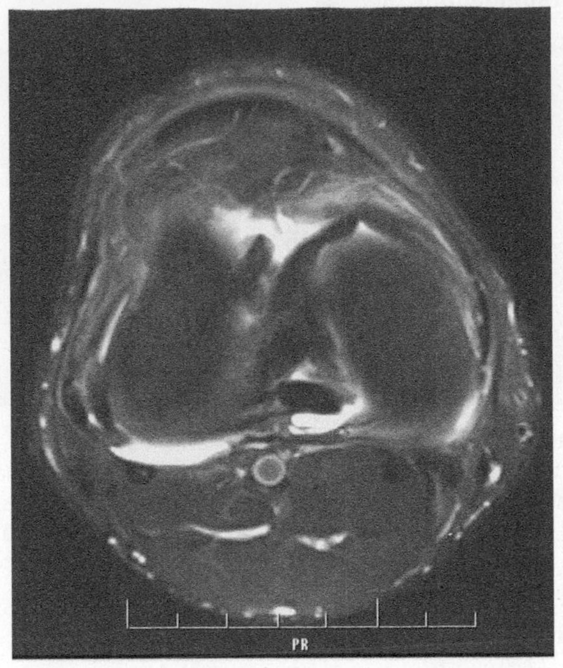

1. What are the imaging features of this entity?

2. What is the management?

3. What are the possible configurations of a flap tear?

4. What are common associated injuries in the presence of a medial meniscal tear?

5. What are the clinical features of a meniscal tear?

Bucket-handle tear of medial meniscus 1721

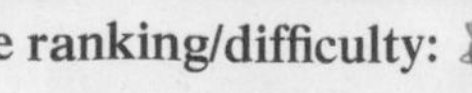

Case ranking/difficulty: **Category:** Trauma

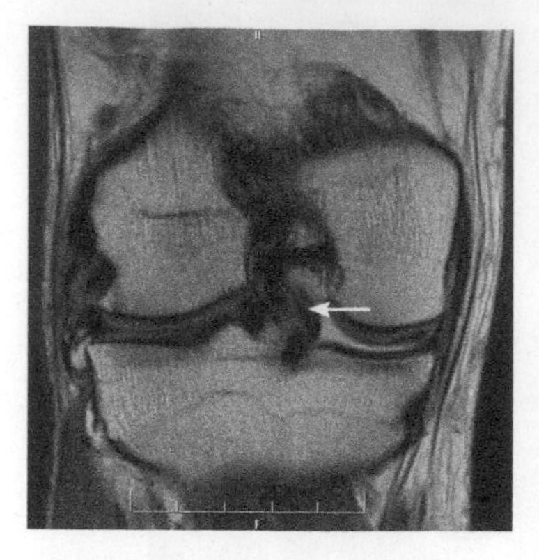

Diminutive appearance of medial meniscus in conjunction with a meniscal flap in the intercondylar notch.

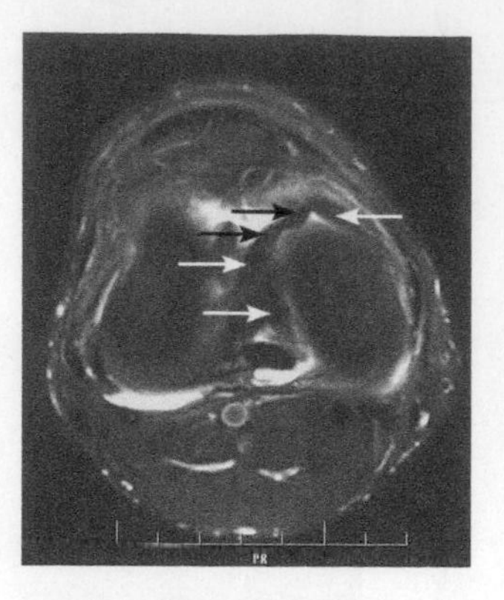

Axial PD FS image demonstrates bucket-handle tear of medial meniscus, which has flipped anterolaterally to lie in the intercondylar notch.

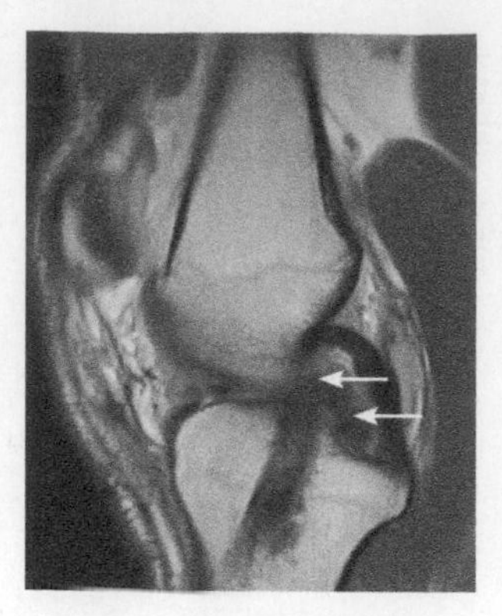

Different patient. "Double-PCL" sign is seen because of the bucket-handle lying adjacent to the native PCL fragment in the intercondylar notch. Incidental note is made of an ACL reconstruction graft.

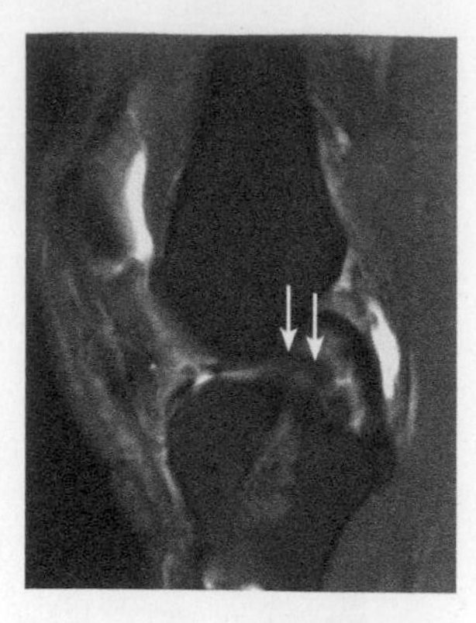

Additional sagittal view of bucket-handle meniscal flap within the intercondylar notch.

Answers

1. Bucket-handle tears are displaced longitudinal tears attached at 2 points to the preserved portion of meniscus. The flipped portion of the meniscus (bucket-handle) may lie in the intercondylar notch, or may flip anteriorly or posteriorly to lie over the residual portion of meniscus. As such, there may be a reduced thickness of either the anterior or posterior horn and a "double-PCL" sign. Bucket-handle tears can be very difficult to diagnose, unless they are actively sought by the reporting radiologist.

2. A bucket-handle tear invariably needs repair, because if left untreated, the tear leads to instability and locking. Repair is done arthroscopically in the overwhelming majority of cases.

3. Displaced radial tears are also known as "parrot-beak" tears because of their morphological appearance. A longitudinal tear attached at two sites with a displaced flap, is a bucket-handle tear. A horizontal tear may also be displaced.

4. ACL, PCL, lateral meniscal, MCL, LCL, and posterolateral corner injuries are associated with medial meniscal injuries. Fractures and bone contusions are also found in association with meniscal injuries.

5. Meniscal injury may lead to pain and instability. Locking is particularly associated with flipped or displaced meniscal tears.

Pearls

- A bucket-handle tear is an important radiological diagnosis as it directly affects orthopaedic management.
- Systematic scrupulous review of knee MRI images is essential to prevent this injury from being missed.
- Absent or reduced thickness of meniscal horns with apparent increase in thickness of the other horn, loss of the bow-tie appearance, or increased soft tissue within the intercondylar notch should raise the index of suspicion for this diagnosis.
- Axial and coronal images are extremely useful adjuncts to make the diagnosis. The entire bucket-handle may be seen on an axial image, although with a typical 4-mm slice thickness, the axial images should not be relied upon exclusively as these tears may be missed. On a coronal image, the only 2 significant structures that should be visible within the intercondylar notch are the ACL and PCL. Any extra soft tissue in the notch is suspicious for a flap or displaced meniscal tear.

Suggested Readings

Engstrom BI, Vinson EN, Taylor DC, Garrett WE Jr, Helms CA.. Hemi-bucket-handle tears of the meniscus: appearance on MRI and potential surgical implications. *Skeletal Radiol.* 2012;41(8):933-938.

Takayama K, Matsushita T, Matsumoto T, Kubo S, Kurosaka M, Kuroda R. The double ACL sign: an unusual bucket-handle tear of medial meniscus. *Knee Surg Sports Traumatol Arthrosc.* 2011;19(8):1343-1346.

Venkatanarasimha N, Kamath A, Mukherjee K, Kamath S. Potential pitfalls of a double PCL sign. *Skeletal Radiol.* 2009;38(8):735-739.

History of skiing injury, treated with surgical repair

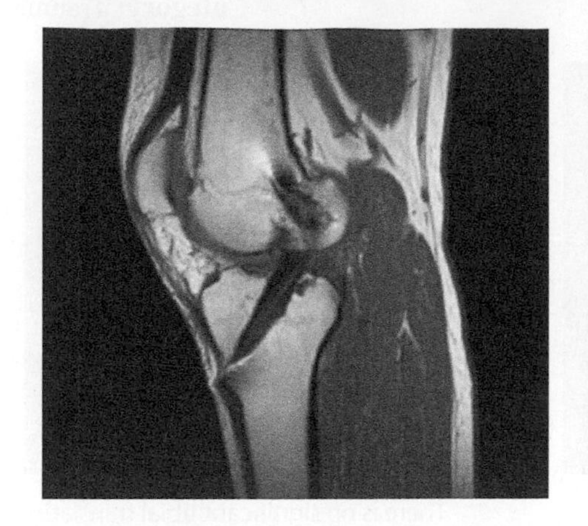

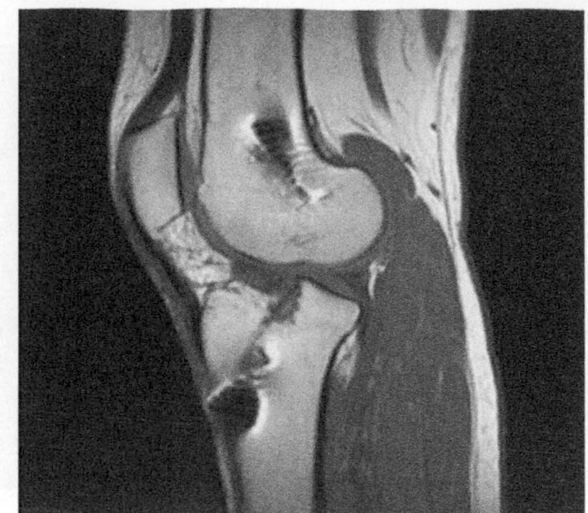

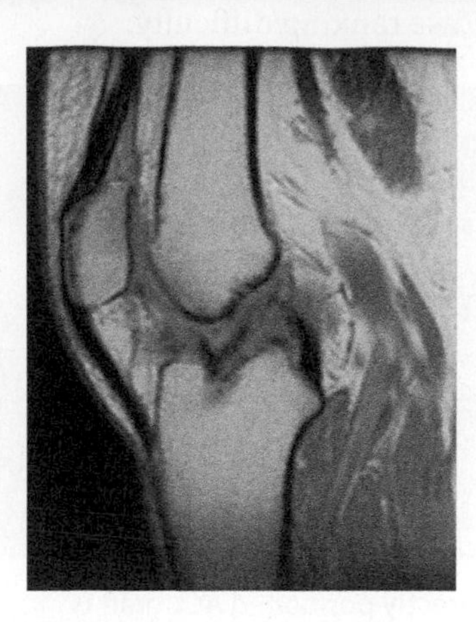

1. What is the structure depicted?

2. Which tendons are commonly used as grafts in the procedure shown?

3. What should be evaluated on MRI with this entity?

4. What injuries are associated with the structure shown?

5. What is the mechanism of initial injury leading to the appearances shown?

ACL reconstruction

114

Case ranking/difficulty: 

Category: Trauma

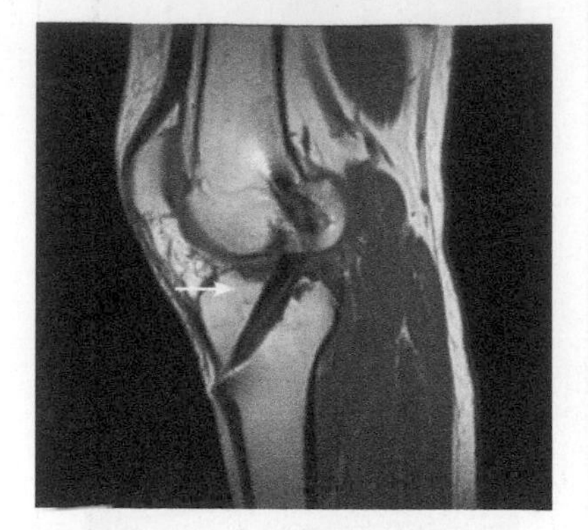

Correctly positioned ACL graft is shown.

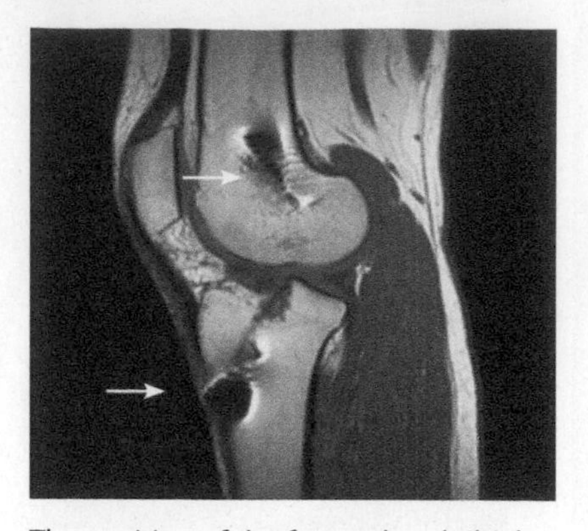

The position of the femoral and tibial tunnels can be well visualized on sagittal sequences.

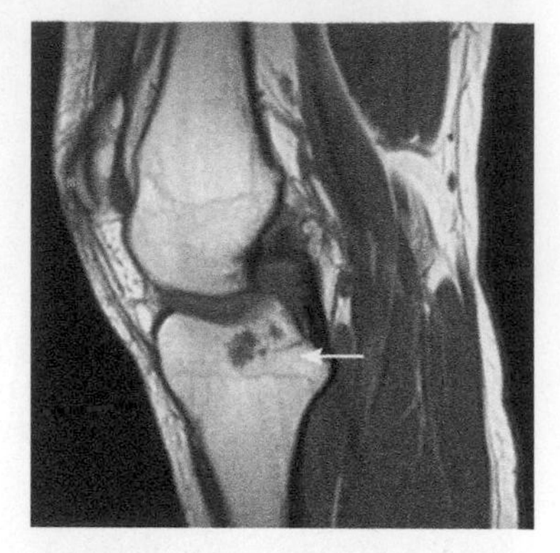

There is no significant tibial translation postoperatively confirming the presence of a functioning graft.

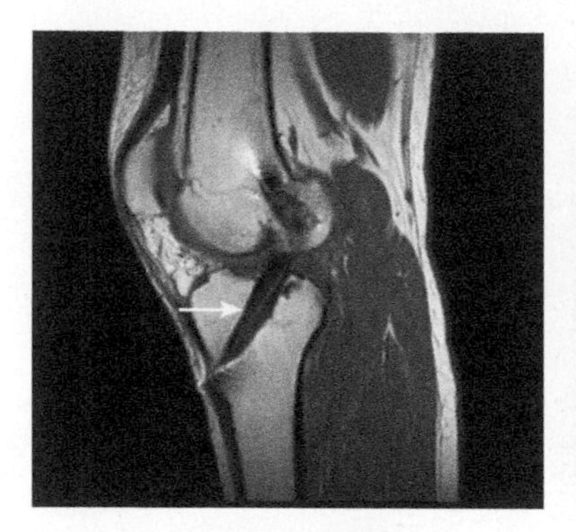

Oblique orientation of graft simulates the normal anatomical direction of the native ACL.

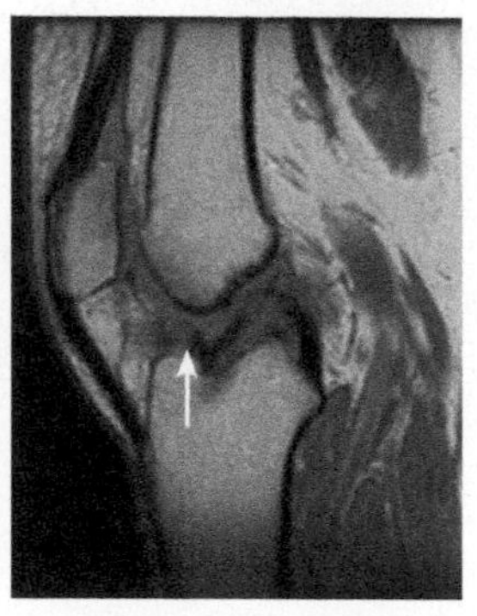

Anterior arthrofibrosis produces the characteristic "cyclops" lesion and may prevent full extension.

Answers

1. ACL reconstruction is performed using a semimembranosus-gracilis or bone-patellar tendon-bone allograft.
2. The choice of tendon graft is not as critical as correct graft placement. However, the most commonly used tendons are the patellar, hamstring, and tibialis anterior tendons.
3. A postoperative MRI should comment on the femoral and tibial tunnel positions, the integrity of the graft, signal within the tunnel, presence of roof impingement, and of course all the other normal structures which may be the source of the patient's pain.
4. ACL injuries occur from a pivot-shift mechanism. This is often associated with injuries to the MCL, PCL, LCL, medial and lateral menisci, and posterolateral as well as posteromedial corner.
5. Pivot shift injuries are strongly associated with rupture of the ACL.

Pearls

- Artefact from screw fixation and lack of a normal striated ACL appearance should raise the possibility of a previous ACL reconstruction.
- The two most common grafts are the bone-patellar tendon-bone graft and the semimembranosus-gracilis hamstring tendon graft.
- The source of the graft is suggested by a defect in the relevant portion of the hamstring musculature, or by a central defect in the patellar tendon ± patella.
- The graft should be carefully evaluated to ensure full continuity to exclude retear.
- The position of the tunnel, integrity of the graft, and presence of arthrofibrosis, infection or intercondylar roof impingement should be commented on when reporting an MRI scan post ACL reconstruction.
- Arthrofibrosis produces a characteristic "cyclops" lesion when occurring anterior to the ACL graft. Essentially, it is a form of nodular fibrosis, which may produce a mechanical block to knee extension that may include entrapped native ACL fibers.
- ACL reconstruction is often accompanied by partial meniscectomy, as meniscal injuries commonly occur with the classical pivot-shift mechanism of ACL injury. Hence, careful evaluation of menisci is essential to differentiate meniscal retears from normal postoperative menisci in these patients.

Suggested Readings

Ho-Fung VM, Jaimes C, Jaramillo D. MR imaging of ACL injuries in pediatric and adolescent patients. *Clin Sports Med.* 2011;30(4):707-726.

Naraghi AM, Gupta S, Jacks LM, Essue J, Marks P, White LM. Anterior cruciate ligament reconstruction: MR imaging signs of anterior knee laxity in the presence of an intact graft. *Radiology.* 2012;263(3):802-810.

Sudden pain in shoulder after lifting heavy load

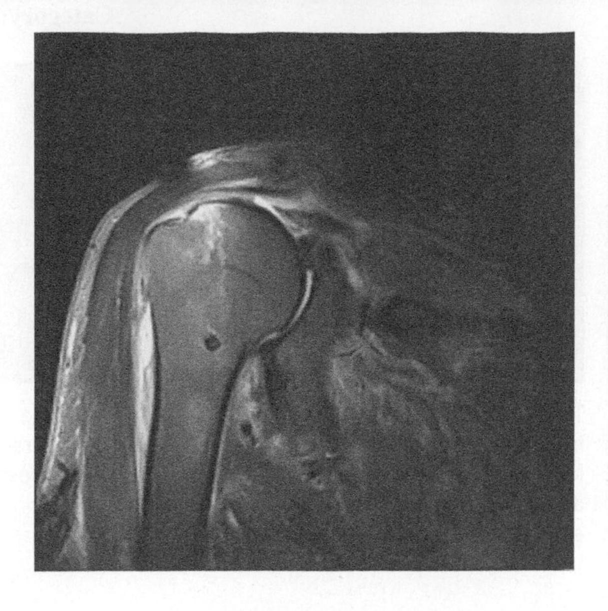

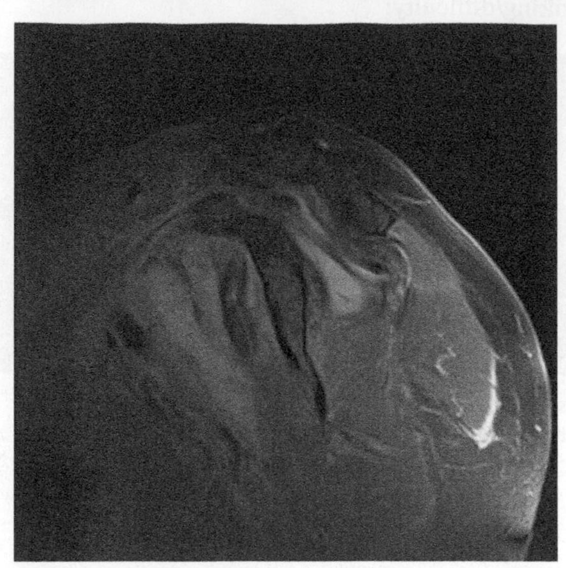

1. What is the main structure that is torn?

2. What are the imaging features relevant to this entity?

3. Which imaging modalities can be used to diagnose this entity?

4. What is the distinction between a massive full-thickness cuff tear and a small full-thickness tear?

5. Which groups of people are most susceptible to this injury?

Massive rotator cuff tear 1700

Case ranking/difficulty: 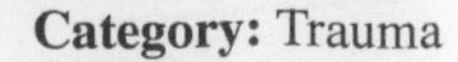 **Category:** Trauma

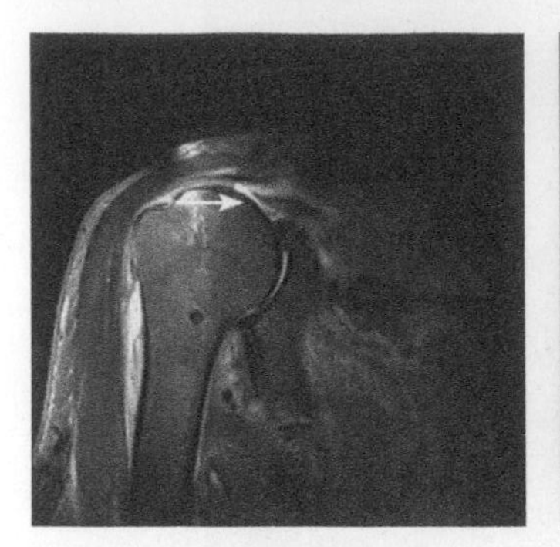

Retracted supraspinatus tendon with massive full-thickness cuff tear.

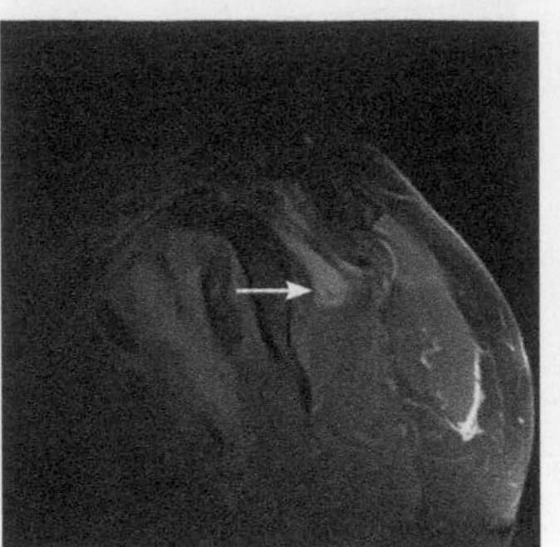

Tear involving supra- and infraspinous fossa of scapula on sagittal images, and hence extending to the infraspinatus tendon.

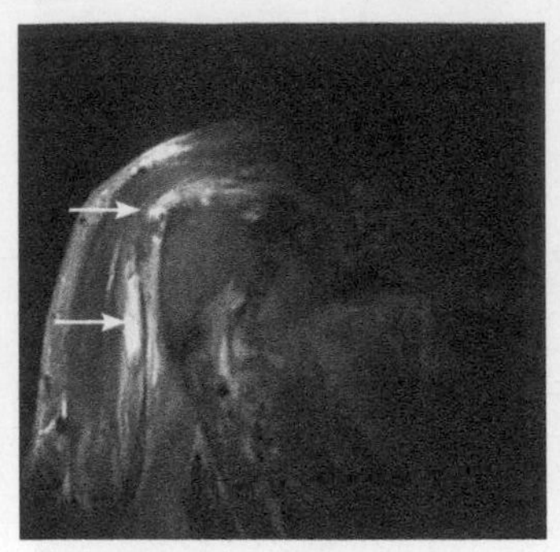

There is discontinuity of the intra-articular portion of the long head of biceps tendon and a large effusion suggestive of extension of the tear to involve the rotator interval structures.

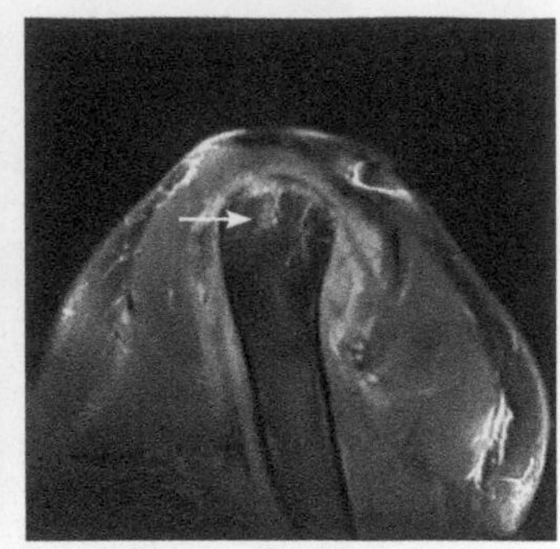

Marrow edema in the posterolateral humeral head is consistent with a severe traumatic injury.

Answers

1. Most tears involve the supraspinatus tendon. They may extend a variable distance to involve the infraspinatus posteriorly or subscapularis tendon anteriorly.
2. A full-thickness tear will result in fluid tracking into the subacromial subdeltoid bursa and the long head of biceps tendon sheath, as it is intra-articular. A defect in the tendon leads to a sonographic "window" to the underlying hyaline cartilage, which will appear hyperechoic as a result of being uncovered.
3. Ultrasound and MRI are the imaging modalities of choice for assessing the rotator cuff. The advantages of ultrasound are its ease, relative cost-effectiveness, and ability to guide percutaneous injections. The advantages of MRI are its reproducibility and independence from the skill of the operator.
4. A full-thickness tear by definition must extend from the bursal surface to the articular surface. However, not all full-thickness tears involve the full width of the supraspinatus tendon. A massive tear is greater than 5 cm in width. It therefore involves the whole width of the supraspinatus (3 cm), but also extends for a variable distance posteriorly (infraspinatus) or anteriorly (subscapularis).
5. Massive cuff tears are most common in elderly patients in whom relatively trivial injuries can extend to involve much of the rotator cuff. In these patients the underlying tendons are degenerate and therefore susceptible to injury. Young elite athletes may have cuff tears, but in general they are small or moderate in size as the tendons are in a better condition and well vascularized.

Pearls

- The rotator cuff can be evaluated with ultrasound or MRI.
- A full-thickness tear extends from the bursal surface to the articular surface.
- A full-thickness tear may extend posteriorly into the infraspinatus, or sometimes anteriorly to involve the subscapularis. The latter will necessarily involve disruption of the biceps anchor in the rotator interval.
- Key information for the surgeon includes size and depth of tear, shape of acromion, and presence of fatty atrophy of supraspinatus muscle belly.

Suggested Readings

Iagulli ND, Field LD, Hobgood ER, Ramsey JR, Savoie FH. Comparison of partial versus complete arthroscopic repair of massive rotator cuff tears. *Am J Sports Med.* 2012;40(5):1022-1026.

Kim JR, Cho YS, Ryu KJ, Kim JH. Clinical and radiographic outcomes after arthroscopic repair of massive rotator cuff tears using a suture bridge technique: assessment of repair integrity on magnetic resonance imaging. *Am J Sports Med.* 2012;40(4):786-793.

Yamaguchi H, Suenaga N, Oizumi N, Hosokawa Y, Kanaya F. Will preoperative atrophy and Fatty degeneration of the shoulder muscles improve after rotator cuff repair in patients with massive rotator cuff tears? *Adv Orthop.* 2012;2012(2012):195876.

Injured right arm doing pushups

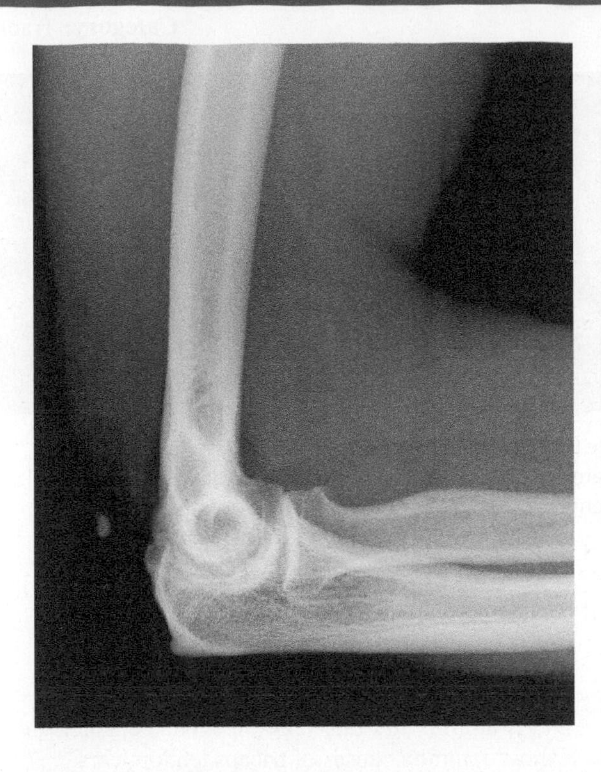

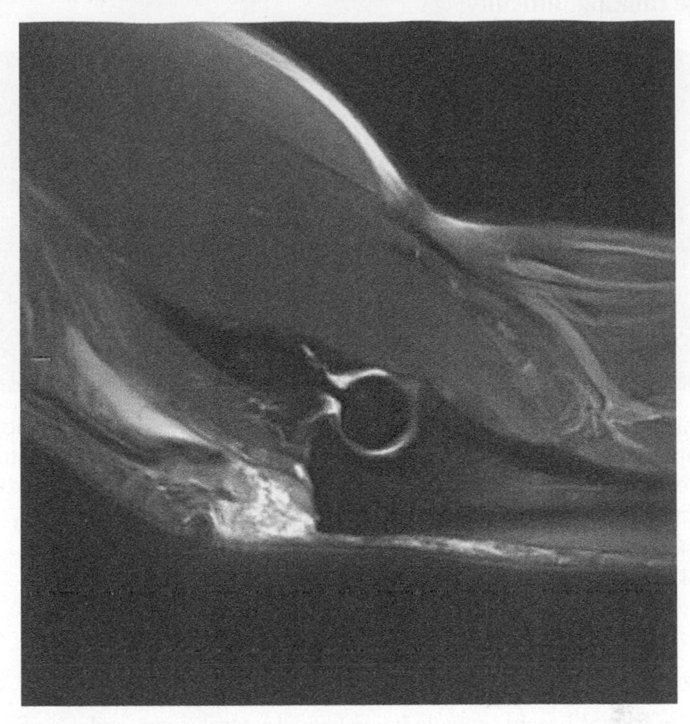

1. What is the anatomy of the involved structure?

2. What are risk factors for injuries involving this structure?

3. What is the differential diagnosis?

4. What is the most common anatomic location for this injury?

5. What is the epidemiology of this injury?

Triceps tendon tear **1467**

Case ranking/difficulty: 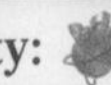

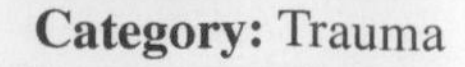
Category: Trauma

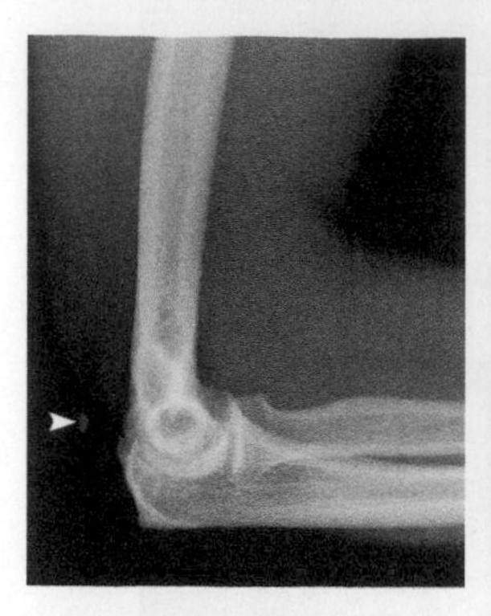

Lateral elbow radiograph demonstrates a small avulsion fracture fragment projecting over the soft tissues at the posterior aspect of the elbow (*arrowhead*).

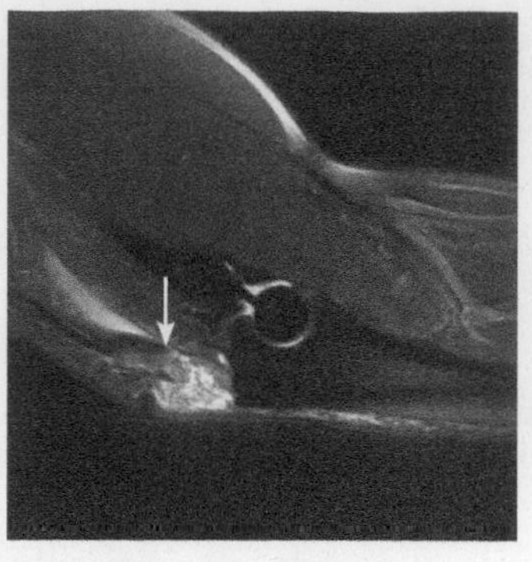

The distal triceps tendon is completely ruptured from its insertion onto the olecranon (*arrow* shows retracted end).

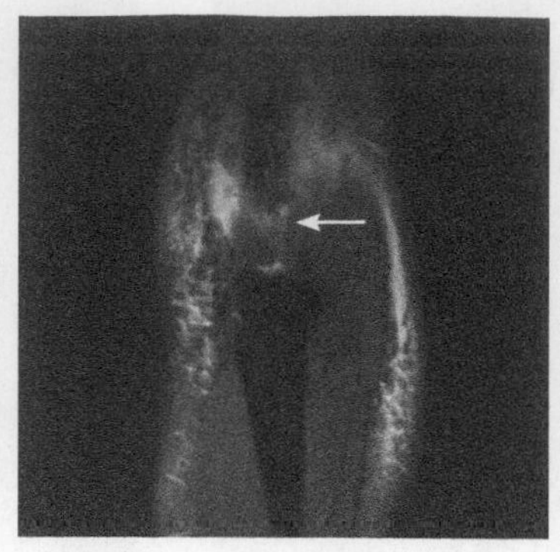

A complete triceps tear is again demonstrated (*arrow* shows retracted end).

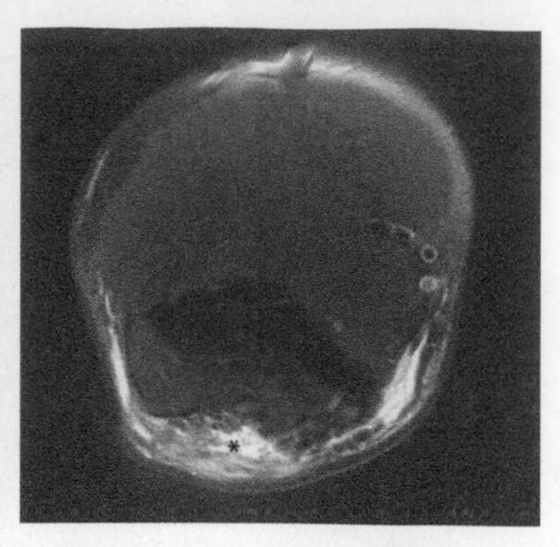

A gap is demonstrated in the expected location of the distal triceps tendon (*asterisk*).

Answers

1. The triceps brachii muscle has 3 heads: lateral, long, and medial.
2. Weightlifting, steroid use, olecranon bursitis, local steroid injection, and hyperparathyroidism are all risk factors.
3. Tendinosis, musculotendinous junction strain, olecranon bursitis, and olecranon fracture are in the differential diagnosis for triceps tendon tear.
4. The osseous insertion onto the olecranon process is the most common site of triceps tendon tear, and they are most commonly partial tears.
5. Triceps tendon tears are more common in males than females by a ratio of 4:1. The average age of these patients is approximately 46 years, and is rare in children.

Pearls

- The triceps brachii is composed of long, lateral, and medial heads.
- The 3 heads form a single tendon distally, which inserts onto the olecranon process of the ulna.
- Tears of the triceps tendon are rare. They occur most often in the distal portion of the tendon, and are more common in males than in females. A small avulsion fracture may be seen.
- Partial tears are more common than complete tears.
- Athletic injuries and falls onto outstretched hands are the most common causes of triceps tendon tears.
- Risk factors include anabolic steroid use, local steroid injection, olecranon bursitis, and hyperparathyroidism.
- Complete tears are generally treated surgically.
- Partial tears involving less than 50% of the tendon are often managed nonsurgically.

Suggested Readings

Koplas MC, Schneider E, Sundaram M. Prevalence of triceps tendon tears on MRI of the elbow and clinical correlation. *Skeletal Radiol.* 2011;40(5):587-594.

Yeh PC, Dodds SD, Smart LR, Mazzocca AD, Sethi PM. Distal triceps rupture. *J Am Acad Orthop Surg.* 2010;18(1):31-40.

Sudden pain behind the heel after exercising

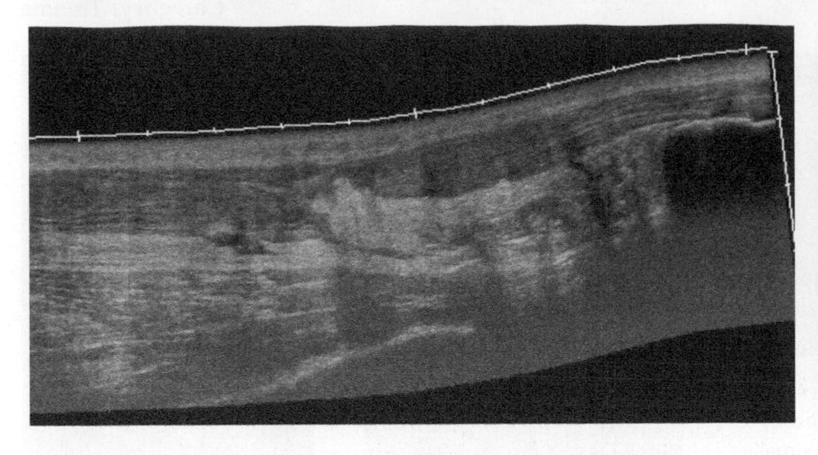

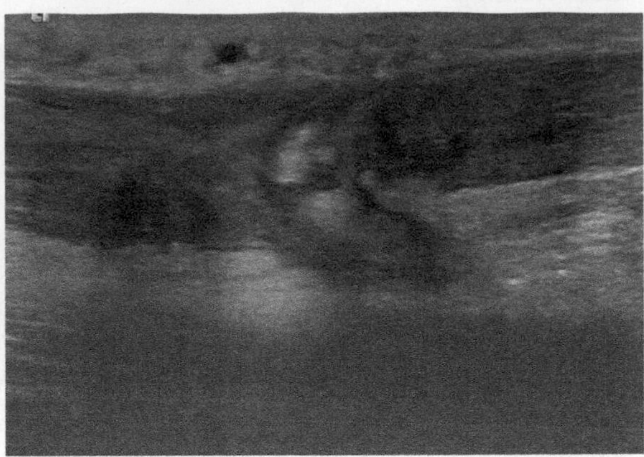

1. What are the ultrasound findings?

2. What are the risk factors for this condition?

3. Which location in the tendon has an increased propensity for tears?

4. What is the classification of this injury?

5. What are the differential diagnoses for acute calf pain?

Achilles tendon tear 1598

Case ranking/difficulty:

Category: Trauma

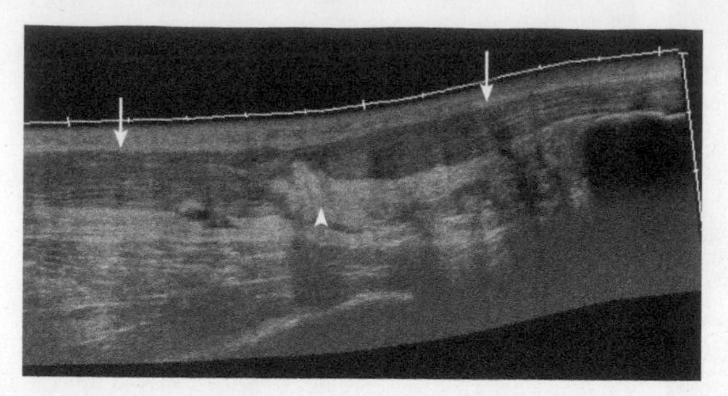

Longitudinal image shows a high-grade partial tear of the Achilles tendon with hemorrhage and Kager fat herniation (*arrowhead*) into the tendon gap, with the normal fibrillary tendon proximally and distally (*arrows*).

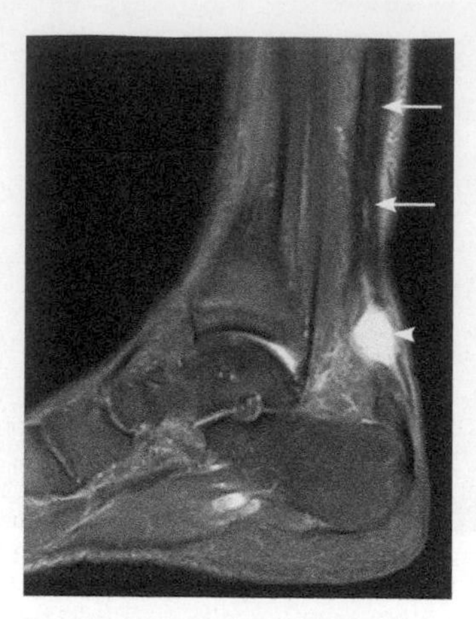

Full-thickness tear in another patient (*arrowhead*), with tendinosis in the retracted proximal tendon (*arrows*).

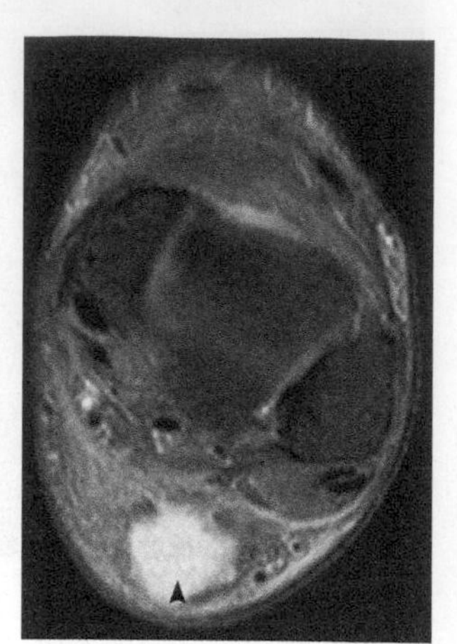

Full-thickness tear in the axial plane.

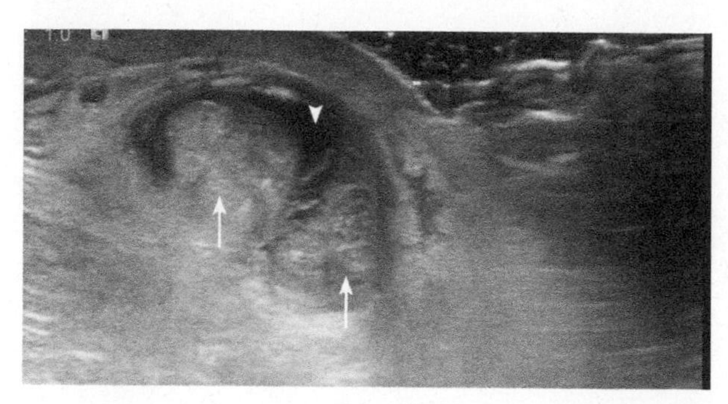

Transverse image showing high-grade partial tear of the Achilles tendon (*arrowhead*) with echogenic tendon peripherally (*arrows*).

Answers

1. Increased echogenicity in the tendon altering the normal echogenic fibrillary pattern reflects a full-thickness Achilles tendon tear. The echogenicity reflects a combination of hemorrhage and herniation of Kager fat into the gap created by the tear.
2. The risk factors including chronic tendinosis, trauma, repeated microtrauma, diabetes, rheumatoid arthritis, systemic lupus erythematosus, gout, and fluoroquinolone antibiotics.
3. The typical location of Achilles tendon tears is approximately 2 to 6 cm proximal to its calcaneal insertion—the critical zone, or area of relative hypovascularity.
4. Achilles tears are divided into 4 groups:
   - Type 1: Partial ruptures less than 50% tendon thickness
   - Type 2: Complete rupture with a gap less than 3 cm
   - Type 3: Complete rupture with a gap of 3 to 6 cm
   - Type 4: Complete rupture with a gap greater than 6 cm
5. Plantaris rupture, soleus rupture, and medial and lateral head of gastrocnemius ruptures are included in the differential for acute calf pain.

Pearls

- Achilles tendon tears commonly occur in young athletes, such as squash and badminton players.
- Risk factors include hyperparathyroidism, gout, previous steroid injections, and fluoroquinolone intake.
- The typical location is 2 to 6 cm proximal to the calcaneal insertion—the critical zone or area of relative hypovascularity.
- The tear can be partial or full thickness.
- Ultrasound shows increased echogenicity of the tear, because of blood and herniation of Kager fat into the defect. There is loss of the normal fibrillary pattern, with posterior acoustic shadowing from the torn tendon edges (refraction artifact).
- The distance of the torn tendon should be measured in both neutral and in equinus position, as this enables the surgeon to decide on the management plan.
- Treatment options include equinus plaster or surgical repair including fascial augmentation. Both options carry their own risks and benefits.

Suggested Readings

Cannon LB, Hackney RG. Operative shortening of the elongated defunctioned tendoachilles following previous rupture. *J R Nav Med Serv.* 2003;89(3):139-141.

Hartgerink P, Fessell DP, Jacobson JA, van Holsbeeck MT. Full- versus partial-thickness Achilles tendon tears: sonographic accuracy and characterization in 26 cases with surgical correlation. *Radiology.* 2001;220(2):406-412.

Fall and injury to right knee

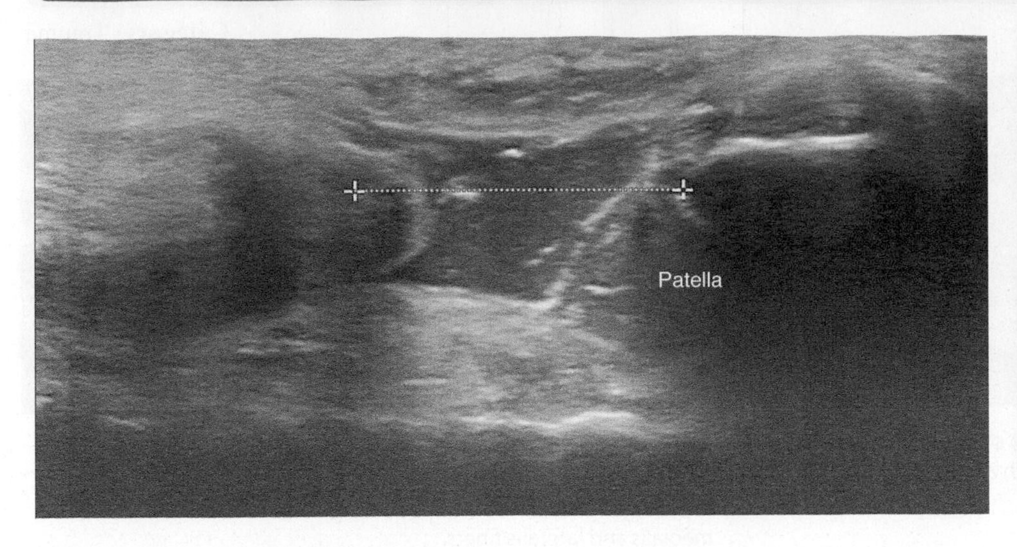

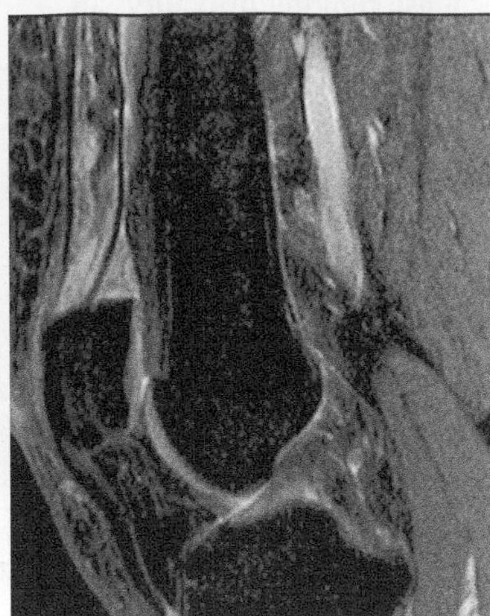

1. What are the ultrasound findings?

2. What are the MRI findings in a different patient, but with a similar condition?

3. What are the types of partial tear?

4. What are the risk factors for this entity?

5. What percentage of this injury are complete ruptures?

Quadriceps tendon rupture 1400

Case ranking/difficulty: **Category:** Trauma

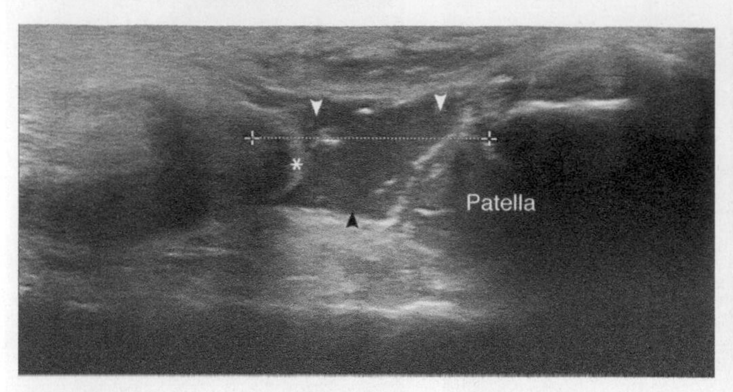

Ultrasound image (longitudinal plane) showing a complete rupture of the quadriceps tendon, with a fluid gap (*arrowheads*). *Asterisk* is the retracted tendon edge.

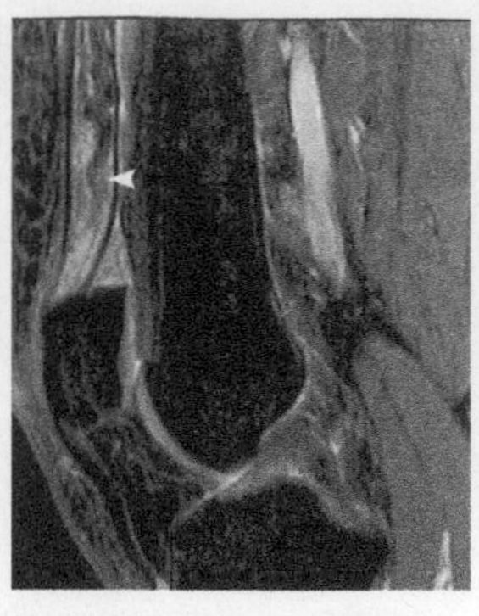

Another patient with a partial quadriceps rupture involving the vastus medialis and lateralis fibers.

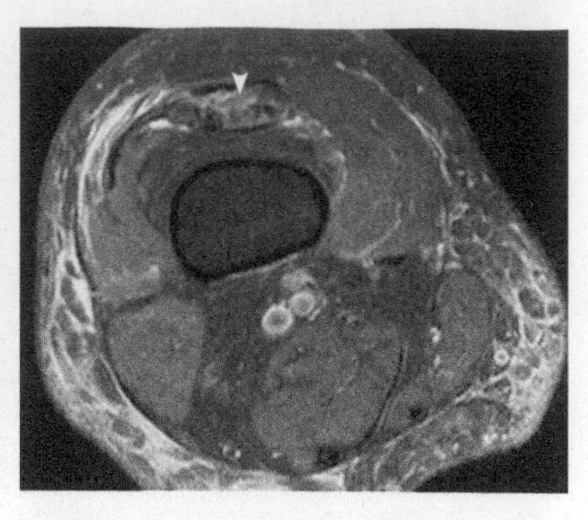

Partial rupture of the quadriceps tendon.

Answers

1. This ultrasound image demonstrates a complete rupture of the quadriceps tendon, with hematoma formation.
2. There is a partial thickness rupture of the quadriceps tendon. This is demonstrated with increased signal within the tendon, and with partial tendon discontinuity.
3. Depending on the laminar involvement, partial quadriceps tendon ruptures are further subdivided into 3 types:

   a superficial laminar rupture comprises a rectus femoris tendon rupture, an intermediate rupture is made up of vastus medialis and vastus lateralis tendon rupture, and the deepest rupture is a vastus intermedius rupture.
4. The risk factors include congenital or atrophic weak tendon, previous surgeries of the tendon, steroid injections, diabetes, infection, tumor, hyperparathyroidism, gout, chronic renal failure, and leukemia.
5. Of all of quadriceps tendon ruptures, 25% are complete.

Pearls

- Quadriceps tendons ruptures are more common than patellar tendon ruptures. They are more common in males.
- They are either partial or complete. In the young adult, quadriceps ruptures are usually partial, and in the elderly, the ruptures are usually complete. Only 25% of all ruptures are complete.
- The presentation is usually pain and inability to straight-leg raise.
- Plain radiographs in a complete tear can show a decrease in the Insall-Salvati ratio (ratio of the length of the patella tendon to length of the patella) or patella baja. Normal is 0.8 to 1.2.
- Ultrasound is the investigative modality of choice because of the ability to dynamically scan.
- MRI shows the discontinuity of the tendon with increased signal on T2 fat-saturated images. Hematoma is seen depending on the time of the injury. Anatomical knowledge helps to differentiate the type of laminar rupture.

Suggested Readings

Mahlfeld K, Mahlfeld A, Kayser R, Franke J, Merk H. Ultrasonography as a diagnostic tool in cases of quadriceps tendon rupture [in German]. *Ultraschall Med.* 1999;20(1):22-25.

Yu JS, Petersilge C, Sartoris DJ, Pathria MN, Resnick D. MR imaging of injuries of the extensor mechanism of the knee. *Radiographics.* 1994;14(3):541-551.

Zeiss J, Saddemi SR, Ebraheim NA. MR imaging of the quadriceps tendon: normal layered configuration and its importance in cases of tendon rupture. *AJR Am J Roentgenol.* 1992;159(5):1031-1034.

Painful swelling of the thumb, history of recent trauma

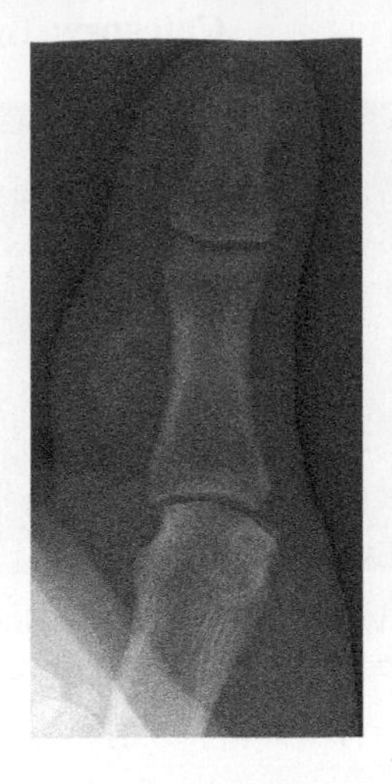

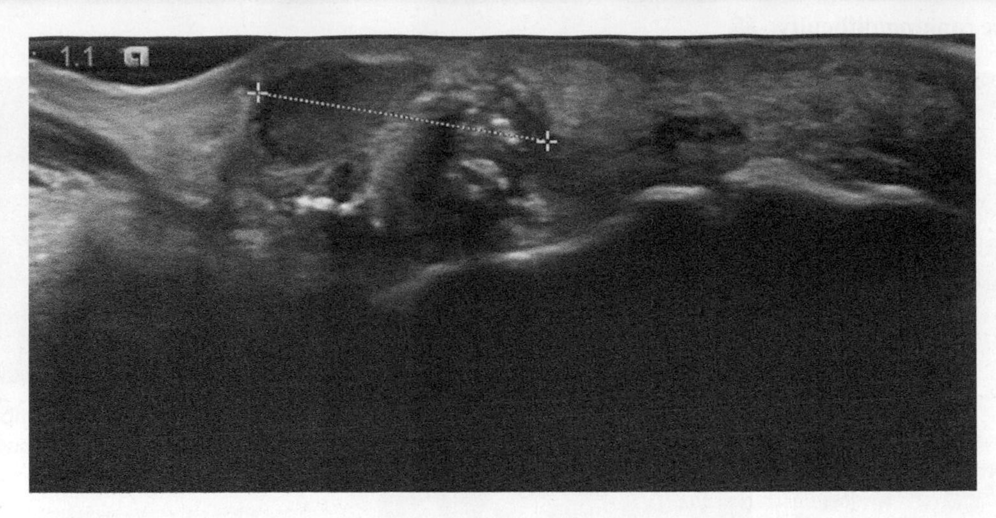

1. What are the imaging findings?

2. What are the different types of myositis ossificans?

3. What is the differential diagnosis?

4. What is the cnhancement pattern after intravenous contrast?

5. Surgical resection is always curative. True or False?

Myositis ossificans circumscripta 1542

Case ranking/difficulty:

Category: Trauma 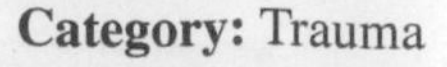

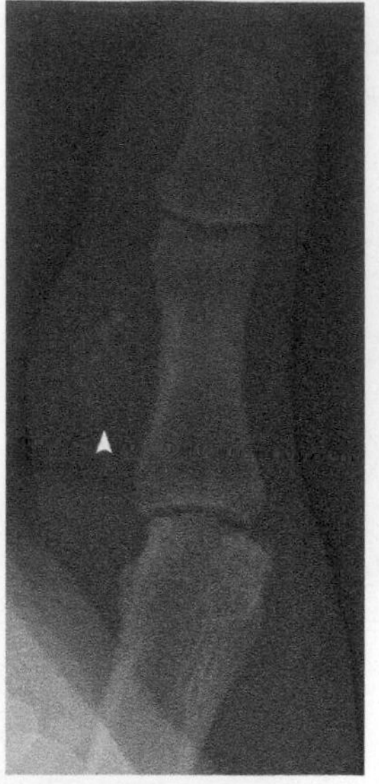

Ossification in the soft tissues at the ulnar aspect of the proximal phalanx of the thumb.

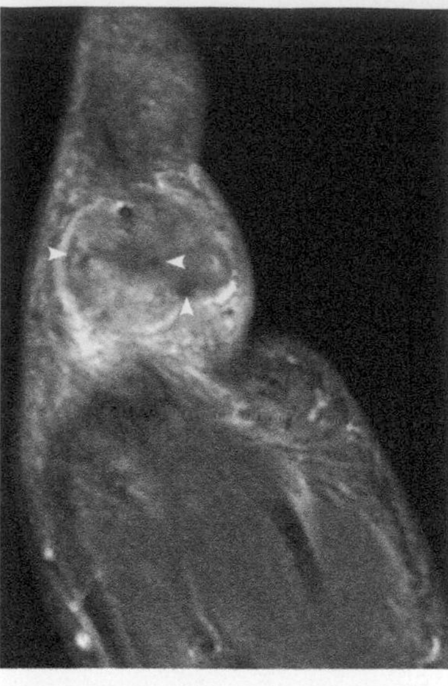

Peripheral high signal intensity in the new bone formation. Scattered foci of calcification (*arrowheads*).

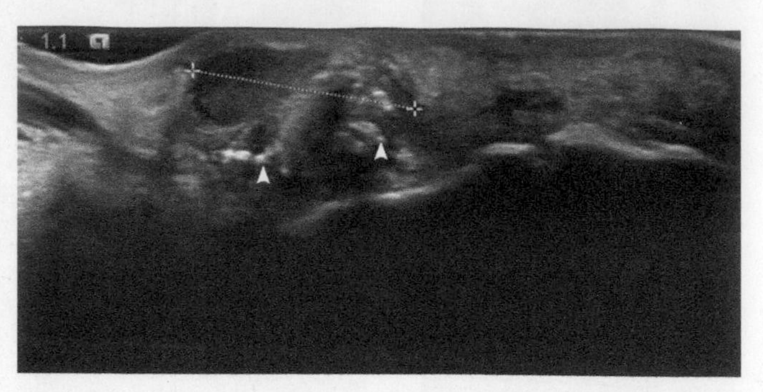

Soft-tissue ossification in the thumb with echogenic shadowing foci compatible with calcification (*arrowheads*).

Answers

1. Extraosseous calcifications, calcification on the periphery with central lucency, and fat-density line separating the lesion from bone. Soft-tissue mass on ultrasound with echogenic foci of calcification.
2. The types of myositis ossificans includes myositis ossificans progressiva, post-traumatic myositis ossificans, non-traumatic myositis ossificans, panniculitis ossificans, and fibro-osseous pseudotumor of the digit.
3. The differential diagnoses include rhabdomyosarcoma, malignant fibrous histiocytoma, parosteal osteosarcoma, synovial sarcoma, and chondrosarcoma.

   In the early phase of myositis ossificans, it is difficult to differentiate from the above conditions even histologically.
4. Contrast enhancement in the early stages can be quite dramatic, raising the concern for a sarcoma. However, there is a gradual decrease in size, edema, and enhancement over a period of several months, and mature myositis ossificans does not enhance.
5. False. Early resection can lead to recurrence. Resection is best performed after 6 months, after maturation of the ossification.

Pearls

- Myositis ossificans is heterotopic ossification that is usually post-traumatic; however, there is no history of trauma in paraplegics or in the congenital fatal form.
- The early phase may not demonstrate any bone, calcification, or mass on plain radiographs. Progressive calcification occurs over a 2- to 6-week period, and the typical dense peripheral calcification occurs by 2 months. In the following 4 months, it becomes denser and smaller.
- CT scan shows a peripherally calcified mass with central lucency. Unlike a sarcoma, lesions decrease in size after 4 to 6 months. A well-defined fat plane demarcates bone and mass.
- MRI: In the early phase, the mass is ill-defined with isointense signal to muscle on T1-weighted images, with heterogenously high central signal intensity and peripheral high T2 signal and edema. Contrast enhancement can also be prominent at this stage.
- In the later phase, there is low signal intensity at the peripheral aspect of the lesion on T1- and on T2-weighted images, and there is intermediate to high signal intensity on T2-weighted images in the central aspect of the lesion. At this stage, there is usually no contrast enhancement.

Suggested Readings

Kransdorf MJ, Meis JM, Jelinek JS. Myositis ossificans: MR appearance with radiologic-pathologic correlation. *AJR Am J Roentgenol.* 1991;157(6):1243-1248.

Lacout A, Jarraya M, Marcy PY, Thariat J, Carlier RY. Myositis ossificans imaging: keys to successful diagnosis. *Indian J Radiol Imaging.* 2012;22(1):35-39.

Tyler P, Saifuddin A. The imaging of myositis ossificans. *Semin Musculoskelet Radiol.* 2010;14(2):201-216.

Painful shoulder

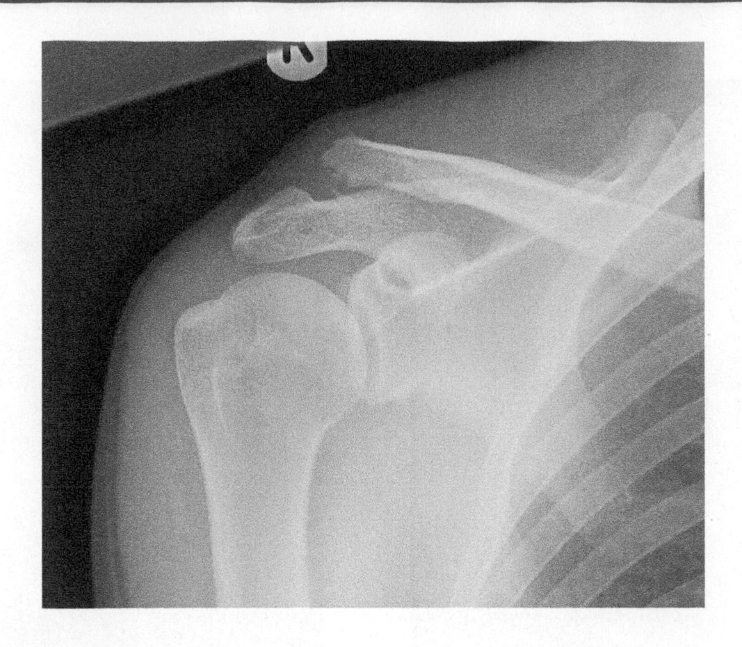

1. What are the radiographic findings?

2. What are the expected MRI findings?

3. What are the differential diagnoses?

4. What is the likely diagnosis?

5. What are the high-risk sports associated with this condition?

Post-traumatic osteolysis of the clavicle 1552

Case ranking/difficulty: **Category:** Trauma

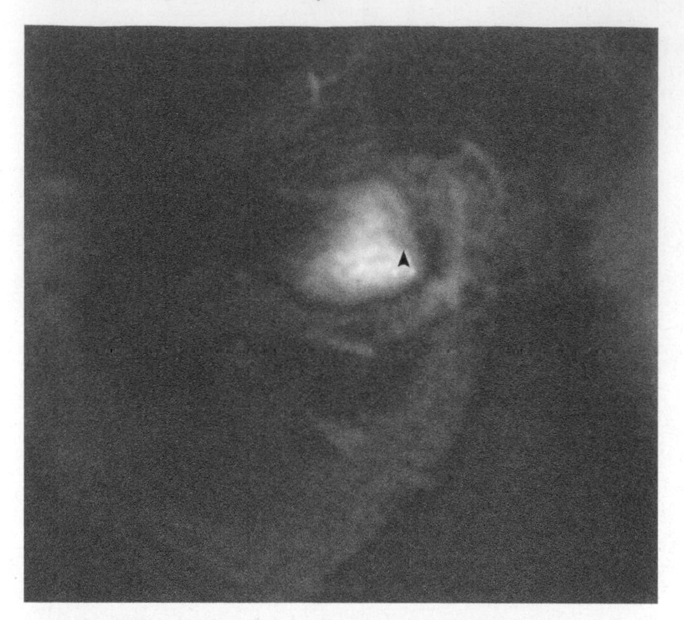

Another patient with post-traumatic osteolysis. Note the intense edema and subchondral fracture line (*arrowhead*). Although described in post-traumatic osteolysis, this fracture can also be seen in painful bone marrow edema syndrome.

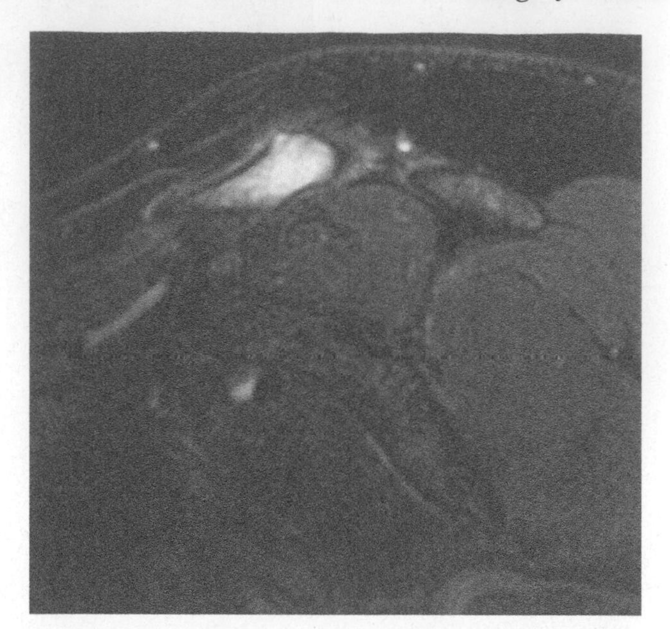

Intense clavicle edema.

Answers

1. There is osteolysis of the distal end of clavicle, AC joint effusion, clavicular erosion, and grade 2 AC joint separation.
2. There is usually bone marrow edema at the distal end of clavicle and acromion, AC joint effusion, subchondral cysts, erosions and there may be a subchondral fracture line. However, it has been suggested that an insufficiency fracture in the distal clavicle may be a sequela of painful bone marrow edema syndrome, rather than post-traumatic osteolysis.
3. Metastasis, rheumatoid arthritis, scleroderma, hyperparathyroidism, and post-traumatic osteolysis of the distal end of clavicle.
4. Post-traumatic osteolysis of the distal end of clavicle
5. Judo, swimming, and heavy weight lifting are the sports commonly associated with post-traumatic osteolysis, as well as all contact sports.

Pearls

- Post-traumatic osteolysis of the clavicle is a synovial based progressive and destructive process, leading to erosions, subchondral cysts, and destruction of the distal end of the clavicle.
- The main cause is repetitive trauma from falling, injury, heavy weight lifting, swimming, and contact sports.
- There is typically AC joint effusion and soft-tissue swelling, subchondral cysts, and possibly subchondral insufficiency fractures, which are better seen on MRI.
- Bone scintigraphy shows increased isotope uptake.
- Differentials include metastasis, hyperparathyroidism, connective tissue disorder, and rheumatoid arthritis.
- Treatment options include anti-inflammatory drugs, steroid injections, and, in rare cases, resection of the distal end of clavicle.
- Prognosis is usually good as this is a self-limiting condition, with typical resolution after 1 to 2 years.

Suggested Readings

de la Puente R, Boutin RD, Theodorou DJ, Hooper A, Schweitzer M, Resnick D. Post-traumatic and stress-induced osteolysis of the distal clavicle: MR imaging findings in 17 patients. *Skeletal Radiol.* 1999;28(4):202-208.

Kim HK, Crotty E. Post-traumatic osteolysis of the distal clavicle. *Pediatr Radiol.* 2010;40(5):784.

Shiota E. Post-traumatic and stress-induced osteolysis of the distal clavicle. *Skeletal Radiol.* 2002;31(5):311.

Right ankle pain and swelling for 3 months

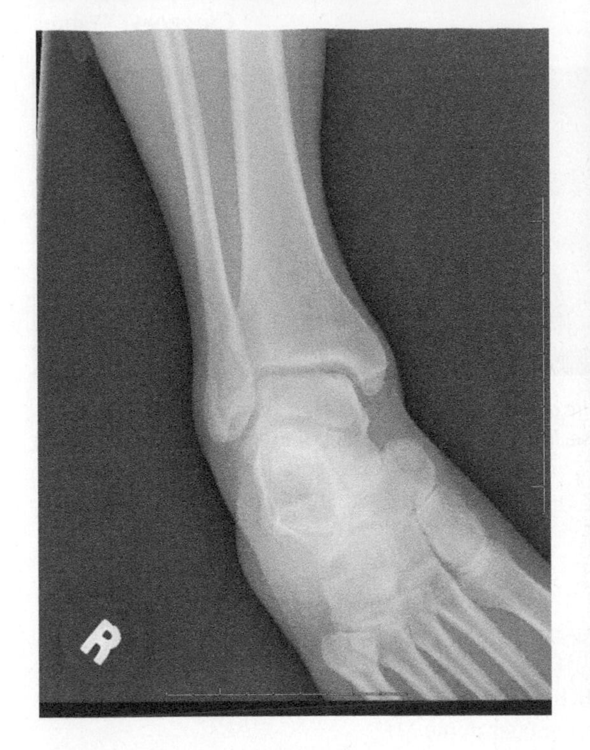

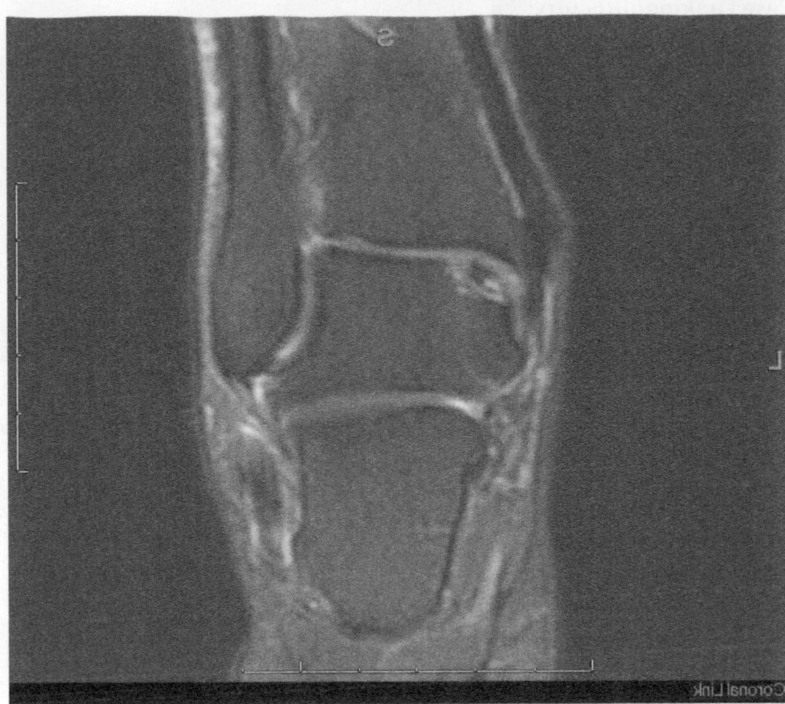

1. Where are the most common locations for this lesion in the talar dome?

2. How often are these lesions bilateral?

3. Are these lesions more common in males or females?

4. What factors are believed to cause or contribute to the development of these lesions?

5. What findings correctly describe a stage IV lesion?

Osteochondral lesion of talar dome 1529

Case ranking/difficulty: 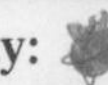

Category: Trauma

A defect is present at the medial aspect of the talar dome containing an osseous fragment (*black arrow*), consistent with an osteochondral lesion.

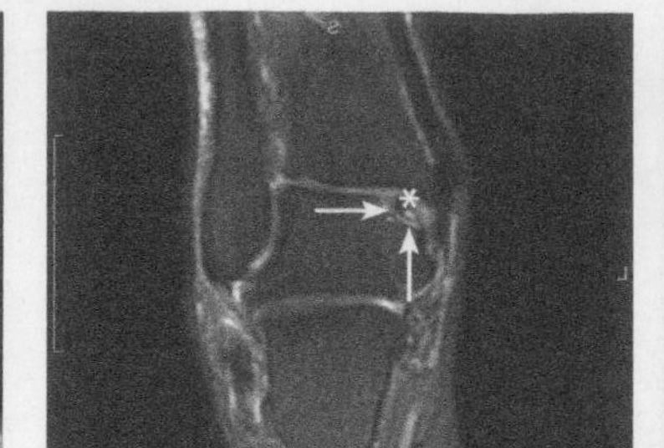

A cleft of hyperintense T2 signal (*white arrows*) is visible between the osseous fragment (*asterisk*) and the parent bone, consistent with an unstable osteochondral lesion. The fragment is T2 hypointense.

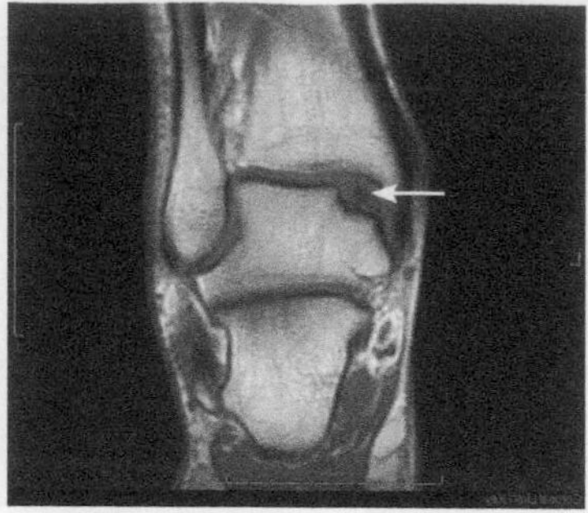

The fragment (*white arrow*) is T1 and T2 hypointense, indicating necrosis.

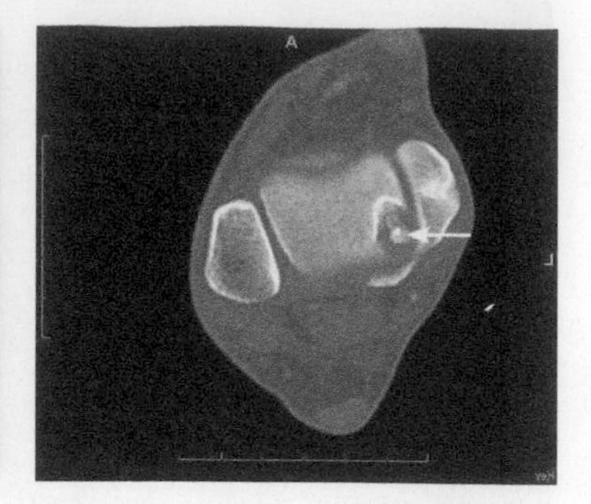

A defect is present at the medial aspect of the talar dome containing an osseous fragment (*white arrow*), consistent with an osteochondral lesion.

Answers

1. The most common locations of osteochondral lesions of the talus are at the medial central (40%), posteromedial (20%), and lateral central (20%) aspects of the dome. The anterolateral aspect accounts for (10%), with the remaining 10% occurring elsewhere.
2. Osteochondral lesions of the talus are bilateral in 10% of cases.
3. Female-to-male ratio is 1.2:1.
4. Multiple causative factors have been suggested, including acute or old trauma, repetitive microtrauma, osteonecrosis caused by systemic metabolic conditions, degenerative arthropathy, and genetic predisposition.
5. A stage IV osteochondral lesion of the talus is characterized by a completely detached osteochondral fragment that is displaced from the donor site.

Pearls

- Osteochondral lesions of the talus are common, occurring after up to 6% of ankle sprains.
- Osteochondral lesions can result in chronic ankle pain, decreased activity level, and osteoarthritis.
- Stage I osteochondral lesions are characterized by abnormality of the subchondral bone; the articular cartilage may be thickened, but is intact.
- Stage II lesions are characterized by breach of the articular cartilage and a partly detached osteochondral fragment.
- Stage III lesions are characterized by a completely detached osteochondral fragment within the donor site of the talar dome.
- Stage IV lesions are characterized by a completely detached osteochondral fragment displaced from the donor site or rotated within the defect.
- Treatment depends on the symptoms and the stability of the lesion. Larger, unstable symptomatic lesions may be treated with a variety of surgical techniques including subchondral drilling, chondrocyte transplantation, and osteochondral autograft transfer system (OATS).
- Large subchondral cysts (>1 cm) with intact cartilage may also be unstable and symptomatic. These may be treated with retrograde drilling (from the sinus tarsi) and packing with autograft or allograft.

Suggested Readings

Orr JD, Dawson LK, Garcia EJ, Kirk KL. Incidence of osteochondral lesions of the talus in the United States military. *Foot Ankle Int.* 2011;32(10):948-954.

Rosenberg ZS, Beltran J, Bencardino JT. From the RSNA Refresher Courses. Radiological Society of North America. MR imaging of the ankle and foot. *Radiographics.* 2000;20 Spec No:S153-S179.

History of bilateral knee pain

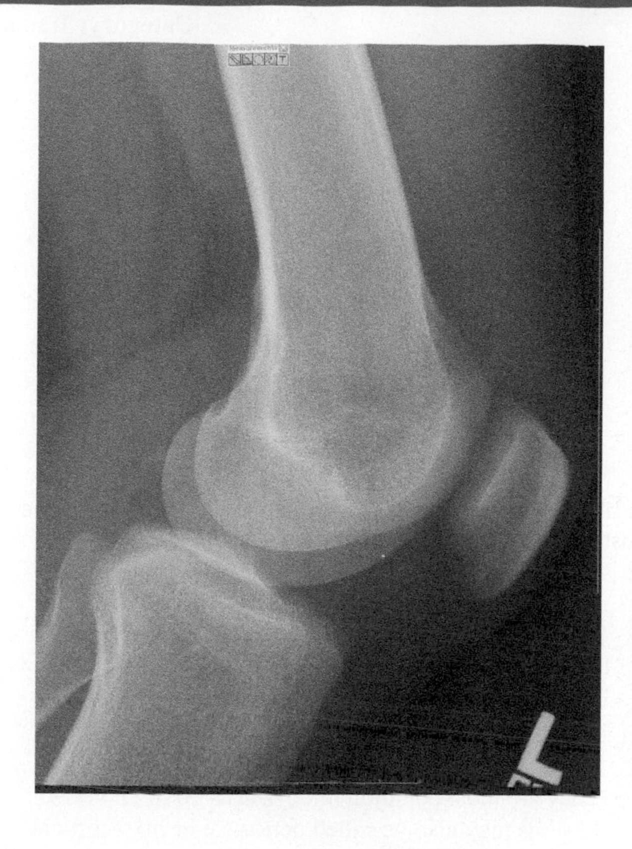

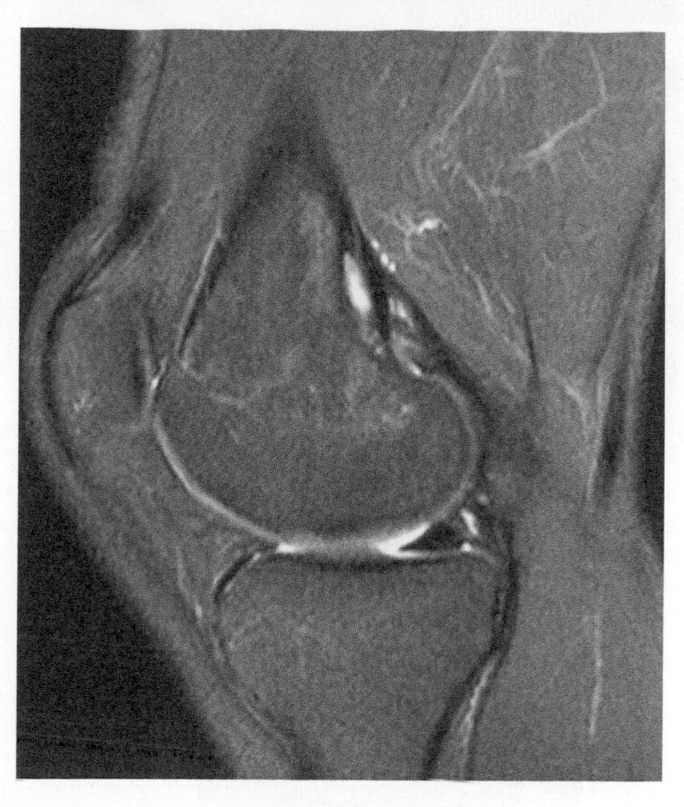

1. What are the radiographic findings?

2. What entities are included in the differential diagnosis?

3. What are the typical MRI features of this lesion?

4. What is the presumed etiology of the lesion?

5. What is a posterior distal femoral metaphyseal stripe?

Cortical desmoid (cortical avulsive injury) 1464

Case ranking/difficulty: 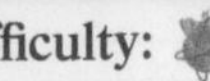

Category: Trauma 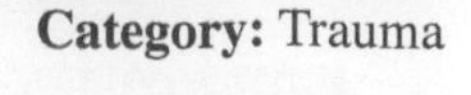

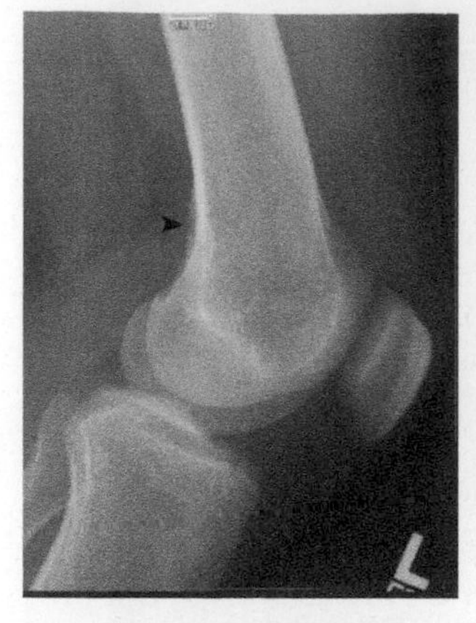

There is mild erosive change in the posterior left medial femoral condyle.

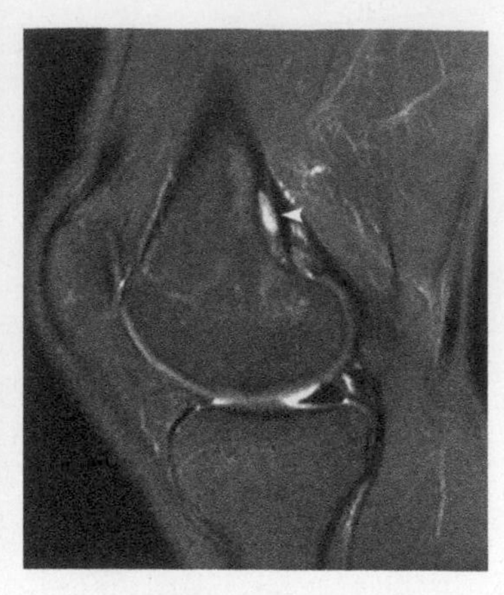

Lesion is T2 hyperintense, but there is no cortical destruction or bone marrow edema.

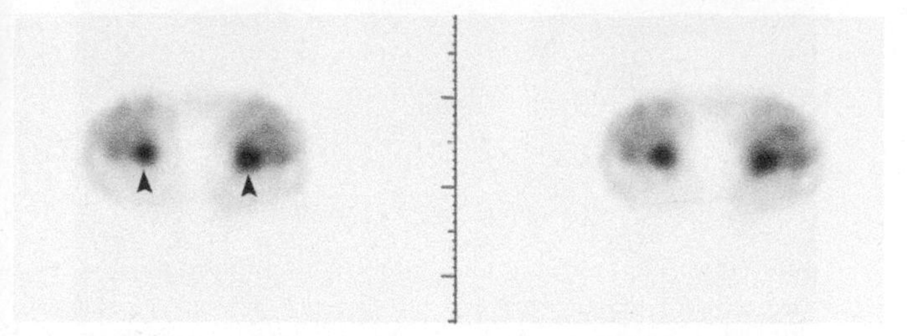

Axial SPECT image shows increased uptake of ^{99m}Tc-MDP in the posterior medial femoral condyles bilaterally.

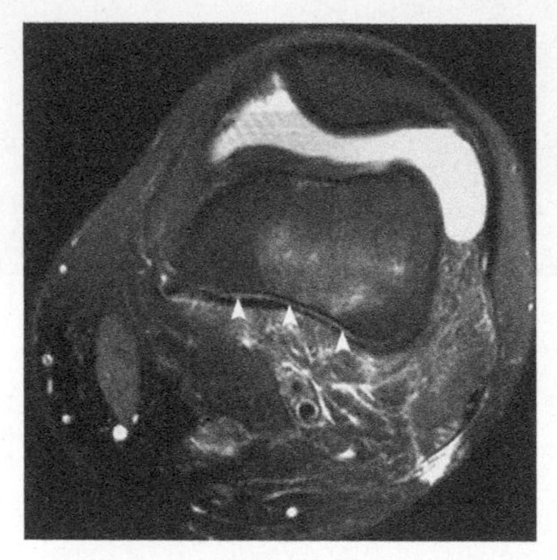

Posterior distal femoral metaphyseal stripe in another patient (*arrowheads*).

Answers

1. Erosive changes in the posterior left medial femoral condyle with mild cortical irregularity in the posterior right femoral condyle. No periosteal reaction or mineralization is seen.

2. Fibrous cortical defect, cortical desmoid, parosteal osteosarcoma, and a posterior distal femoral metaphyseal stripe.

3. The lesions are T1 hypointense and T2 hyperintense with a hypointense rim. Periosteal reaction and soft-tissue edema are seen in the more acute stages. Mineralization may also be present.

4. Traction at the medial gastrocnemius or adductor magnus attachments.

5. A posterior distal femoral stripe is normal fibrovascular tissue located between the posterior femoral cortex and the periosteum. It is more extensive than a cortical desmoid, and located under the entire posterior periosteum.

Pearls

- Cortical desmoids (cortical avulsive injury) are traction or tug lesions located in the posterior medial supracondylar distal femur.
- They are most common in boys ages 10 to 15 years.
- Lesions may also be called periosteal or juxtacortical desmoids, distal femoral condyle irregularity, or cortical avulsive injury.
- Radiological findings depend on the acuity of the lesion.
- Early stage lesions show cortical irregularity, periosteal reaction and possible erosions on plain films. MRI will show a lesion that is T1 hypointense, and T2 hyperintense with bone marrow and soft-tissue edema, and periosteal reaction.
- Later-stage lesions will show a more defined cortex and no periosteal reaction on radiographs, with resolution of the edema and periosteal reaction on MRI, and a more defined cortical rim.
- This is a "do not touch" lesion, hence biopsy is not indicated.

Suggested Readings

Gould CF, Ly JQ, Lattin GE, Beall DP, Sutcliffe JB. Bone tumor mimics: avoiding misdiagnosis. *Curr Probl Diagn Radiol.* 2008;36(3):124-141.

Vieira RL, Bencardino JT, Rosenberg ZS, Nomikos G. MRI features of cortical desmoid in acute knee trauma. *AJR Am J Roentgenol.* 2011;196(2):424-428.

Chronic wrist pain

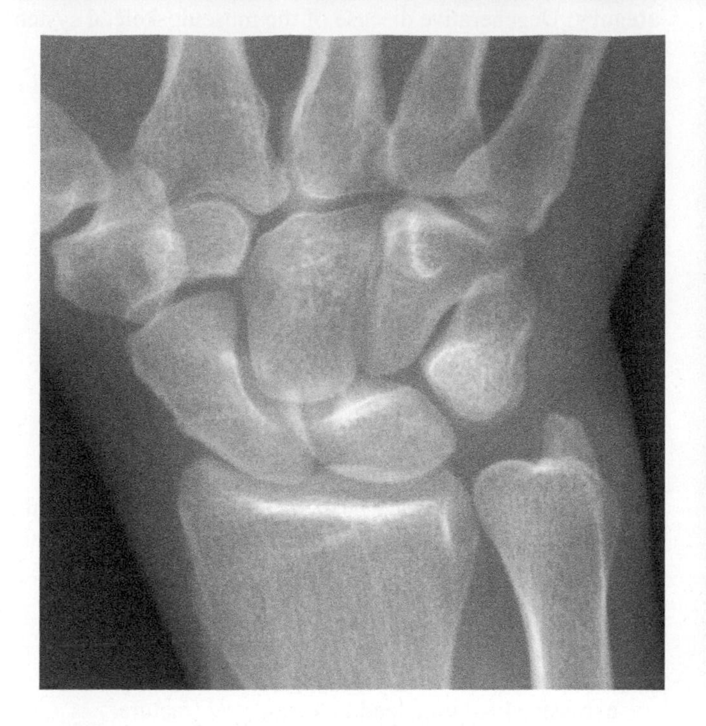

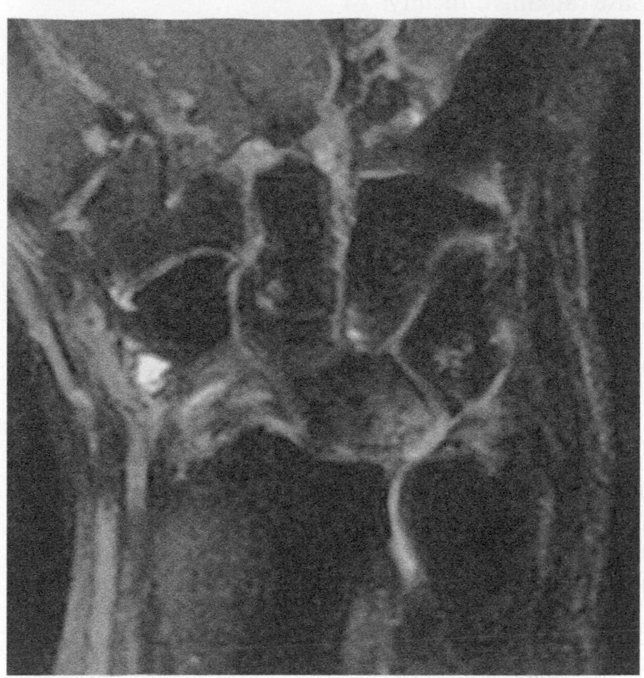

1. What are the imaging findings?

2. How does ulnar variance change with positioning?

3. How does the load across the wrist increase with 1 mm of positive ulnar variance?

4. What are the most appropriate imaging modalities when planning surgical management?

5. What is the cause of ulnar styloid impaction?

Ulnar impaction syndrome 2367

Case ranking/difficulty:

Category: Degenerative disease of the musculoskeletal system

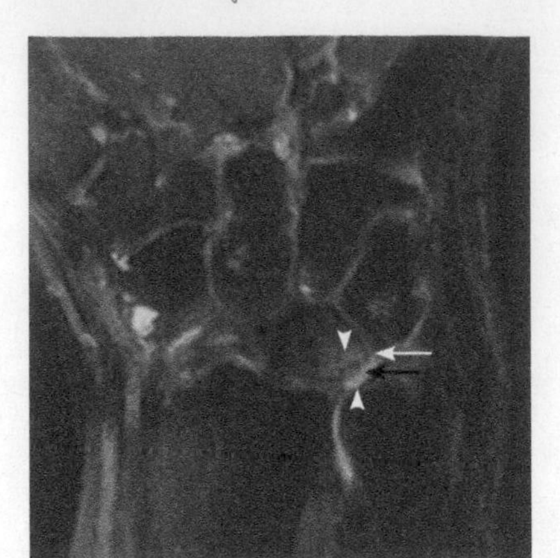

Edema in the lunate with cystic change (*distal arrowhead*), with lunotriquetral ligament partial tear (*white arrow*). Triangular fibrocartilage (TFC) tear (*proximal arrowhead*), and chondromalacia of the lunate and distal ulna (*black arrow*).

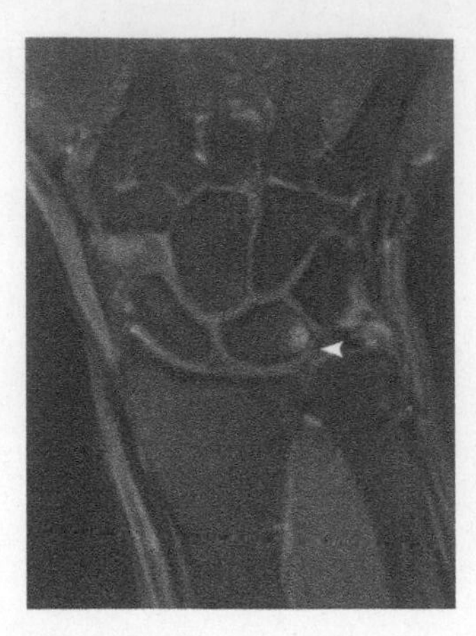

Another patient with positive ulnar variance and partial tear of the TFC (*arrowhead*), with edema and cystic change in the lunate.

Answers

1. There is positive ulnar variance on the plain films. MRI shows edema and cystic change in the ulnar aspect of the lunate and radial aspect of the triquetrum, tear of the central triangular fibrocartilage, and a partial lunotriquetral ligament tear, with chondromalacia of the distal ulna and lunate.

2. Ulnar variance increases with pronation and with gripping. Consequently, films should be obtained in the neutral position. However, preoperative planning often requires pronation and gripping to assist in the choice of surgical procedure.

3. Normally the ulna only accepts approximately 20% of the load across the wrist. With just a 1-mm increase in ulnar variance, this load increases by 25%.

4. Radiographs are the first step in assessing the cause of ulnar-sided wrist pain. Preoperative planning should be done in both the neutral position and in pronation, as well as with gripping.

   MRI is required to assess the triangular fibrocartilage and the lunotriquetral ligament, as well as the degree of ulnar and lunate chondromalacia. In select cases, MR or CT arthrography is required to better define the degree of chondromalacia, the extent of triangular fibrocartilage tearing, and the integrity of the ulnocarpal and lunotriquetral ligaments.

5. Ulnar styloid impaction is caused by an excessively long ulnar styloid process, which will lead to impaction of the process on the triquetrum. Subsequent ulnar styloid and triquetral chondromalacic changes can occur, as can lunotriquetral ligament instability. Rarely, a single excessive load may lead to a triquetral fracture.

   Non-union of an ulnar styloid process fracture may also lead to ulnocarpal impaction, although this is not typically included in the category of "ulnar styloid impaction."

Pearls

- Ulnar impaction syndrome is caused by a positive ulnar variance.
- MRI may show edema and cystic change in the ulnar aspect of the lunate, the radial aspect of the triquetrum, and chondromalacic changes in these bones, as well as in the distal ulna. The lunotriquetral ligament is often torn, as well as the triangular fibrocartilage.
- If there is ulnar impaction because of an elongated ulnar styloid or fracture non-union, the changes are usually confined to the triquetrum, distal ulna, and lunotriquetral ligament.
- Ulnar styloid impaction and ulnocarpal impaction may co-exist.

Suggested Readings

Cerezal L, del Piñal F, Abascal F, García-Valtuille R, Pereda T, Canga A. Imaging findings in ulnar-sided wrist impaction syndromes. *Radiographics.* 2004;22(1):105-121.

Cerezal L, del Piñal F, Abascal F. MR imaging findings in ulnar-sided wrist impaction syndromes. *Magn Reson Imaging Clin N Am.* 2004;12(2):281-299, vi.

Chronic ankle pain

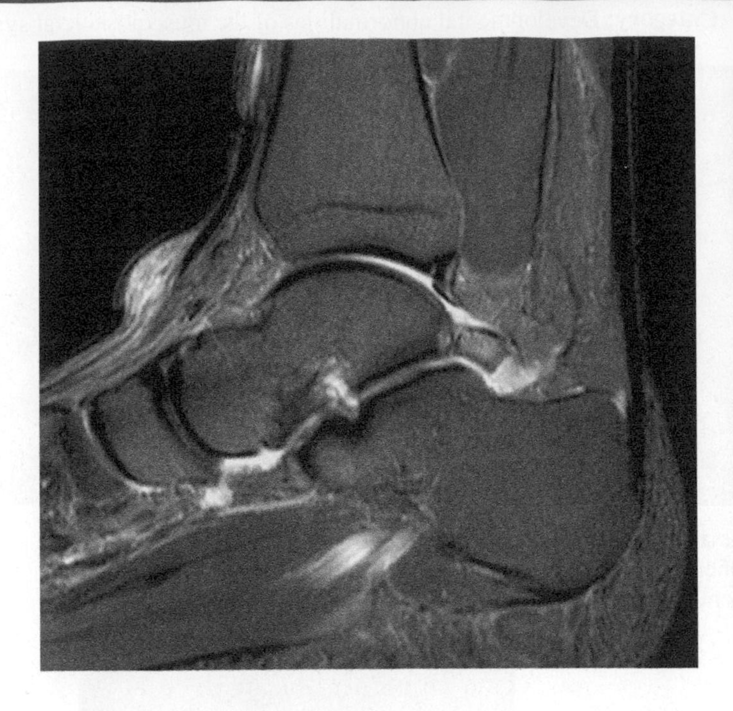

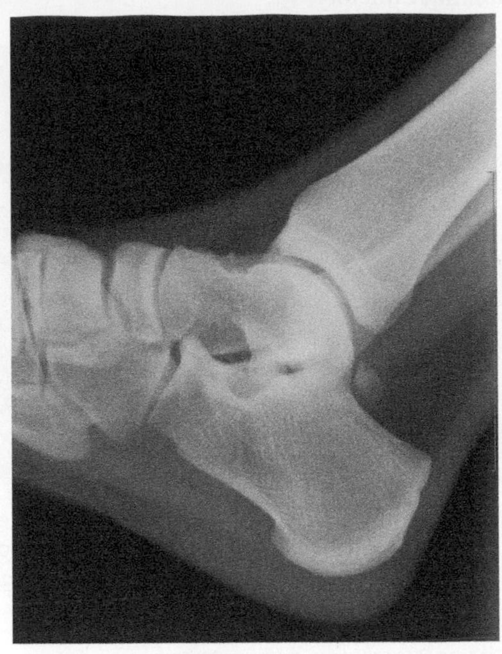

1. What are the radiographic findings?
2. What are the MRI findings?
3. What is the diagnosis?
4. What are contributory factors for this entity?
5. What ankle movement results in a greater risk of this entity?

Os trigonum syndrome 1287

Case ranking/difficulty: 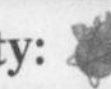 **Category:** Developmental abnormalities of the musculoskeletal system

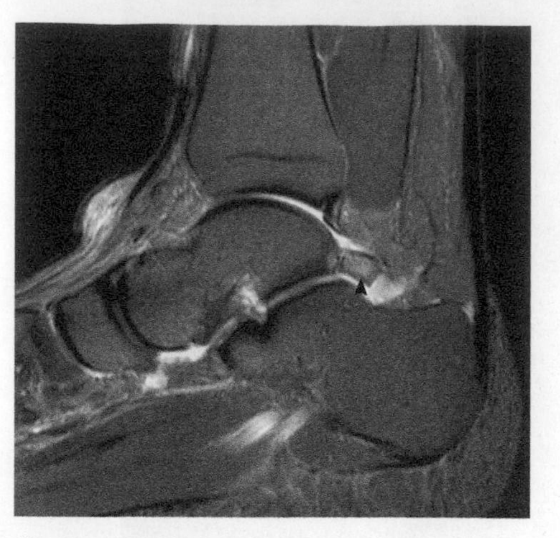

Os trigonum marrow edema (*arrowhead*), soft-tissue edema, and joint effusion.

Edema is also seen in the posterior talofibular ligament (*arrowhead*). Os trigonum edema (*arrow*) is seen.

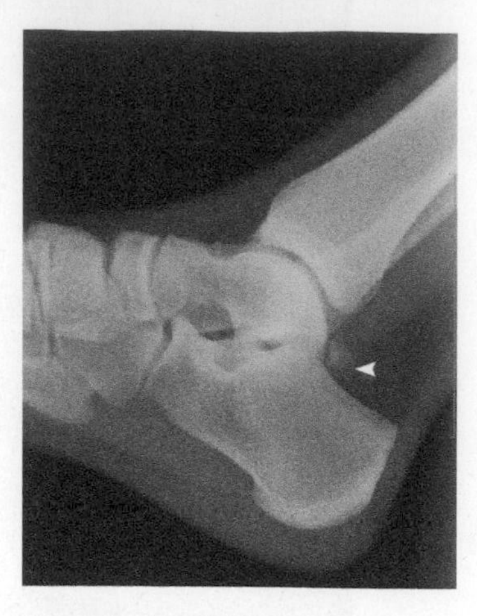

Large os trigonum.

Answers

1. A large os trigonum is demonstrated.
2. MRI shows a large os trigonum with bone marrow edema in the os trigonum and soft tissues.
3. Posterior ankle impingement syndrome secondary to an os trigonum.
4. Stieda process (lateral process) of the talus, prominent superior and posterior aspect of calcaneus, os trigonum, a posterior intermalleolar ligament, and downward sloping posterior slip of the tibia are the main contributory factors for posterior ankle impingement syndrome.
5. Repetitive plantar flexion is the main contributory factor for posterior impingement.

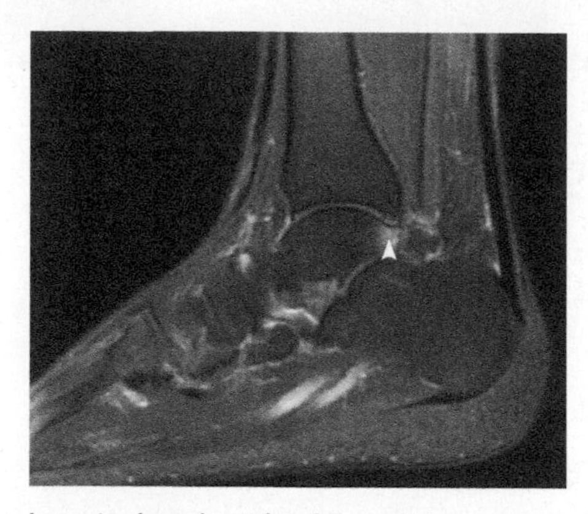

Marrow edema in the talar side of the os trigonum synchondrosis (another patient).

Pearls

- The os trigonum is an ossification center at the posterior aspect of the talus, which fails to fuse with the talus in 7% to 14% of individuals. It is bilateral in 1% to 4% of individuals.
- Os trigonum syndrome is classically seen in ballet dancers, but can also occur in athletes who participate in sports with repetitive plantar flexion of the ankle.
- It is a part of posterior impingement syndrome, where repetitive plantar flexion leads to pain and limitation of movement.
- Posterior impingement can be caused by other bony abnormalities such as a prominent Stieda process, downward slope of the posterior lip of the tibia and a prominent process of the calcaneus.
- Posterior impingement can also be caused by the inconstant posterior intermalleolar ligament.
- Lateral plain film shows the os trigonum and other osseous abnormalities.
- T1-weighted images confirm the presence of the bony abnormality, and T2-weighted images will show bone and soft-tissue edema and a possible disruption of the synchondrosis. Associated flexor hallucis longus tenosynovitis is often seen.

Suggested Readings

Fiorella D, Helms CA, Nunley JA. The MR imaging features of the posterior intermalleolar ligament in patients with posterior impingement syndrome of the ankle. *Skeletal Radiol.* 1999;28(10):573-576.

Karasick D, Schweitzer ME. The os trigonum syndrome: imaging features. *AJR Am J Roentgenol.* 1996;166(1): 125-129.

Lee JC, Calder JD, Healy JC. Posterior impingement syndromes of the ankle. *Semin Musculoskelet Radiol.* 2008;12(2):154-169.

Twisted ankle several years ago, chronic ankle pain

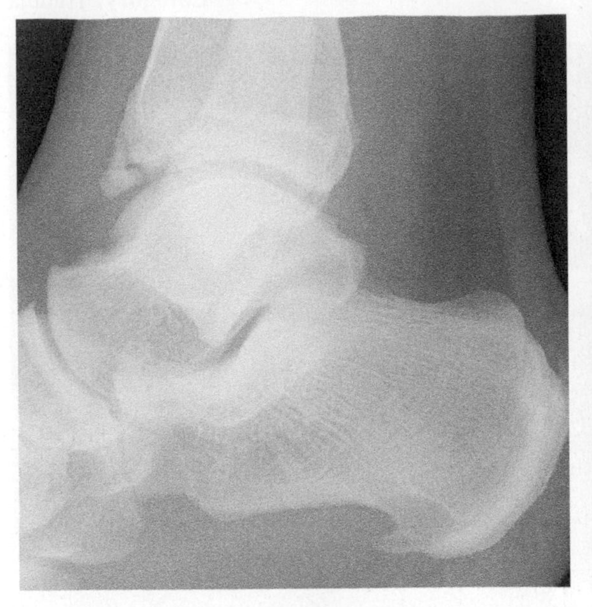

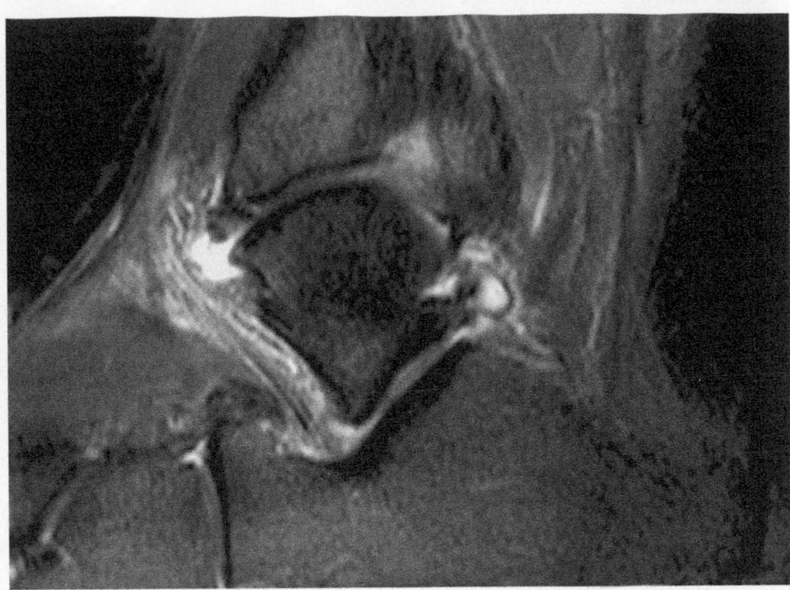

1. What are the radiographic findings?

2. What are the MRI findings?

3. What is the diagnosis?

4. What sports are commonly related to this entity?

5. What are the signal characteristics of the capsular changes?

Anterior impingement syndrome of ankle 1199

Case ranking/difficulty: 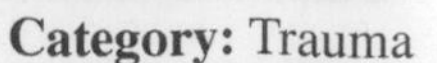 **Category:** Trauma

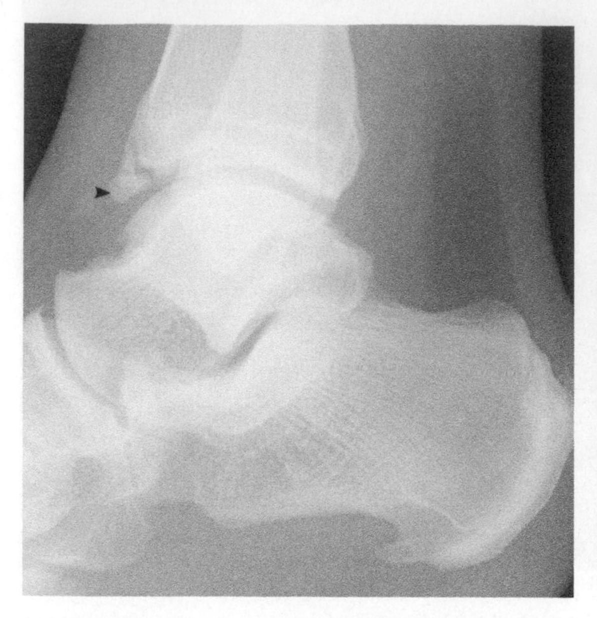

Large anterior spur formation, which may be a partially detached osteophyte or old fracture.

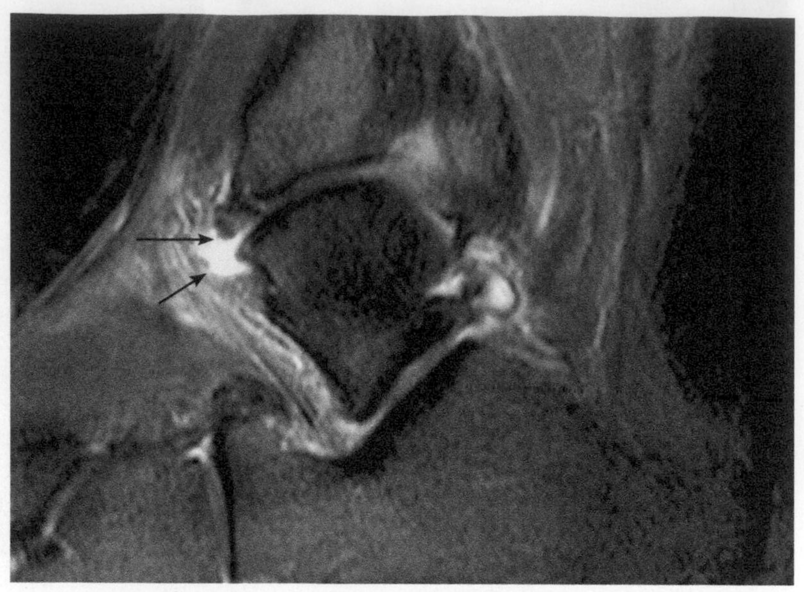

Arrows showing anterior osteophyte (*long arrow*) with thickening of the anterior capsule of the ankle (*inferior arrow*). Minimal effusion and edema is noted.

Answers

1. Anterior spur or old fracture at the tibial plafond and talus (not shown).
2. There is thickening of the anterior joint capsule with fibrosis and scarring. There is also edema of the tibial spur and soft-tissue edema with an effusion.
3. The constellation of findings are consistent with anterior impingement syndrome.
4. Repetitive forced dorsiflexion in ballet dancers and soccer players are the major sports-related causes of anterior impingement.
5. Synovial thickening shows low T1 signal and low-to-intermediate T2 signal intensity.

Pearls

- Anterior impingement of ankle is caused by repeated trauma during sports requiring dorsiflexion of the ankle, such as football and ballet.
- Repeated trauma leads to cartilage damage and early degenerative changes, fibrosis, and spur formation.
- Radiographs shows a spur on the anterior and inferior aspect of the tibia and corresponding talus.
- An angle of less than 60 degrees between the tibial and talar spurs suggests impingement.
- MRI shows thickening of the anterior joint capsule, with bone marrow edema. In some cases, early degenerative changes are evident.
- Treatment include analgesics and anti-inflammatory drugs. Arthroscopy and open excision may be required in some cases.

Suggested Readings

Masciocchi C, Catalucci A, Barile A. Ankle impingement syndromes. *Eur J Radiol.* 1998;27 Suppl 1:S70-S73.

Robinson P, White LM. Soft-tissue and osseous impingement syndromes of the ankle: role of imaging in diagnosis and management. *Radiographics.* 2002;22(6):1457-1469; discussion 1470-1471.

Schweitzer ME. Magnetic resonance imaging of the foot and ankle. *Magn Reson Q.* 1993;9(4):214-234.

Shoulder pain

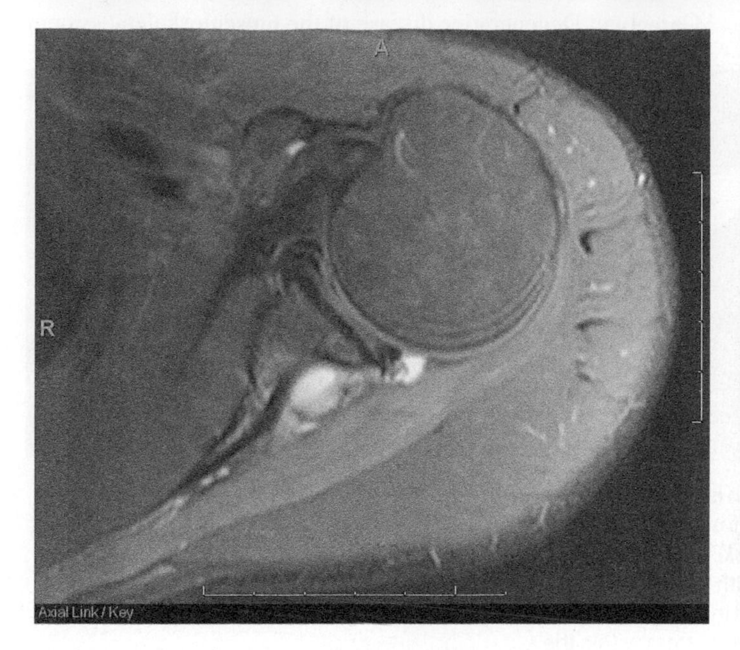

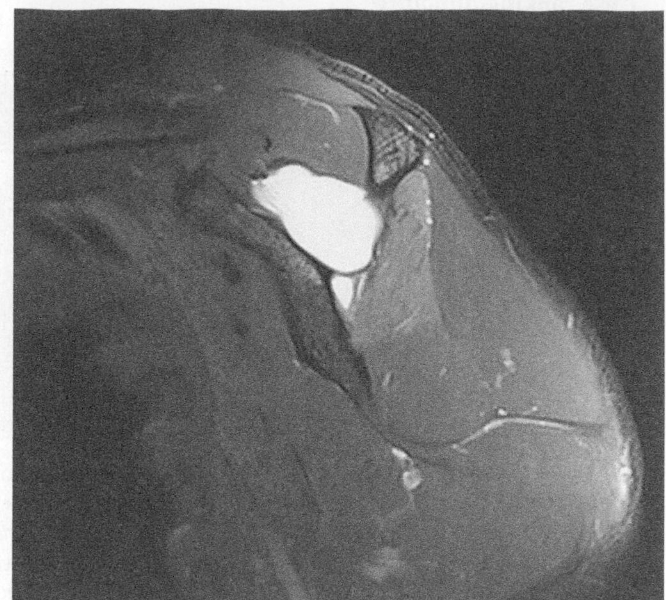

1. What muscle demonstrates abnormal signal intensity?

2. What is the most likely etiology of the muscle edema?

3. What additional findings are present?

4. The suprascapular nerve receives contributions from which nerve roots?

5. What are recognized causes of suprascapular neuropathy?

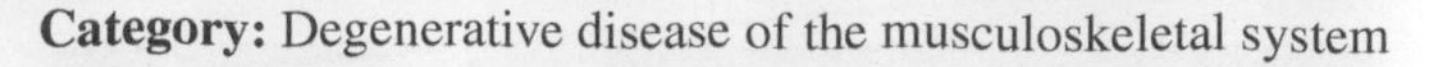

Paralabral cyst with infraspinatus denervation 1530

Case ranking/difficulty: **Category:** Degenerative disease of the musculoskeletal system

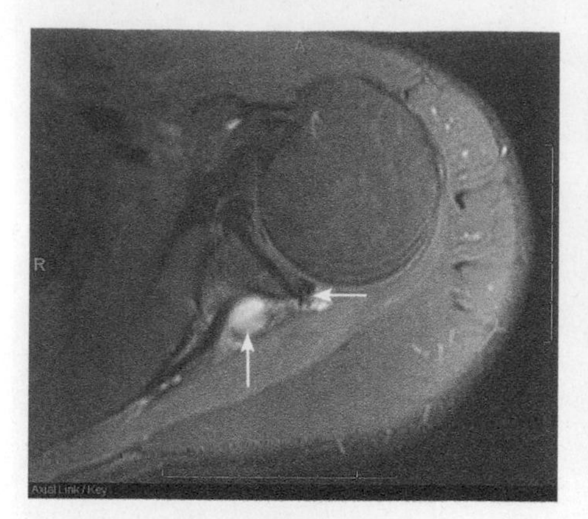

A posterior glenoid labral tear is demonstrated (*thin white arrow*), as well as an adjacent paralabral cyst extending medially (*thick white arrow*).

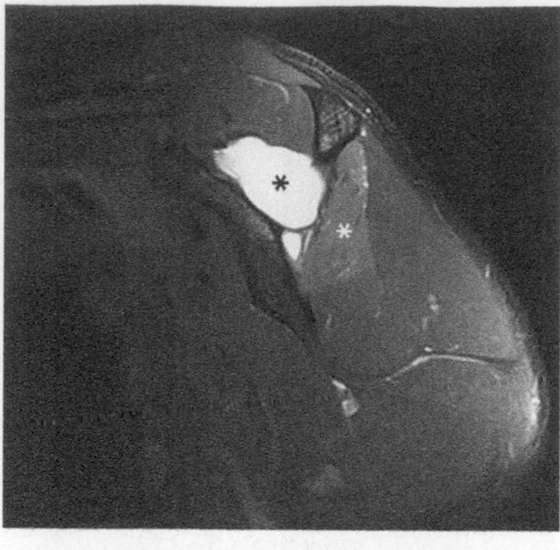

A large cystic lesion is demonstrated in the suprascapular fossa and spinoglenoid notch (*black asterisk*). This cystic lesion was continuous with the paralabral cyst demonstrated in the figure on extreme left. Edema pattern within the infraspinatus muscle is apparent (*white asterisk*) because of subacute denervation.

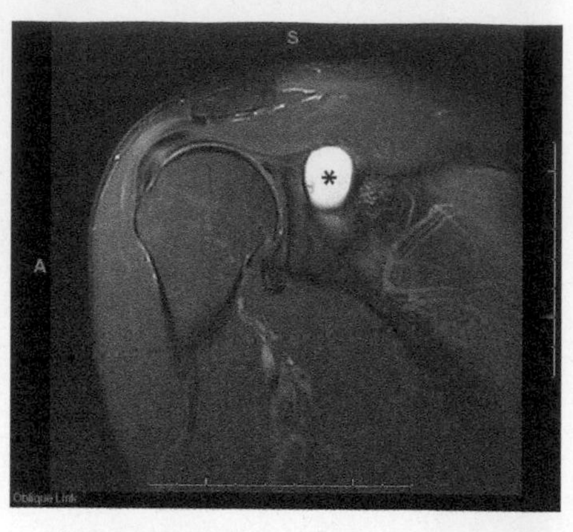

A large cystic lesion is demonstrated in the spinoglenoid notch (*black asterisk*).

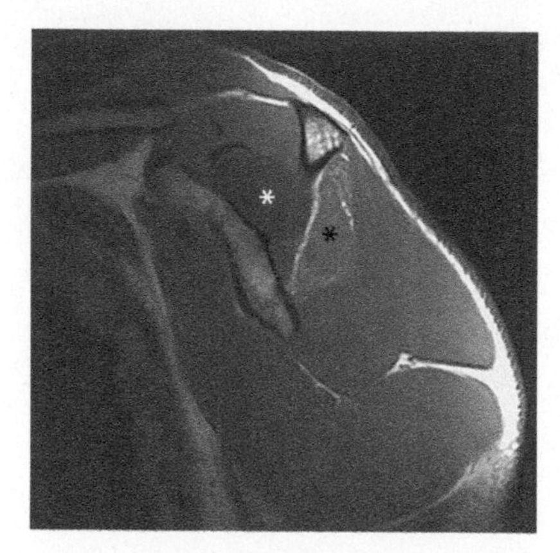

Cyst is seen in the suprascapular fossa and spinoglenoid notch (*white asterisk*). Disproportionate fatty atrophy of the infraspinatus muscle is apparent (*black asterisk*) because of denervation.

Answers

1. There is increased T2 signal intensity within the infraspinatus muscle consistent with an edema pattern.
2. Suprascapular neuropathy caused by compression by a cyst in the spinoglenoid notch is the most likely etiology.
3. In addition to edema pattern within the infraspinatus muscle, a posterior glenoid labral tear and an adjacent paralabral cyst are depicted.
4. The suprascapular nerve arises from the upper trunk of the brachial plexus from the C5 and C6 nerve roots. There is a variable contribution of fibers from C4.
5. Ganglion or paralabral cysts, hematoma, scapular fractures, and overhead sports are all contributory.

Pearls

- The suprascapular nerve arises from the upper trunk of the brachial plexus, from the C5 and C6 nerve roots; C4 variably contributes fibers.
- The suprascapular nerve provides motor innervation to the supraspinatus and infraspinatus muscles.
- It is susceptible to entrapment at the suprascapular and spinoglenoid notches.
- Compression of the nerve at the suprascapular notch affects both the supraspinatus and infraspinatus muscles.
- Compression of the nerve at the spinoglenoid notch affects the infraspinatus muscle only.
- Common causes of suprascapular nerve compression include paralabral cysts, ganglion cysts, hematomas, and other mass lesions.
- Scapular fractures, traction caused by repetitive overhead motion including overhead sports, and traction caused by large retracted rotator cuff tears are additional causes of suprascapular neuropathy.

Suggested Readings

Lee BC, Yegappan M, Thiagarajan P. Suprascapular nerve neuropathy secondary to spinoglenoid notch ganglion cyst: case reports and review of literature. *Ann Acad Med Singapore.* 2007;36(12):1032-1035.

Piasecki DP, Romeo AA, Bach BR, Nicholson GP. Suprascapular neuropathy. *J Am Acad Orthop Surg.* 2009;17(11):665-676.

Athlete with pain on lateral aspect of elbow

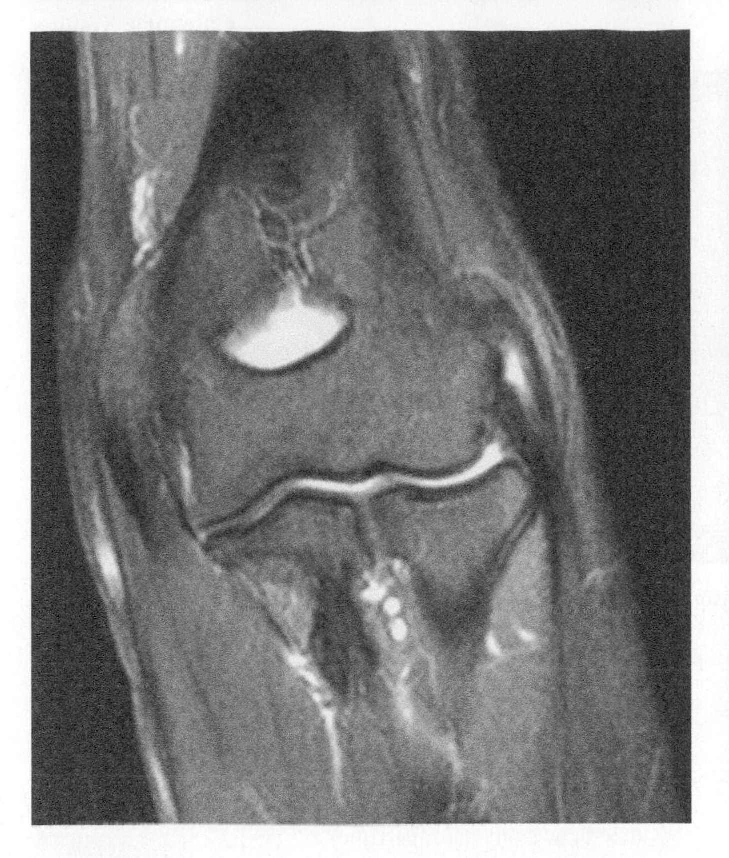

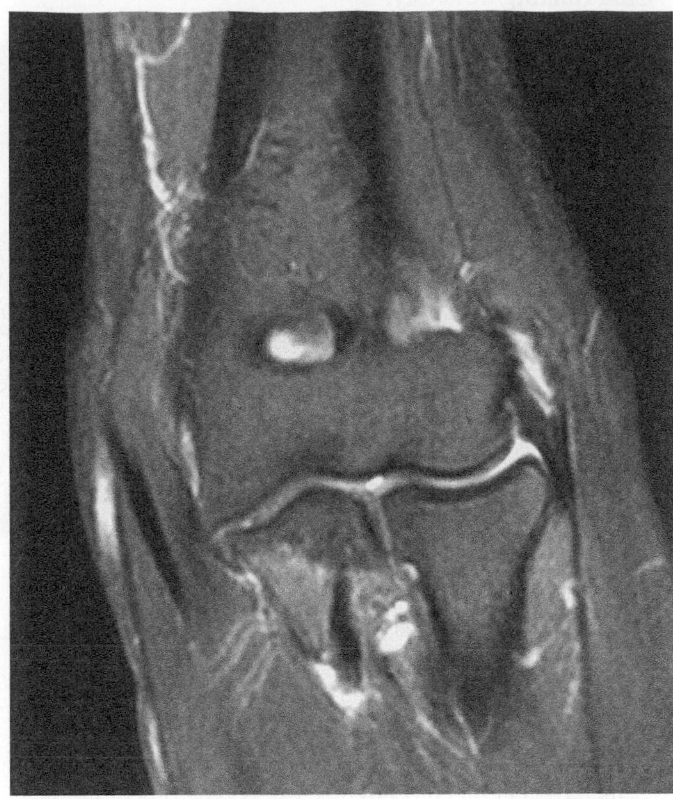

1. What is the differential diagnosis of this condition?

2. What is the tendon most commonly affected in this condition?

3. What are the imaging modalities of choice for this condition?

4. Which patient groups are predisposed to this condition?

5. What treatments may be used?

Lateral epicondylitis 209

Case ranking/difficulty:

Category: Trauma

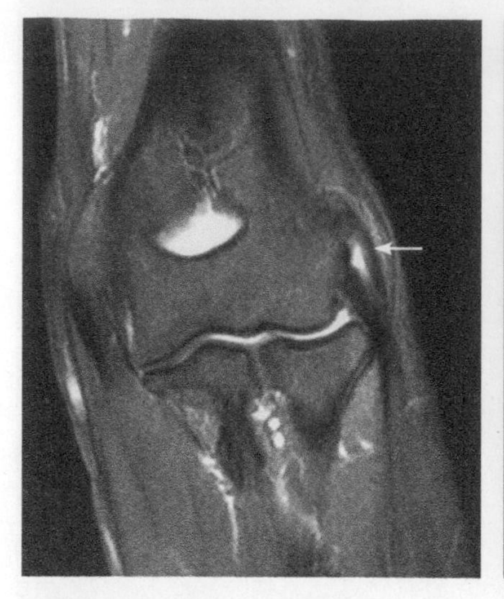

High signal within extensor tendon origin at lateral epicondyle consistent with ECRB tendinosis and partial tear.

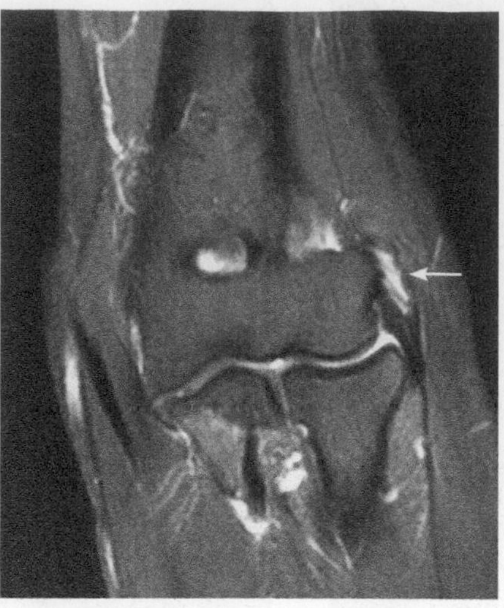

High signal within extensor tendon origin at lateral epicondyle consistent with ECRB tendinosis and partial tear.

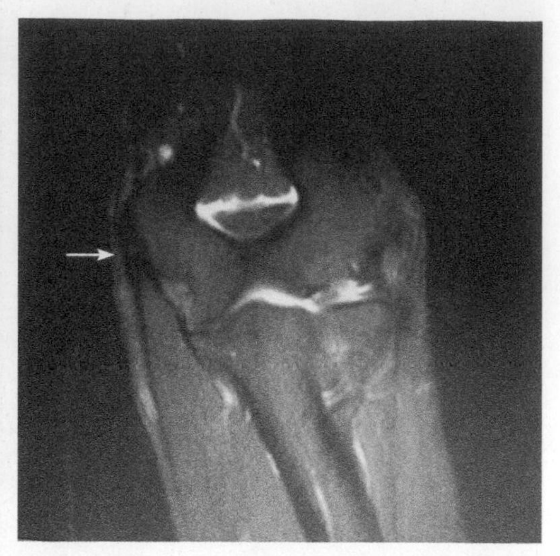

Normal appearances of the medial epicondyle and common flexor origin.

Answers

1. Differential diagnosis of lateral-sided elbow pain includes lateral epicondylitis, osteochondritis of the capitellum, posterior interosseous nerve entrapment syndrome, and cervical radiculopathy.
2. Most cases are caused by tendinosis or microtears of ECRB.
3. Ultrasound and MRI can both be used for imaging lateral epicondylitis. Ultrasound is the preferred imaging modality as it is dynamic and can guide percutaneous therapy.
4. Activities that result in excessive extension of the wrist are particularly prone. As the name "tennis elbow" suggests, this includes tennis players, but more frequently it affects people using computers, doing manual work, and musicians.
5. There are many treatments that may be used for the treatment of lateral epicondylitis, including physiotherapy, ECRB tendon decompression, lateral epicondyle decortication, and anti-inflammatory medication.

Pearls

- Lateral epicondylitis is a very common pathology affecting individuals who are predisposed to overuse of their extensor tendons, for example, tennis players, typists, and musicians.
- The most common pathological finding is tendinosis of the extensor carpi radialis brevis (ECRB) tendon, 1 to 2 cm from the insertion.
- The process is extra-articular hence an elbow effusion is not an associated feature and arthrography plays no role in diagnosis.
- Ultrasound is the investigative modality of choice for diagnosis and for guiding percutaneous treatment.
- MRI is an equivalent modality for diagnosis and will show edema within the common extensor origin.
- The preferred imaging planes for evaluation with MRI are axial and coronal, ideally using T1 and STIR sequences.

Suggested Readings

Bernardino Saccomanni. Corticosteroid injection for tennis elbow or lateral epicondylitis: a review of the literature. *Curr Rev Musculoskelet Med.* 2010;3(1-4):38-40.

Lattermann C, Romeo AA, Anbari A, et al. Arthroscopic debridement of the extensor carpi radialis brevis for recalcitrant lateral epicondylitis. *J Shoulder Elbow Surg.* 2010;19(5):651-656.

Worsening ankle pain

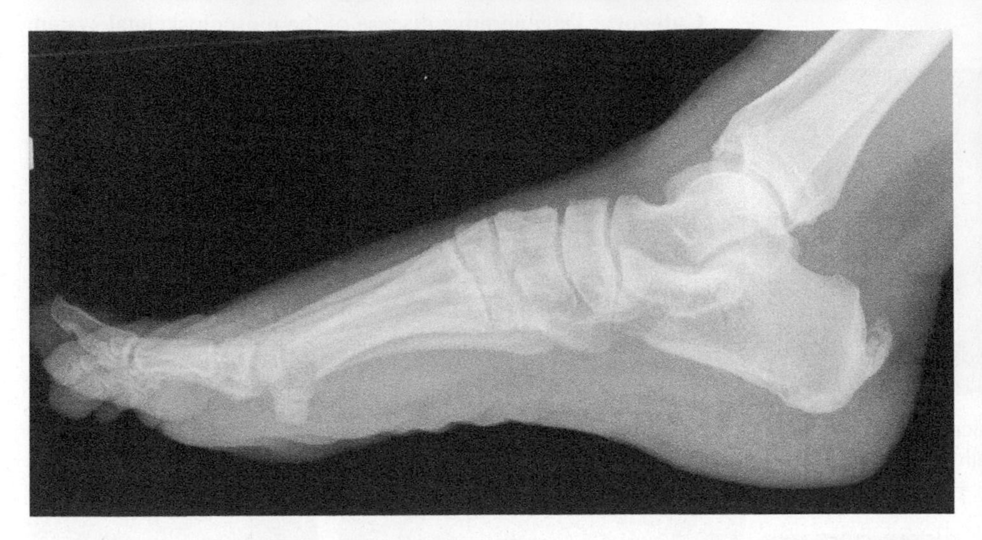

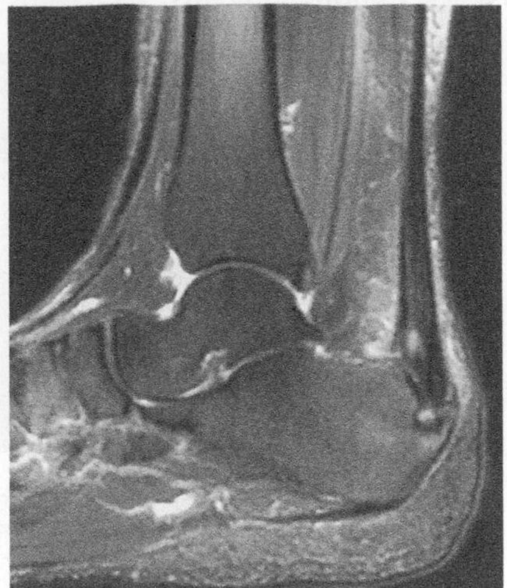

1. What features characterize this condition?

2. What is the most common age group affected by this condition?

3. What conditions are included in the differential diagnosis?

4. What is the most common surgical management in refractory cases?

5. What MRI criteria are used to determine Achilles tendinosis?

Haglund syndrome 1321

Case ranking/difficulty:

Category: Degenerative disease of the musculoskeletal system

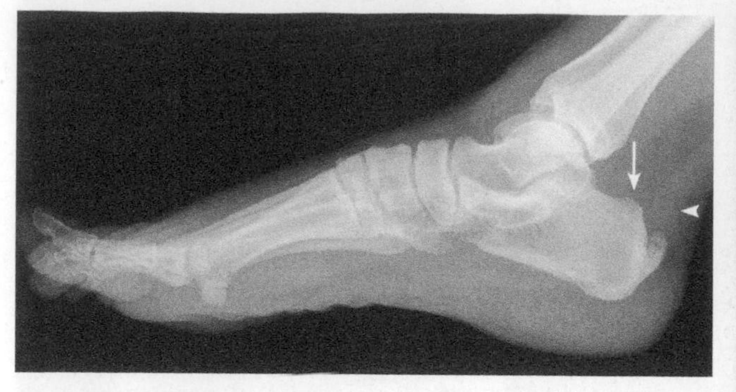

There is a prominent posterior superior calcaneus (*arrow*), with a posterior calcaneal enthesophyte and mild thickening of the distal Achilles tendon (*arrowhead*).

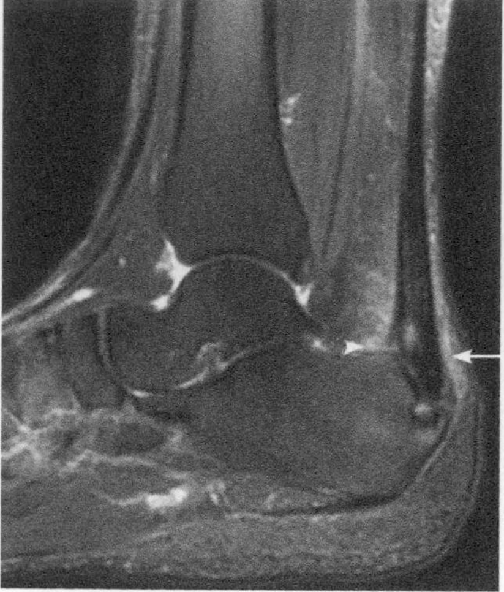

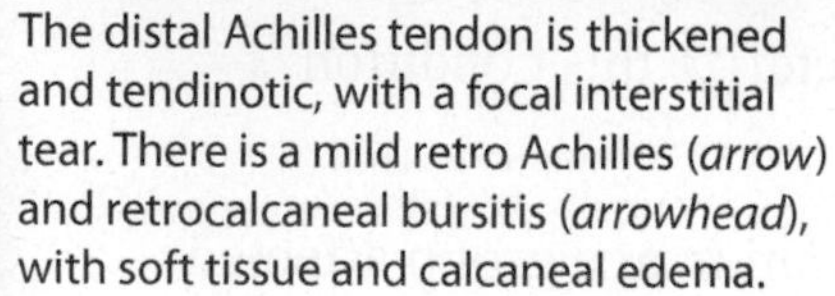

The distal Achilles tendon is thickened and tendinotic, with a focal interstitial tear. There is a mild retro Achilles (*arrow*) and retrocalcaneal bursitis (*arrowhead*), with soft tissue and calcaneal edema.

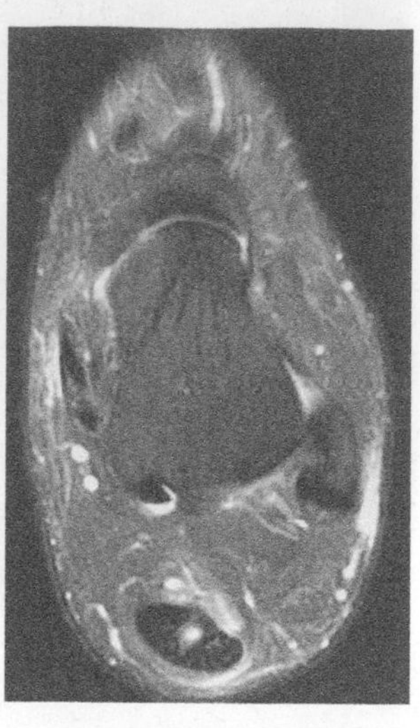

There is a convex contour of the distal Achilles consistent with tendinosis, and a focal interstitial tear.

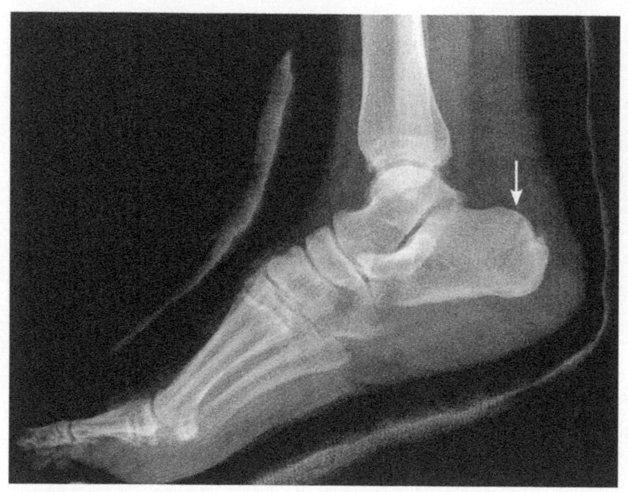

This has been treated with posterior superior calcaneal exostectomy.

Answers

1. Haglund syndrome is characterized by Achilles tendinosis, retrocalcaneal bursitis, retro Achilles bursitis, and a prominent posterior superior calcaneus.
2. The most common age group in Haglund syndrome is 20 to 35 years.
3. The usual differential for patients with bursitis and posterior ankle pain is reactive (Reiter) arthritis and rheumatoid arthritis.
4. The most common surgical management in refractory Haglund syndrome is calcaneal exostectomy.
5. Achilles tendinosis is characterized by a convex rather than flat or concave contour on axial MR images, increased T2 signal but without fluid signal, and a maximum AP measurement greater than 8 mm on axial images. Associated Kager fat pad edema may be seen, but is not required to make the diagnosis.

Pearls

- Haglund syndrome is most common in young females.
- High heel shoes (pumps) are implicated in the etiology.
- Prominent posterior superior calcaneus (pump bump) is a causative factor in the retrocalcaneal and retro Achilles bursitis, and the Achilles tendinosis.
- MRI shows a prominent posterior superior calcaneus with retrocalcaneal or retro Achilles bursitis, Achilles tendinosis, and Kager fat pad edema.
- Treatment is conservative. In refractory cases, calcaneal exostectomy is indicated.

Suggested Readings

Haglund P. Beitrag zur Klinik der Achillessehne. *Orthop Chir.* 1927;49:49-58.

Stephen MM. Haglund's deformity and retrocalcaneal bursitis. *Orthop Clin North Am.* 1994;25(1):41-46.

Pain on abduction of shoulder

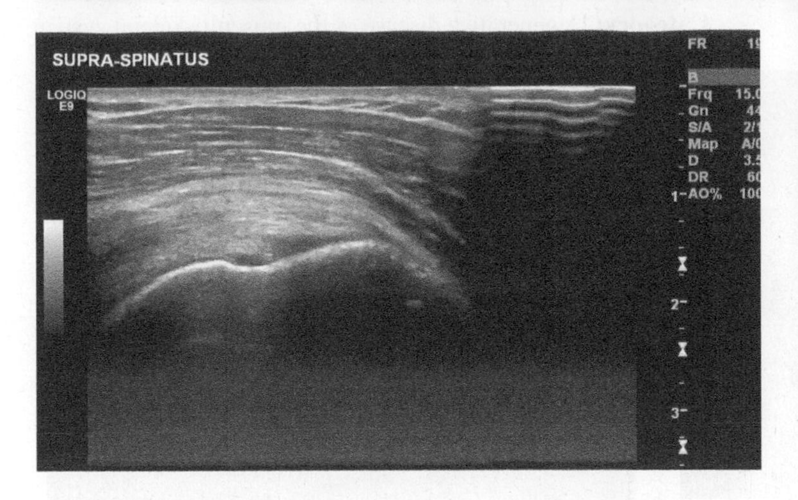

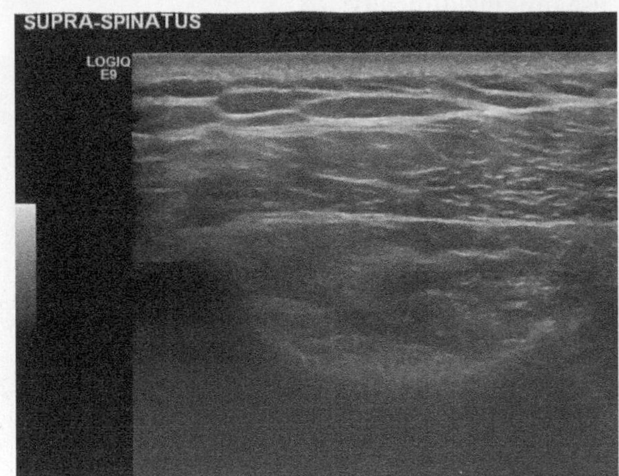

1. What is said to be the normal thickness of the affected structure visualized in the figure on the left?

2. What are the treatment options for this entity?

3. What are the advantages of ultrasound over MRI in rotator cuff imaging?

4. How can a diagnosis of this entity be made on ultrasound?

5. What is an acceptable regime for percutaneous injection therapy?

Subacromial subdeltoid bursitis 1723

Case ranking/difficulty: 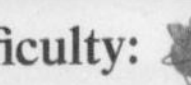 **Category:** Degenerative disease of the musculoskeletal system

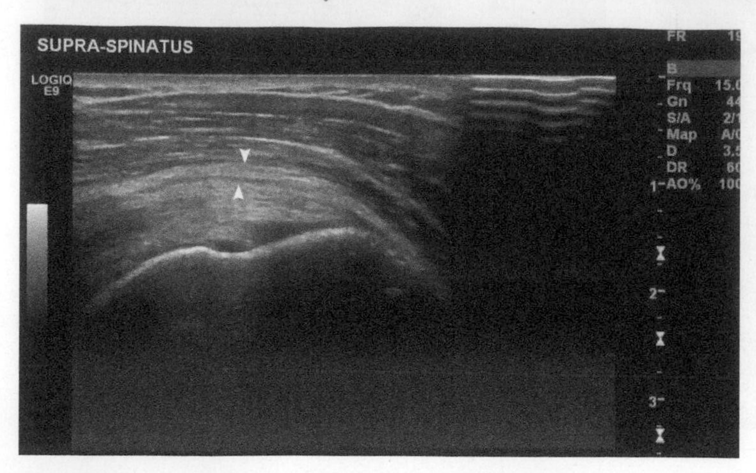

Marked thickening of the hyperechoic bursal walls is demonstrated.

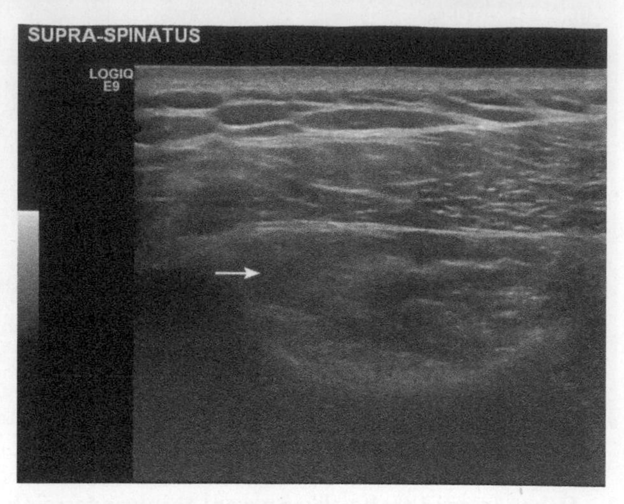

Fatty infiltration and atrophy of supraspinatus caused by tendinosis and disuse secondary to pain.

Answers

1. The normal thickness of the subacromial bursa is up to 2 mm. The majority of bursae measuring more than 3 mm may be thickened, consistent with bursitis.

2. The correct order of treatment is with oral anti-inflammatory medication for a period of weeks, as well as physiotherapy, followed by cortisone injection if resistant. Subacromial decompression may be required if other measures fail, especially if AC joint osteophytes or a type 3 or downward-sloping acromion is the cause of the subacromial impingement.

3. Ultrasound is the imaging modality of choice for assessment of the rotator cuff. It is operator-dependent, but with adequate training a sensitivity in excess of 95% can be obtained for the detection of rotator cuff tears. In addition, image-guided therapy can be administered at the same visit, including subacromial bursal injections.

4. Subacromial subdeltoid bursitis can be reliably diagnosed on ultrasound when characteristic features of bursal thickening and excess fluid are seen in conjunction with subacromial impingement on dynamic examination. There is often bunching of the bursa as it comes into contact with the inferior surface of the acromion. The presence of osteophytes may further place a mechanical block to full abduction.

   Synovitis in the anterior interval and restriction of all movements is characteristic of frozen shoulder, which is in the clinical differential.

5. Most authorities believe that the combination of long-acting local anaesthetic, for example bupivacaine, in combination with 40 mg of corticosteroid in a depot preparation, is the most efficacious.

   The total volume injected should be approximately 5 to 10 mL to enable the medication to disperse throughout the bursa.

Pearls

- Supraspinatus tendinosis, subacromial subdeltoid bursitis and partial or full-thickness degenerative cuff tears are inter-related and have the same basic pathology.
- Ultrasound is the investigative modality of choice as it can also guide percutaneous treatment.
- Excess fluid and thickening of the walls of the bursa are the hallmarks on ultrasound.
- Subacromial subdeltoid bursal thickening of greater than 3 mm is suggestive, but not specific for bursitis.

Suggested Readings

White EA, Schweitzer ME, Haims AH, et al. Effect of specific exercise strategy on need for surgery in patients with subacromial impingement syndrome: randomised controlled study. *BMJ.* 2012;344(344):e787.

White EA, Schweitzer ME, Haims AH. Range of normal and abnormal subacromial/subdeltoid bursa fluid. *J Comput Assist Tomogr*. 2006;30(2):316-320.

Severe pain in lateral hip

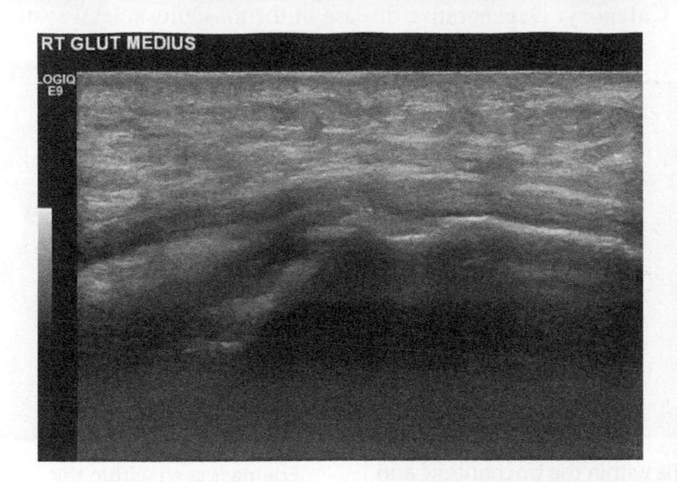

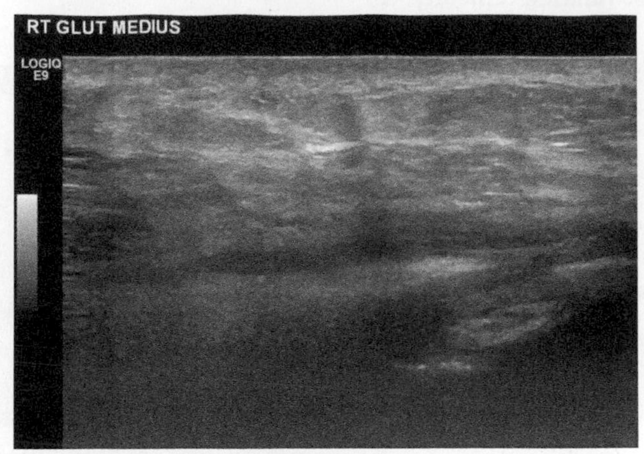

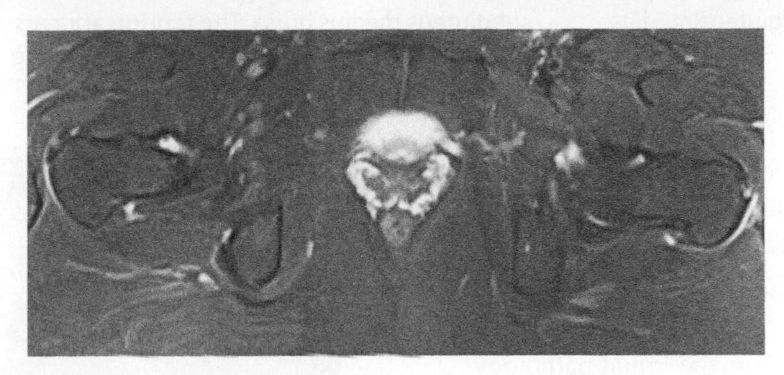

1. What is the differential diagnosis of lateral hip pain?

2. What tendons are implicated in this condition?

3. What are the imaging features of this entity?

4. What are the common treatments for this entity?

5. What are the complications of a trochanteric bursa steroid injection?

Trochanteric bursitis 1724

Case ranking/difficulty: 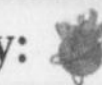

Category: Degenerative disease of the musculoskeletal system

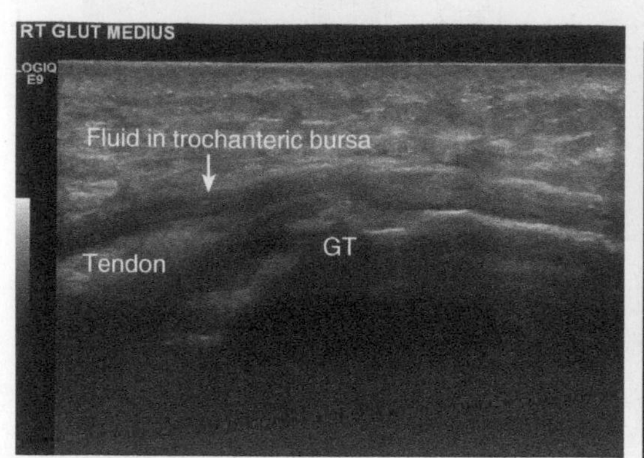

Fluid in trochanteric and subgluteus medius bursae. Intact, but severely attenuated gluteus medius tendon shown.

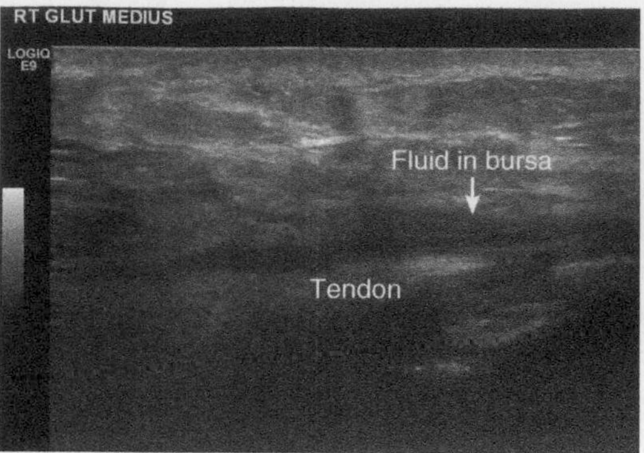

Extensive edema within the trochanteric and subgluteus medius bursa. The tendon appears intact, although may be attenuated in keeping with a partial tear.

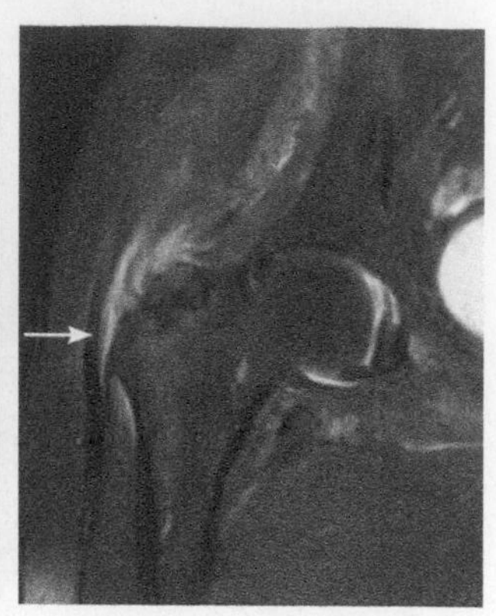

Edema is seen within the trochanteric bursa.

Answers

1. Lumbar nerve root irritation, "true" trochanteric bursitis, hip osteoarthritis and a gluteus medius tendon tear can all give lateral hip pain clinically.
2. Gluteus medius tendinopathy is often the cause of greater trochanteric pain. There may be secondary trochanteric bursitis, although the initial pathology is often gluteus medius tendinopathy or tendon tears. As the gluteus minimus tendon also attaches onto the greater trochanter, tendinopathy or tear may contribute to greater trochanteric pain.
3. Greater trochanteric pain syndrome, more simplistically termed *trochanteric bursitis*, is diagnosed by ultrasound or MRI.

   Both modalities may demonstrate fluid within the trochanteric and subgluteus medius bursae, gluteus medius tendinopathy, and greater trochanter enthesophytes.

   Ultrasound has the advantage of guiding percutaneous injection.
4. Surgery plays no real role in the condition. Corticosteroid injection, abductor strengthening and physical therapy is effective in relieving the symptoms of greater trochanteric pain syndrome.
5. Possible side effects are infection, allergy, and local and systemic effects of steroid. The most troublesome local side effects are fat necrosis and skin atrophy.

Pearls

- Trochanteric bursitis is probably more accurately termed *greater trochanteric pain syndrome*.
- The etiology is often secondary to tendinosis/partial tears of the gluteus medius or minimus tendon insertions.

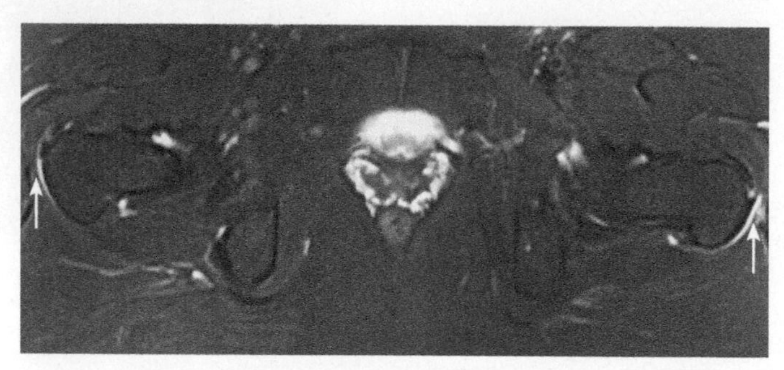

There is bilateral trochanteric edema and mild gluteus medius tendinosis, which is a common finding.

- Ultrasound or MRI can be used for diagnosis, although ultrasound can be used to guide therapeutic bursal injections.
- A distinction should be made between "true" trochanteric bursitis and subgluteus medius or minimus bursitis. These smaller bursae lie deep to the gluteus medius and minimus respectively.
- Depending on where the pathology is centered, the appropriate bursa should be targeted with an injection.

Suggested Readings

Kong A, Van der Vliet A, Zadow S. MRI and US of gluteal tendinopathy in greater trochanteric pain syndrome. *Eur Radiol.* 2007;17(7):1772-1783.

Tibor LM, Sekiya JK. Differential diagnosis of pain around the hip joint. *Arthroscopy.* 2008;24(12):1407-1421.

Walker P, Kannangara S, Bruce WJ, Michael D, Van der Wall H. Lateral hip pain: does imaging predict response to localized injection? *Clin Orthop Relat Res.* 2007;457(457):144-149.

Pain in lower calf

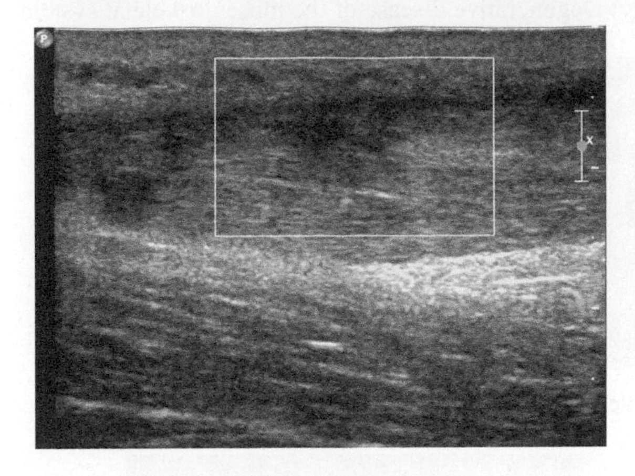

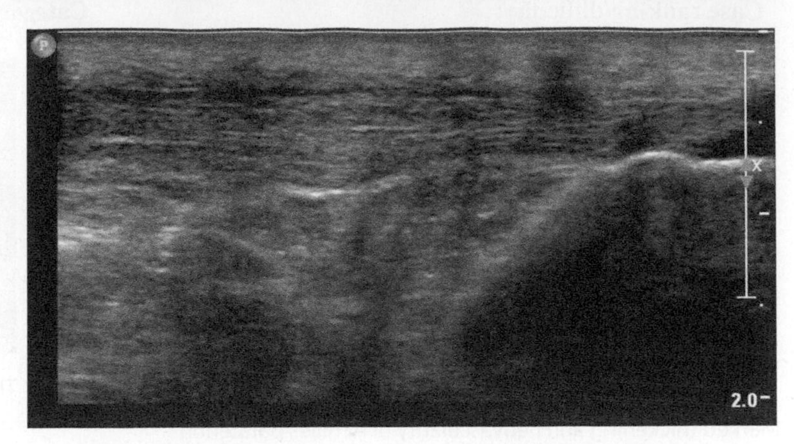

1. What is the differential diagnosis?

2. What is the imaging modality of choice for this entity?

3. What are the MRI features of this entity?

4. What are the predisposing factors for this condition?

5. What are the possible treatments for this condition?

Case ranking/difficulty:

Category: Degenerative disease of the musculoskeletal system

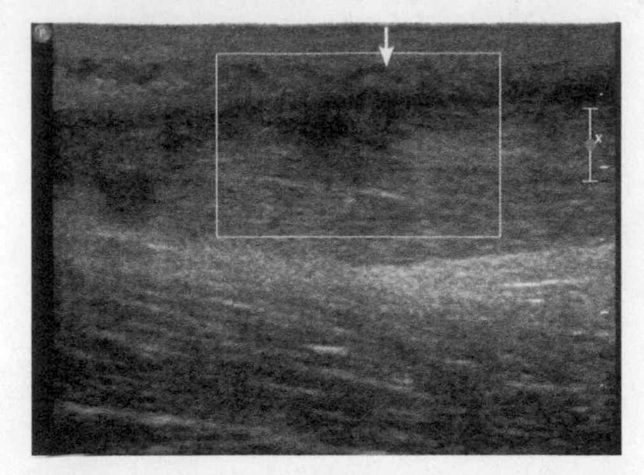

Marked thickening and neovascularity of Achilles paratenon on color Doppler imaging.

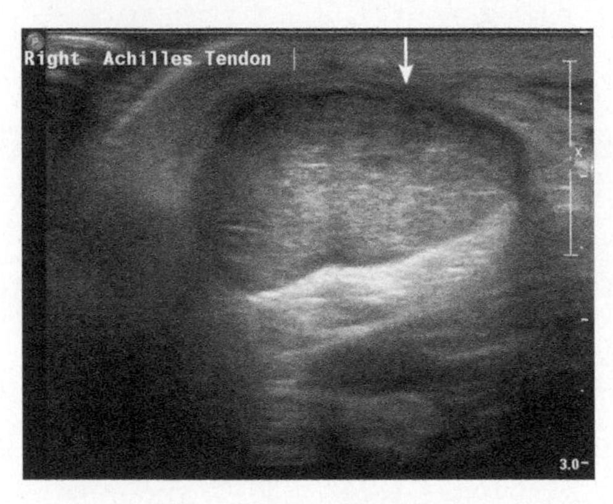

Axial images demonstrate increase diameter of tendon as a result of thickened paratenon superficially.

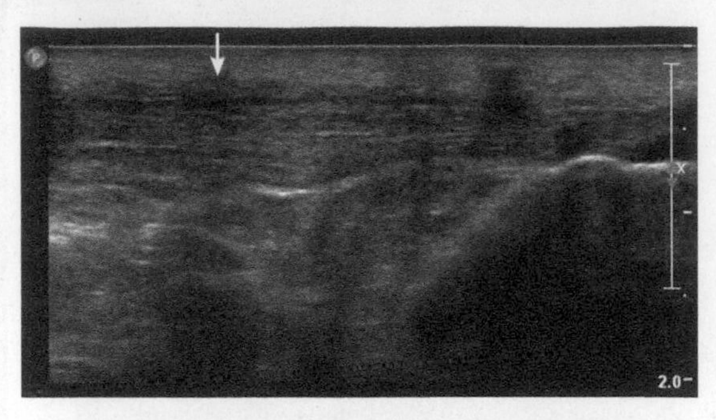

Thickening and loss of reflectivity of paratenon.

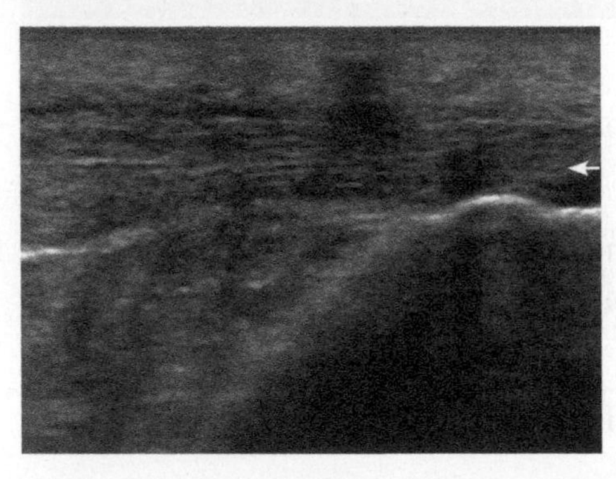

There is no fluid in the retrocalcaneal bursa, no enthesophytes at the calcaneal insertion, and no significant insertional tendinosis, which are important negative findings.

Answers

1. The differential diagnosis of this entity is between a paratenonitis and a noninsertional tendinopathy. As the paratenon is focally thickened, there is probably only one real diagnosis.
2. Ultrasound is the preferred mode of tendon assessment and guides percutaneous therapy, for example, high-volume injection and paratenon stripping.
3. On MRI, the thickened Achilles paratenon will be seen as an area of low T1 and high STIR signal, remote from the calcaneal insertion.
4. Running, excessive walking, and poor footwear are the most important factors for Achilles tendon disorders, including paratenonitis.
5. Fluoroquinolones, for example, ciprofloxacin, should be stopped as they are associated with Achilles tendon rupture. Steroid injection is contraindicated for similar reasons. There are many other treatments, for example, extracorporeal shock wave therapy, autologous blood/platelet-rich plasma injection, and high-volume injection, although few of these are based on robust evidence.

Pearls

- The Achilles tendon does not have a synovial sheath, but instead has a paratenon.
- Distinction should be made between Achilles tendinosis, Achilles tendon tears (partial or full thickness), and paratenonitis.
- Ultrasound is the gold-standard imaging modality for Achilles tendon assessment as it allows dynamic assessment and guides percutaneous management.
- Focal thickening of the paratenon between the MTJ and calcaneal insertion is associated with neovascularity and compression tenderness on ultrasound in this condition.

Suggested Readings

Naidu V, Abbassian A, Nielsen D, Uppalapati R, Shetty A. Minimally invasive paratenon release for non-insertional Achilles tendinopathy. *Foot Ankle Int.* 2009;30(7):680-685.

Tan SC, Chan O. Achilles and patellar tendinopathy: current understanding of pathophysiology and management. *Disabil Rehabil.* 2008;30(20-22):1608-1615.

Testa V, Capasso G, Benazzo F, Maffulli N. Management of Achilles tendinopathy by ultrasound-guided percutaneous tenotomy. *Med Sci Sports Exerc.* 2002;34(4):573-580.

Hand numbness

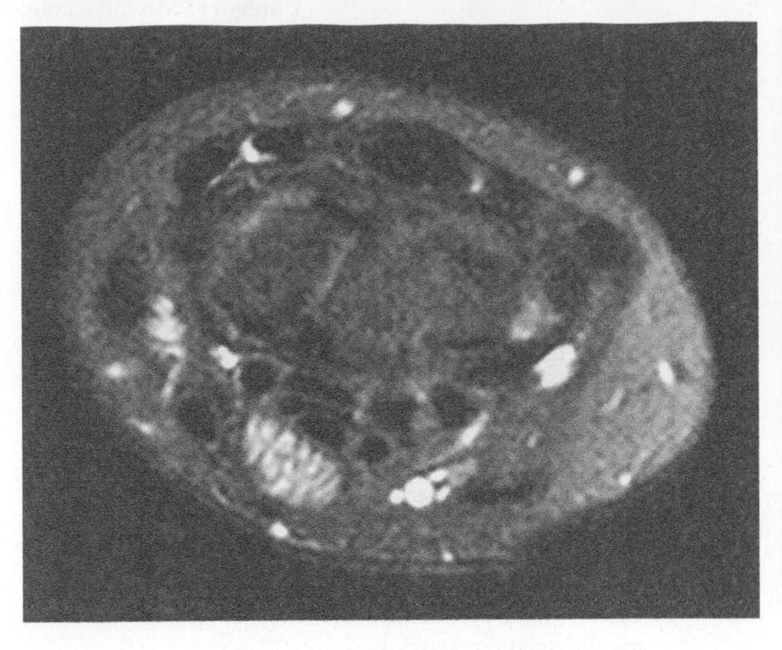

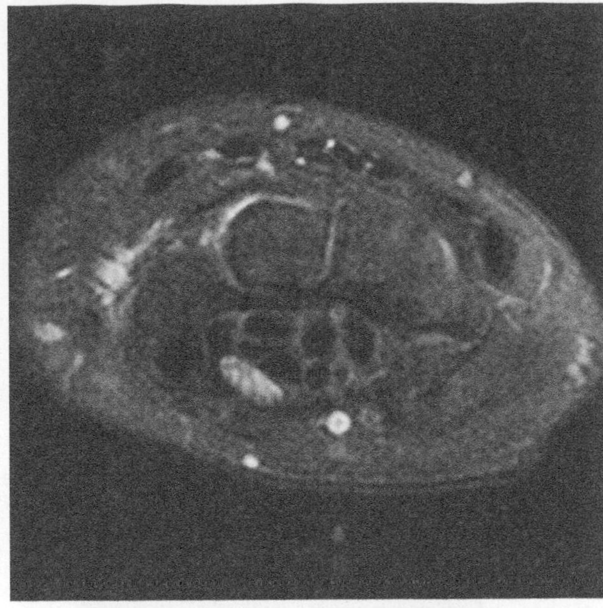

1. What is the most common peripheral neuropathy affecting the upper extremity?

2. What are the contents of the carpal tunnel?

3. What are causes of this entity?

4. What are the locations at which the median nerve may become entrapped in the upper extremity?

5. In what demographic group is this condition most common?

Carpal tunnel syndrome (median neuritis) 1531

Case ranking/difficulty: **Category:** Miscellaneous

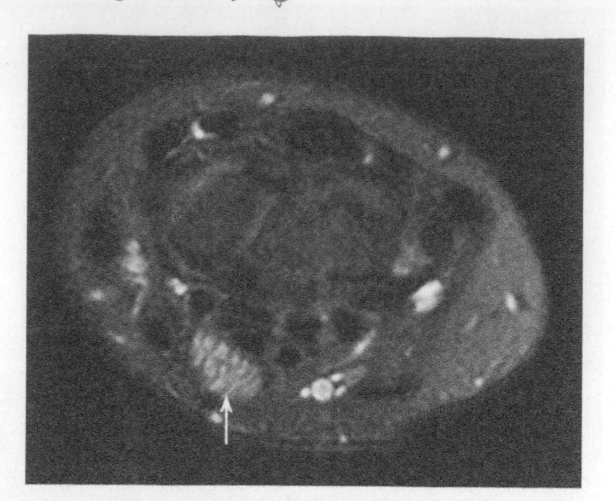

The median nerve proximal to the carpal tunnel demonstrates enlargement and increased signal intensity (*arrow*).

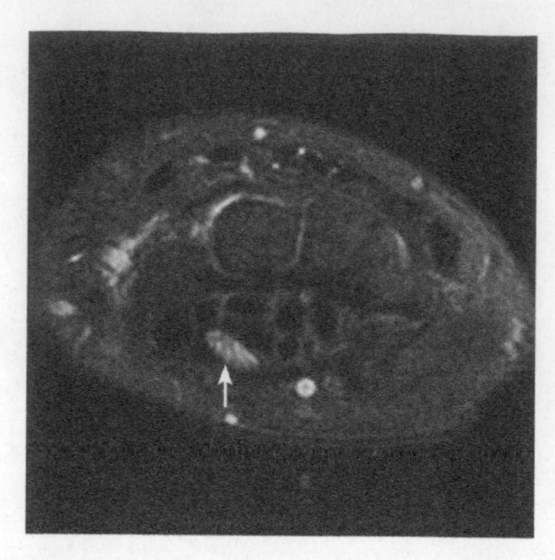

Similar findings, although to a lesser degree, at the proximal carpal tunnel.

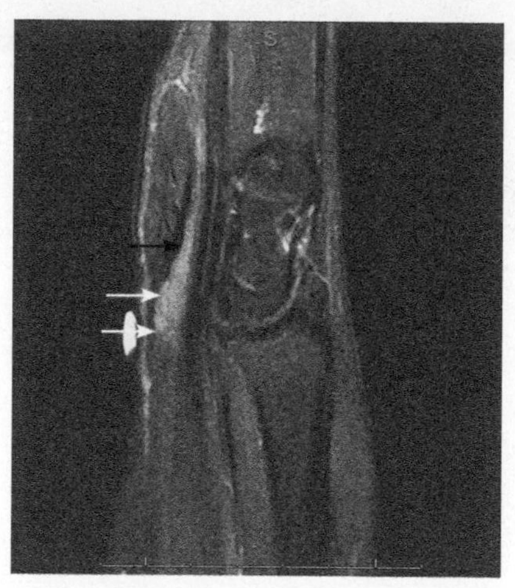

The nerve is enlarged proximal to the carpal tunnel and within the proximal aspect of the carpal tunnel (*proximal arrows*). It becomes flattened within the distal aspect of the carpal tunnel (*distal arrow*).

Answers

1. Carpal tunnel syndrome is the most common peripheral neuropathy affecting the upper extremity.
2. The median nerve, flexor digitorum superficialis and profundus tendons (8 tendons), and flexor pollicis longus tendon lie within the carpal tunnel.
3. Diabetes mellitus, pregnancy, hypothyroidism, and ganglion cysts are known causes of carpal tunnel syndrome.
4. Potential locations of median nerve entrapment include the supracondylar process of the distal humerus, between the humeral and ulnar heads of the pronator teres muscle, and beneath the flexor retinaculum at the wrist (carpal tunnel syndrome).
5. Carpal tunnel syndrome occurs most commonly in middle-aged females.

Pearls

- Carpal tunnel syndrome results from compression of the median nerve within the carpal tunnel at the wrist.
- The carpal tunnel is a fibro-osseous canal at the volar aspect of the wrist extending to the proximal palm.
- Carpal tunnel syndrome is most commonly idiopathic but may result from ganglion cysts, vascular malformations, lipomas, neurofibromas, fibrolipomatous hamartomas, and tenosynovitis of the flexor tendons within the carpal tunnel. Systemic causes are contributory.
- Typical MRI findings include enlargement of the median nerve just proximal to and within the proximal aspect of the carpal tunnel, flattening within the distal aspect of the tunnel, and hyperintensity of the nerve on fluid-sensitive sequences. There is usually contrast enhancement.
- Diffusion tensor imaging (DTI) shows promise for the early detection of median neuritis.

Suggested Readings

Linda DD, Harish S, Stewart BG, Finlay K, Parasu N, Rebello RP. Multimodality imaging of peripheral neuropathies of the upper limb and brachial plexus. *Radiographics.* 2010;30(5):1373-1400.

Yao L, Gai N. Median nerve cross-sectional area and MRI diffusion characteristics: normative values at the carpal tunnel. *Skeletal Radiol.* 2009;38(4):355-361.

Chronic heel pain

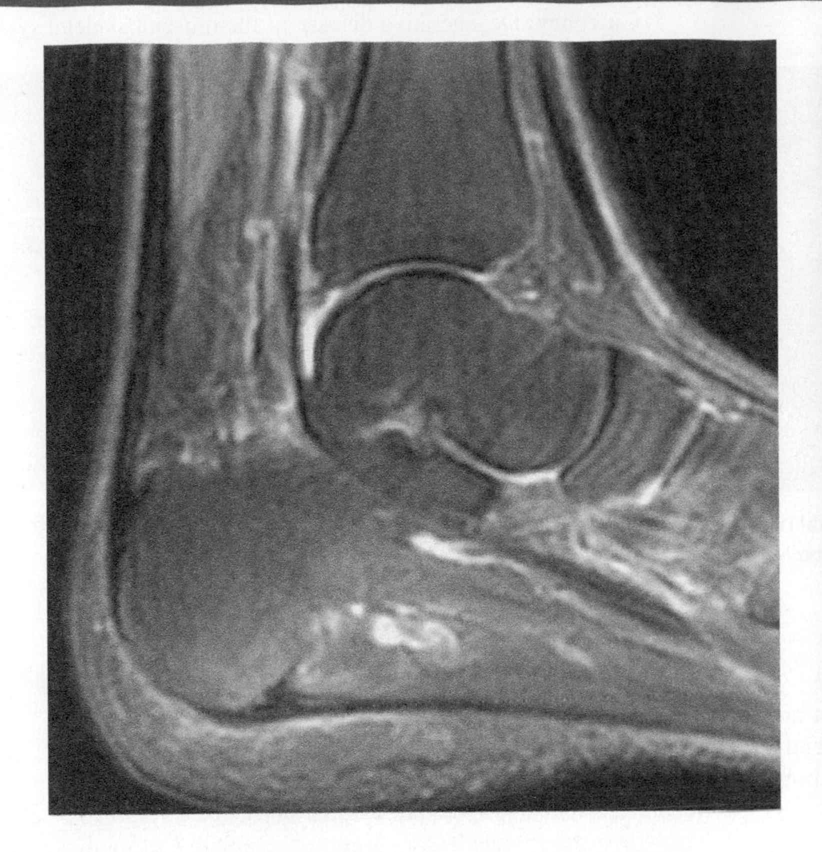

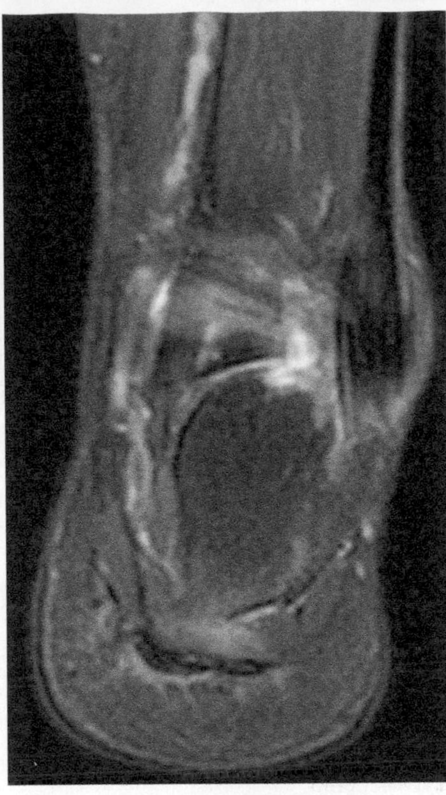

1. What are the imaging findings?

2. What is the differential for the findings?

3. What is the most prevalent finding in MR imaging of this condition?

4. What is the relevance of a calcaneal osteophyte in this condition?

5. What is the treatment for this condition?

Plantar fasciitis 1331

Case ranking/difficulty:

Category: Degenerative disease of the musculoskeletal system

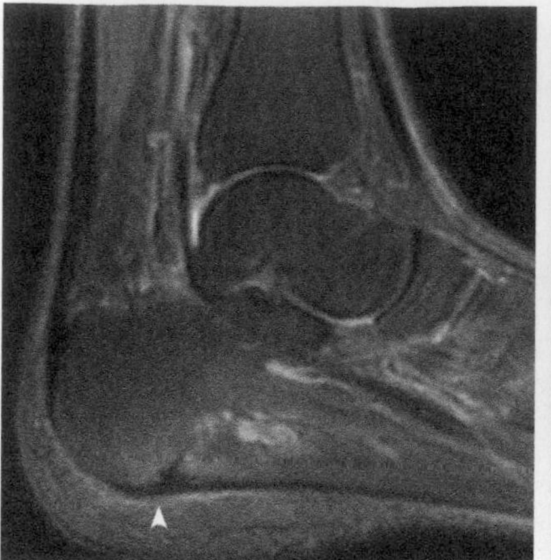

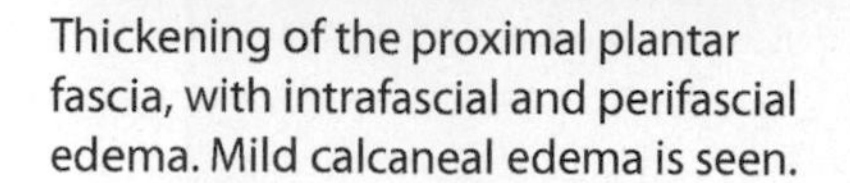

Thickening of the proximal plantar fascia, with intrafascial and perifascial edema. Mild calcaneal edema is seen.

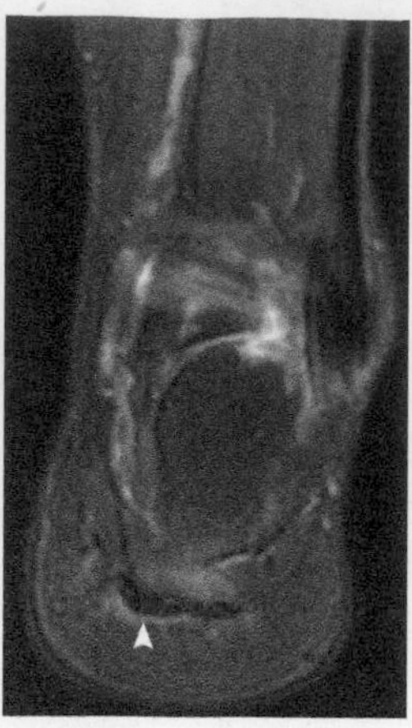

The central band of the fascia is mainly involved.

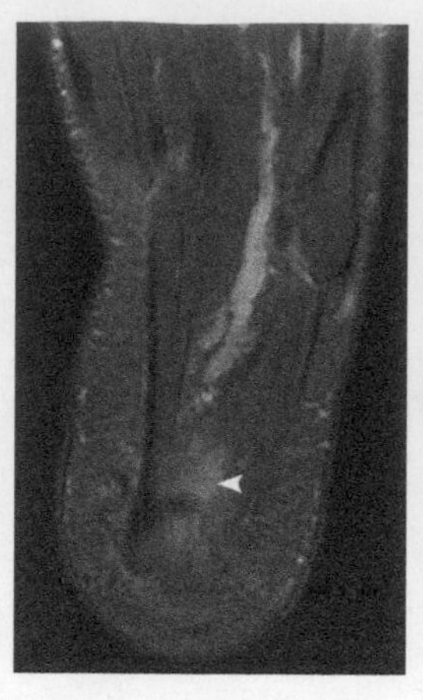

Perifascial edema is well seen.

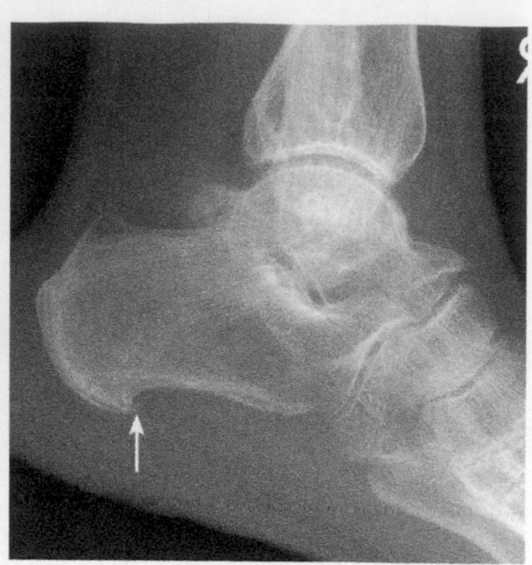

Typical large calcaneal enthesophyte in another patient.

Answers

1. There is a thickened proximal plantar fascia measuring more than 4 mm in thickness, with intrafascial and perifascial edema and associated calcaneal bone marrow edema.

2. Edema within and surrounding a thickened proximal plantar fascia can be seen in both plantar fasciitis and recent steroid injections of the fascia. In fascial rupture, there would be discontinuity of the fascia. A plantar fibroma or clear cell sarcoma would have a mass-like appearance.

3. In order of prevalence of MR findings for plantar fasciitis, edema in the soft tissues plantar to the fascia is the most prevalent, followed by edema in the soft tissues deep to the fascia, then edema within the fascia, calcaneal edema, and, finally, thickening of the fascia.

4. Of asymptomatic patients, 25% have a calcaneal spur and there is no direct relationship to fasciitis. Some believe the spur may arise as a consequence of fascitis. The spur is not located at the calcaneal attachment of the plantar fascia.

5. Conservative management for plantar fasciitis is NSAIDs, with or without concomitant steroid injections. Fasciotomy may be indicated in patients who do not respond to conservative management.

   Excision of the calcaneal spur has not been proven to be effective, although some patients may have some symptomatic relief.

Pearls

- The plantar fascia has 3 main bands: the medial, central, and lateral bands, with the central band being the largest and most important.
- The plantar fascia is contiguous with the Achilles tendon in children, but that communication is lost with increasing age.
- Plantar fasciitis typically involves the proximal central band.
- Chronic repetitive trauma is the most likely etiology.
- Calcaneal spurs are seen in 25% of asymptomatic patients, and is likely not a causative factor in plantar fasciitis.
- MRI features include perifascial edema, intrafascial edema, calcaneal bone marrow edema, and thickening of the plantar fascia.

Suggested Readings

Narváez JA, Narváez J, Ortega R, Aguilera C, Sánchez A, Andía E. Painful heel: MR imaging findings. *Radiographics*. 2000;20(2):333-352.

Theodorou DJ, Theodorou SJ, Farooki S, Kakitsubata Y, Resnick D. Disorders of the plantar aponeurosis: a spectrum of MR imaging findings. *AJR Am J Roentgenol.* 2001;176(1):97-104.

Diffuse bone pain

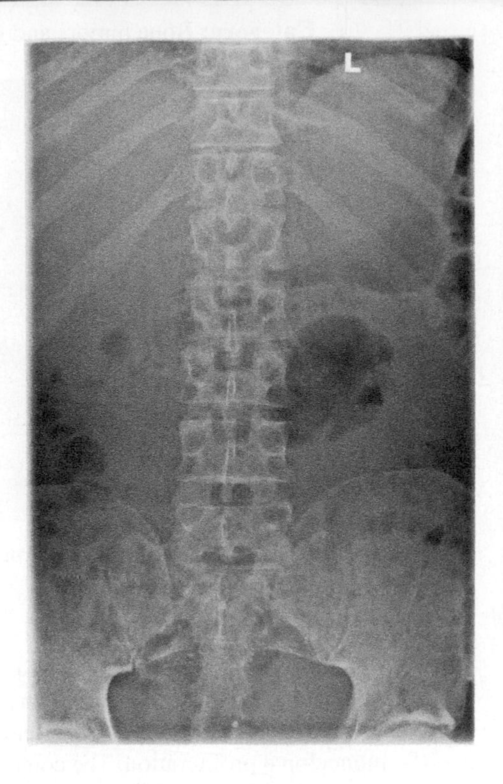

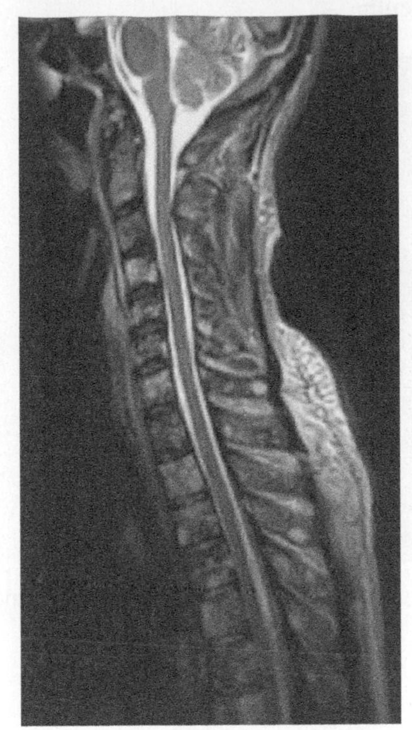

1. What are the imaging features of this entity?

2. What are the complications of this disease?

3. This disease is caused by clonal proliferation of which type of cell?

4. What are risk factors for this condition?

5. What are the possible treatments?

Multiple myeloma 1725

Case ranking/difficulty:

Category: Bone tumors and marrow abnormalities

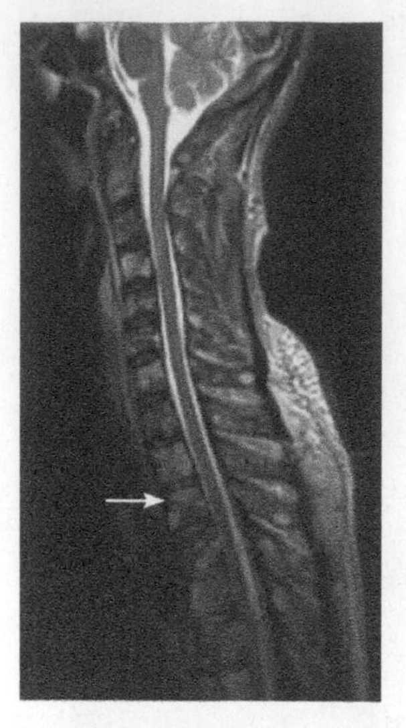

Diffuse marrow replacement seen in cervical spine as high signal intensity lesions on STIR sequences.

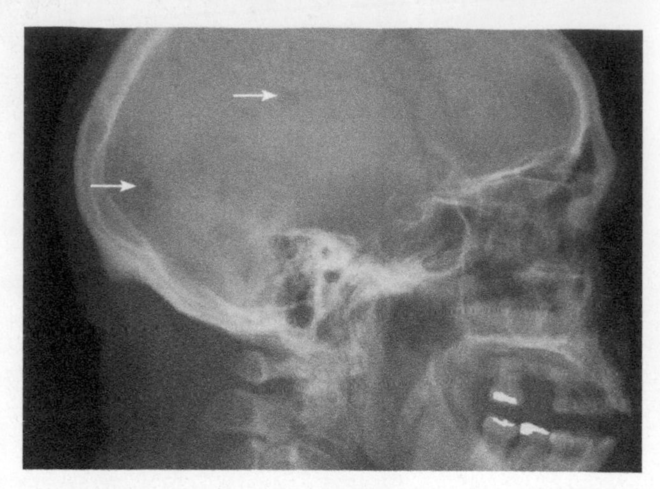

Lytic lesions are present in the skull, a common site for multiple myeloma.

Answers

1. MRI is the most sensitive test for myeloma. Marrow infiltration by myeloma results in low T1 marrow signal, although the STIR signal can be variable.

   Pathological fractures result from the weakening of bone as a consequence of lytic lesions.

   Myeloma has typically low uptake on radionuclide scans; however, a lesion may show increase uptake in the presence of a pathological fracture.

2. Myeloma does not cause thrombocytosis. As a consequence of marrow infiltration by plasma cells, thrombocyte production is reduced leading to thrombocytopenia.

   Secondary amyloidosis can cause effects in multiple organs, including liver, kidneys, and lungs.

   Cord compression can result from spinal deposits with epidural soft-tissue masses. Pathological fractures are relatively common.

3. Monoclonal proliferation of plasma cells results in multiple myeloma. The immunoglobulin light chains are detected in the serum and urine (Bence-Jones protein), which forms the basis of laboratory diagnosis.

4. There are no known risk factors for multiple myeloma. There is no known genetic predisposition, with mutations acquired, rather than hereditary. Hence it is extremely rare in persons younger than 40 years of age.

5. Stem cell transplantation offers the best chance of disease remission, although stem cell transplantation often cannot be tolerated in the elderly who tend to have the disease. There is no possibility of cure with surgery, as the disease, by definition, is a systemic disorder of plasma cell monoclonal proliferation. The complications of bone pain, hypercalcemia and pathological fracture can be treated.

Pearls

- Multiple myeloma is the most common primary bone tumor. It must always be considered in the differential diagnosis of multiple lytic lesions, especially in the appropriate age group (older than age 50 years).
- A skeletal survey is often performed to stage the extent of the disease.
- MRI is however the gold standard where resources permit, as the full extent of marrow replacement can be appreciated, as well as any associated soft-tissue components.
- Complications of myeloma include pathological fracture, making it is as important to highlight to the clinician sites prone to fracture as it is to comment on the presence of established fractures.

Suggested Reading

Li SD, Wang YF, Qi JY, Qiu LG. Clinical features of bone complications and prognostic value of bone lesions detected by X-ray skeletal survey in previously untreated patients with multiple myeloma. *Indian J Hematol Blood Transfus.* 2010;26(3):83-88.

Anterior knee pain

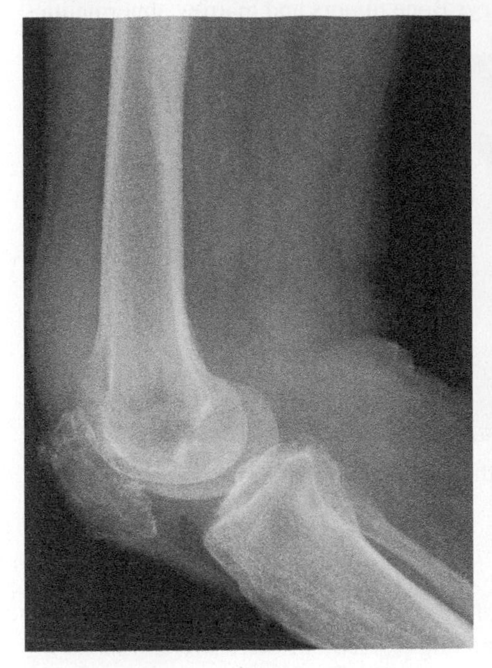

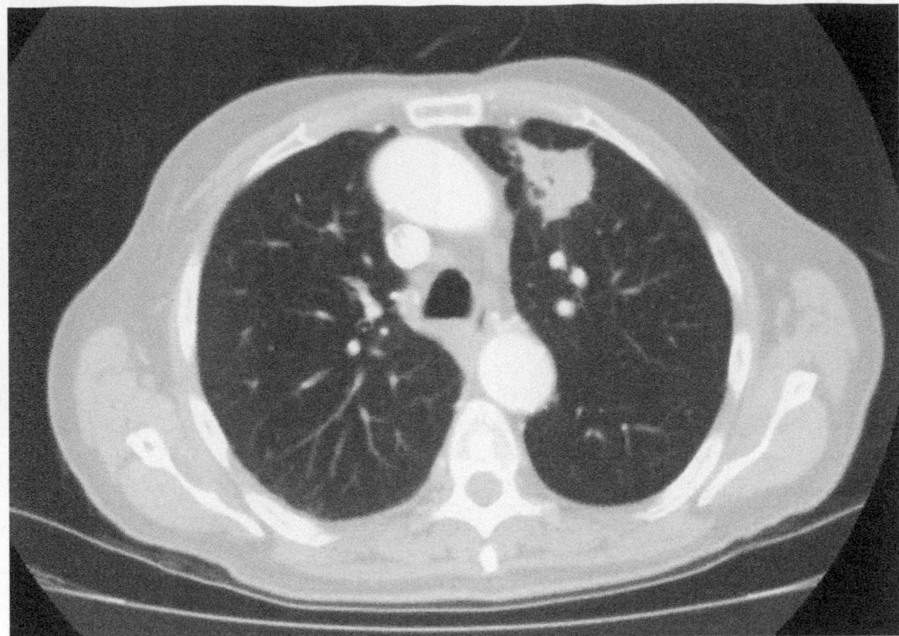

1. What are the radiographic and CT scan findings?

2. What are the differential diagnoses for the patella lesion?

3. What is the likely diagnosis?

4. What are the most common causes for this entity?

5. The patella has a very good blood supply. True or False?

Lung metastasis within the patella 1553

Case ranking/difficulty:

Category: Bone tumors and marrow abnormalities

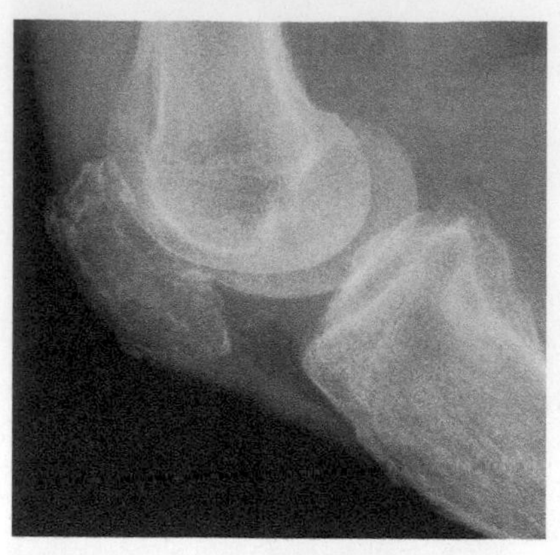

Magnified view of the patella showing the destructive lucent lesion.

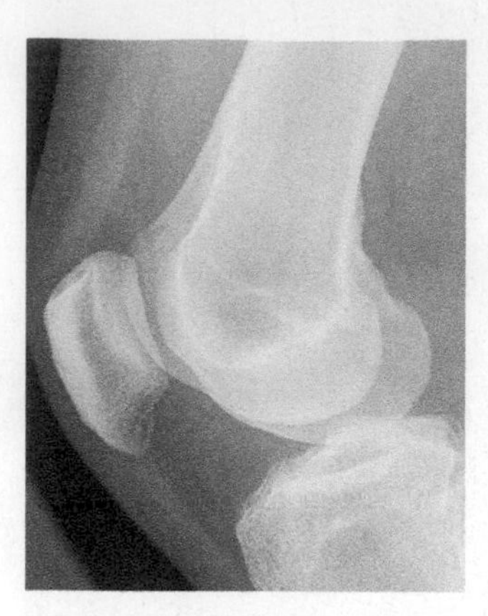

Normal patella.

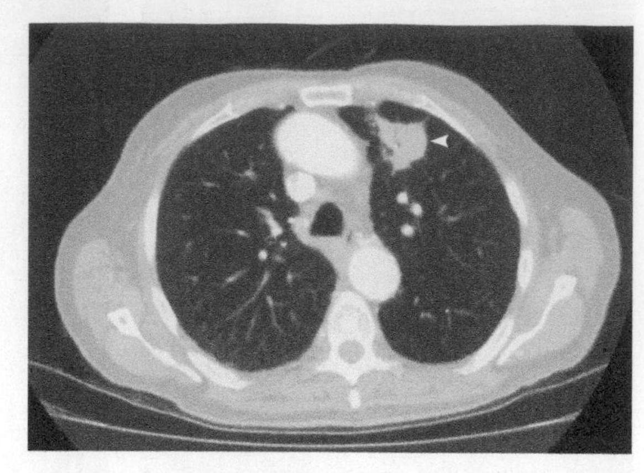

Mass in the left lung, which is the primary tumor.

Answers

1. A lucent destructive lesion of the patella is the main diagnostic finding. The CT scan shows a lung mass.
2. The differential diagnosis includes metastasis, lymphoma, melanoma, infection, and chondrosarcoma.
3. The likely diagnosis, given a lung mass and destructive bone lesion, is a solitary metastasis to the patella.
4. The most common primaries for patella metastasis are lung and breast cancers. However, other primaries, such as melanoma and bowel cancer, have been reported.
5. False. The patella has a poor blood supply, and therefore metastasis to the patella is rare.

Pearls

- Metastasis to the patella is rare because of its poor vascularity as a sesamoid bone.
- When considering anterior knee pain with a lucent bone lesion, patellar bone metastasis should be considered as one of the rare causes.
- The majority of the cases in the literature are metastasis from lung or breast primaries. The imaging features typically show a destructive lucent lesion of the patella, with no internal matrix.
- The differential diagnosis includes chondrosarcoma, lymphoma, malignant melanoma, and infection.

Suggested Readings

Choi YS, Yoon YK, Kwak HY, Song IS. Patellar metastasis from a squamous cell carcinoma of the larynx. *AJR Am J Roentgenol.* 2000;174(6):1794-1795.

Codreanu I, Zhuang H, Alavi A, Torigian DA. Patellar metastasis from lung adenocarcinoma revealed by FDG PET/CT. *Clin Nucl Med.* 2012;37(6):623-624.

Urvoy P, Mestdagh H, Butin E, Lecomte-Houcke M, Maynou C. Patellar metastasis from a large bowel adenocarcinoma. *Acta Orthop Belg.* 1993;59(4):409-411.

3-month history of generalized bony pain

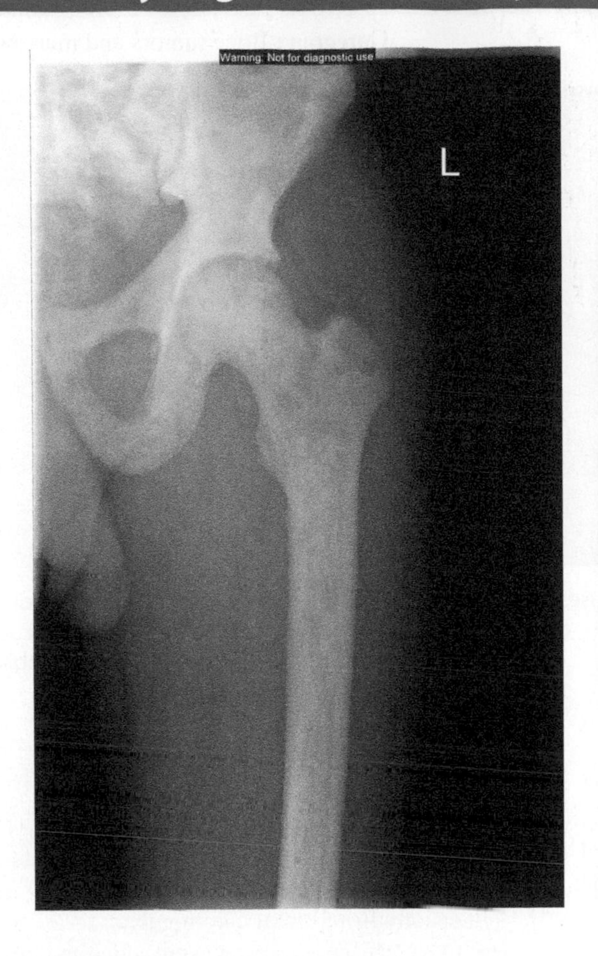

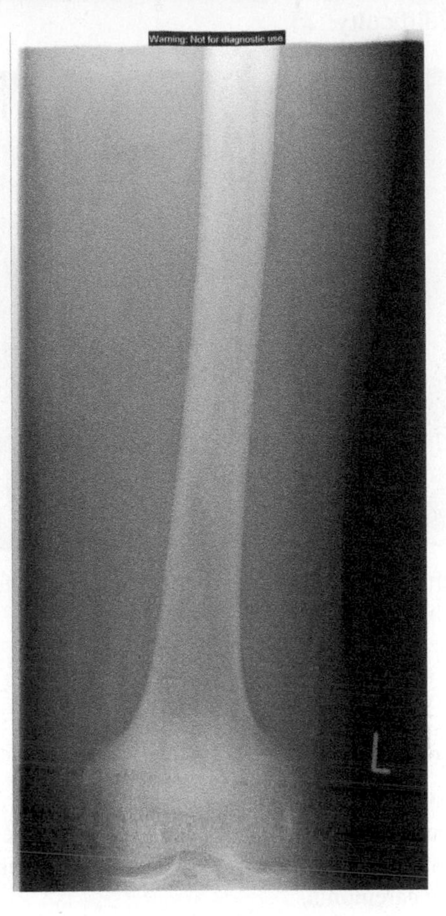

1. What is the most likely diagnosis in this patient?

2. What is the most appropriate initial management?

3. Which solid-organ malignancies may present with these bony appearances?

4. What is the appropriate treatment for this condition?

5. What conditions may have identical appearances?

Diffuse sclerotic metastases (prostatic carcinoma) 104

Case ranking/difficulty: **Category:** Bone tumors and marrow abnormalities

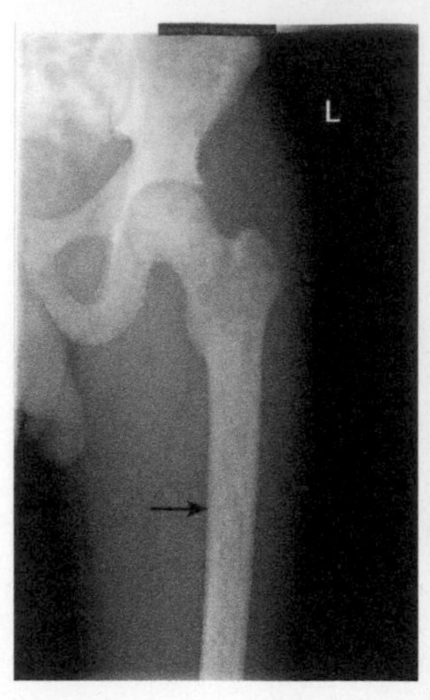

Diffuse sclerosis throughout left femur and pelvis.

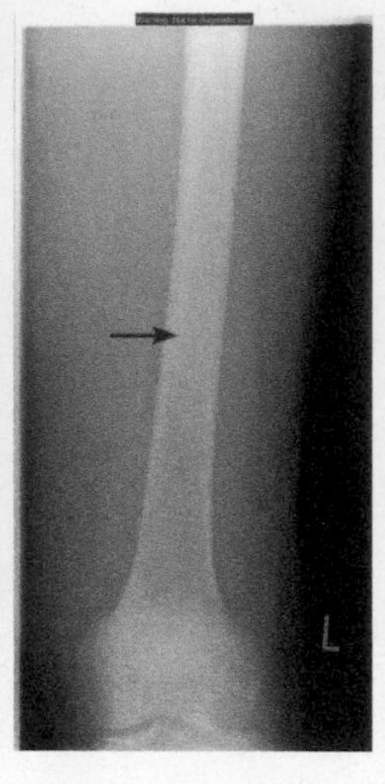

Diffuse sclerosis is seen in the left femur consistent with sclerotic metastases.

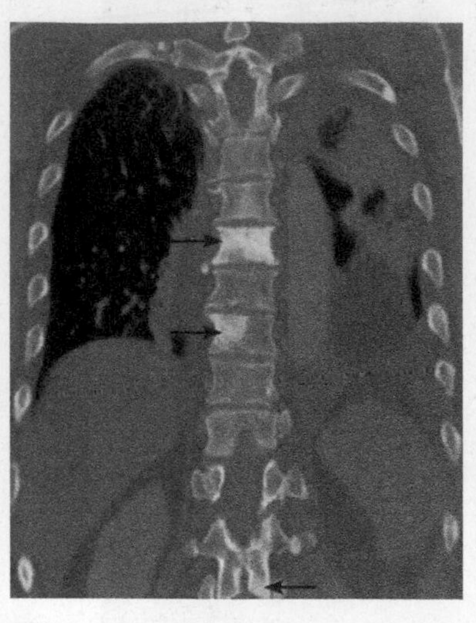

Diffuse sclerotic vertebral metastases.

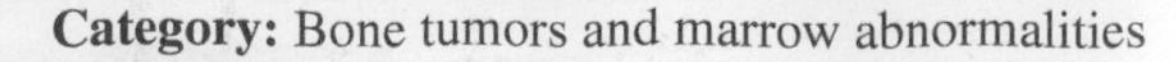
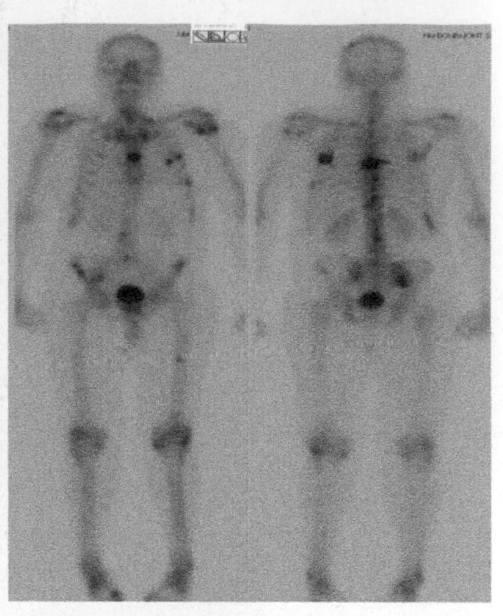

Multifocal increased uptake on a technetium bone scan demonstrates the full extent of the osteoblastic metastases.

Answers

1. The common sclerotic metastases are from prostate, breast, colorectal, and lung carcinoma. There is no real differential in an elderly patient with a rising PSA other than prostatic carcinoma.
2. A bone scan with urological referral is most appropriate for a patient with diffuse sclerotic lesions and a rising PSA. A technetium bone scan is cheap and very sensitive in the detection of osteoblastic metastases. Other modalities, for example, SPECT or PET-CT, would be needlessly expensive when the diagnosis is in little doubt.
3. Breast, prostate, and colorectal carcinoma are the most common osteoblastic skeletal metastases. Lung and renal cell carcinoma have lytic metastases.
4. Metastatic prostate cancer could be appropriately managed with palliation, radiotherapy for local or skeletal complications, hormonal therapy, or chemotherapy. However, radical curative surgery is not appropriate.
5. Breast and prostatic carcinoma metastases can have identical appearances. Other causes for diffuse sclerosis, for example, sickle cell disease, may look similar although the patient demographics would be very different. Osteopetrosis has a more uniformly sclerotic appearance and is very rare in comparison.

Pearls

- Generalized osteosclerosis in an adult is often secondary to metastatic disease. In a male, this is usually from prostate carcinoma. In a female, this is usually from breast carcinoma.
- Other causes are rarer and are suggested by other imaging features, for example, fluorosis—enthesopathy; sickle cell disease—H-shaped vertebrae; osteopetrosis—age and Erlenmeyer flask deformity.
- The axial skeleton is involved first with prostatic metastases.
- Progressive sclerosis is not easy to monitor on imaging studies when comparison of treatment response is sought. For this purpose, serum PSA is an appropriate test, as changes from the baseline can be used to better monitor the response to therapy.
- Bone scans, plain radiographs, CT scans, and MRI scans can all be used to demonstrate the extent of disease. Technetium-99 radionuclide scans are still first line investigations for mapping the extent of disease, although they may lack specificity, being positive in other instances, for example, post-trauma and infection.

Suggested Readings

Feydy A, Carlier R, Vallée C, et al. Imaging of osteosclerotic metastases [in French]. *J Radiol.* 1995;76(9):561-572.

Hackländer T, Scharwächter C, Golz R, Mertens H. Value of diffusion-weighted imaging for diagnosing vertebral metastases due to prostate cancer in comparison to other primary tumors [in German]. *Rofo.* 2006;178(4):416-424.

Incidental finding on radiograph of finger

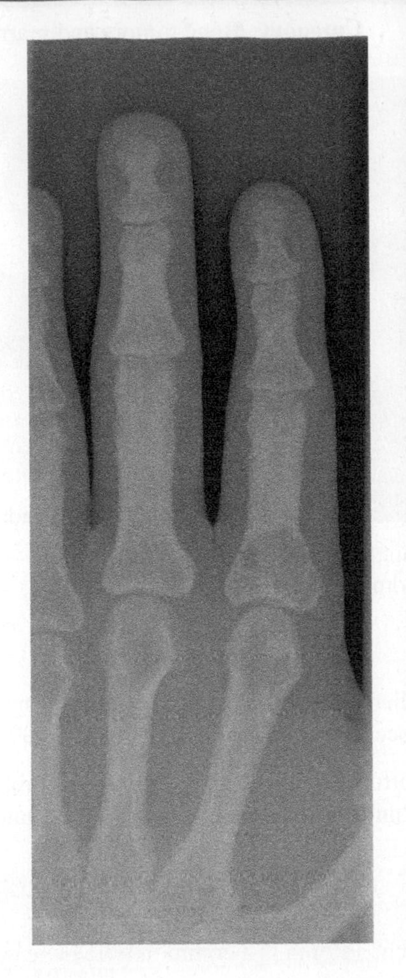

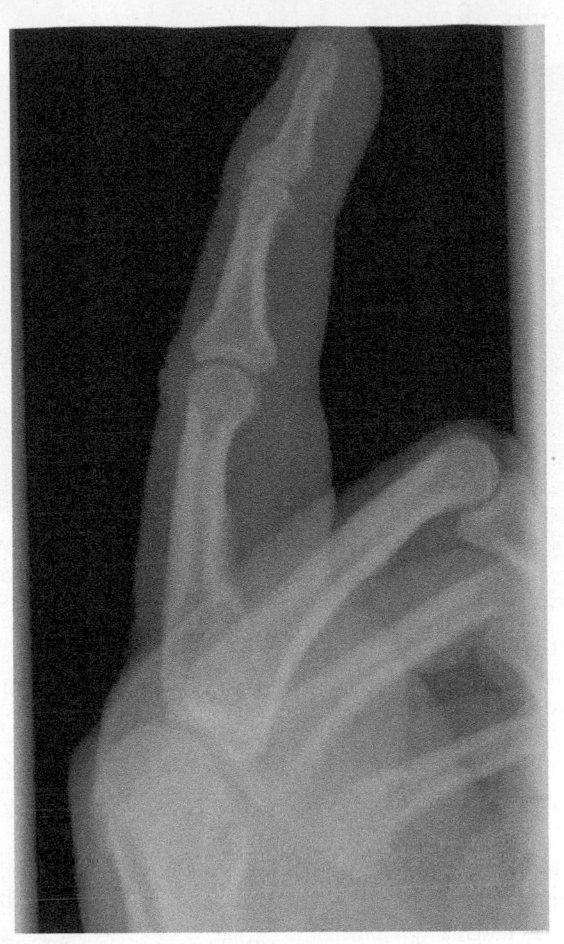

1. What are the characteristic features of this entity?

2. What is the differential diagnosis of this lesion?

3. What are the most common locations for this entity?

4. How may this lesion present?

5. What is the association of this entity in combination with cutaneous angiomata?

Enchondroma 1973

Case ranking/difficulty:

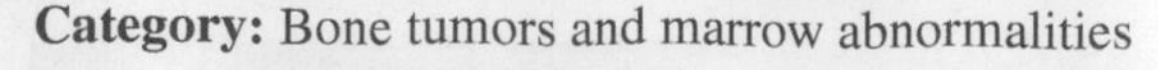

Category: Bone tumors and marrow abnormalities

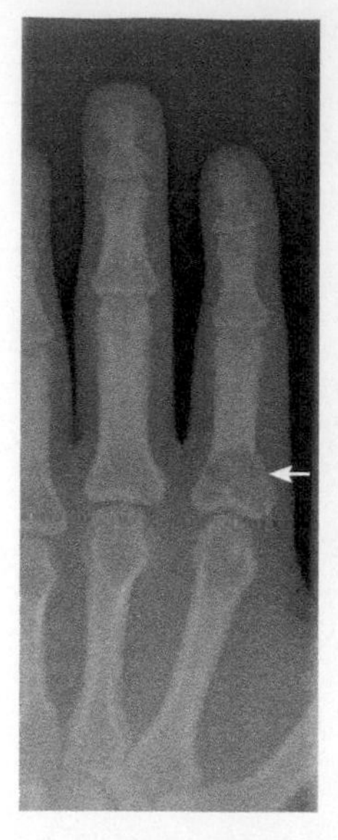

Expansile lytic lesion at base of proximal phalanx with no cortical destruction or periosteal reaction.

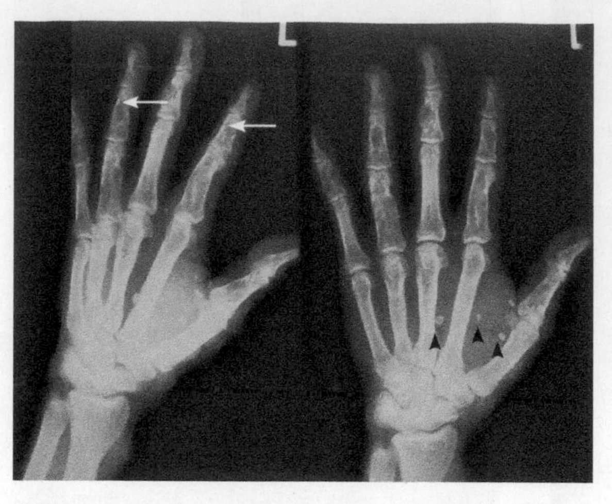

Diffuse enchondromatosis in conjunction with multiple hemangiomata—a condition called Maffucci syndrome. *Arrows,* enchondromata; *arrowheads,* calcified phleboliths consistent with hemangiomata.

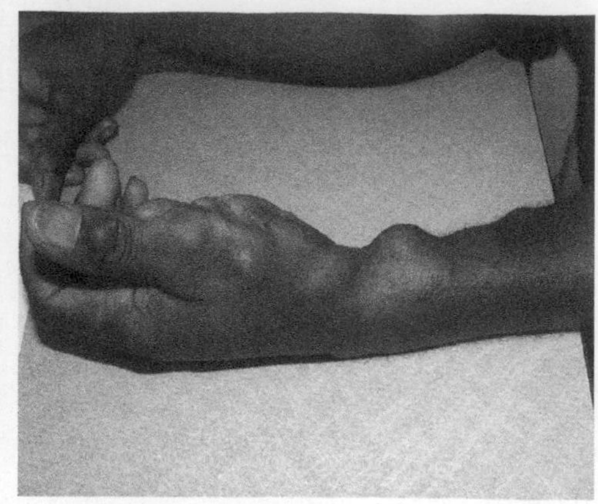

A patient with Maffucci syndrome.

Answers

1. Enchondromata are found in bones that ossify from cartilage; skull bones and the clavicle ossify directly from a membranous matrix.

   Benign features are the hallmarks of this tumor: periosteal reaction is only seen with fracture or sarcomatous transformation.

   As they are often located in the small bones of the hand, they are liable to pathological fracture with trauma to the fingers.

   The most common age is 10 to 25 years.

   The combination of fibrous dysplasia and precocious puberty is McCune-Albright syndrome. Maffucci syndrome is the association of multiple enchondromata and hemangiomata.

2. Lytic bone lesions, such as fibrous dysplasia and simple bone cysts, may be mistaken for an enchondroma. However, aggressive features such as the periosteal reaction seen with osteosarcoma and osteomyelitis are not typical.

3. The most common sites are the long bones of the hands and feet and about the knee. The proximal femur is possible, but less common than the distal femur.

4. They are often discovered as incidental findings, either presenting as a swelling, or after a fracture.

5. Ollier disease is hereditary multiple enchondromatosis. It occurs in approximately 1 in 100,000 individuals.

   Maffucci syndrome is the genetic condition characterized by multiple enchondromatosis and cutaneous angiomata.

Pearls

- Enchondroma is a common lytic bone tumor.
- The overall appearances are of a benign bone lesion, with a narrow zone of transition, no periosteal reaction, no associated soft tissue mass (although see Maffucci syndrome below).
- Increased pain, cortical destruction or periosteal reaction should alert the radiologist to the complications of fracture or sarcomatous transformation.
- Multiple enchondromatosis is the clinical syndrome of Ollier disease and carries a high risk of sarcomatous transformation (approximately 25% of cases).
- The combination of multiple enchondromata and hemangiomata is Maffucci syndrome, a rare genetic syndrome that has an even higher risk of neoplastic transformation from an enchondroma (approximately 30% to 35% of patients).
- Patients with these syndromes should have periodic systemic screening for malignancy.

Suggested Readings

Eisenberg RL. Bubbly lesions of bone. *AJR Am J Roentgenol.* 2009;193(2):W79-W94.

Vanel D, Ruggieri P, Ferrari S, et al. The incidental skeletal lesion: ignore or explore? *Cancer Imaging.* 2009;9 Spec No A:S38-S43.

Slow-growing mass in the buttocks and constipation

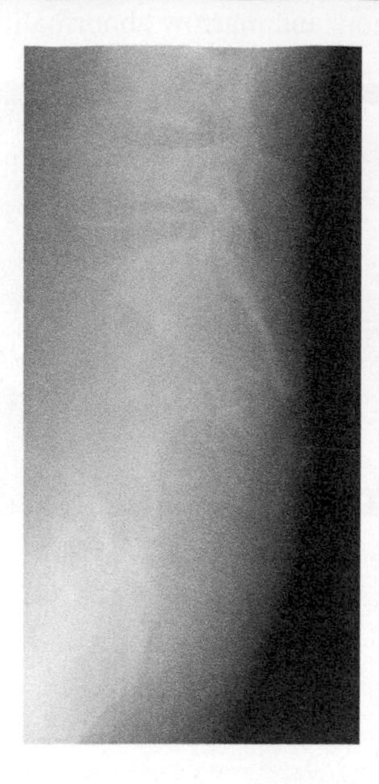

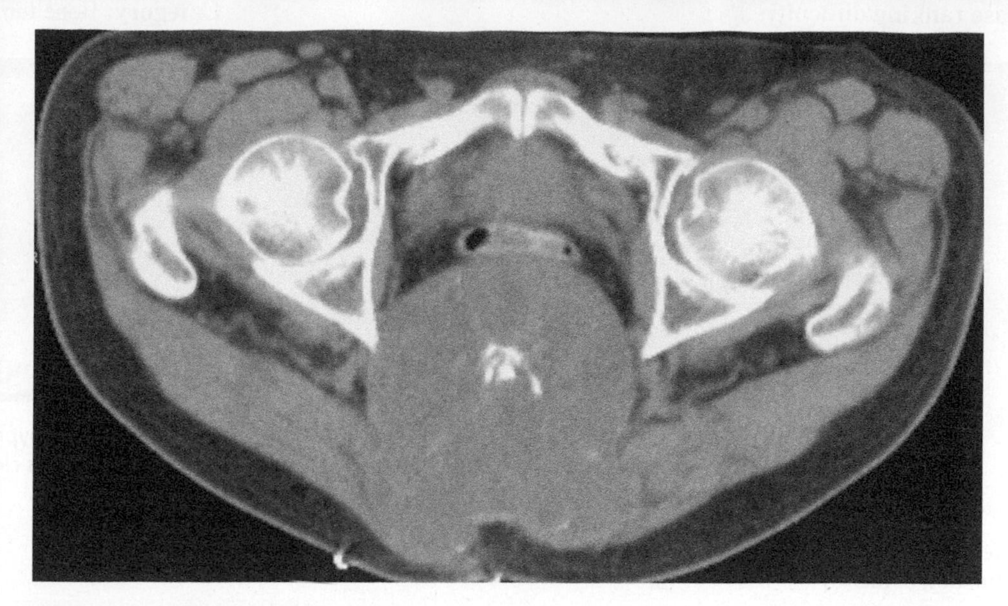

1. What are the radiograph and CT findings?
2. Which entities are included in the differential diagnosis?
3. What is the most likely diagnosis?
4. What is the most common location for these tumors?
5. What percentage of these lesions show calcification?

Chordoma 1412

Case ranking/difficulty: 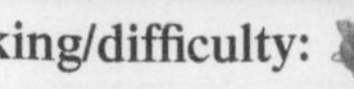 **Category:** Bone tumors and marrow abnormalities

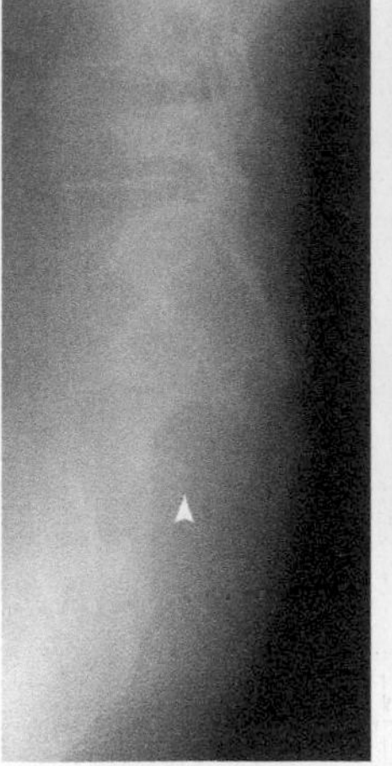

There is complete destruction of the lower sacrum and coccyx. Calcification can faintly be seen (*arrowhead*).

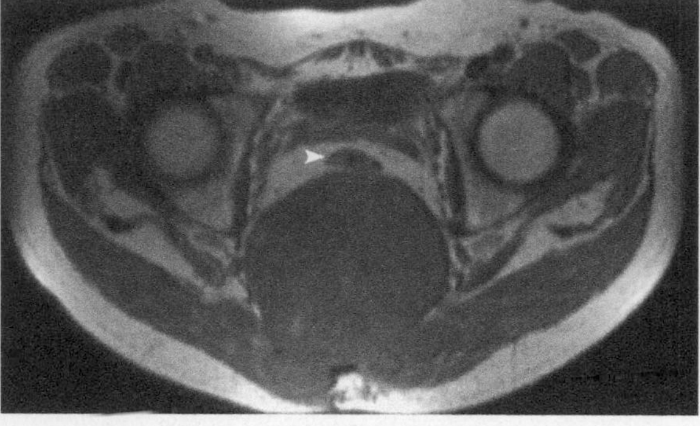

There is a large mass with T1 hyperintense foci suggesting hemorrhage arising from the sacrum, with destruction of the sacrum and coccyx. The rectum is displaced anteriorly (*arrowhead*).

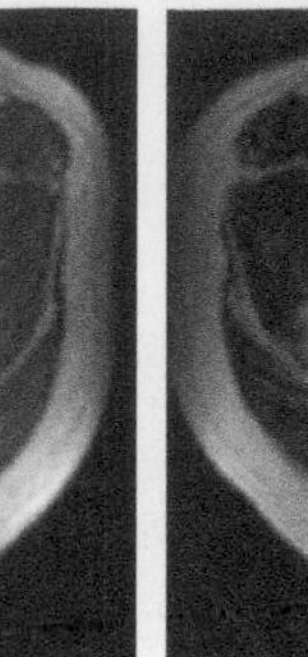

Heterogenous T2 hyperintense mass is seen. The gluteal extension is clearly seen (*arrowhead*).

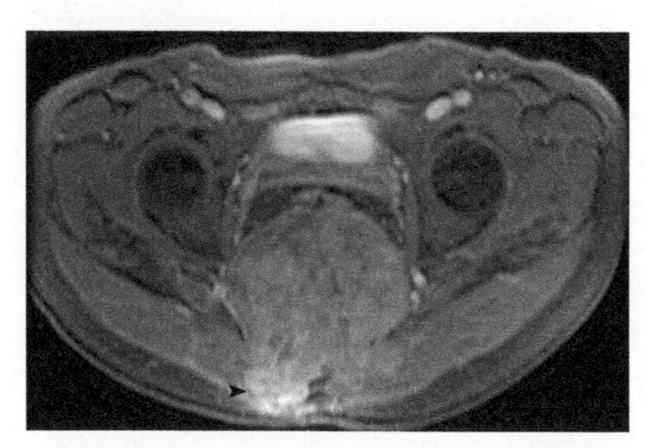

There is heterogenous enhancement of the mass, with gluteal extension especially on the right (*arrowhead*).

Answers

1. The lower sacrum is destroyed, with a soft-tissue mass that contains calcification and bone fragments. The rectum is displaced anteriorly.
2. Chordoma, chondrosarcoma, metastasis, plasmacytoma, lymphoma, and giant cell tumor are differentials.
3. Based on the location, appearance, and pattern of calcification, the most likely diagnosis is a chordoma.
4. The sacrococcygeal region is the most common location for chordomas.
5. 30-40% of chordomas calcify.

Pearls

- Chordomas are tumors arising from notochordal remnants.
- They occur most commonly in the sacrococcygeal region (50%), clivus (30%), and spine (15%) especially at C2.
- Lesions are locally aggressive, and have a high tendency to recur.
- Calcifications are seen in 30% to 40% of tumors.
- Lesions are large at diagnosis, usually greater than 8 cm.
- Multiple sacral and coccygeal segments are destroyed at the time of diagnosis.
- MRI is used to assess the local spread as follows:
  - Proximal extension to bone and spinal canal;
  - Distal lateral extensions to gluteus maximus, hamstrings, sciatic nerve, and sciatic notch;
  - Anterior extension to rectum and retroperitoneal lymph nodes;
  - Posterior extension to the subcutaneous fat.

Suggested Readings

Meyer JE, Lepke RA, Lindfors KK, et al. Chordomas: their CT appearance in the cervical, thoracic and lumbar spine. *Radiology.* 1984;153(3):693-696.

Wetzel LH, Levine E. Pictorial essay. MR imaging of sacral and presacral lesions. *AJR Am J Roentgenol.* 1990;154(4):771-775.

Limp

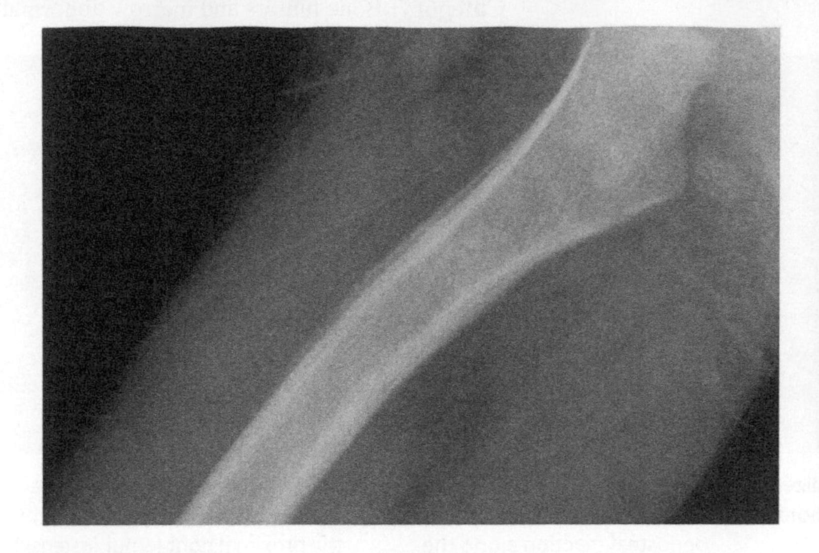

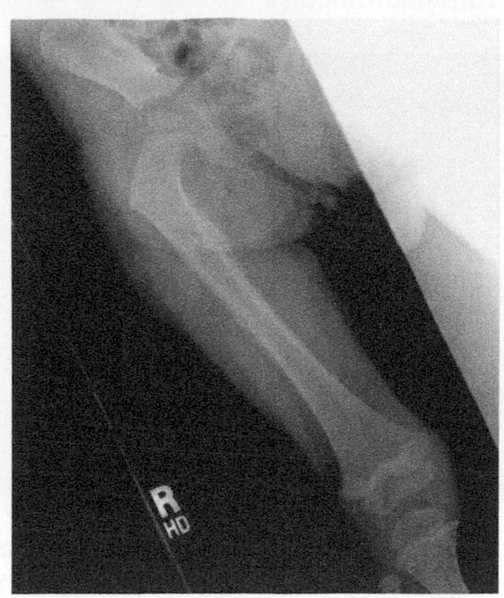

1. What are the 2 most common sites of primary bone disease in this entity?

2. What are the 2 most common sites of metastasis in this disease?

3. How does this entity typically present?

4. This entity is common in African American and Asian populations. True or False?

5. What neoplasms belong in the family to which this entity belongs?

Ewing sarcoma 1839

Case ranking/difficulty:

Category: Bone tumors and marrow abnormalities

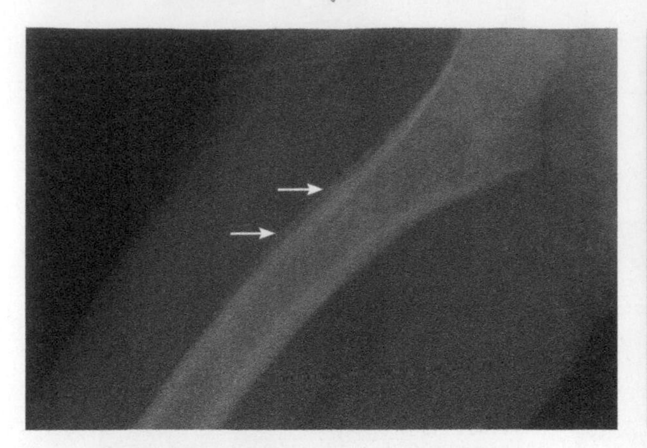

Lateral radiograph of the femur demonstrates localized periosteal reaction (*arrows*) along the proximal femoral shaft.

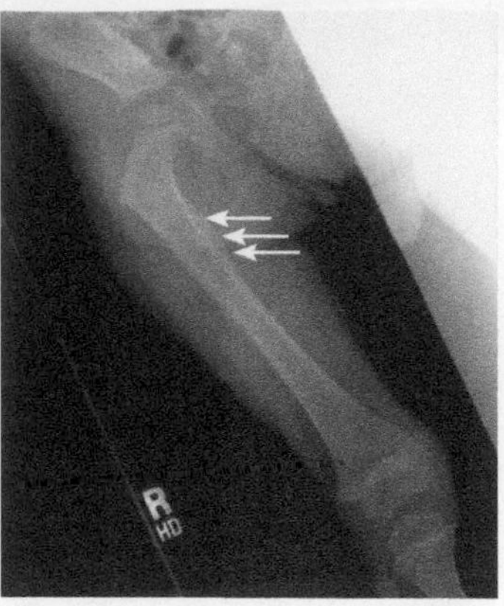

Frontal radiograph of the femur demonstrates diffuse lamellated periosteal reaction along the proximal femoral shaft, thick medially (*arrows*).

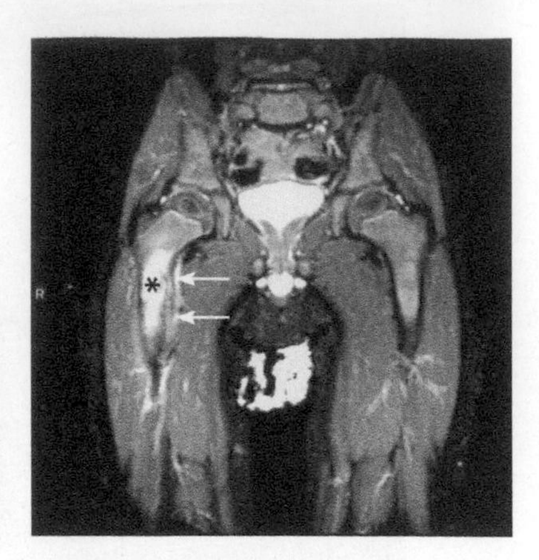

MRI demonstrates hyperintense signal within the medullary cavity of the proximal right femur (*asterisk*), as well as abnormal hyperintense signal overlying the cortex (*arrows*) which reflects the periosteal reaction and extraosseous component.

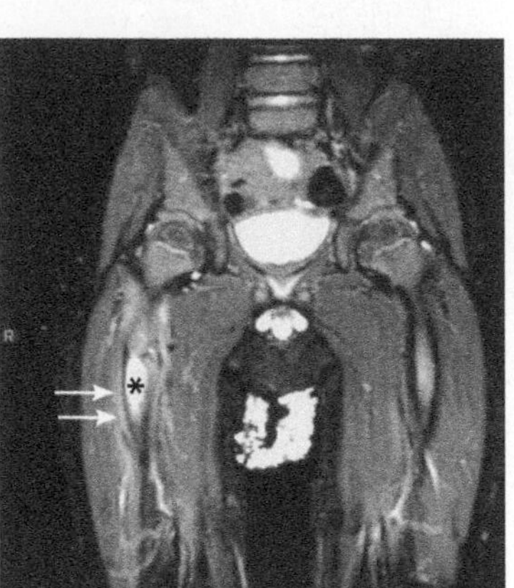

Similar findings are demonstrated.

Answers

1. The most common sites of primary bone disease in Ewing sarcoma are the pelvis and the lower extremity.
2. Lung and bone are the most common sites of metastasis.
3. Ewing sarcoma typically presents as localized pain and swelling for weeks to months, sometimes incorrectly attributed to trauma. Fever and systemic symptoms are associated with advanced disease.
4. Ewing sarcoma is most common in whites, and is very uncommon in African American and Asian populations.
5. The Ewing sarcoma family of tumors (ESFT) includes Ewing sarcoma of bone, extraskeletal Ewing sarcoma, peripheral primitive neuroectodermal tumor (PNET), and malignant, small, round, blue cell tumors of the thoracopulmonary region (Askin tumors).

Pearls

- Ewing sarcoma is a member of the small, round, blue cell group of tumors.
- It constitutes 10% of bone sarcomas.
- It typically occurs in individuals ages 5 to 25 years, and is rare in persons older than age 30 years.
- The lesions are osteolytic, with a permeative pattern and periosteal reaction that may be thin, lamellated, or Codman type.
- The associated soft-tissue mass often appears disproportionately larger than the degree of bone destruction, as is typical for all small, round, blue cell tumors.
- Ewing sarcoma typically presents as localized pain and swelling for weeks to months, sometimes incorrectly attributed to trauma.
- The most common sites of primary bone disease include the pelvis and the diaphysis and metaphyseal-diaphyseal region of long bones, including the femur and tibia.
- Lung and bone are the most common sites of metastasis.
- Twenty-five percent of patients have metastatic disease at diagnosis, which carries a poor prognosis.

Suggested Readings

Bloem JL, Bluemm RG, Taminiau AH, van Oosterom AT, Stolk J, Doornbos J. Magnetic resonance imaging of primary malignant bone tumors. *Radiographics.* 1987;7(3):425-445.

Moser RP, Davis MJ, Gilkey FW, et al. Primary Ewing sarcoma of rib. *Radiographics.* 1990;10(5):899-914.

Pain and swelling of lower leg

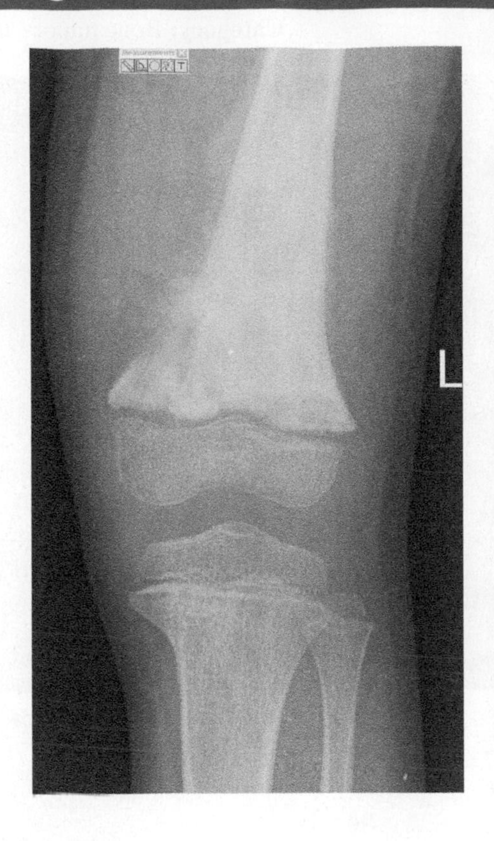

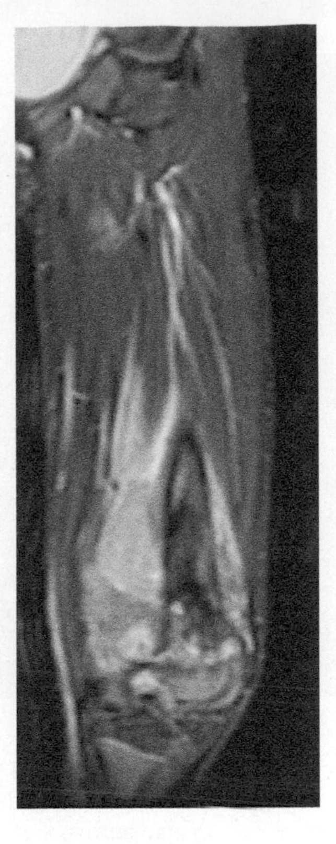

1. What are the radiograph findings?

2. What are the MRI findings, and what is the diagnosis?

3. What MRI sequence is most useful in assessing the longitudinal extent of the lesion?

4. Which MRI sequence is most sensitive for evaluating the longitudinal extent of tumor?

5. What MRI sequence is most sensitive in assessing for transepiphyseal extension?

Osteosarcoma: conventional type 1414

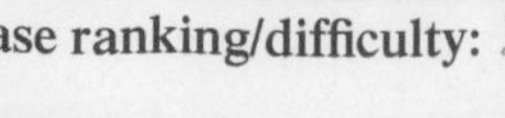

Case ranking/difficulty: **Category:** Bone tumors and marrow abnormalities

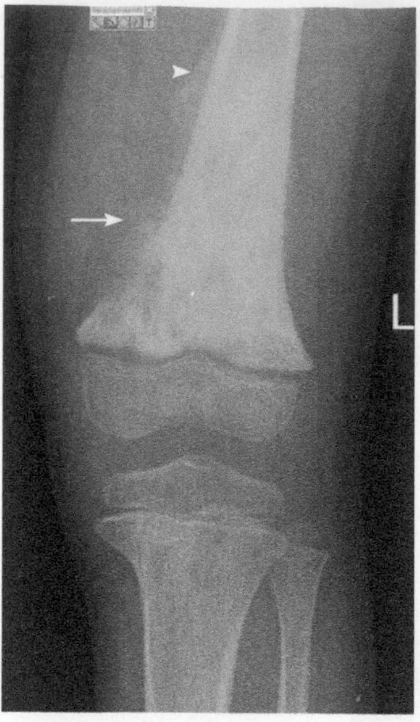

Extensive sclerosis, cortical destruction and aggressive periosteal reaction with a "sunburst" (*arrow*) and "Codman triangle" (*arrowhead*) pattern.

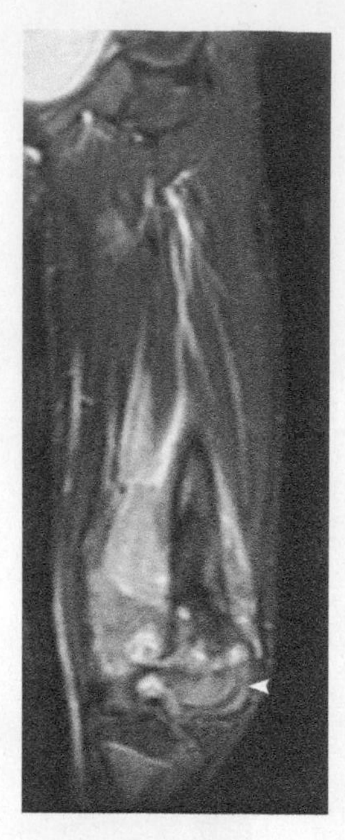

STIR images show the extensive bone marrow edema in the metadiaphysis and tumor extension into the epiphysis (*arrowhead*).

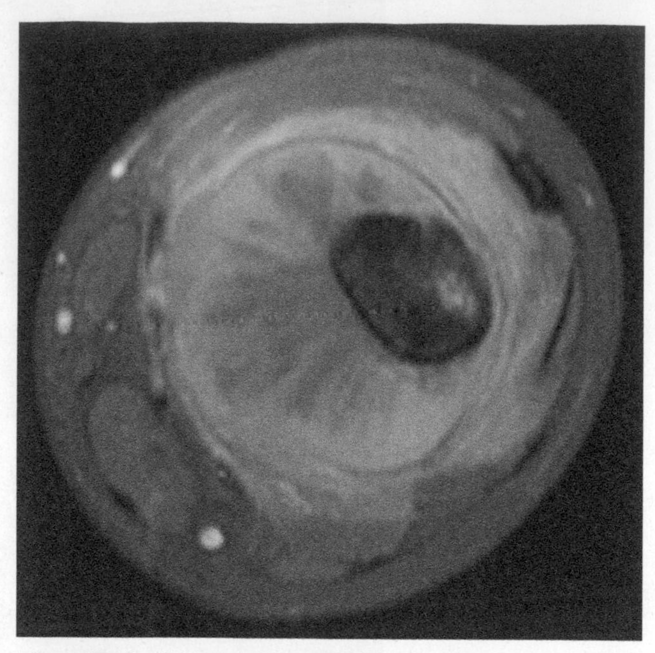

Mineralized soft-tissue mass with enhancement.

Answers

1. There is osteosclerosis with cortical destruction, tumor osteoid matrix, and aggressive periosteal reaction.
2. There is cortical destruction with a soft-tissue mass and transepiphyseal extension, but no transarticular extension. No skip lesions are seen. The diagnosis is osteosarcoma.
3. T1-weighted images are the most useful in assessing the longitudinal extent of osteosarcomas.
4. Although T1-weighted images are the most useful sequence in routine imaging, dynamic contrast-enhanced (DCE) MRI can detect tumor extending up to 3.5 cm beyond what is detectable on conventional sequences, and is the most sensitive sequence. However, the time and cost required to obtain DCE MR images limits its usefulness.
5. T1-weighted sequence is slightly more specific, but the STIR sequence is more sensitive in evaluating for transepiphyseal extension.

Pearls

- Osteosarcomas are the most common primary bone neoplasm following plasma cell myeloma.
- Conventional osteosarcomas are the most common form of osteosarcomas.
- The distal femur followed by the proximal tibia are the most common locations.
- Plain films typically show a lesion with mixed lucency and sclerosis, cortical destruction, soft-tissue mass, and aggressive periosteal reaction, including the Codman triangle and a sunburst pattern.
- Tumor osteoid may be seen in the mass.
- MRI is useful for the degree of osseous involvement, transepiphyseal extension, and neurovascular bundle compromise.
- Transepiphyseal extension occurs in up to 70% of cases.
- The relationship to neurovascular structures and muscular compartment involvement is important to determine.
- Bone scans are useful for the detection of bone and pulmonary metastases.

Suggested Readings

Hoffer FA, Nikanorov AY, Reddick WE, et al. Accuracy of MR imaging for detecting epiphyseal extension of osteosarcoma. *Pediatr Radiol.* 2000;30(5):289-298.

White LM, Kandel R. Osteoid-producing tumors of bone. *Semin Musculoskelet Radiol.* 2000;4(1):25-43.

Incidental finding in a 45-year-old male

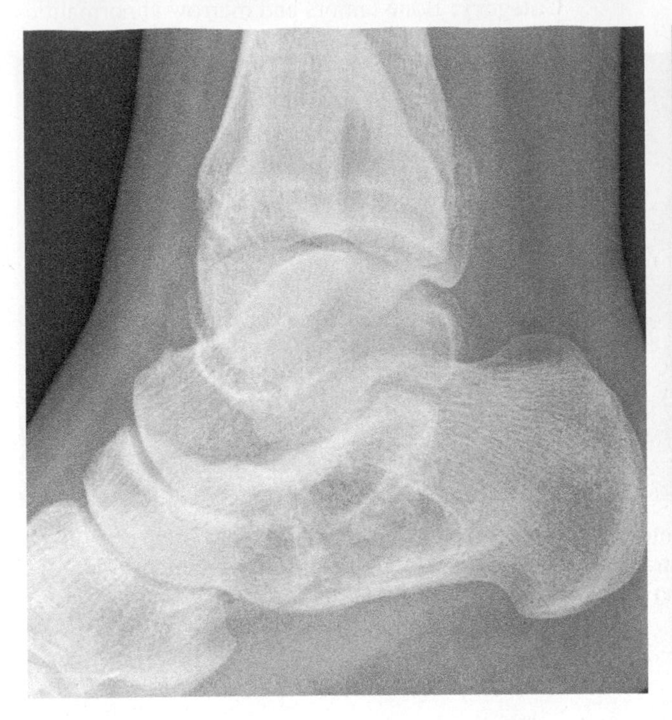

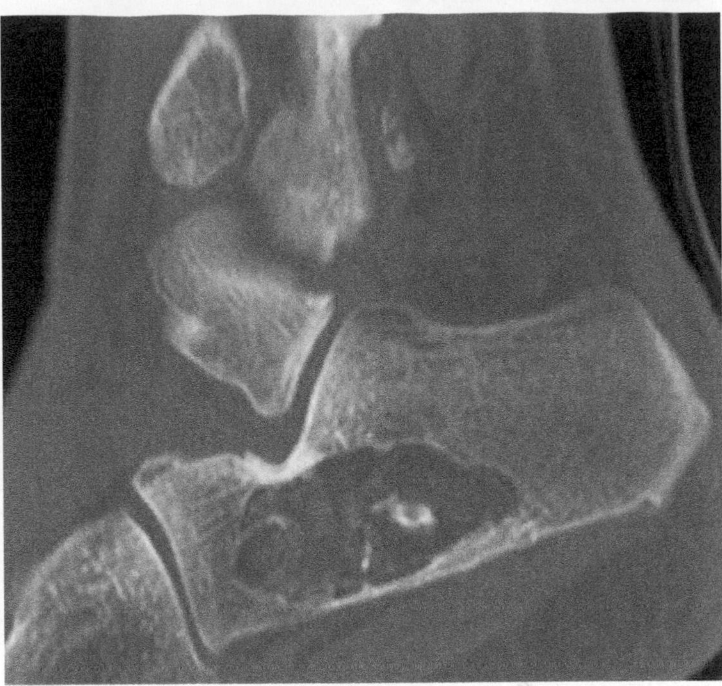

1. What are the radiographic findings?

2. What is the pathognomic radiographic finding of this condition?

3. What are the typical MRI features?

4. What are the differential diagnoses?

5. The lesion frequently undergoes malignant transformation. True or False?

Calcaneal lipoma 1404

Case ranking/difficulty:

Category: Bone tumors and marrow abnormalities

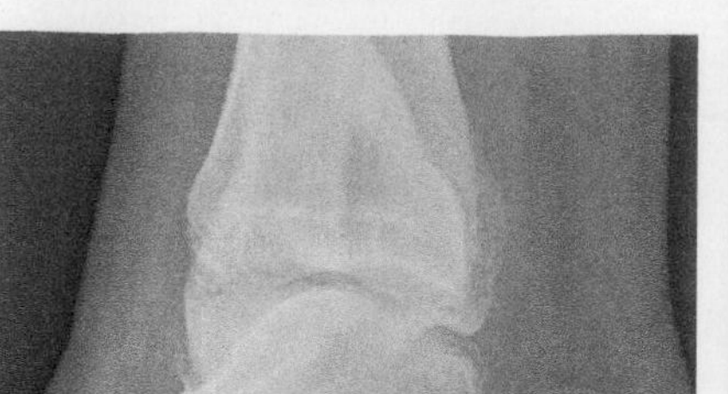

Lucent lesion with "bull's-eye" appearance and central calcification (*arrow*).

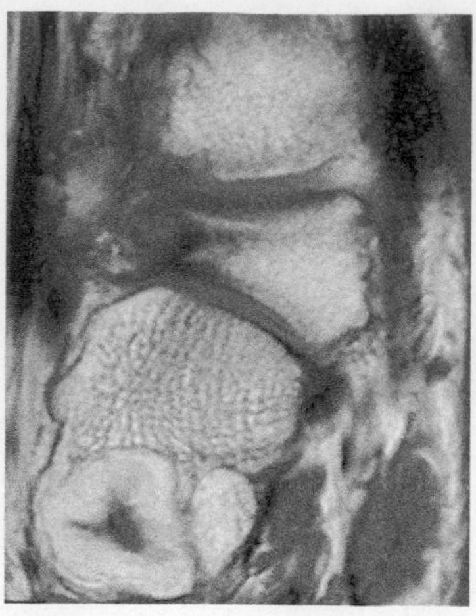

Well-defined high T1-signal intensity intraosseous lesion, with central low signal intensity corresponding to calcification and fat necrosis.

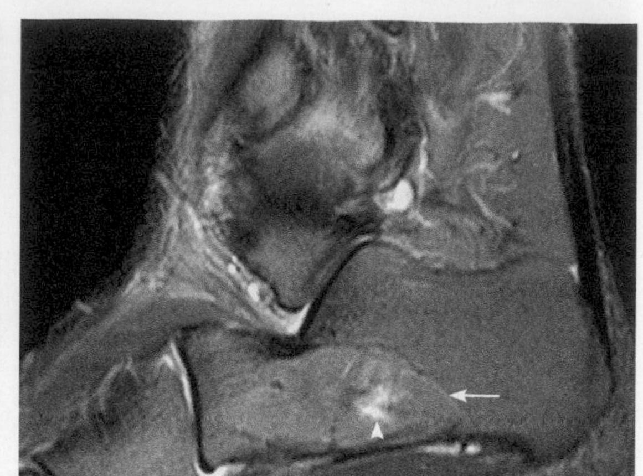

Complete saturation of fat within the lesion on STIR sequence (*arrow*). Central signal hyperintensity is a result of fat necrosis (*arrowhead*).

Answers

1. There is a nonaggressive lucent lesion of the calcaneus, with central calcification and peripheral sclerosis.
2. Lucent lesion with central high-density calcification, gives the appearance of a "bull's eye."
3. There is usually a high T1-, low T2-signal intensity lesion with similar features to fat, and with complete saturation on fat saturated images. There is no contrast enhancement. Central T2 hyperintensity is a result of fat necrosis.
4. The differential diagnoses includes osteonecrosis of the calcaneus, simple bone cyst, and calcaneal pseudotumor. The latter is the result of a relative paucity of trabeculae in the neck of the calcaneus, giving a cyst-like appearance.
5. False. There is very little risk of malignant transformation or recurrence.

Pearls

- Intraosseous lipoma is a benign tumor composed of mature fat located in the proximal femur intertrochanteric region, calcaneus, tibia, and ilium.
- Milgram classified this lesion according to the presence and degree of viable or necrotic fat within the lesion.
- On radiographs calcaneal lipomas have a typical "bull's-eye" appearance with a lucent matrix and central calcification. On MRI, there are typical features of a lipomatous lesion with high signal intensity on T1-weighted images that completely saturates on fat-saturated images, and central T2 hyperintensity caused by fat necrosis in some cases.
- The differential diagnosis include pseudotumor, simple bone cyst, osteonecrosis, aneurysmal bone cyst, and osteonecrosis.
- No treatment is needed if asymptomatic, and the lesion typically disappears spontaneously.
- Curettage and bone grafting for symptomatic lesions is suggested.

Suggested Readings

Genchi V, Scialpi M, Scarciolla G, Dimauro F, Trigona A. Intraosseous lipoma of the calcaneus. Characterization with computerized tomography and magnetic resonance in a case [in Italian]. *Radiol Med.* 2005;99(1-2):86-88.

Regi L, Panzarola P, Pazzaglia G, Barzi F. Intraosseous lipoma of the calcaneus. Report of a case identified with magnetic resonance [in Italian]. *Radiol Med.* 1994;87(5):701-704.

Schulz T, Prietzel T, Bier T, Mühlig K, Schmidt F. An intraosseous lipoma of the calcaneus [in German]. *Rofo.* 1999;170(3):324-325.

Right hip pain

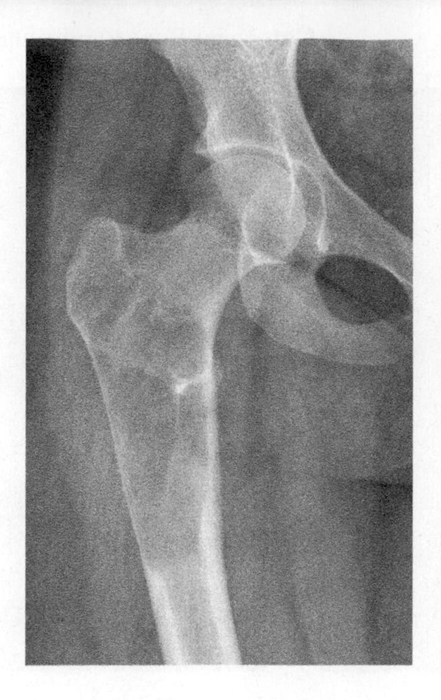

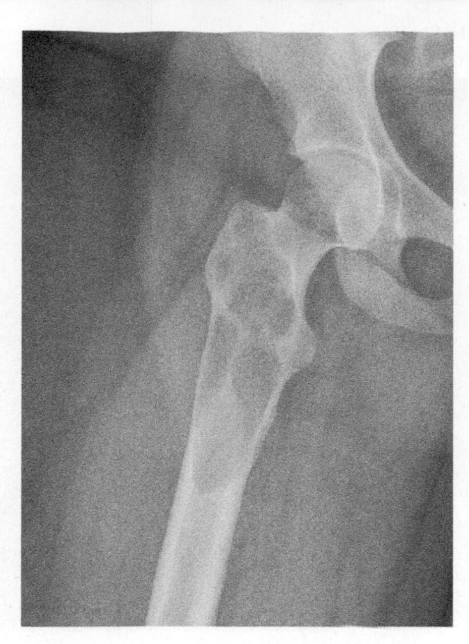

1. What radiologic features are seen in this lesion?
2. What does the differential diagnosis include?
3. What would be the next most appropriate study?
4. What is the natural history of this lesion?
5. Regarding treatment options, what is usually appropriate?

Unicameral bone cyst 1325

Case ranking/difficulty: 

Category: Bone tumors and marrow abnormalities

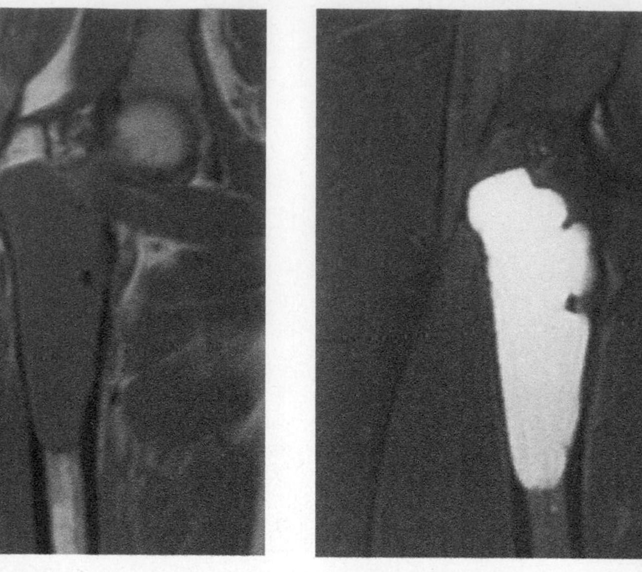

Hypointense lesion with no cortical breakthrough or solid component.

Well-defined mildly expansile lesion that is of fluid signal intensity.

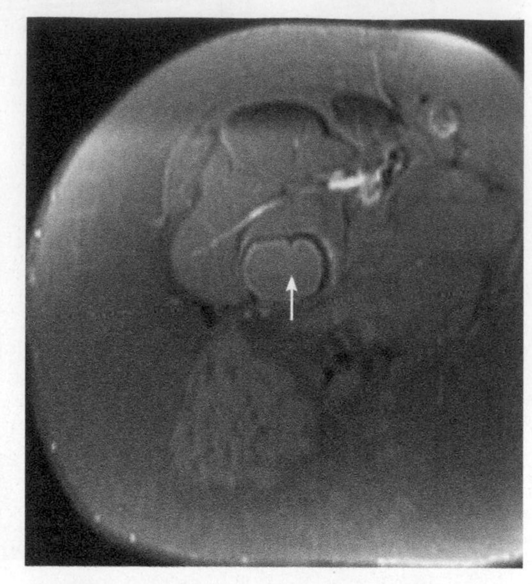

Peripheral rim enhancement but no solid component. A fluid–fluid level is seen (*arrow*).

Answers

1. There is a well-defined lucent lesion with coarse internal trabeculae and no internal matrix, and a sclerotic rim is not demonstrated. There are no aggressive features.
2. The lesion has no aggressive features to suggest a telangiectatic osteosarcoma. The expansion in an aneurysmal bone cyst is more marked and typically eccentric. Fibrous dysplasia is certainly possible, but the margins tend to be more sclerotic. An intraosseous lipoma is also possible, but these typically do not cause expansion and there may be central dystrophic calcification. A unicameral bone cyst (UBC) is most likely.
3. Comparison with prior studies is always useful when evaluating a newly discovered bone lesion, to assess for any interval change and rate of growth (if any). An MRI would be the next most appropriate study.
4. Although spontaneous resolution of a UBC is typical, a pathologic fracture may occur if there is significant cortical thinning. Growth of the host bone may cause the lesion to appear to migrate into the diaphysis.
5. UBCs can resolve spontaneously and require only observation if there is no risk for pathological fracture. If the patient is symptomatic, or if there is a pathologic fracture or risk of one, treatment options include intralesional injection of methylprednisolone acetate and curettage with bone grafting. Intramedullary rodding can also be performed.

Pearls

- Well-defined lucent lesion with mild expansion and cortical thinning.
- Occurs in the growing bone, typically in patients ages 5 to 20 years.
- Pathologic fractures may occur. "Fallen fragment" and "trapdoor" signs occur with a displaced fragment into the cavity.
- "Rising bubble" sign can be seen in patients with a UBC and pathologic fracture. This is a bubble of air in the nondependent part of the lesion, indicating it is not solid.
- No aggressive features, such as soft-tissue mass, cortical breakthrough, or periosteal reaction.
- Periosteal reaction can occur if there is a pathologic fracture.

Suggested Readings

Farber JM, Stanton RP. Treatment options in unicameral bone cysts. *Orthopedics.* 1990;13(1):25-32.

Jordanov MI. The "rising bubble" sign: a new aid in the diagnosis of unicameral bone cysts. *Skeletal Radiol.* 2009;38(6):597-600.

Pain and discomfort in left leg

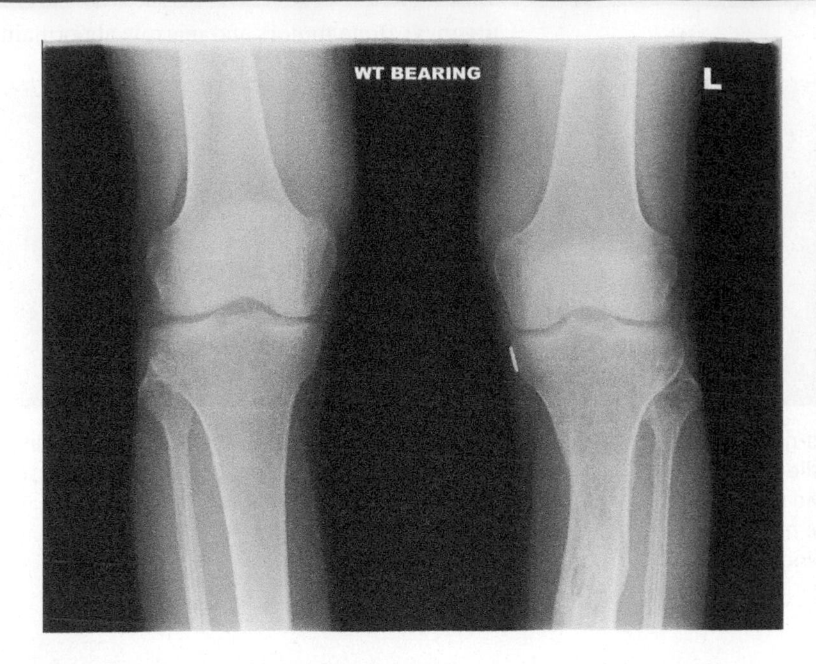

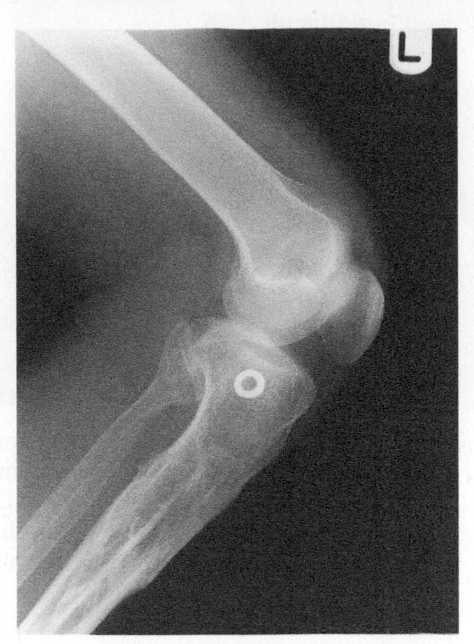

1. What is the differential diagnosis of this abnormality in a pediatric patient?
2. What is the association of endocrine abnormalities and skin pigmentation with this condition termed?
3. What are the radiographic features of this condition?
4. What is the most common age group for this condition?
5. Which bones are frequently involved in this condition?

Fibrous dysplasia

Case ranking/difficulty: 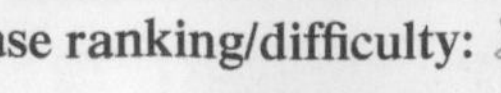

Category: Bone tumors and marrow abnormalities

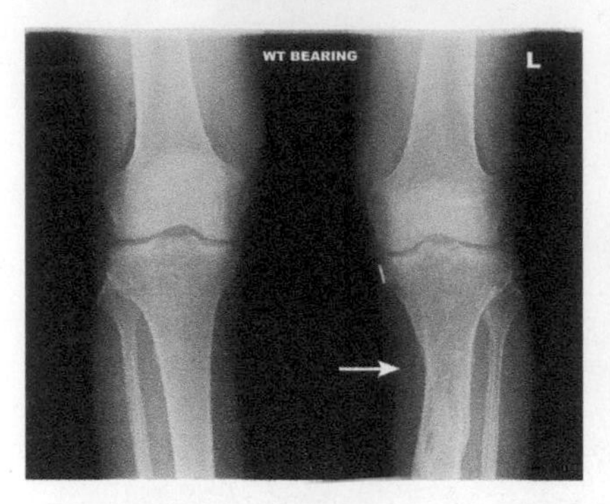

Expansile lytic lesion with a ground glass matrix in the proximal tibia.

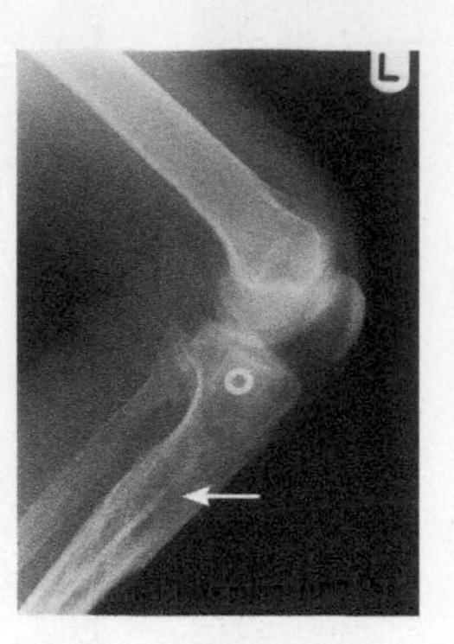

Ground-glass matrix, expansile lytic lesion in tibia. Old pathological fracture has resulted in modelling deformity.

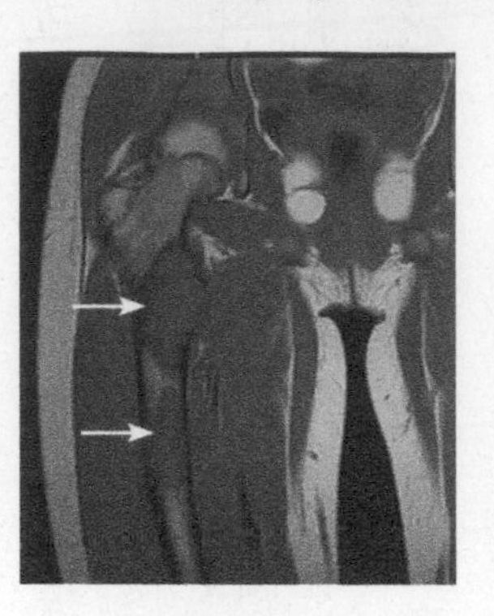

Large, well-defined lesions of low T1 signal in proximal femur.

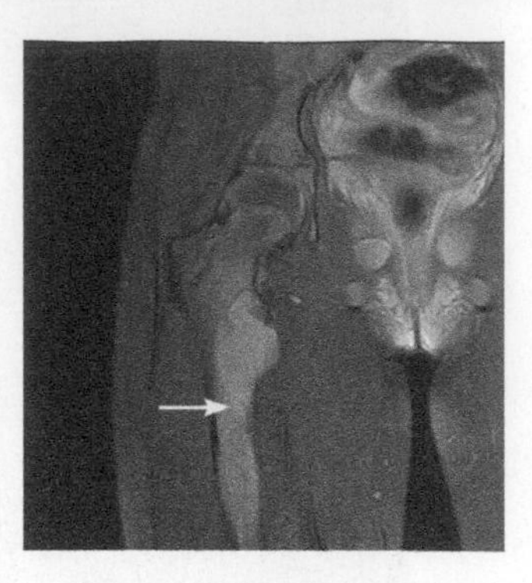

Lesions are of corresponding high signal on fat-suppressed images.

Answers

1. The differential diagnosis for a primary bone tumor depends on the patient's age. Large expansile lytic lesions in children include aneurysmal bone cysts and fibrous dysplasia. Giant cell tumor is subarticular and occurs in the third and fourth decades of life. Chondrosarcoma is not common in childhood.

2. Polyostotic fibrous dysplasia with precocious puberty and café-au-lait spots occurs in 4% of cases. It is much more frequent in females than in males (9:1).

3. Fibrous dysplasia is a nonaggressive condition, although there is a very small risk of sarcomatous transformation in the polyostotic form of the disease. However, extensive bony involvement in the polyostotic form can result in deformity and pain, with pathological fractures common. A shepherd's crook deformity is seen in the proximal femur, and angulation with remodelling is frequently seen in other long bones too.

4. Fibrous dysplasia most commonly presents in the first and second decades of life.

5. The most common bones to be involved with fibrous dysplasia are the femur, tibia, ribs, skull, and pelvis.

Pearls

- Fibrous dysplasia is a rare but important differential diagnosis of expansile lytic lesions in the first and second decades.
- There are monostotic (80%) and polyostotic (20%) forms of the disease.
- The lesions have a characteristic ground-glass matrix.
- The risk of malignant transformation is very small, but higher in the polyostotic form of the disease (1%).
- Plain radiography, CT, MRI, and bone scans may all be used in the diagnosis and follow-up of fibrous dysplasia.
- Increased activity on a bone scan, or periosteal reaction seen on CT or MRI may be useful in determining the activity of individual lesions in polyostotic fibrous dysplasia.
- McCune-Albright syndrome is the constellation of polyostotic fibrous dysplasia with precocious puberty and café-au-lait skin pigmentation.
- Mazabraud syndrome is the rare association of single or multiple intramuscular myxomas with fibrous dysplasia.

Suggested Readings

Faucherre M, Pazár B, So A, Aubry-Rozier B. Clinical images: polyostotic fibrous dysplasia. *Arthritis Rheum.* 2011;63(9):2616.

Lädermann A, Stern R, Ceroni D, De Coulon G, Taylor S, Kaelin A. Unusual radiologic presentation of monostotic fibrous dysplasia. *Orthopedics.* 2008;31(3):282.

Park SK, Lee IS, Choi JY, et al. CT and MRI of fibrous dysplasia of the spine. *Br J Radiol.* 2012;85(1015):996-1001.

History of longstanding deformity

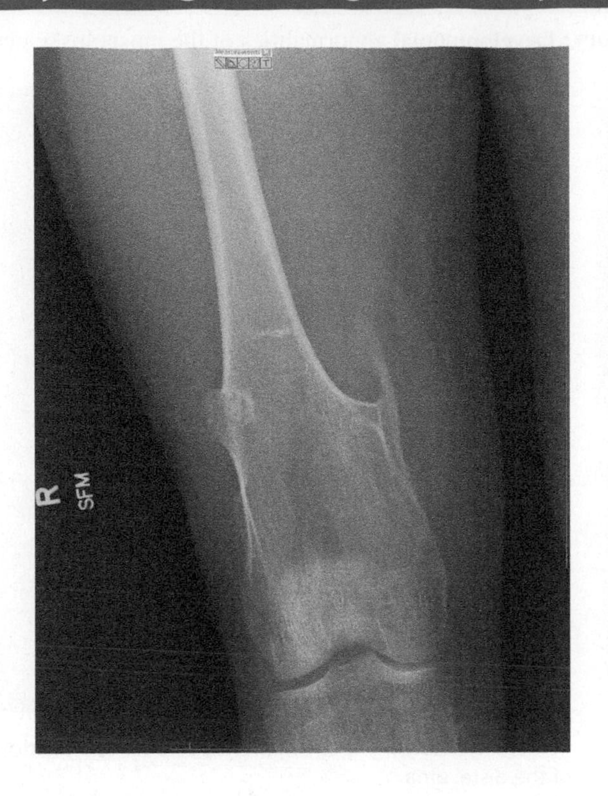

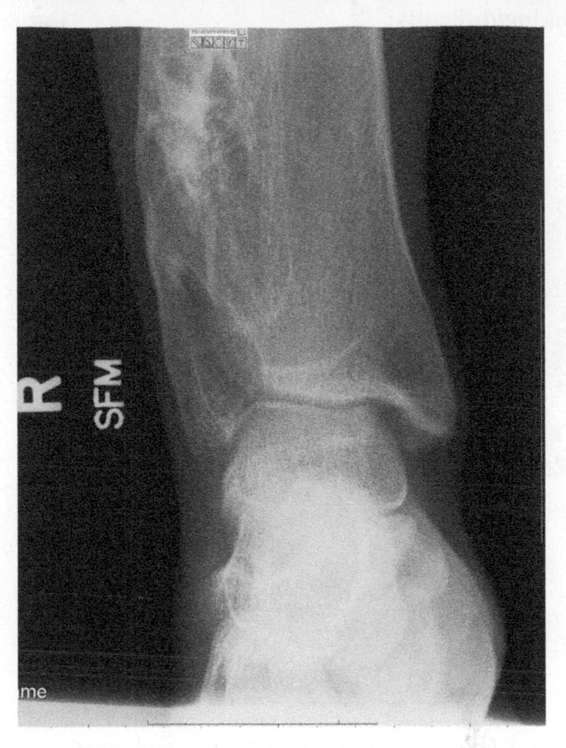

1. What are the plain radiograph findings?

2. What is the most likely diagnosis?

3. What are the sources of pain in this condition?

4. What are the radiological features that suggest malignant transformation?

5. What is the estimated lifetime risk of malignant transformation, and to what type of tumor?

Multiple hereditary exostoses 1338

Case ranking/difficulty:

Category: Developmental abnormalities of the musculoskeletal system

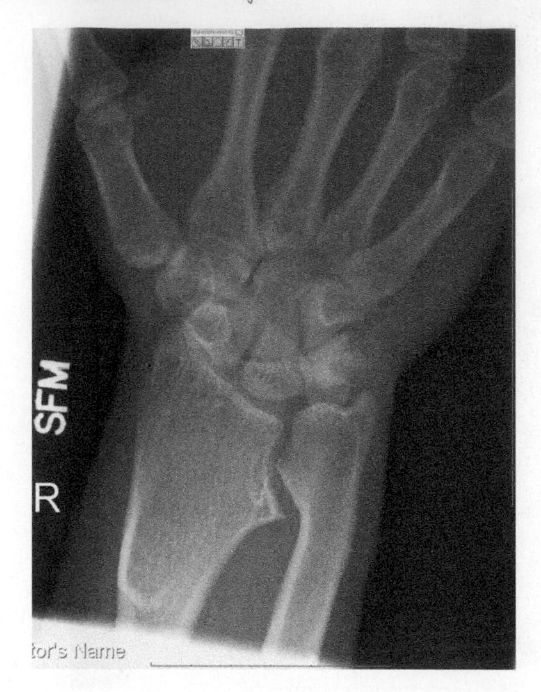

Madelung deformity, with multiple osteochondromas.

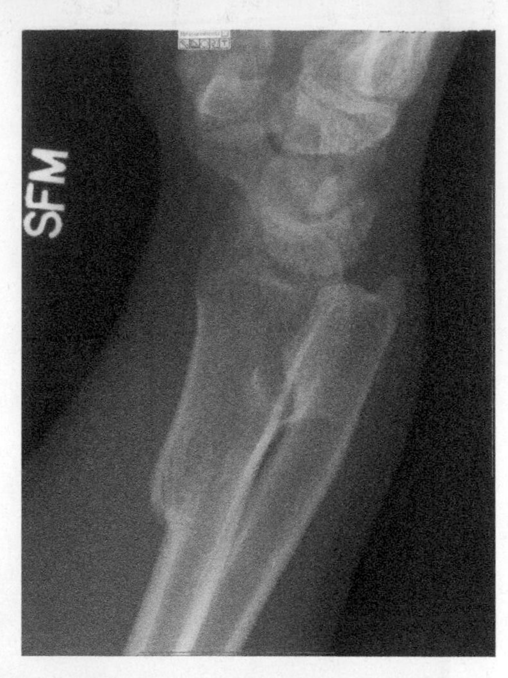

Madelung deformity with apparent posterior subluxation of the distal ulna.

Answers

1. The long bones are undertubulated, with multiple osseous lesions that are located in the metaphyses. There is both medullary and cortical continuity with the host bone.
2. The presence of a generalized dysplasia with multiple osteochondromas are consistent with the diagnosis of multiple hereditary exostoses. Osteochondromas can be seen in tuberous sclerosis, but there are no cysts or sclerosis to support this diagnosis.
3. New onset of pain should always raise the concern of malignant transformation. Other causes for pain include bursae formation, impingement on nerves, or a fracture.
4. Increased uptake of radiopharmaceutical on bone scan after skeletal maturity and dispersion of the calcified cartilage cap on radiographs are suggestive of malignant transformation.

   On MRI, cartilage cap thickness of greater than 2 cm in adults and 3 cm in children, as well as an indistinct cartilage cap, is suspicious for sarcomatous transformation.
5. The risk of sarcomatous transformation is difficult to estimate, but has been quoted to be between 3% and 25% in multiple hereditary exostoses (MHE), and much less in isolated osteochondromas. When sarcomatous transformation does occur, it is usually to a chondrosarcoma.

Pearls

- Multiple hereditary exostoses is inherited as an autosomal dominant condition.
- Radiographs can show general dysplasia, with a metaphyseal lesion that has a cortex and medullary cavity contiguous with the native bone, and an orientation of the lesion away from the joint.
- MRI will show a cartilage cap that is less than 1 cm in an adult and less than 2 cm in children. Growth or indistinctness of the cap raises the concern for malignant transformation.
- Pain may be caused by malignant transformation, bursa formation, or impingement on nerves.
- The risk of sarcomatous degeneration is difficult to estimate but has been stated to be 3% to 25% in MHE, the risk increasing with the number of lesions.
- Management is conservative, unless the patient is symptomatic, has deformity, or there is malignant transformation. Then surgery is required.

Suggested Readings

Epstein DA, Levin EJ. Bone scintigraphy in hereditary multiple exostoses. *AJR Am J Roentgenol.* 1978;130(2):331-333.

Murphey MD, Choi JJ, Kransdorf MJ, Flemming DJ, Gannon FH. Imaging of osteochondroma: variants and complications with radiologic-pathologic correlation. *Radiographics.* 2000;20(5):1407-1434.

Pain in the heel

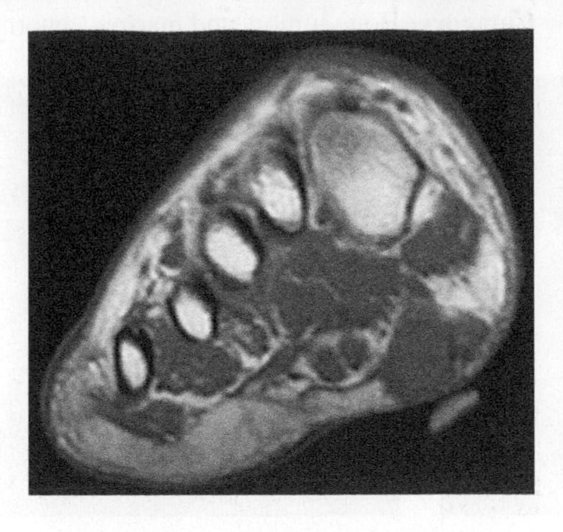

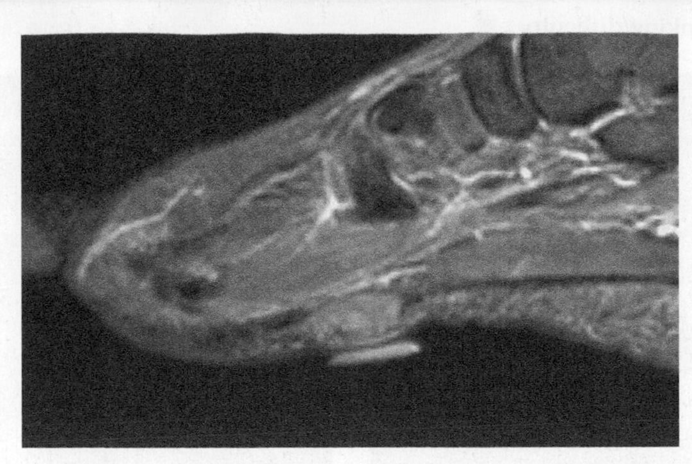

1. What are the MRI findings?

2. What is the likely diagnosis?

3. What may you expect to see after IV contrast administration?

4. What are the typical T2 characteristics of these lesions?

5. What is the management for these lesions?

Plantar fibroma 1453

Case ranking/difficulty: 

Category: Bone tumors and marrow abnormalities

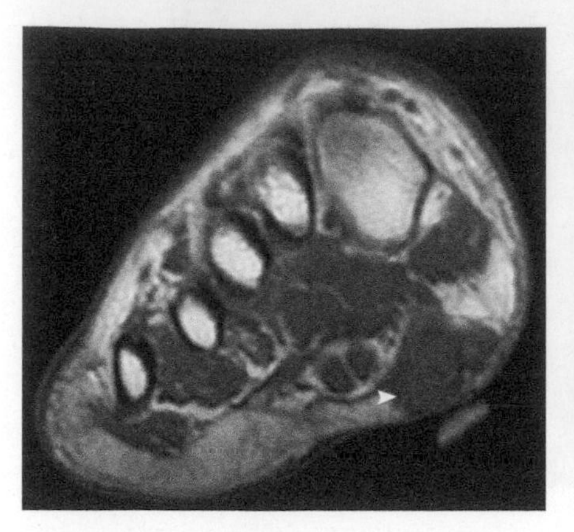

T1 hypointense soft-tissue mass attached to the plantar fascia.

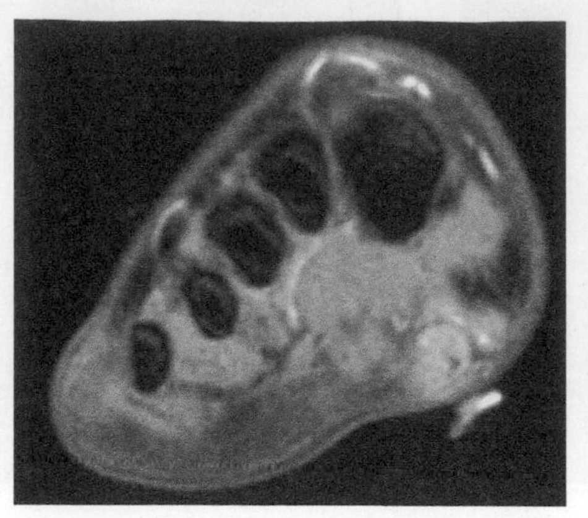

Precontrast image.

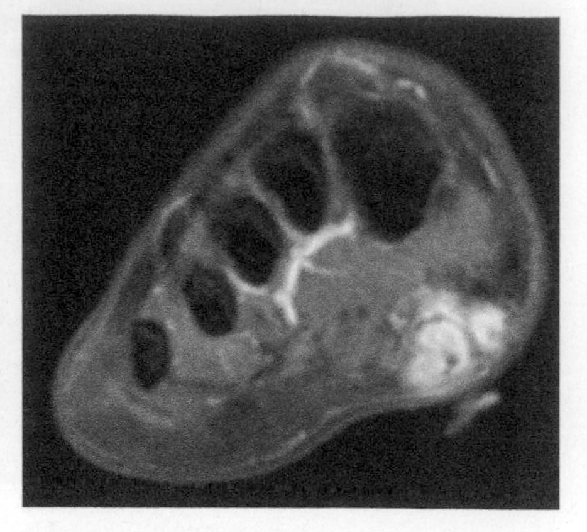

There is intense enhancement after intravenous contrast.

Answers

1. There is a soft-tissue mass attached to the plantar fascia that is predominantly T1 hypointense and T2 hyperintense. The deep margins appear mildly infiltrative.
2. The MRI appearance is consistent with a plantar fibroma.
3. The lesions typically enhance after contrast, and the adjacent normal fascia may also enhance (fascial tail sign).
4. The T2 signal is variable, with cellular early lesions appearing T2 hyperintense and more mature collagenous lesions appearing T2 hypointense. Mixed signal characteristics are often seen. There is increased signal on T2 fat-suppression sequences.
5. Plantar fibromas are typically treated conservatively with footwear modification and orthotics. Intralesional steroids are also helpful. Local excision with wide margins is reserved for large infiltrative lesions.

Pearls

- Plantar fibromas are histologically similar to palmar fibromas, and together they form the superficial fibromatoses.
- Lesions are multiple in 33%, bilateral in 30% to 50% and concomitant with palmar fibromas in 10% to 65% of cases.
- Unlike in palmar fibromas, contractures do not develop.
- Ultrasound shows hypoechoic to isoechoic soft-tissue lesions attached to the plantar aponeurosis with increased Doppler flow.
- MRI shows lesions that are T1 hypointense with mild to significant enhancement after contrast.
- T2 signal is variable, with early more cellular lesions T2 hyperintense, and more mature collagenous lesions are T2 hypointense.
- Lesions tend to recur, especially immature cellular T2 hyperintense lesions. Therefore wide excision is needed if surgery is performed. Surgery is only performed for infiltrative, large, symptomatic lesions.

Suggested Readings

Dinauer PA, Brixey CJ, Moncur JT, Fanburg-Smith JC, Murphey MD. Pathologic and MR imaging features of benign fibrous soft-tissue tumors in adults. *Radiographics.* 2009;27(1):173-187.

Robbin MR, Murphey MD, Temple HT, Kransdorf MJ, Choi JJ. Imaging of musculoskeletal fibromatosis. *Radiographics.* 2009;21(3):585-600.

Painful knee

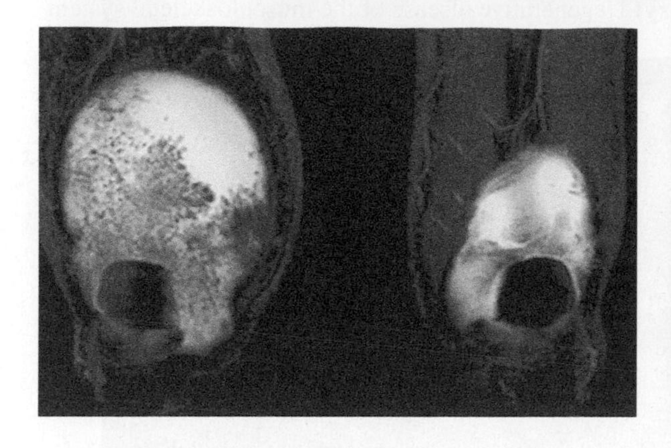

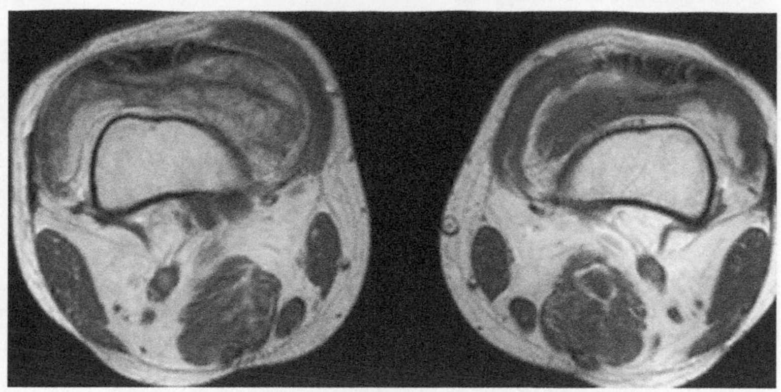

1. What are the MRI findings?

2. What are the differential diagnoses?

3. What is the modality of choice in diagnosing this entity?

4. What is the treatment for this entity?

5. What is the risk of recurrence after treatment?

Lipoma arborescens of knee 1447

Case ranking/difficulty: 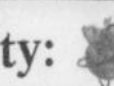

Category: Degenerative disease of the musculoskeletal system

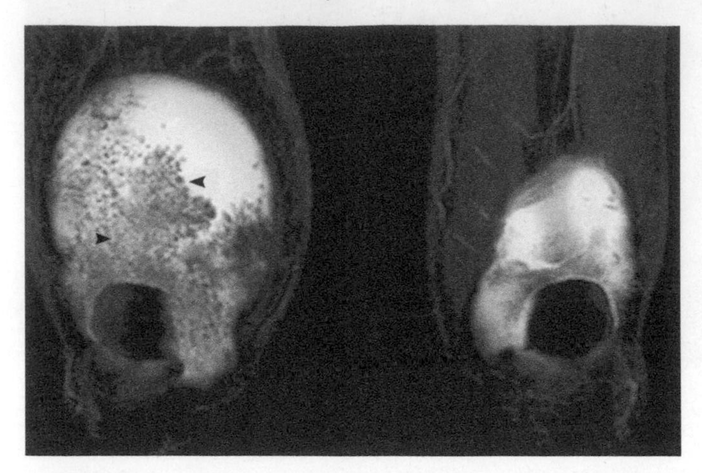

Extensive synovial proliferations that are fat saturated on STIR images.

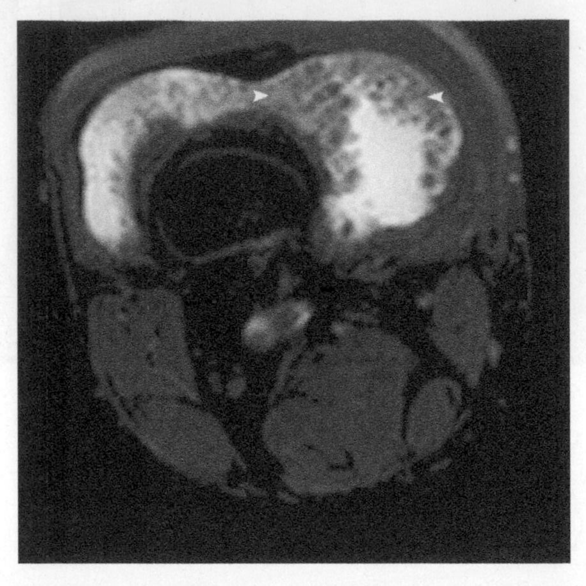

Extensive synovial proliferations that are fat saturated on STIR images.

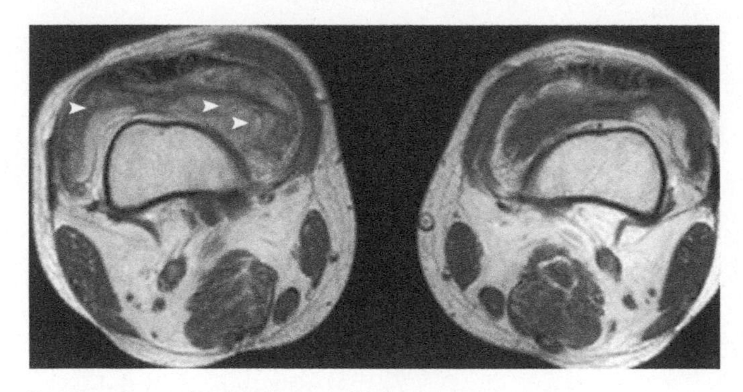

T1 hyperintensity consistent with fat.

Answers

1. There are fat signal intensity synovial projections that are suppressed on fat-saturated sequences, with chemical shift artifact. There is no susceptibility artifact of these synovial projections to suggest pigmented villonodular synovitis (PVNS).
2. PVNS, synovial chondromatosis, rheumatoid arthritis, synovial hemangioma, and lipoma arborescens are differentials for a soft, boggy swelling of the suprapatellar pouch. Other differential diagnoses include amyloid arthropathy and xanthomata.
3. MRI is the investigative modality of choice.
4. Arthroscopic or open synovectomies are the main treatment options. Intra-articular injection of steroids and ^{90}Y have also been utilized.
5. There have been no reported cases of recurrence in the literature.

Pearls

- Lipoma arborescens is a result of frond-like projections of fat in the suprapatellar bursa. It is a rare disorder of unknown etiology.
- The normal synovium is replaced by lipomatous cells. Clinically, it presents as slow-growing swelling and joint effusion. Pain is inconstant.
- Ultrasound can show the hyperechogenic frond-like projections, which can be seen to be mobile on dynamic scanning.
- MRI is the investigative modality of choice. It shows high T1- and low T2-signal intensity, synovial, frond-like, villous projections that are completely suppressed on fat-saturated images. There may be associated joint effusion. These projections may show chemical shift artifact at the fat–fluid interface.

Suggested Readings

Feller JF, Rishi M, Hughes EC. Lipoma arborescens of the knee: MR demonstration. *AJR Am J Roentgenol.* 1994;163(1):162-164.

Vilanova JC, Barceló J, Villalón M, Aldomà J, Delgado E, Zapater I. MR imaging of lipoma arborescens and the associated lesions. *Skeletal Radiol.* 2003;32(9):504-509.

History of trauma and left hip pain

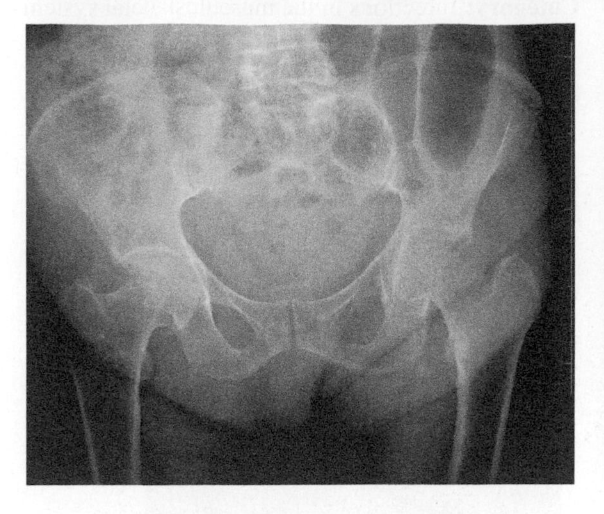

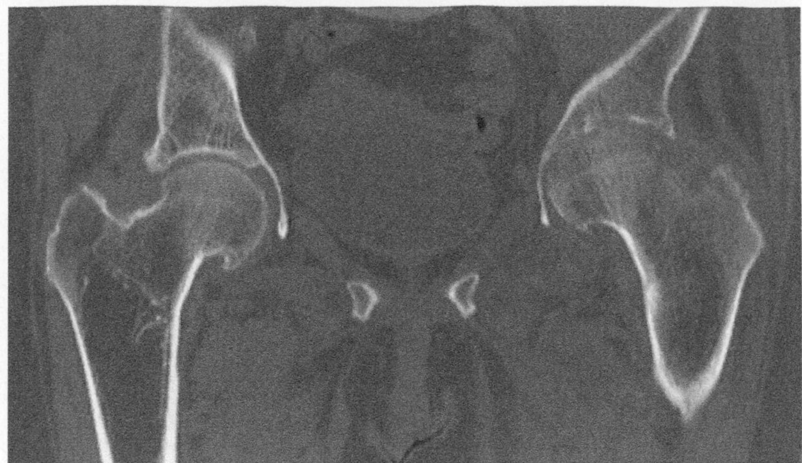

1. What are the radiograph findings?

2. What is the likely diagnosis?

3. What constitutes the Phemister triad?

4. In what condition is the Phemister triad seen?

5. How is the definitive diagnosis of this condition made?

Septic arthritis of the hip 1533

Case ranking/difficulty:

Category: Infections in the musculoskeletal system

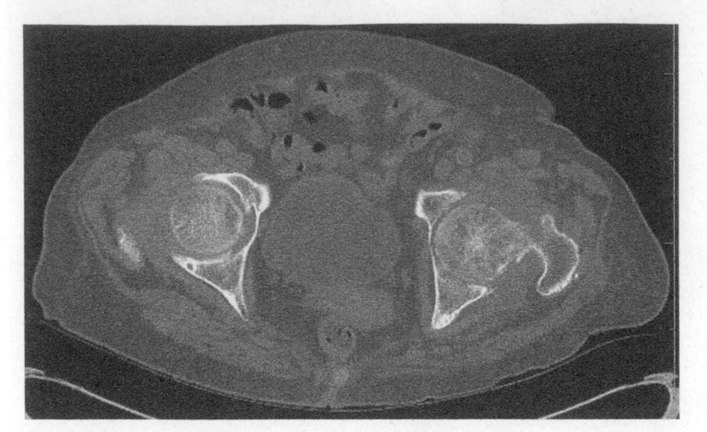

Joint effusion and erosions in the left hip.

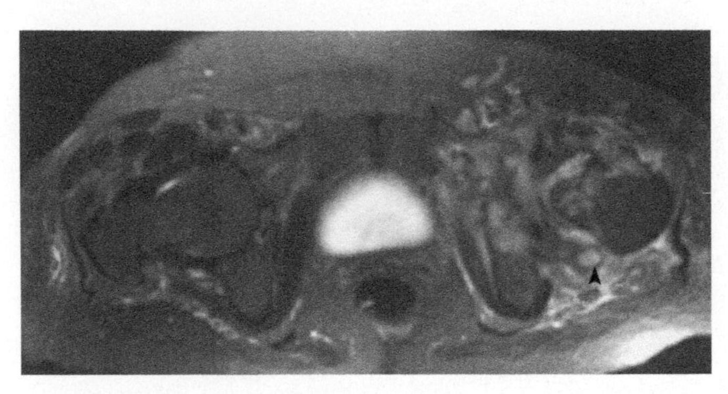

Extensive periarticular inflammatory change, and posterior fluid collection (*arrowhead*).

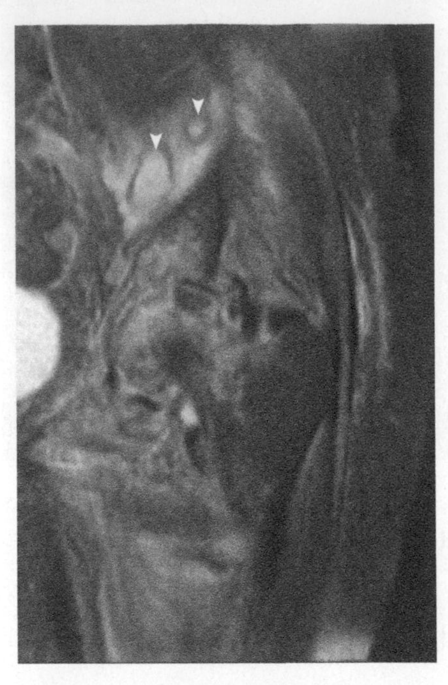

Extensive hip bone marrow edema, effusion, erosions, and fluid collections in the iliacus (*arrowheads*).

Answers

1. The joint space is narrowed, with periarticular osteoporosis and erosions.
2. The findings of a unilateral destructive arthritis is most suggestive of septic arthritis.
3. The Phemister triad is gradual joint space narrowing, marginal erosions, and periarticular osteoporosis.
4. The Phemister triad is seen in tuberculous arthritis.
5. The definitive and most appropriate diagnostic test for a septic arthritis is joint aspiration.

Pearls

- Septic arthritis may be pyogenic or nonpyogenic.
- Pyogenic arthritis is typically caused by *Staphylococcus aureus*.
- Nonpyogenic causes include TB and viral and fungal organisms.
- Patients older than age 65 years are most commonly affected, especially those with comorbidities such as rheumatoid arthritis, SLE, and diabetes. Children younger than age 2 years also are often affected.
- Radiographs initially will show soft-tissue swelling, loss of fat planes, and joint effusion. Periarticular osteoporosis is then seen, with loss of the cartilage leading to joint space narrowing. Cortical destruction then follows.
- TB will result in the Phemister triad, which is periarticular osteoporosis, marginal erosions, and gradual joint space narrowing.
- MRI is useful in the early stages, but is nonspecific. Changes will include bone and soft-tissue edema, with a joint effusion. Intraosseous and soft-tissue abscesses also may be seen. Finally, cortical destruction may be seen.
- Definitive diagnosis is made with joint aspiration.

Suggested Readings

Averill LW, Hernandez A, Gonzalez L, Pena AH, Jaramillo D. Diagnosis of osteomyelitis in children: utility of fat-suppressed contrast-enhanced MRI. *AJR Am J Roentgenol.* 2009;192(5):1232-1238.

Miller TT, Randolph DA, Staron RB, Feldman F, Cushin S. Fat-suppressed MRI of musculoskeletal infection: fast T2-weighted techniques versus gadolinium-enhanced T1-weighted images. *Skeletal Radiol.* 1997;26(11):654-658.

Localized pain and swelling in left thigh

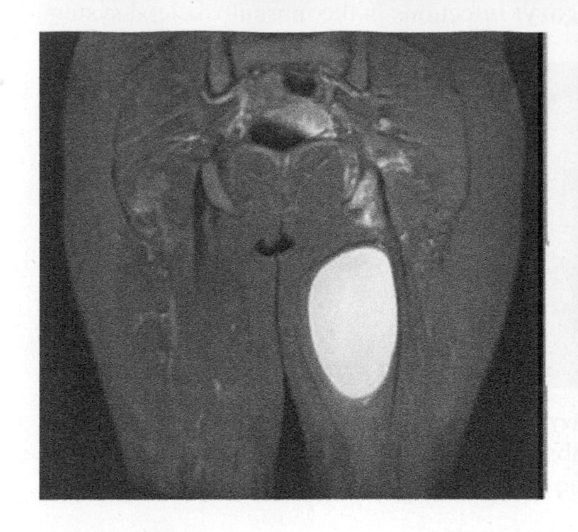

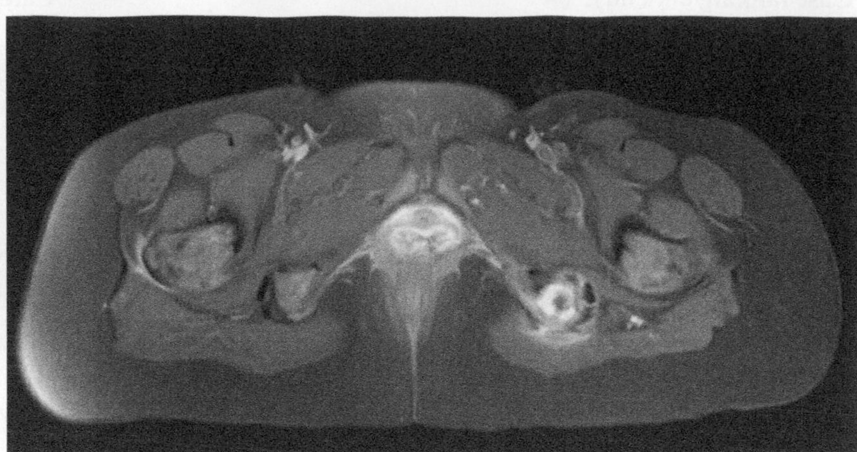

1. What is the differential diagnosis?
2. What drug(s) are commonly used in the treatment of this condition?
3. Which patient groups are at risk of this entity?
4. What imaging modalities are appropriate for diagnosis?
5. What is the affected structure in the figure on the right?

Case ranking/difficulty:

Category: Infections in the musculoskeletal system

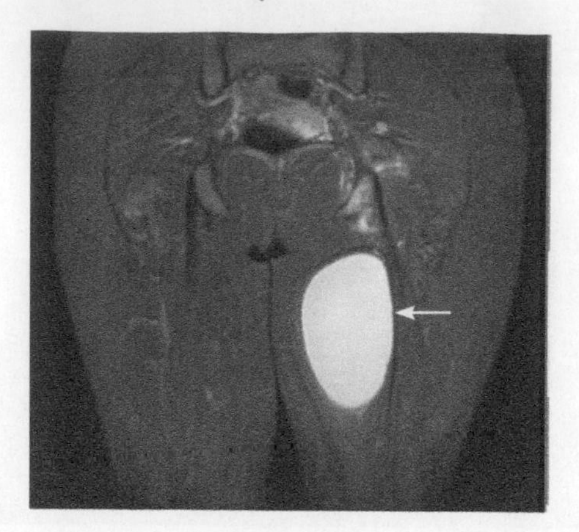

Tuberculous abscess within left hamstring muscles.

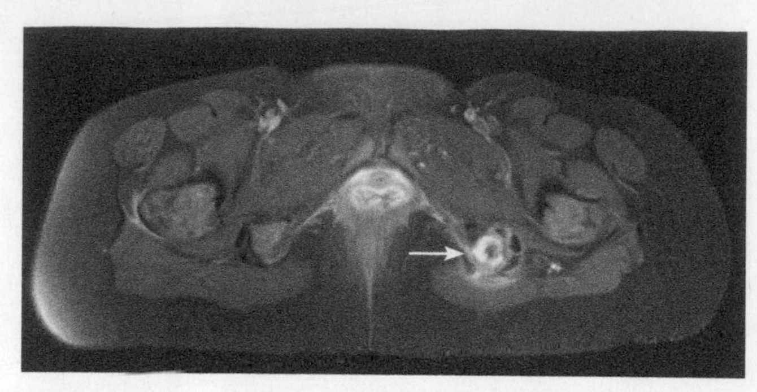

There is enhancement proximally to the level of the left ischial tuberosity. The abscess has tracked along the fascial planes of the left hamstring (biceps femoris) muscles.

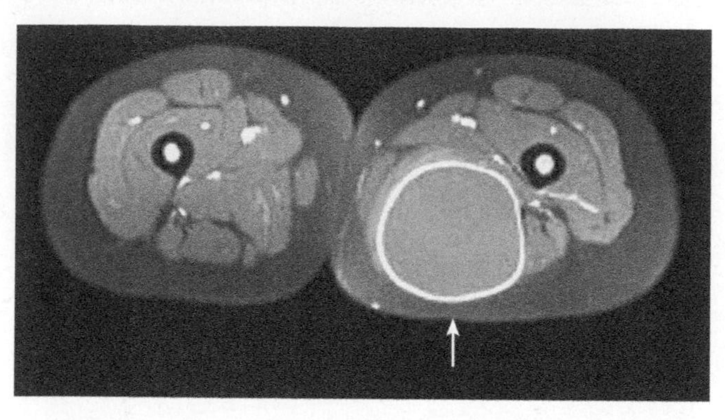

Rim-enhancing abscess within hamstring muscles postgadolinium administration.

Answers

1. A tuberculous abscess is also termed a *cold (nonpyrogenic) abscess*. An infected hematoma may have similar appearances, although one would expect a history of trauma. Rim-enhancement is not a typical feature of a sarcoma.
2. First-line treatment for TB involves 3 or 4 drugs, including ethambutol, isoniazid, rifampicin, pyrazinamide, and streptomycin.
3. The disease is rife in Africa and Asia, and among certain immigrant populations in developed countries, where living conditions may be suboptimal.
4. Ultrasound and MRI are the investigative modalities of choice for imaging abscesses. CT may also be used. Ultrasound has the advantage of guiding percutaneous aspiration. MRI enables an overall impression of disease extent to be reliably obtained.
5. The biceps muscles insert into the ischial tuberosity. Pathology in the muscles therefore can track proximally to the ischium and pelvis.

Pearls

- Tuberculous abscess must be considered in the differential diagnosis of a painful mass in populations which may be susceptible, for example, HIV, immunocompromised, Asian, and African patient groups.
- MRI is the investigative modality of choice for evaluating tuberculous abscesses as any potential bony involvement can be assessed, as well as determining the full extent of disease.
- Gadolinium-enhanced MRI is useful for demonstrating rim-enhancement, a feature often distinguishing it from a hematoma, sarcoma, or other soft-tissue mass.
- Ultrasound is of particular use in guiding percutaneous aspiration.
- Workup should include ESR, CXR, WCC, and, ultimately, aspiration for AFBs and microscopy and culture.
- A combination of extended antituberculous therapy plus incision and drainage is often required to treat an established cold abscess.

Suggested Readings

Sabat D, Kumar V. Primary tuberculous abscess of rectus femoris muscle: a case report. *J Infect Dev Ctries.* 2009;3(6):476-478.

Tonolini M, Campari A, Bianco R. Common and unusual diseases involving the iliopsoas muscle compartment: spectrum of cross-sectional imaging findings. *Abdom Imaging.* 2012;37(1):118-139.

Severe back pain

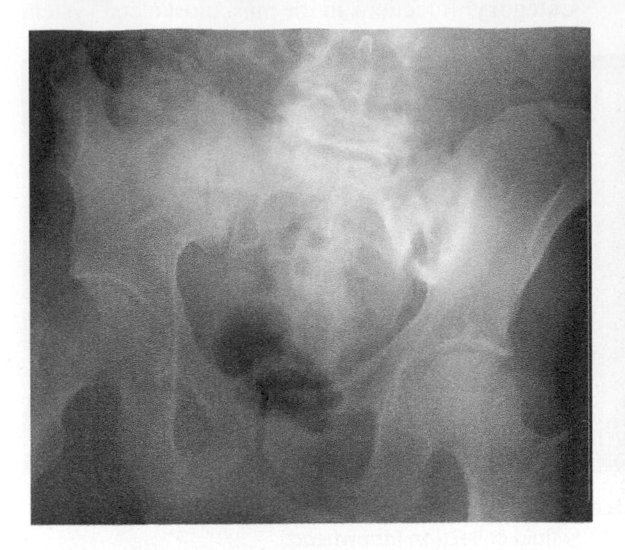

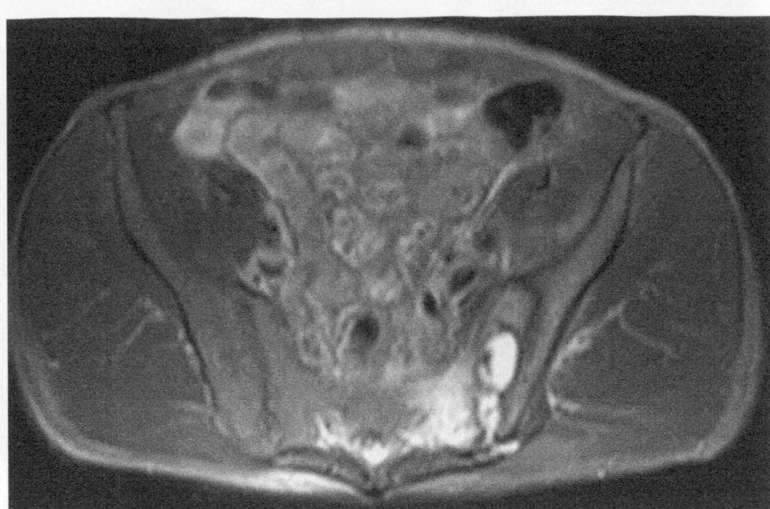

1. What are the radiograph findings?

2. What are the MRI findings?

3. What conditions are included in the differential?

4. What are the most useful techniques on MRI of this condition?

5. What is the most appropriate treatment?

Infectious sacroiliitis 1347

Case ranking/difficulty:

Category: Infections in the musculoskeletal system

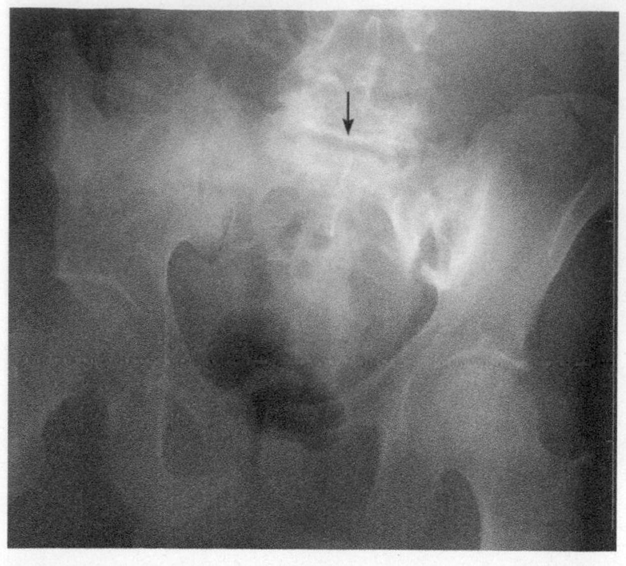

There is erosion of the left sacroiliac joint with surrounding sclerosis. Additional changes of L5-S1 discitis are noted (*arrow*).

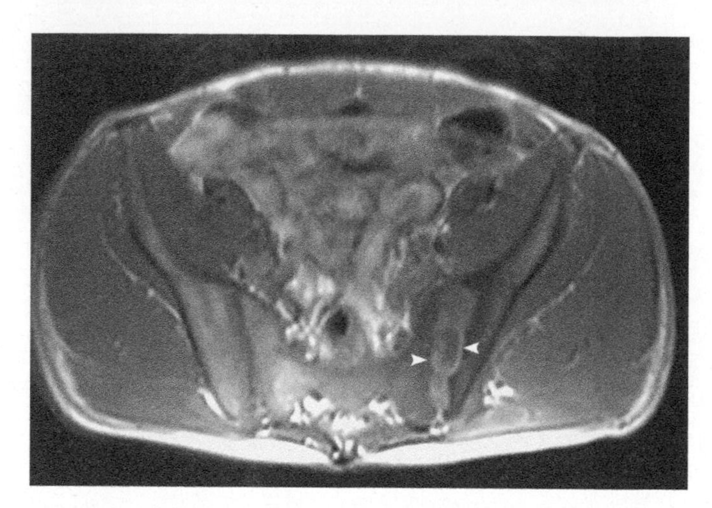

Synovial thickening is appreciated on precontrast images.

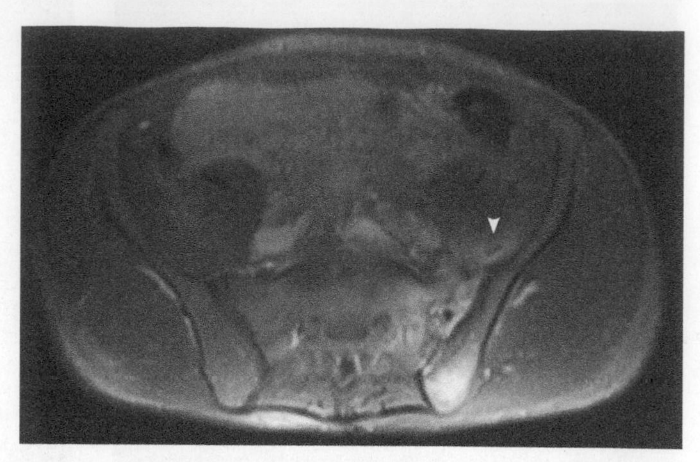

There is enhancement in and around the SI joint with a small periarticular fluid collection (*arrowhead*).

Answers

1. The classic features of infectious sacroiliitis are demonstrated with erosions, periarticular sclerosis, and joint space widening in the left sacroiliac joint. This patient also had an infectious discitis at L5-S1. He was an intravenous drug user.
2. There is periarticular bone and soft tissue edema, joint effusion, erosions, and a soft-tissue abscess.
3. Ankylosing spondylitises is a bilateral symmetric arthritis affecting both SI joints. The seronegative arthritides are bilateral and asymmetric. A unilateral destructive arthritis is most likely infectious.
4. A STIR sequence is very useful in the early detection of a sacroiliitis. T1 images with contrast are useful especially for the detection of associated periarticular soft-tissue fluid collections. Diffusion tensor imaging has also been described as useful in the early detection of active sacroiliitis.
5. Typical management for infectious sacroiliitis is intravenous antibiotics, with percutaneous or open drainage of any associated significant fluid collections.

Pearls

- Infectious sacroiliitis is typically a unilateral arthritis.
- It is more common in children and adolescents.
- Intravenous drug users have a higher incidence than the average patient population.
- Erosions, joint space widening, and surrounding sclerosis are typical on plain films. Eventual ankylosis may occur.
- MRI is more sensitive for the early detection of sacroiliitis, especially using a STIR sequence.
- T1 fat-saturated images after contrast will help to delineate periarticular and soft-tissue abscesses.
- Diffusion tensor imaging has been suggested as a useful modality for the early detection of sacroiliitis.

Suggested Readings

Bellussi A, Busi Rizzi E, Schininà V, De Santis A, Bibbolino C. STIR sequence in infectious sacroiliitis in three patients. *Clin Imaging.* 2002;26(3):212-215.

Bollow M, Braun J, Hamm B, et al. Early sacroiliitis in patients with spondyloarthropathy: evaluation with dynamic gadolinium-enhanced MR imaging. *Radiology.* 1995;194(2):529-536.

Chronic bilateral hand and wrist pain

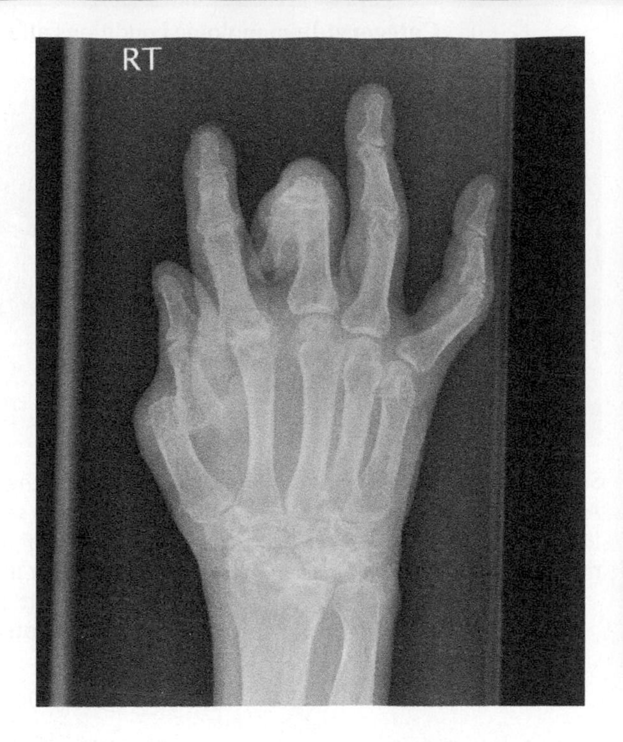

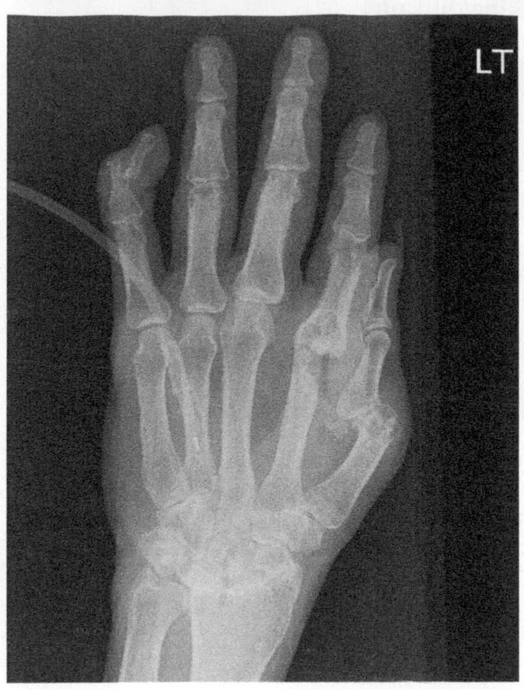

1. What is the classic presentation of this entity?

2. In this entity, where in the bone do osseous erosions tend to occur first?

3. What are the systemic manifestations of this disease?

4. Which imaging modality is the most sensitive for detecting early manifestations of this disease?

5. What are the typical MRI findings in this entity?

Rheumatoid arthritis 1381

Case ranking/difficulty:

Category: Immunologic conditions affecting bone

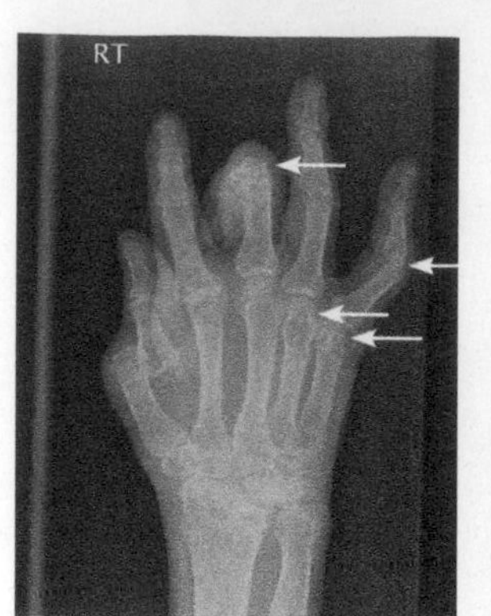

Marked joint space narrowing with multiple subluxations/ dislocations are noted. Multiple erosions are present (*arrows*).

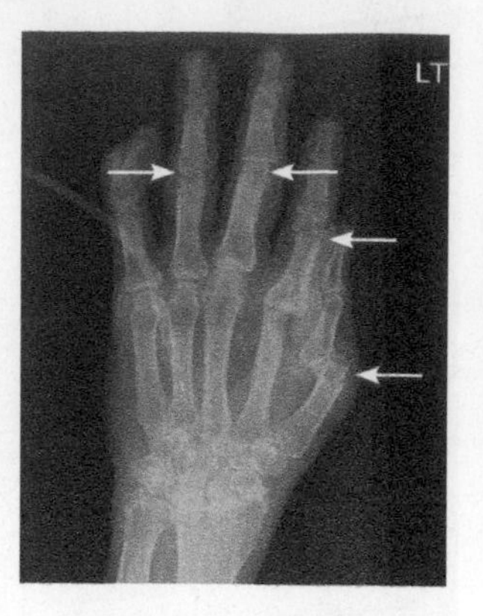

Marked joint space narrowing with multiple subluxations/ dislocations are again noted. Multiple erosions are present (*arrows*).

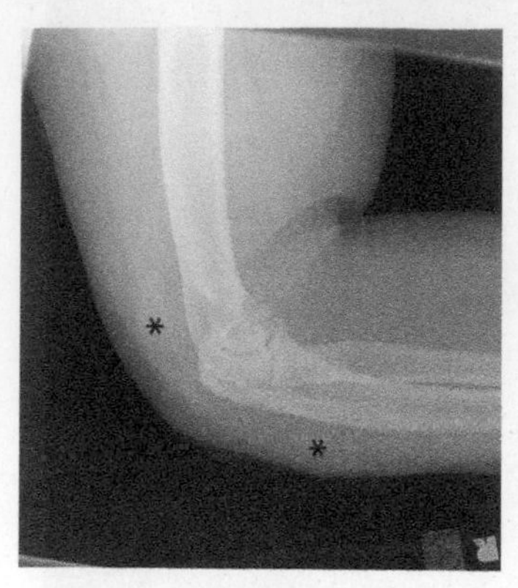

Soft-tissue swelling posteriorly. Areas of soft-tissue nodularity (*asterisks*) compatible with rheumatoid nodules are present.

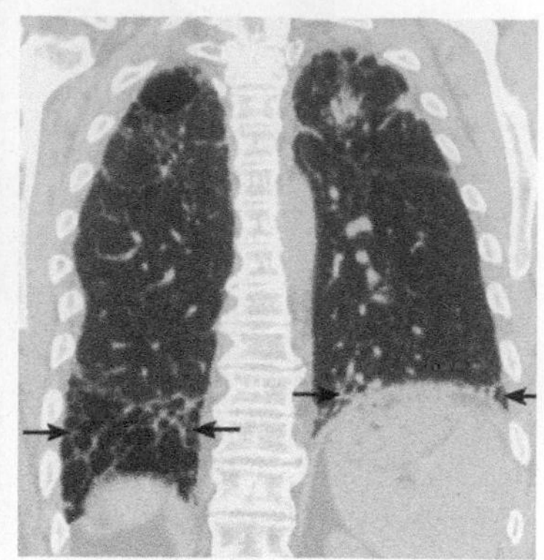

Coronal CT image of the lungs at lung window settings demonstrates bibasilar fibrotic changes, right greater than left (*arrows*). Incidental left upper lobe confluent fibrosis is noted.

Answers

1. Rheumatoid arthritis is classically a bilaterally symmetric arthritis of 3 or more joints, often in the hand.
2. The "bare area" of bone at synovial joints—the area located near the joint capsule insertion and not covered by articular cartilage—lies in direct contact with the inflamed synovium and tends to be affected by erosions first.
3. Vasculitis, anemia, lymphadenopathy, pericarditis, and cardiovascular disease are some systemic manifestations.
4. MRI is the most sensitive imaging modality for detecting early manifestations of rheumatoid arthritis.
5. Pannus, effusions, tenosynovitis, and bone erosions are among the typical MRI findings seen in rheumatoid arthritis.

Pearls

- Rheumatoid arthritis is the most common inflammatory arthritis, affecting between 0.5% and 1% of the population.
- Females are affected 2 to 3 times more often than males.
- Rheumatoid arthritis is classically a bilaterally symmetric arthritis of 3 or more joints; involvement of the wrists, metacarpophalangeal joints, and proximal interphalangeal joints is characteristic.
- It is primarily a disease of the synovium, affecting the synovial joints and tendon sheaths.
- Imaging findings may include synovitis, tenosynovitis, tendinitis, joint effusions, bone marrow edema, paraarticular osteoporosis, bone erosions, cartilage loss, joint space narrowing, joint deformities, and ankylosis.
- Radiography has traditionally been used to assess rheumatoid arthritis; it depicts the later manifestations of disease, including erosions, joint space narrowing, and joint deformities.
- MRI is more sensitive for the earlier manifestations of disease, including hyperemia, synovitis, effusions, and bone marrow edema.

Suggested Readings

Sommer OJ, Kladosek A, Weiler V, Czembirek H, Boeck M, Stiskal M. Rheumatoid arthritis: a practical guide to state-of-the-art imaging, image interpretation, and clinical implications. *Radiographics.* 2005;25(2):381-398.

Villeneuve E, Emery P. Rheumatoid arthritis: what has changed? *Skeletal Radiol.* 2009;38(2):109-112.

Pain. History of a chronic condition, diagnosed at age 12

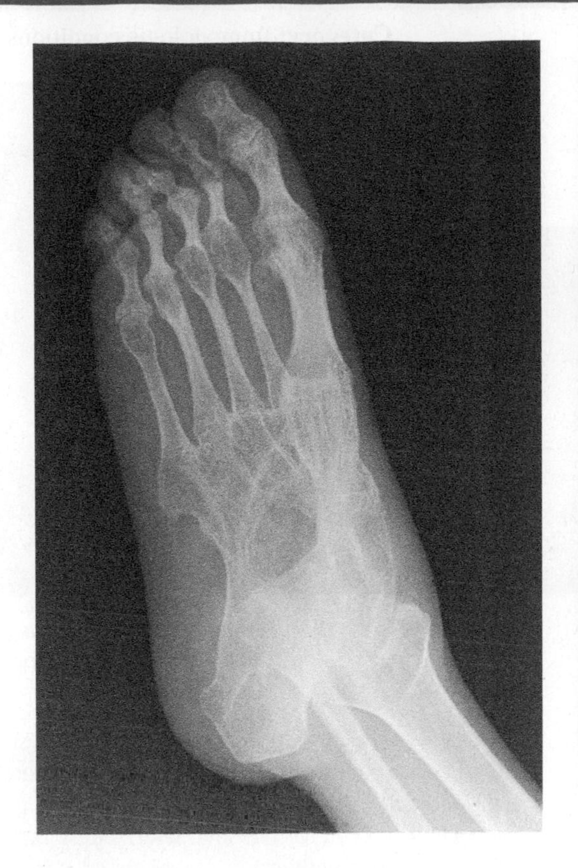

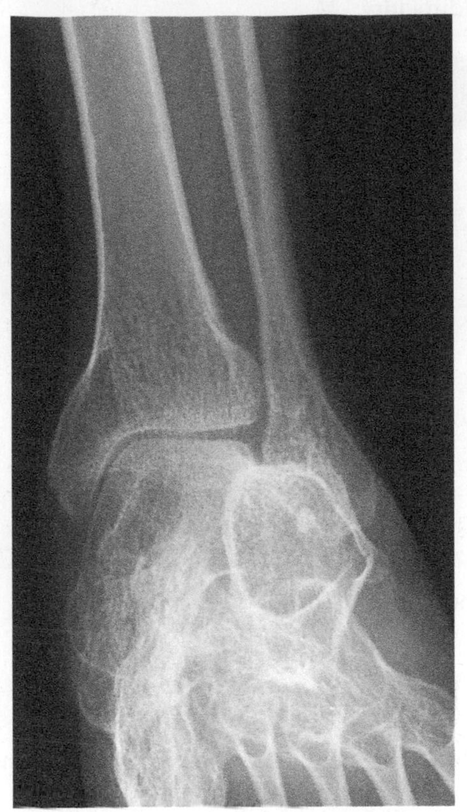

1. What are the radiographic findings?

2. What is the differential diagnosis, and what is the most likely diagnosis?

3. What are the major forms of this condition, using the American College of Rheumatology (ACR) criteria?

4. The pauciarticular type of this condition typically affects which joints?

5. What are radiologic features of this condition?

Juvenile idiopathic arthritis 1380

Case ranking/difficulty:

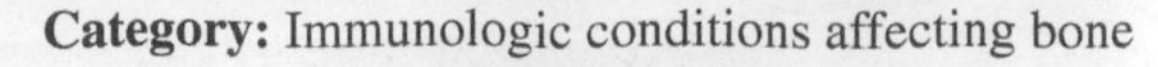

Category: Immunologic conditions affecting bone

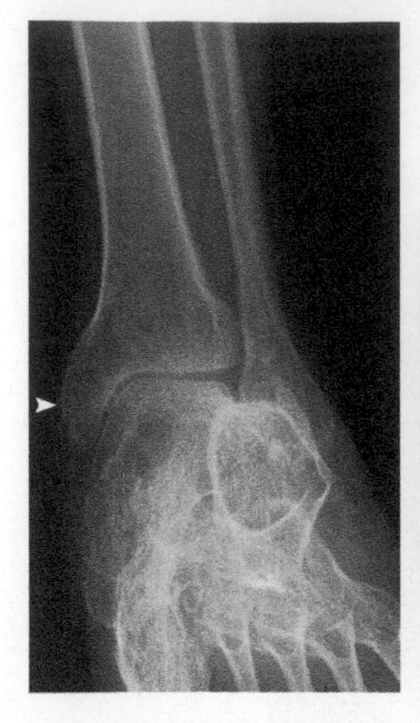

There is enlargement of the tibial epiphysis.

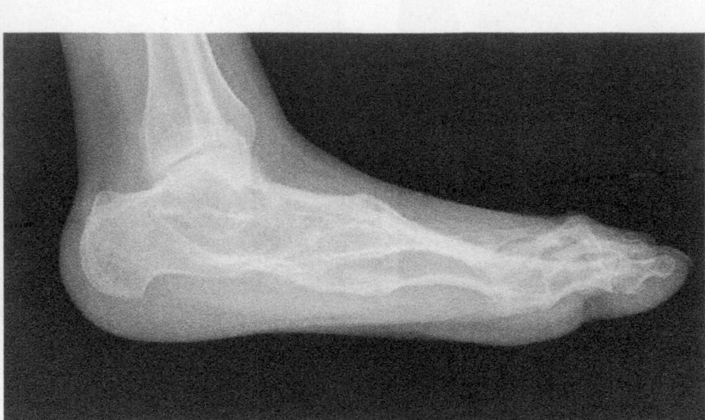

Subtalar joint ankylosis is seen.

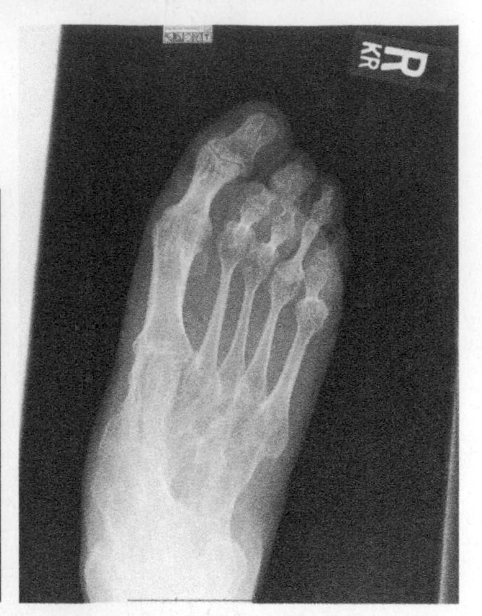

Right foot also shows extensive bony ankylosis and osteopenia.

Answers

1. Bony ankylosis and joint deformity are the predominant features on these radiographs. Mild epiphyseal overgrowth is also demonstrated.
2. Extensive bony ankylosis can be seen in juvenile idiopathic arthritis (JIA), and ankylosing spondylitis. There is no spine or SI joint involvement to suggest ankylosing spondylitis. The most likely diagnosis is JIA.
3. The 3 major types of JIA recognized by the ACR are the polyarticular, pauciarticular, and systemic types.
4. The pauciarticular type typically affects the large joints such as the knees and ankles. The polyarticular type affects the small joints of the hands and feet.
5. Epiphyseal overgrowth, periosteal reaction, soft-tissue swelling, ankylosis, and deformity are all features of JIA. Erosions can be present especially in rheumatoid factor-positive polyarthritis, but are generally a less-prominent feature as compared to adult rheumatoid arthritis.

Pearls

- JIA has 3 main forms: polyarticular, pauciarticular, and systemic.
- Polyarticular form affects the small joints of the hands and feet.
- Pauciarticular form affects larger joints such as knees and ankles.
- The systemic form is characterized by mainly systemic symptoms, with arthralgia, pleuritis, and pericarditis amongst a range of other symptoms.
- Soft-tissue swelling, effusions, and periosteal reaction are typical. Hyperemia may result in overgrowth of the epiphyses.
- Bony ankylosis is characteristic and may affect the small and large joints. Ankylosis is not typically a feature of adult rheumatoid arthritis, except in the cervical spine.
- Ultrasound and MRI are useful in evaluating early changes, and monitoring the response to therapy.

Suggested Readings

Johnson K. Imaging of juvenile idiopathic arthritis. *Pediatr Radiol.* 2006;36(8):743-758.

Johnson K, Wittkop B, Haigh F, Ryder C, Gardner-Medwin JM. The early magnetic resonance imaging features of the knee in juvenile idiopathic arthritis. *Clin Radiol.* 2002;57(6):466-471.

Bilateral foot pain

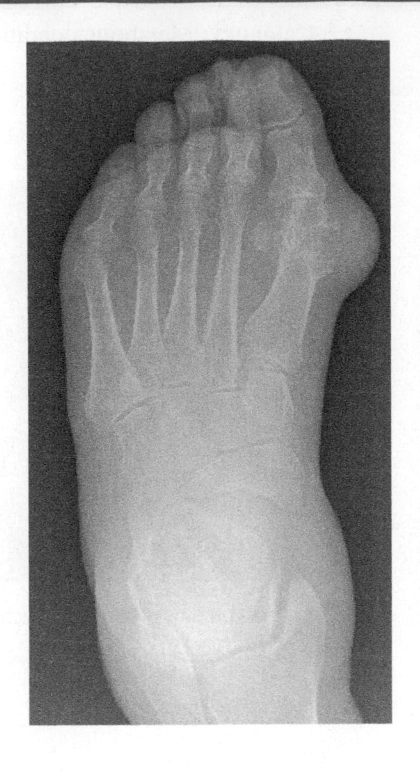

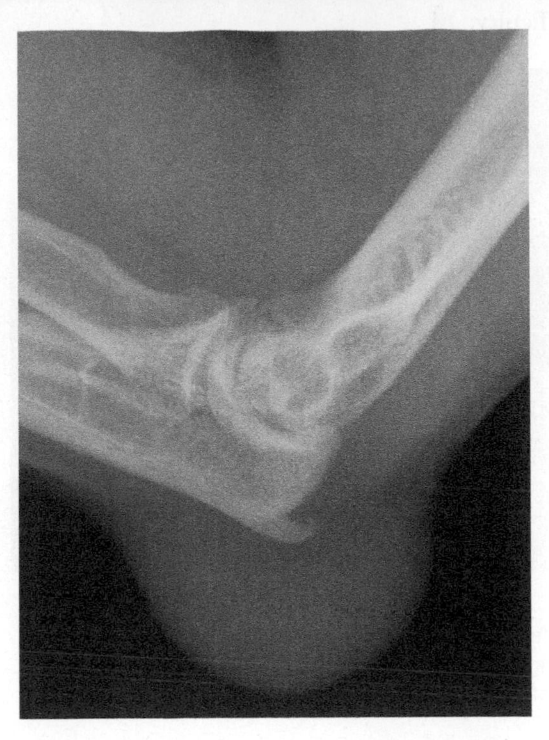

1. What are the relevant imaging findings?

2. What is the most likely diagnosis?

3. What is the treatment of this entity?

4. Soft-tissue involvement of this entity is classically seen in which structures?

5. What are the typical MRI signal characteristics of this entity?

Gout 1330

Case ranking/difficulty:

Category: Metabolic conditions affecting bone

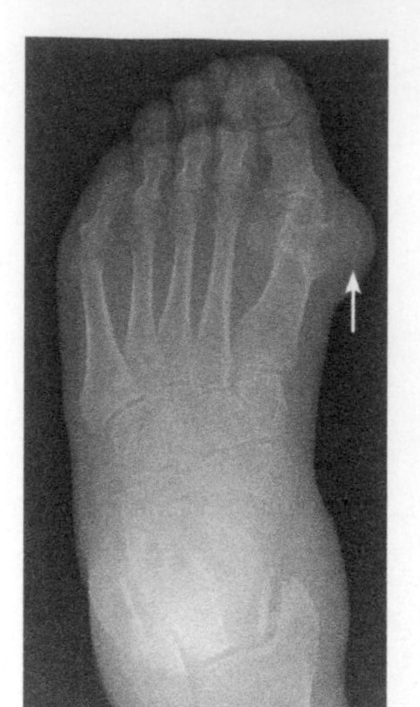

Large juxtaarticular erosions around the left first metatarsophalangeal joint, with calcified soft-tissue tophi.

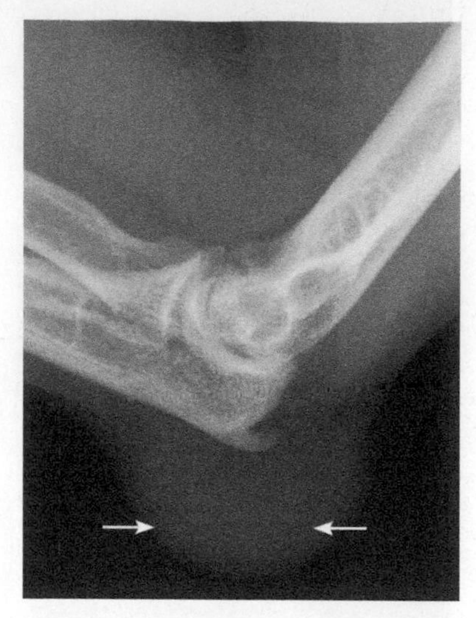

Elbow shows olecranon bursitis.

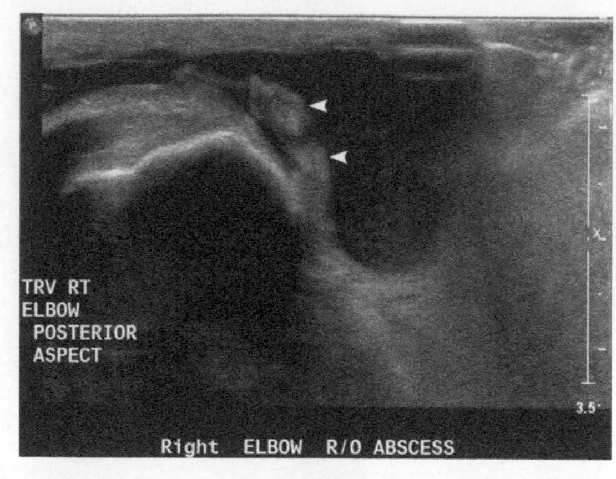

Olecranon bursitis is seen, with echogenic gouty tophi (*arrowheads*).

Answers

1. There are extensive juxtaarticular erosions with overhanging edges primarily centered around the first MTP, with adjacent calcified soft tissue masses. Relative preservation of the joint spaces is noted. There is also an olecranon bursitis.

2. Given the imaging findings, the likely diagnosis is gout. CPPD, septic arthritis, and osteoarthritis would not show calcified soft-tissue masses.

   Multicentric reticulohistiocytosis can also resemble gout, but is rare and has extensive skin manifestations that were not demonstrated.

3. Colchicine and NSAIDs are used for acute attacks in gout, and allopurinol for chronic gouty arthritis. Modification of diet, including avoidance of purine-rich foods and excessive alcohol, is an important component of the management.

4. Although soft-tissue deposition of gouty tophi can occur in any soft tissue, the classic soft-tissue locations are in the pinna of the ear and the olecranon bursae (which is typically bilateral).

5. There is typically T1 hypointensity in gout, but the T2 signal is variable. T2 hyperintensity may occur as a result of edema and the presence of hydrated crystals, but T2 hypointensity may also occur as a result of fibrous tissue deposition and nonhydrated crystals. Contrast enhancement is typical.

Pearls

- Primary gout is a result of inborn error of metabolism of purines and is more common than secondary gout.
- Radiographic features include preservation of mineralization and joint spaces initially, with eventual joint destruction and narrowing.
- Juxtaarticular sharply marginated erosion with overhanging edges are typical.
- Periarticular soft-tissue masses that may contain calcifications are frequently seen. Olecranon bursitis and aural calcification may occur.
- Dual-energy CT shows promise in the noninvasive detection of monosodium urate crystals.

Suggested Readings

Dalbeth N, McQueen FM. Use of imaging to evaluate gout and other crystal deposition disorders. *Curr Opin Rheumatol.* 2009;21(2);124-131.

Paparo F, Fabbro E, Ferrero G, et al. Imaging studies of crystalline arthritides. *Reumatismo.* 2012;63(4):263-275.

Painful hands

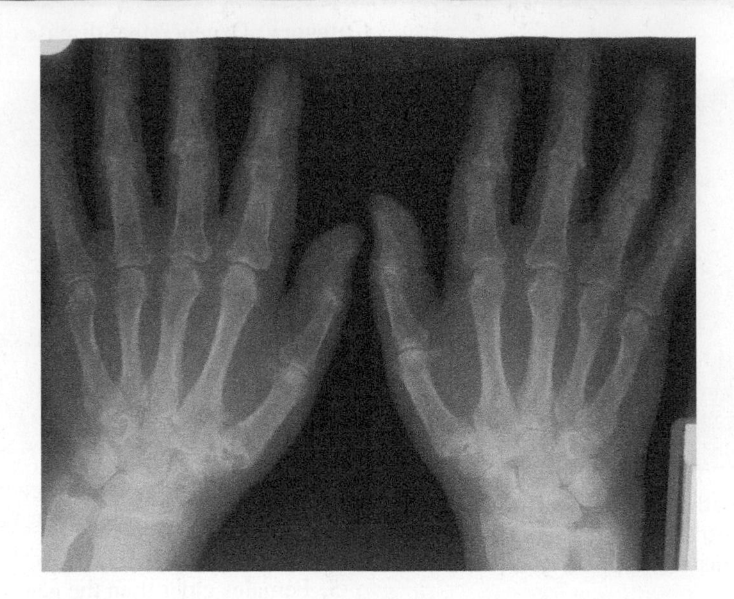

1. What are the radiographic findings?

2. What are the differential diagnoses?

3. What is the most likely diagnosis?

4. What are the associations of this condition?

5. Which patient population is most often affected in this entity?

Erosive Osteoarthritis 1729

Case ranking/difficulty:

Category: Degenerative disease of the musculoskeletal system

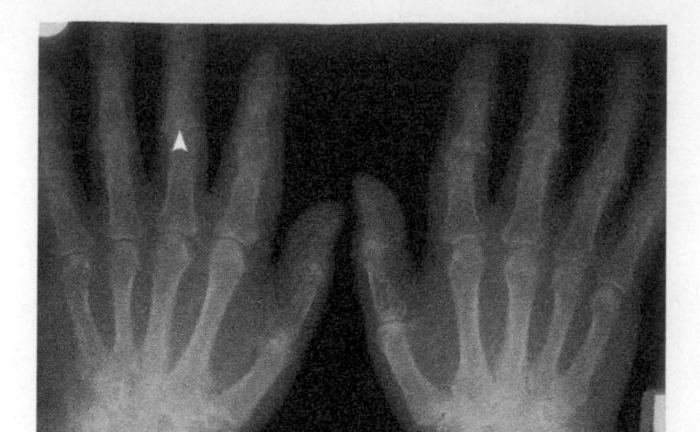

Central erosions and bony proliferative changes, with a seagull appearance (*arrowhead*) suggesting erosive OA. There are also subluxations at the proximal and distal interphalangeal joints.

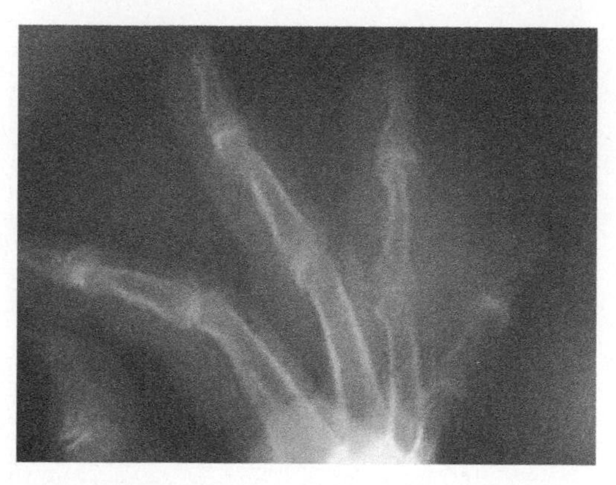

Marked proliferative bone changes affecting the distal interphalangeal joints.

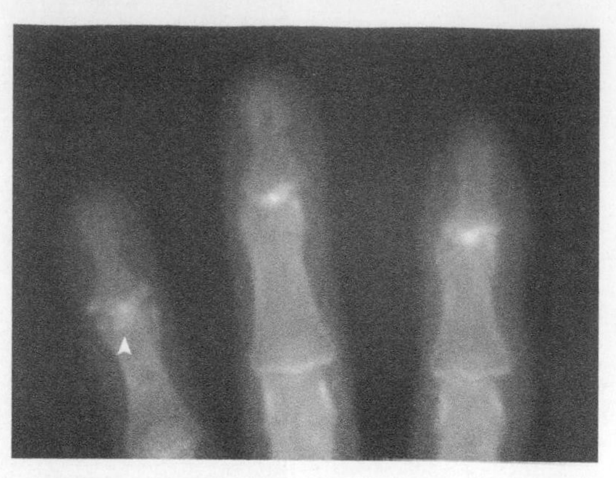

Bony proliferative changes and central erosions in another patient. (Image is provided by Dr. Rajendra Solanki)

Answers

1. Erosions of the proximal and distal interphalangeal joints are noted. These erosions are central with peripheral marginal synovial proliferation and osteophytes, giving a "seagull" or "gullwing" appearance. No erosions of the MCP joints. No subluxation of the joints, but there is proliferative bone changes and joint space narrowing. There is usually a symmetrical bilateral distribution.
2. The main differential diagnoses are rheumatoid arthritis, psoriatic arthritis, erosive osteoarthritis, and crystalline arthropathy.
3. The acute history of swelling, pain, and erythema with a negative rheumatoid factor and "seagull" appearance of central erosions and proliferative bone changes on radiographs, suggests the diagnosis of erosive osteoarthritis.
4. Autoimmune disease, such as autoimmune thyroiditis and Sjögren disease, as well as scleroderma, are associations of erosive osteoarthritis.
5. Females older than the age of 65 years are at least 12 times more often affected than males.

Pearls

- Erosive osteoarthritis is an inflammatory osteoarthritis affecting females, more commonly females who are older than the age of 65 years.
- It typically affects the small joints of the hands such as the proximal, and especially the distal, interphalangeal joints, as well as the first carpometacarpal joint.
- There are central erosions and marginal proliferative changes leading to a seagull or gullwing appearance on plain radiographs, with evidence of joint space narrowing. Ankylosis may be a sequela.
- It has been thought to be associated with other autoimmune diseases such as autoimmune thyroiditis and Sjögren syndrome.
- Conservative treatment is usually sufficient. In a few advanced cases, arthroplasty, arthrodesis, or tendon transfer may be required.

Suggested Readings

Addimanda O, Mancarella L, Dolzani P, et al. Clinical and radiographic distribution of structural damage in erosive and nonerosive hand osteoarthritis. *Arthritis Care Res (Hoboken).* 2012;64(7):1046-1053.

Kortekaas MC, Kwok WY, Reijnierse M, Huizinga TW, Kloppenburg M. In erosive hand osteoarthritis more inflammatory signs on ultrasound are found than in the rest of hand osteoarthritis. *Ann Rheum Dis.* 2012 Jul 20 [Epub ahead of print].

Martel W, Stuck KJ, Dworin AM, Hylland RG. Erosive osteoarthritis and psoriatic arthritis: a radiologic comparison in the hand, wrist, and foot. *AJR Am J Roentgenol.* 1980;134(1):125-135.

Severe pain and deformity in digits with skin changes

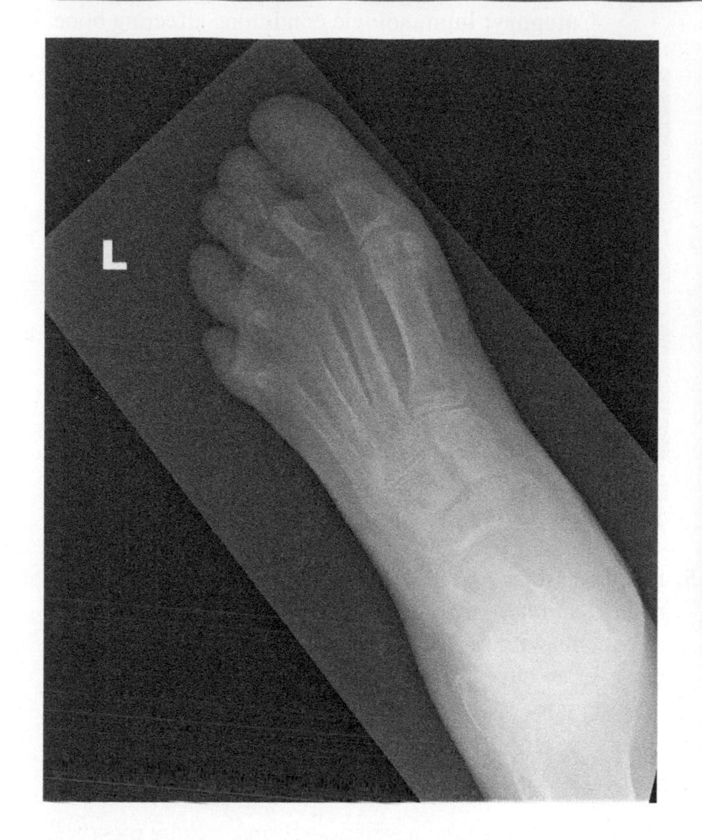

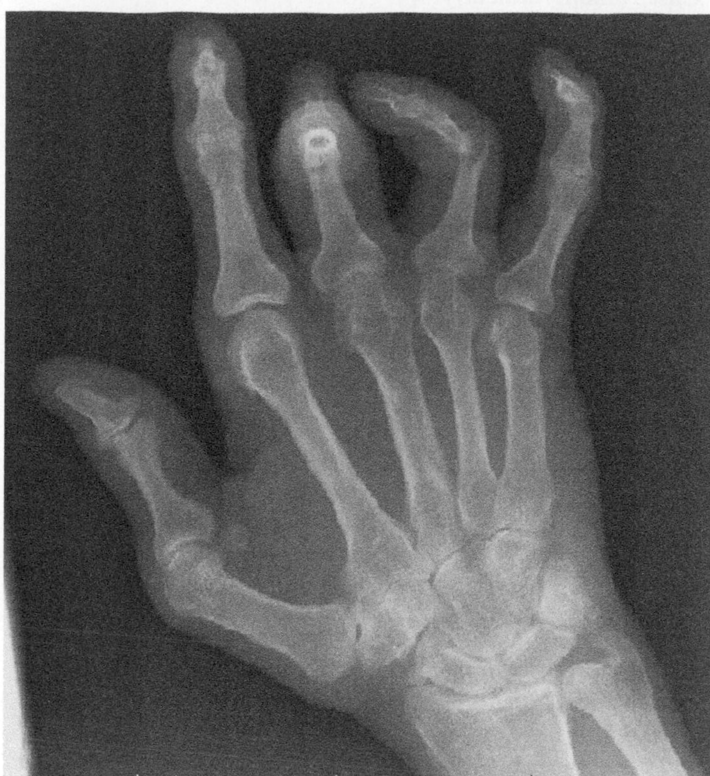

1. What are the clinical features of this condition?

2. What are the imaging features of this condition?

3. What are the possible treatments of this condition?

4. What is the most common pattern of arthritis seen with this condition?

5. What proportion of patients with cutaneous disease have an inflammatory arthritis?

Case ranking/difficulty:

Category: Immunologic conditions affecting bone

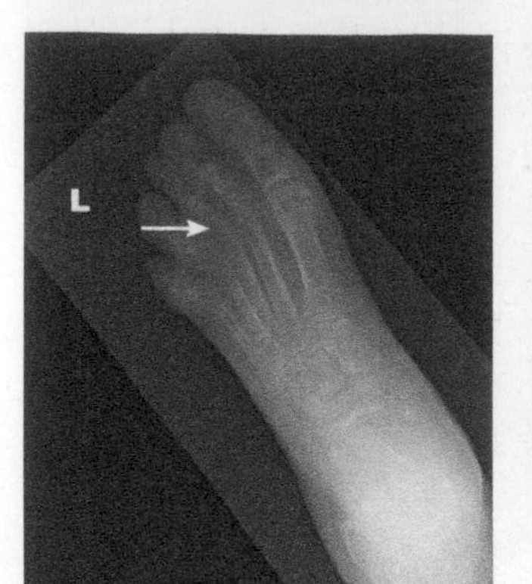

Periarticular erosions and osteopenia.

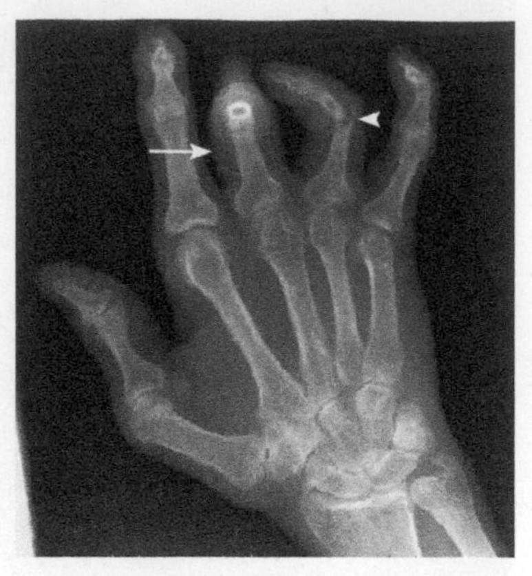

Arthritis mutilans with severe destructive "pencil-in-cup" erosions (*arrowhead*) and extensive soft-tissue swelling termed "sausage digits" (*arrow*).

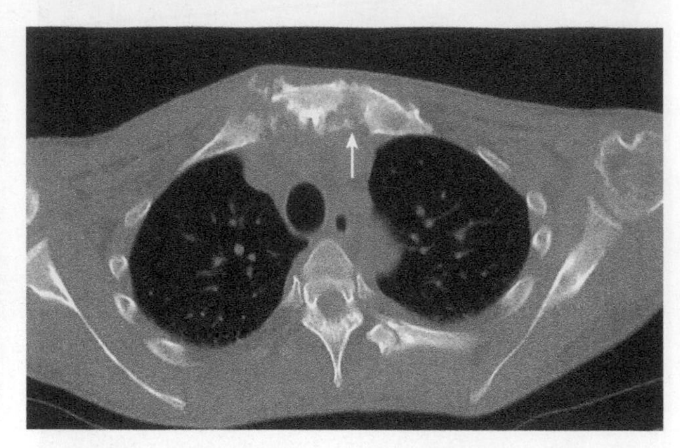

Erosive psoriatic osteitis affecting the sternoclavicular joints. Sclerosis and new bone proliferation are characteristic findings.

Answers

1. The most common forms of psoriatic arthritis are an asymmetric form affecting a few joints only, and a form that resembles rheumatoid arthritis clinically. The presence of dactylitis, enthesitis and nail changes are very suggestive of psoriatic arthritis. Erosions are synovial and therefore periarticular; gout is characterized by juxtaarticular "rat-bite" erosions. Disease that involves the DIP joints alone is typical of psoriatic arthritis, although this textbook description is not as common as the other varieties discussed.

2. Achilles enthesopathy is easily demonstrated on ultrasound as increased color Doppler flow. Reduced bone mineral density is a feature of rheumatoid and psoriatic arthritis, and may relate to increased concentrations of inflammatory cytokines, for example, TNF-α which increase osteoclastic activity. Osteoporosis is compounded by the side effect of use of corticosteroids in these patients.

   Erosions are periarticular in rheumatoid and psoriasis, and juxtaarticular in gout. Calcified synovial loose bodies are found in synovial chondromatosis. TFCC (triangular fibrocartilaginous complex) calcification is a feature of calcium pyrophosphate arthropathy.

3. Methotrexate and azathioprine are classic disease-modifying steroid-sparing antirheumatic drugs (DMARDs). Intra-articular injections have the benefit of avoiding or minimizing severe systemic corticosteroid side effects. Surgery is reserved for severe functionally limiting cases.

4. Contrary to common perception, DIP joint predominant arthritis is actually not the most common form of psoriatic arthritis. An asymmetric pauciarticular arthritis is the most common variety, followed by a symmetric rheumatoid-like pattern.

5. Psoriatic arthritis is a relatively common generalized manifestation of psoriasis, occurring in up to one-third of patients with the skin condition. It is quite possible, however, to have arthritis as the first presentation of the disease, prior to the development of any skin lesions.

Pearls

- Psoriatic arthritis may have many forms, but the most common manifestations are an asymmetric arthritis affecting a few joints, and a seronegative symmetric arthritis, clinically indistinguishable from rheumatoid arthritis.
- The most severe form of psoriatic arthritis is termed *arthritis mutilans*.
- Characteristic features of arthritis mutilans are severe erosions in a "pencil-in-cup" pattern, "sausage digits," and a distribution more distal than a typical rheumatoid pattern.
- "Sausage digits" refers to the sausage-like appearance of dactylitis in some cases of psoriatic arthritis.
- Enthesitis (eg, Achilles) and dactylitis are characteristic of psoriatic arthritis.
- Psoriatic arthritis is one of the most common spondyloarthropathies after primary ankylosing spondylitis.
- Patients are frequently HLA-B27 positive.

Suggested Readings

Amrami KK. Imaging of the seronegative spondyloarthropathies. *Radiol Clin North Am.* 2012;50(4):841-854.

Anandarajah A. Imaging in psoriatic arthritis. *Clin Rev Allergy Immunol.* 2012 Feb 1 [Epub ahead of print].

Cimmino MA, Parodi M, Zampogna G, et al. Magnetic resonance imaging of the hand in psoriatic arthritis. *J Rheumatol Suppl.* 2009;83(83):39-41.

Young male with lower back pain

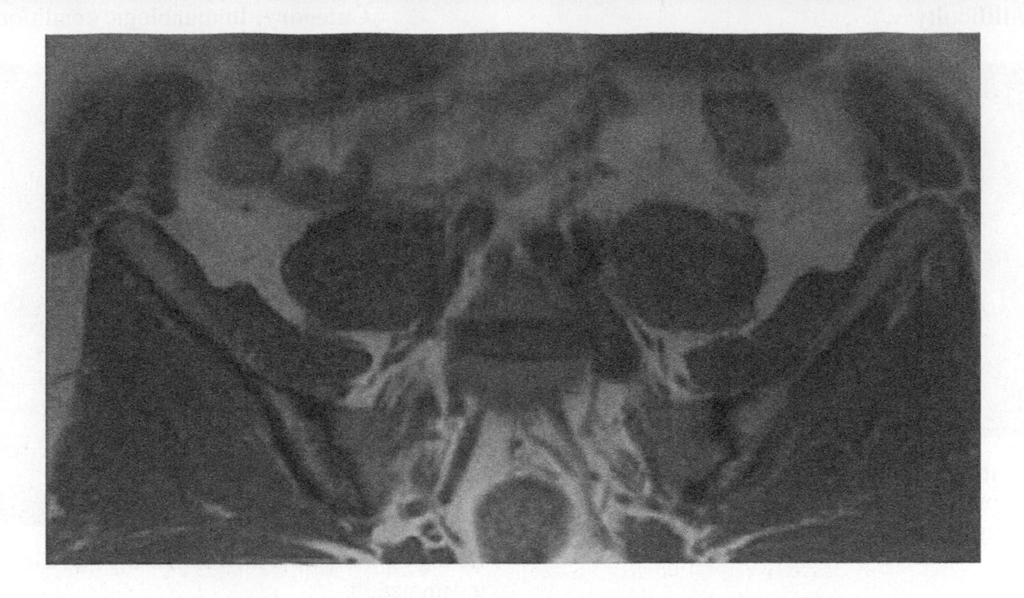

1. What are the imaging features of this entity?
2. What is the differential diagnosis?
3. What type of joint is shown?
4. What are the associations of Crohn disease with this entity?
5. What are the features of this condition that are secondary to inflammatory bowel disease?

Enteropathic sacroiliitis 1837

Case ranking/difficulty:

Category: Immunologic conditions affecting bone

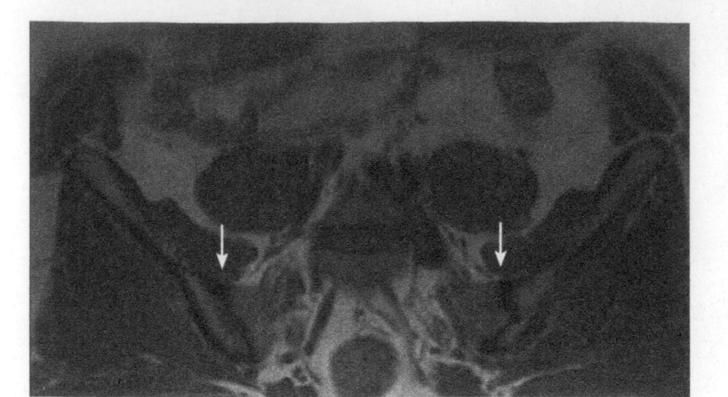

Fused sacroiliac joints with asymmetric low T1 signal on either side of the joint is consistent with sclerosis. The features may represent ankylosing spondylitis or enteropathic arthritis.

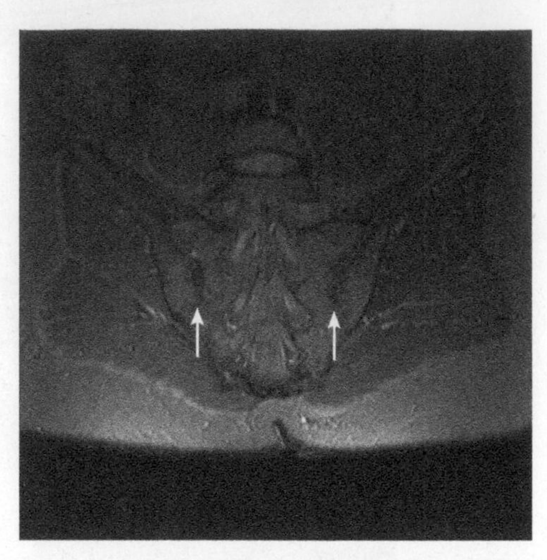

No high STIR signal is seen consistent with a lack of active inflammation.

Answers

1. Sacroiliitis can be detected on plain film radiography, although the most sensitive diagnostic examination is MRI, which can detect subtle changes of early edema.

   Plain films will reveal erosions, sclerosis and joint space loss, although these changes occur later in the course of the disease.

   Osteitis condensans ilii is a radiological diagnosis characterized by symmetrical increased density on the iliac sides of the sacroiliac joints, more common in women.

2. Gout does form part of the differential diagnosis of sacroiliitis, although it could be a rare presentation of the disease. TB and pyogenic osteomyelitis would also cause unilateral sacroiliitis.

   Reactive/psoriatic arthritis classically causes bilateral asymmetrical sacroiliitis and ankylosing spondylitis/ enteropathic arthritis classically causes bilateral symmetrical sacroiliitis.

3. Sacroiliitis related to spondyloarthropathies will affect the lower synovial aspect of the joints first, and these areas should be paid close attention to on imaging studies.

4. There is a weak association with HLA-B27 (in 30% of cases), but there is a strong genetic predisposition to sacroiliitis if sufferers of Crohn disease carry the CARD15 gene polymorphism.

5. Enteropathic sacroiliitis is less frequently associated with positive HLA-B27 (30%) compared to primary ankylosing spondylitis (90%). The sacroiliitis is asymmetrical and seen in 4% of cases. It is independent of the bowel disease status. Crohn has a stronger association with sacroiliitis and spondylitis than ulcerative colitis.

Pearls

- Sacroiliitis is detected most sensitively on a fat-suppressed MRI sequence (eg, STIR).
- The inferior (synovial) portions of the sacroiliac joints typically show the earliest changes of edema.
- Plain films or CT will demonstrate sclerosis and erosions, although these features are seen later in the course of the disease.
- Important distinctions are between unilateral versus bilateral causes and asymmetrical versus symmetrical disease.
- The most common pattern is symmetrical and bilateral disease, characteristic of ankylosing spondylitis.
- Despite the characteristic bilateral and symmetrical distribution, as ankylosing spondylitis is overwhelmingly more prevalent than other inflammatory causes, atypical asymmetrical cases of ankylosing spondylitis are often seen; hence this diagnosis should still be considered.
- Enteropathic sacroiliitis is an important cause of sacroiliitis and should be considered in patients with bowel symptoms in conjunction with pelvic/ sacroiliac pain.
- In these patients, sacroiliitis and spondyloarthropathy may occur before any bowel disease manifestations.

Suggested Readings

Braun J, Golder W, Bollow M, Sieper J, van der Heijde D. Imaging and scoring in ankylosing spondylitis. *Clin Exp Rheumatol.* 2005;20(6 Suppl 28):S178-S184.

Docherty P, Mitchell MJ, MacMillan L, Mosher D, Barnes DC, Hanly JG. Magnetic resonance imaging in the detection of sacroiliitis. *J Rheumatol.* 1992;19(3):393-401.

Chest pain

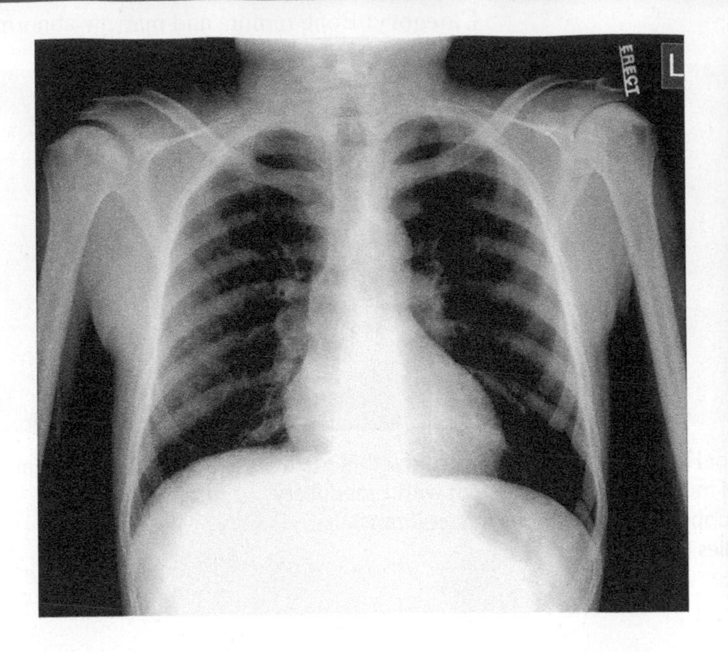

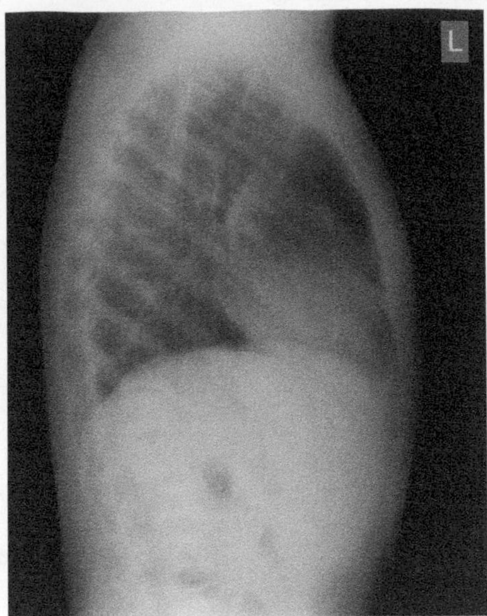

1. What are the musculoskeletal manifestations of this entity?

2. Approximately what percentage of African Americans carry at least 1 gene for this entity?

3. Vertebral endplate softening in this entity gives what appearance?

4. What are the 2 most common organisms implicated in osteomyelitis in patients with this disease?

5. Avascular necrosis is more often bilateral in patients with this entity than in patients who have avascular necrosis from other causes. True or False?

Sickle cell anemia 1544

Case ranking/difficulty: 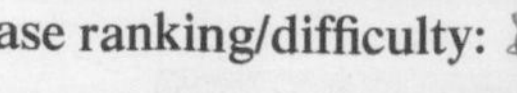

Category: Bone tumors and marrow abnormalities

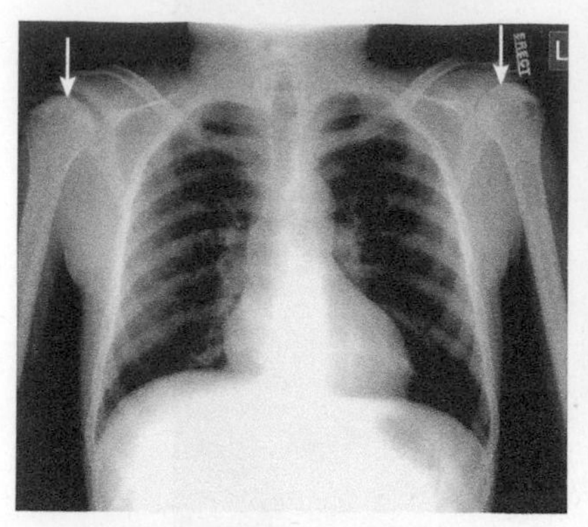

Sclerosis within both humeral heads (*arrows*) consistent with avascular necrosis.

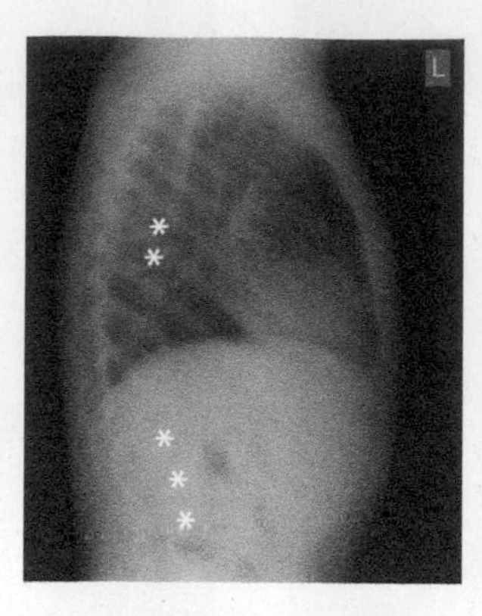

"Fish mouth" or H-shaped deformities of multiple thoracic and upper lumbar vertebral bodies (*asterisks*).

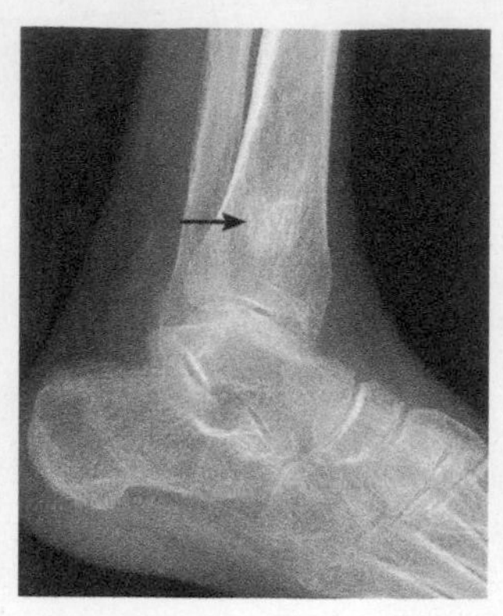

Focal sclerosis within the tibia consistent with a medullary bone infarct (*arrow*).

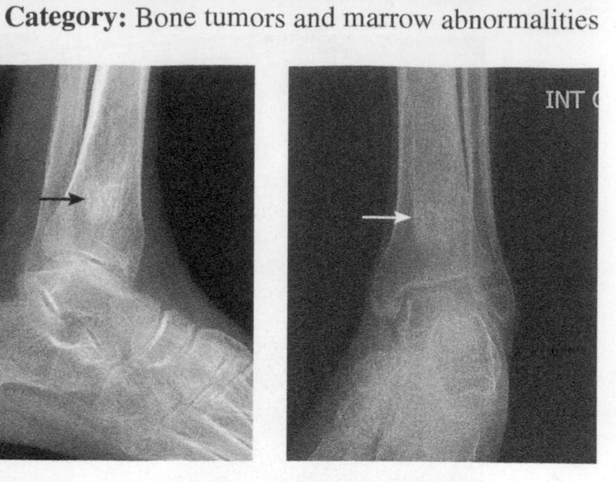

Medullary bone infarct (*arrow*).

Answers

1. Musculoskeletal manifestations of sickle cell anemia include bone infarctions, dactylitis, osteomyelitis, and persistence of hematopoietic red marrow in the appendicular skeleton into adult life.
2. Approximately 8% of African Americans carry the gene for sickle cell hemoglobin, and 0.2% of African Americans have sickle cell anemia.
3. Vertebral endplate softening in sickle cell anemia gives the appearance of "fish mouth" or H-shaped vertebrae.
4. *Staphylococcus aureus* is the most common, followed by *Salmonella*. Other Gram-negative organisms are uncommonly involved; tuberculosis has been reported but is not common.
5. Avascular necrosis, which affects 50% of sickle cell anemia patients by age 35 years, is more often bilateral in sickle cell anemia compared to other causes.

Pearls

- Sickle cell anemia is an autosomal recessive hemoglobinopathy resulting in abnormal morphology of red blood cells.
- Sickle cell disease is more prevalent in individuals of African origin; 8% of African Americans carry the gene for sickle cell hemoglobin resulting in sickle cell trait, and 0.2% have sickle cell anemia.
- The abnormal red blood cells are destroyed at an increased rate, resulting in anemia.
- The cells also aggregate, leading to microvascular occlusion and ischemia or infarction of tissues and organs.
- Avascular necrosis affects 50% of patients by age 35 years, often in the humeral and femoral heads, and is commonly bilateral.
- Infection (osteomyelitis and septic arthritis) is another major complication.
- Classic radiographic features include bone infarcts, dactylitis, H-shaped vertebrae, and changes of extramedullary hematopoiesis.

Suggested Readings

Ejindu VC, Hine AL, Mashayekhi M, Shorvon PJ, Misra RR. Musculoskeletal manifestations of sickle cell disease. *Radiographics.* 2007;27(4):1005-1021.

Lonergan GJ, Cline DB, Abbondanzo SL. Sickle cell anemia. *Radiographics.* 2001;21(4):971-994.

Progressive swelling and pain on the ulnar aspect of the wrist

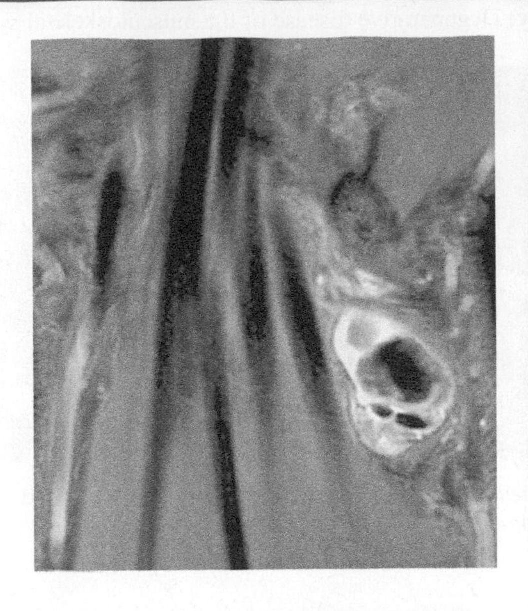

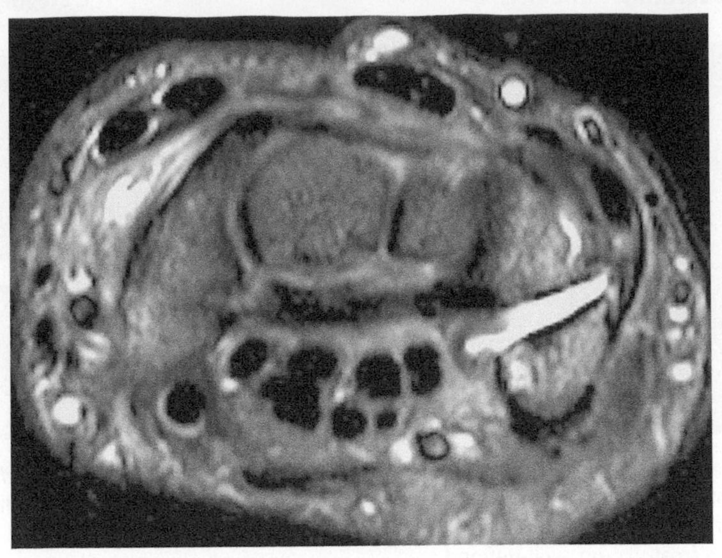

1. What are the expected findings on a radiograph?

2. What are the MRI findings?

3. What is the diagnosis?

4. What are the different types of this entity, and what is the etiology?

5. What are the treatment options?

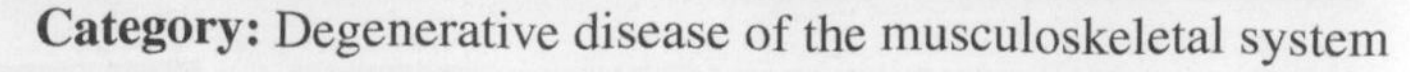

Synovial osteochondromatosis 1450

Case ranking/difficulty: **Category:** Degenerative disease of the musculoskeletal system

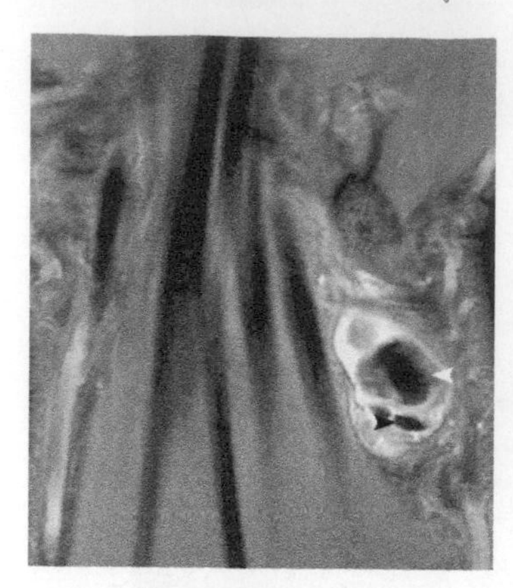

Pisotriquetral joint osteoarthritis with synovial osteochondromatosis. There are multiple small, round, well-defined osteocartilaginous loose bodies.

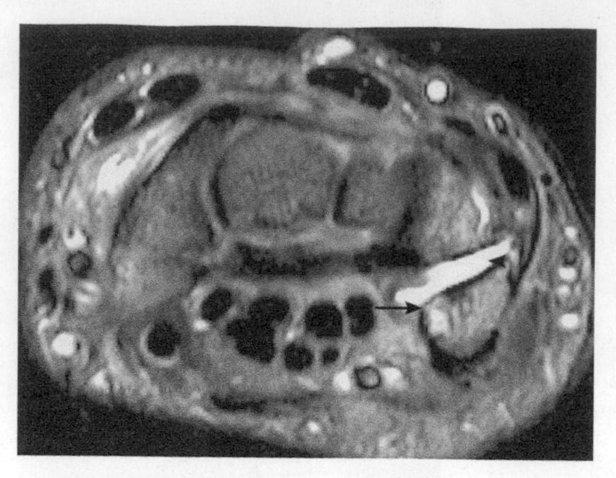

Pisotriquetral (PT) joint effusion (*arrowhead*). Cyst in the pisiform and PT joint osteoarthritic change (*arrow*).

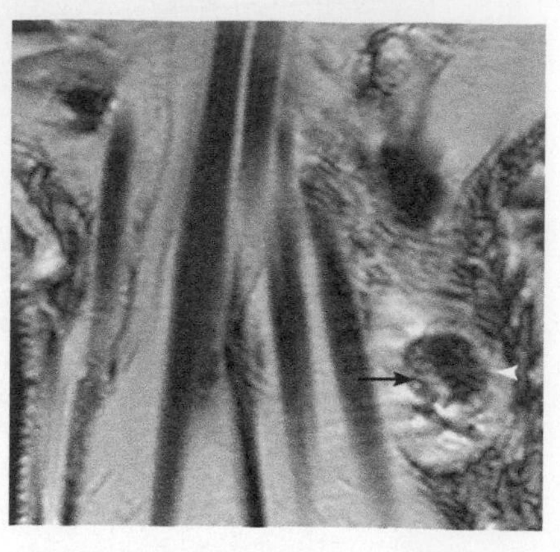

Synovial osteochondral loose body in the pisotriquetral joint.

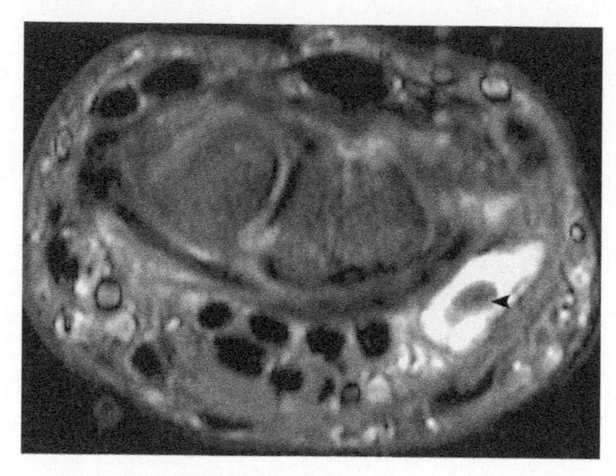

PT joint effusion with synovial osteochondromatosis.

Answers

1. Radiographs would be expected to show multiple loose bodies and degenerative changes within the PT (pisotriquetral) joint.
2. There is synovial hypertrophy (not shown), with multiple osteocartilaginous loose bodies at the PT joint, joint effusion, and PT joint osteoarthritic change.
3. The diagnosis is synovial chondromatosis of the PT joint, with multiple loose bodies and secondary degenerative changes of this joint.
4. Synovial chondromatosis could be primary or secondary, and the underlying pathogenesis is related to synovial metaplasia.
5. Treatment options include synovectomy with excision of the loose bodies, or conservative management in mild cases. Excision of the pisiform has been considered in the treatment of advanced cases.

Pearls

- Synovial osteochondromatosis can be primary or secondary.
- Secondary synovial osteochondromatosis is usually caused by degenerative changes of a joint, most often involving the knee and hip joints. Other etiologies include intra-articular fractures, osteochondritis desiccans, and neuropathic arthritis. These loose bodies are fewer in number and are more likely to be nonuniform compared to primary osteochondromatosis.
- Primary synovial osteochondromatosis (PSO) is a metaplastic process of synovial membranes of joints, bursae and tendons.
- PSO can also lead to secondary degenerative changes.
- PSO rarely affects the pisotriquetral joint. Men are twice as often affected, in the third and fourth decades.
- Plain film shows osteochondral loose bodies and degenerative changes.
- Ball catcher's view might be useful for PT disease. Loose bodies and osteoarthritic changes may be seen.
- MRI will show a joint effusion and multiple uniform loose bodies.
- Management is surgical resection of the synovium and the loose bodies. Surgical excision of the pisiform in extreme cases.

Suggested Readings

Bunn J, Crone M, Mawhinney I. Synovial chondromatosis of the pisotriquetral joint. *Ulster Med J.* 2001;70(2):139-141.

Tudor A, Sestan B, Miletić D, et al. Synovial chondromatosis of the pisotriquetral joint with secondary osteoarthritis: case report. *Coll Antropol.* 2007;31(4):1179–1181.

Right knee pain—history of knee arthroplasty for many years

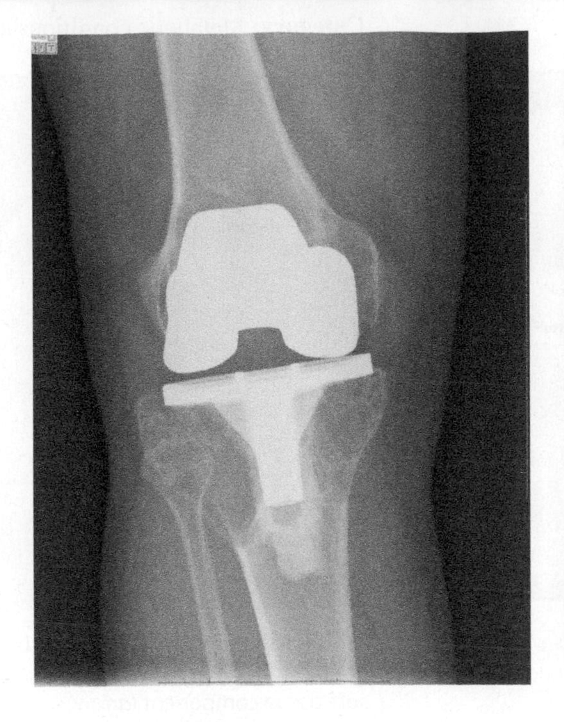

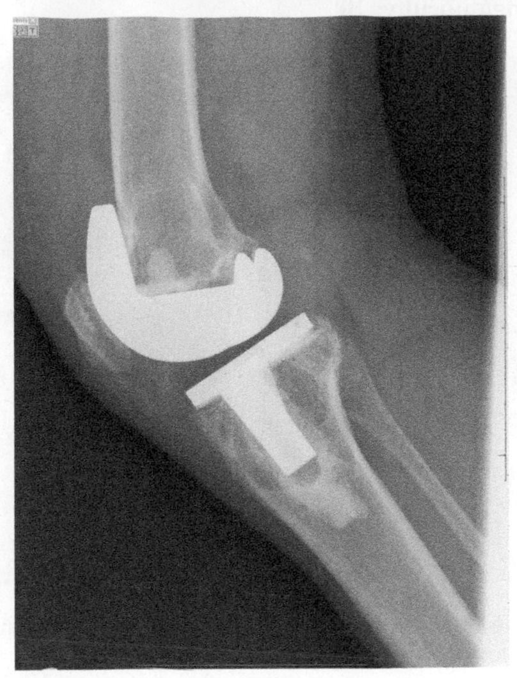

1. What are the radiograph findings?
2. What is the most likely diagnosis?
3. What is the proposed etiology for this condition?
4. What is the next most appropriate study?
5. What is the management for this condition?

Particle disease 1376

Case ranking/difficulty:

Category: Metabolic conditions affecting bone

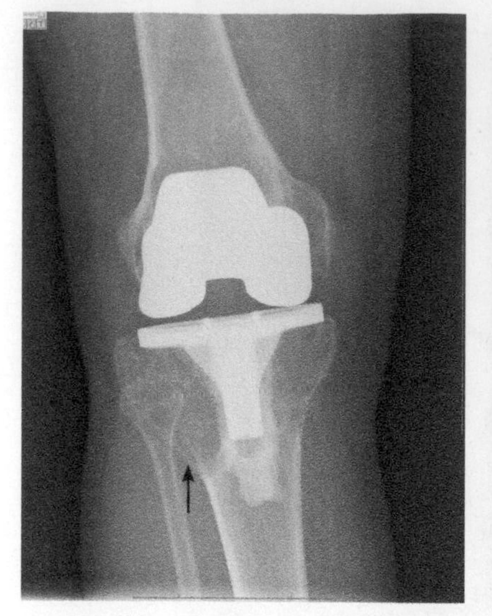

Lucent expansile lesions in the proximal tibia and distal femur are seen around the prostheses.

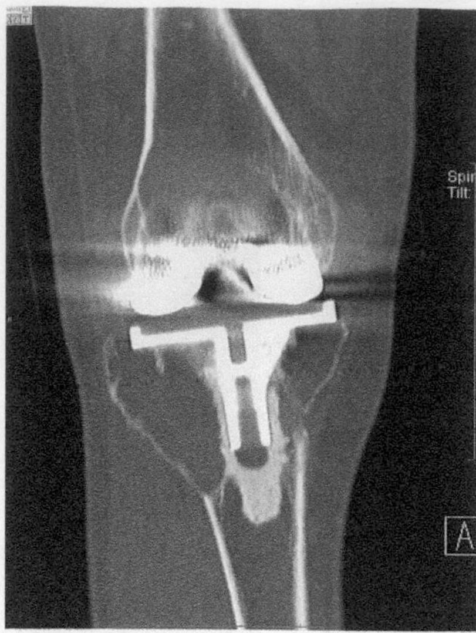

Lucent expansile lesions with cortical thinning.

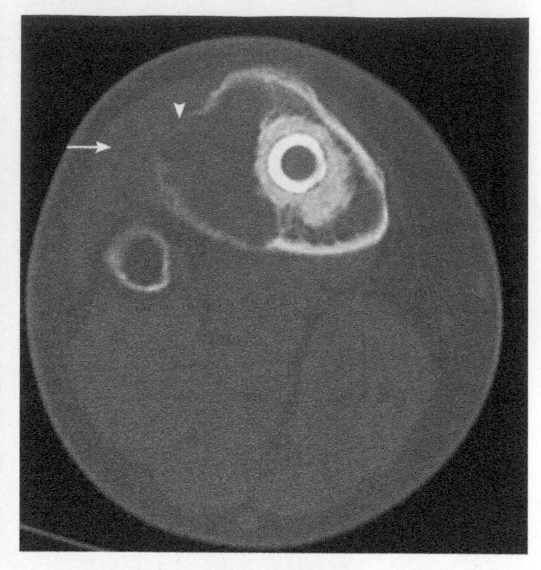

Proximal tibia expansile lesion with cortical breakthrough (*arrowhead*), and extraosseous soft-tissue component (*arrow*).

Answers

1. There are large, well-defined, lucent lesions in the proximal tibia and one in the distal femur. There is mild bony expansion, no matrix, and mild cortical breakthrough laterally.
2. Lucent, expansile, well-demarcated lesions surrounding a prosthesis, with or without cortical breakthrough, are most likely to be particle disease.
3. These findings are classic for particle disease, which is a foreign-body granulomatous reaction to any of the components of a prosthesis including the metal, polyethylene liner or the cement.
4. If particle disease is suspected and infection is not, a CT scan is the next appropriate study to assess the degree of bone loss, and the amount of secondary prosthetic loosening. Additional details provided by CT would include the presence of a pathological fracture.
5. The accepted management for particle disease and a loose prosthesis is revision arthroplasty.

Pearls

- Particle disease is a foreign-body granulomatous reaction to any of the components of a prosthesis, including the metal, cement, or polyethylene liner.
- It presents with lucent, well-defined lesions without sclerotic rims surrounding a prosthesis, with or without bone expansion or cortical breakthrough.
- Lesions may appear aggressive and may be confused with primary or secondary bone tumors. Centering around a prosthesis narrows the differential.
- No matrix is seen in the lesions.
- The lesions typically result in loosening of the prosthesis. The knee is more often affected than the hip.
- Treatment is with revision arthroplasty.

Suggested Readings

Choplin RH, Henley CN, Edds EM, Capello W, Rankin JL, Buckwalter KA. Total hip arthroplasty in patients with bone deficiency of the acetabulum. *Radiographics*. 2008;28(3):771-786.

Otto M. Classification of prosthetic loosening and determination of wear particles [in German]. *Pathologe*. 2008;29 Suppl 2:232-239.

Pain in both knees

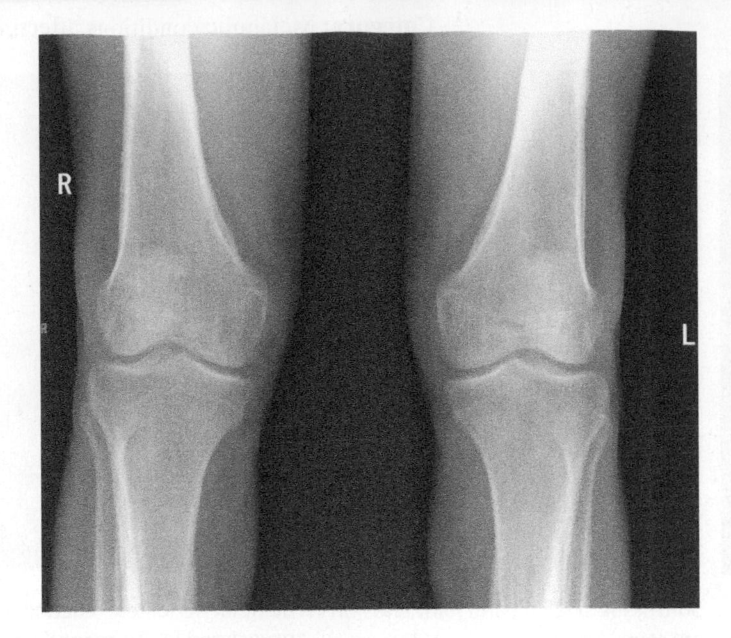

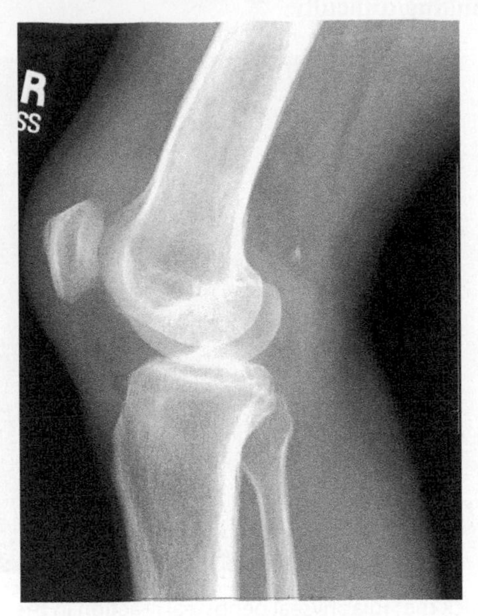

1. What is the finding on the plain radiographs?

2. What is the differential for this finding?

3. What would be the expected finding on a radionuclide bone scan?

4. What are the facts regarding bilaterality and painfulness of this condition?

5. What are the proposed etiologies and associations regarding this condition?

Hypertrophic osteoarthropathy 1323

Case ranking/difficulty:

Category: Metabolic conditions affecting bone

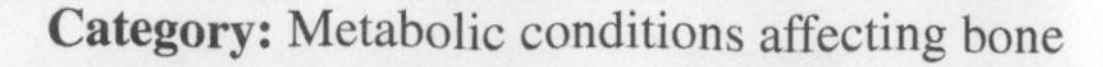

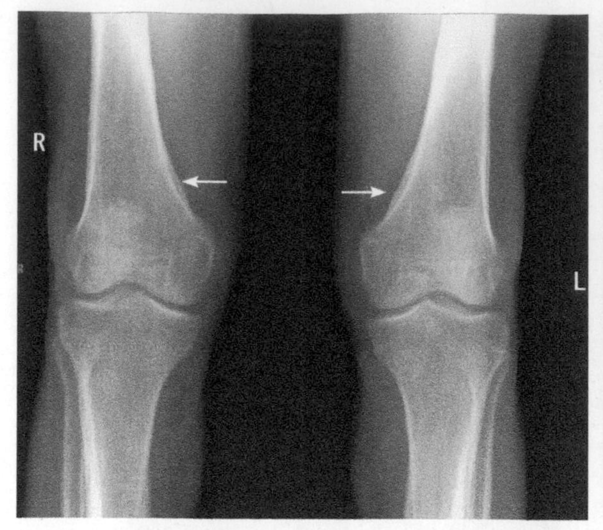

There is thick metadiaphyseal periosteal reaction in the bilateral distal femurs and proximal tibias.

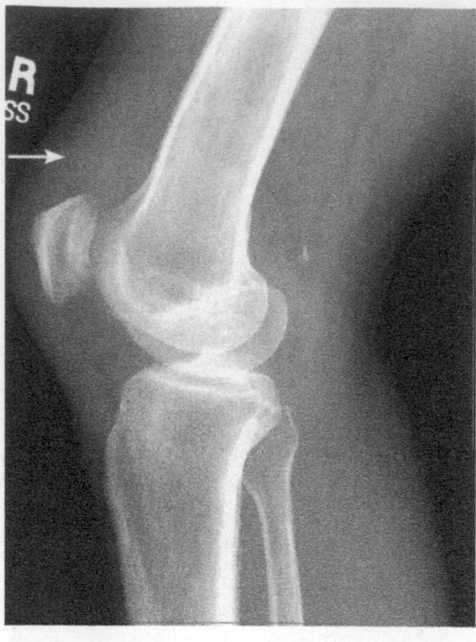

Soft-tissue swelling and joint effusion are seen.

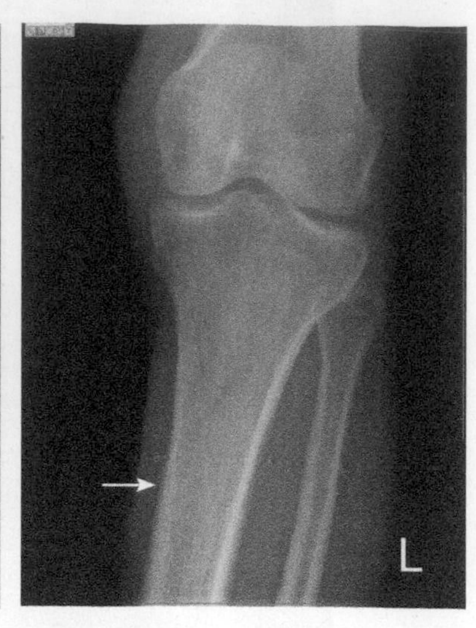

The tibial periosteal reaction is better appreciated in this magnified image.

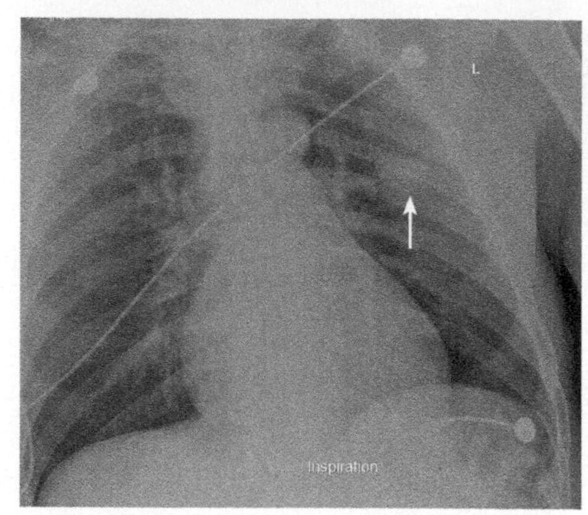

Chest radiograph shows a large tumor in the left lung.

Answers

1. Bilateral thick periosteal reaction, associated soft-tissue swelling, and a small knee effusion are seen.
2. The differential includes hypertrophic osteoarthropathy, pachydermoperiostitis, hypervitaminosis A, chronic venous stasis, and thyroid acropachy. Prolonged Voriconazole antifungal therapy may also induce florid periostitis.
3. Periosteal uptake in hypertrophic osteoarthropathy (HOA) would be expected. Periarticular uptake can also occur as a result of synovitis. The appendicular skeleton is affected most commonly.
4. HOA is a bilateral symmetric painful condition. There is often clinical and later radiologic resolution after removal of the underlying cause.
5. A hormonal theory for HOA is postulated, supported by resolution of clinical and radiologic findings after tumor resection. A neurogenic theory is also postulated, supported by resolution after vagotomy.

   Bronchogenic tumors and inflammatory bowel disease, as well as right-to-left shunts, are leading causes.

Pearls

- Thick bilateral periosteal reaction involving the metadiaphysis is characteristic. The epiphysis is usually spared.
- Soft-tissue swelling and effusion may occur.
- Radionuclide bone scan shows bilateral symmetric metadiaphyseal uptake and periarticular uptake if there is synovitis.
- The presence of this finding on radiographs warrants a chest radiograph or CT to exclude lung neoplasm.
- Symptoms can resolve promptly after tumor resection, followed by radiologic resolution in some cases.
- A neurogenic or hormonal etiology has been proposed, supported by improvement after tumor resection or vagotomy.
- This condition can be differentiated from pachydermoperiostitis by the lack of involvement of the epiphysis and by patient demographics.

Suggested Readings

Jajic Z, Jajic I, Nemcic T. Primary hypertrophic osteoarthropathy: clinical, radiologic, and scintigraphic characteristics. *Arch Med Res.* 2001;32(2):136-142.

Pineda C. Diagnostic imaging in hypertrophic osteoarthropathy. *Clin Exp Rheumatol.* 1993;10 Suppl 7:27-33.

78-year-old male with chest pain

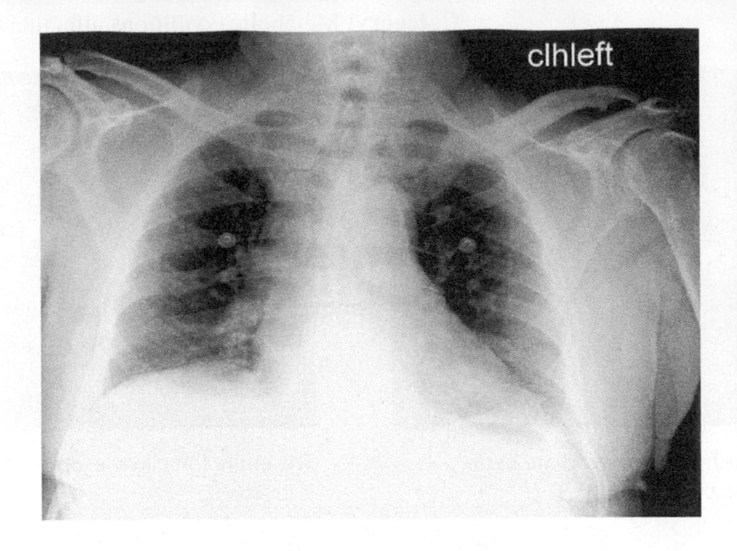

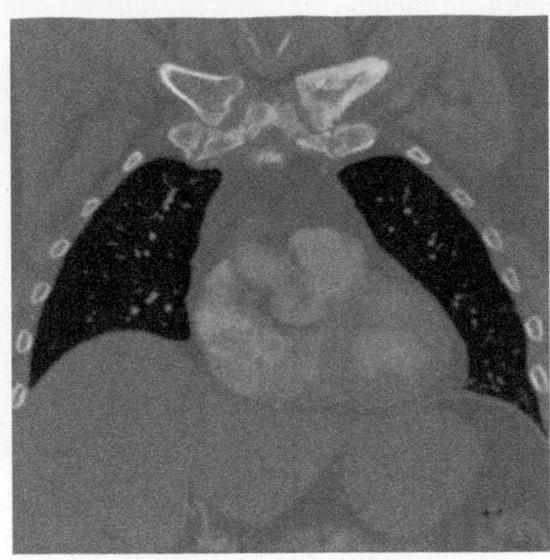

1. What is the most likely process affecting this patient's left clavicle?

2. What are the recognized phases of this disease?

3. Name some descriptive terms used to describe the radiographic findings in this condition?

4. This entity is believed to have a genetic component. True or False?

5. The axial skeleton is commonly affected in this entity. True or False?

Paget disease 1825

Case ranking/difficulty:

Category: Metabolic conditions affecting bone

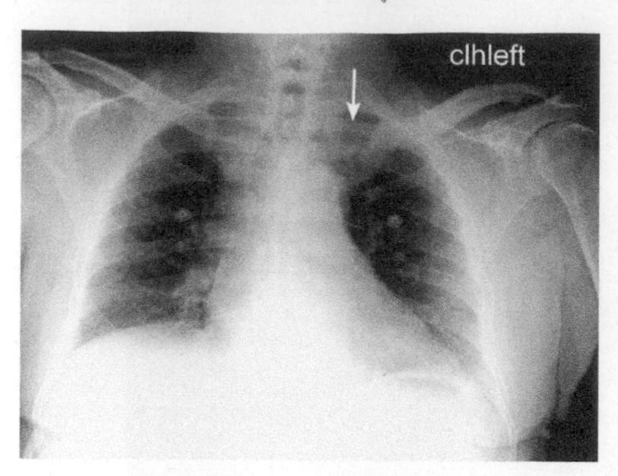

Asymmetric enlargement, sclerosis, and cortical thickening of the left clavicle (*arrow*).

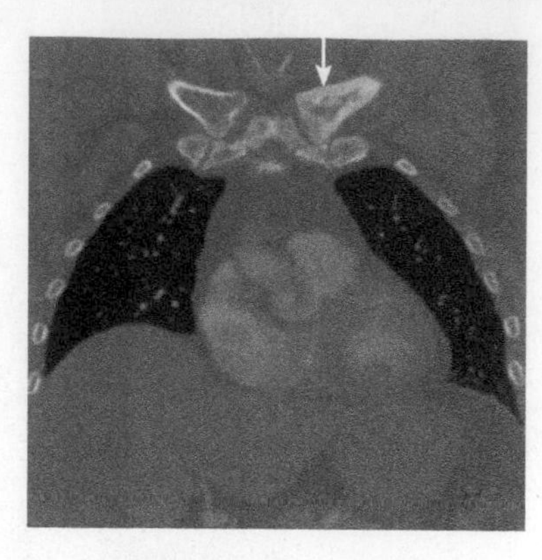

The findings (*arrow*) are better demonstrated on CT.

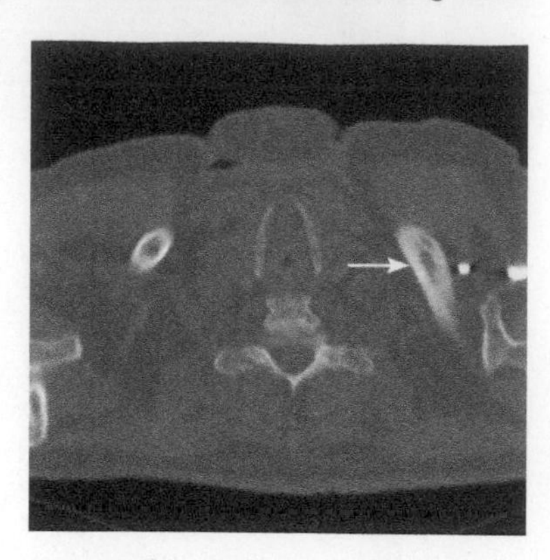

The entire left clavicle (*arrow*) is involved.

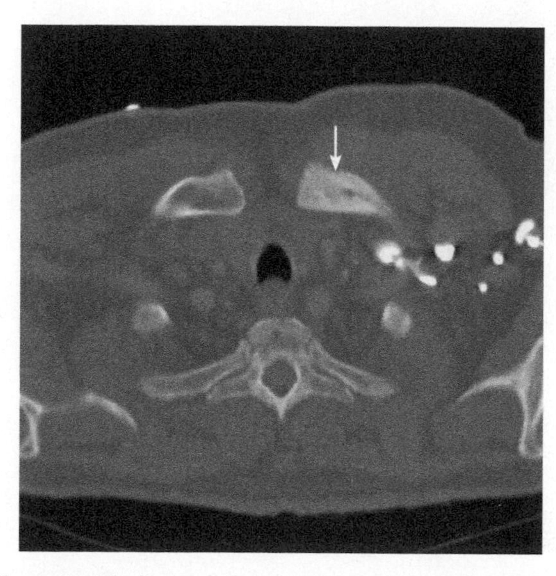

The typical findings are best appreciated medially (*arrow*).

Answers

1. Characteristic features of Paget disease include sclerosis, cortical thickening, trabecular accentuation, and enlargement of the contour of the bone.
2. Paget disease has 3 major phases: lytic, mixed, and blastic.
3. "Flame shaped," "blade of grass," "cotton-wool skull," "osteoporosis circumscripta," and "advancing osteolysis" are descriptive terms used in Paget disease.
4. Paget disease is believed to have a strong genetic component. Latent infection of osteoclasts by a paramyxovirus has also been proposed.
5. Paget disease has a predilection for the axial skeleton. The pelvis is involved in 70% of cases. Other common sites of involvement include the femur (55%), tibia (32%), lumbar spine (53%), and skull (42%).

Pearls

- Paget disease is characterized by excessive, abnormal remodelling of bone resulting in bone which is denser but structurally weaker than normal.
- The prevalence of Paget disease increases with age, especially in persons older than age 40 years, with a slight male preponderance.
- It is most common in the United Kingdom, but is also common in Australia, New Zealand, Western Europe, and the United States.
- An infectious etiology caused by latent infection of osteoclasts by a paramyxovirus has been proposed. There is a strong genetic predisposition as well.
- It is a progressive disorder with 3 major phases: lytic, mixed, and blastic.
- During the late lytic and mixed phases, osteolysis results in lucencies classically described as having a "flame-shaped" or "blade-of-grass" configuration in long bones.
- Sclerosis, cortical thickening, trabecular coarsening, and bone expansion are characteristic findings in the mixed and blastic phases.
- Complications of Paget disease include bone pain, bone deformity, fractures, and sarcomatous degeneration.
- Sarcomatous transformation is manifested by increasing pain and change in the radiologic appearance. The most common malignant transformation is to an osteosarcoma, followed by fibrosarcoma and then chondrosarcoma.

Suggested Readings

Smith SE, Murphey MD, Motamedi K, Mulligan ME, Resnik CS, Gannon FH. From the archives of the AFIP. Radiologic spectrum of Paget disease of bone and its complications with pathologic correlation. *Radiographics.* 2002;22(5):1191-1216.

Theodorou DJ, Theodorou SJ, Kakitsubata Y. Imaging of Paget disease of bone and its musculoskeletal complications: review. *AJR Am J Roentgenol.* 2011;196(6 Suppl):S64-S75.

Failure to thrive

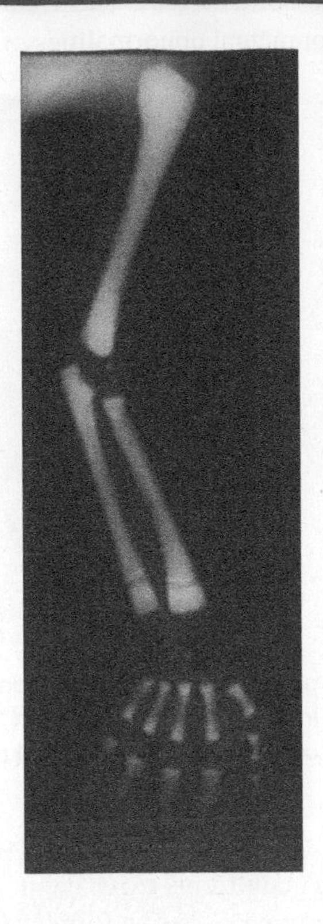

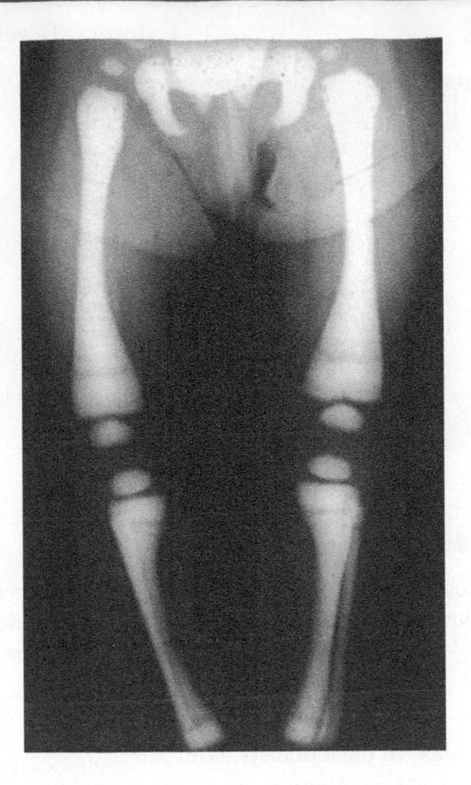

1. What are the pertinent radiologic findings?

2. What conditions are included in the differential, and what is the most likely diagnosis?

3. What is the pathogenesis for this entity?

4. Which form of the disease is most severe?

5. What are some of the complications of this entity?

Osteopetrosis 2310

Case ranking/difficulty: **Category:** Developmental abnormalities of the musculoskeletal system

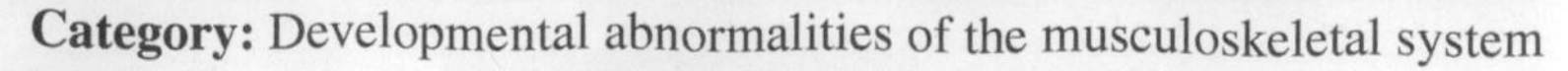

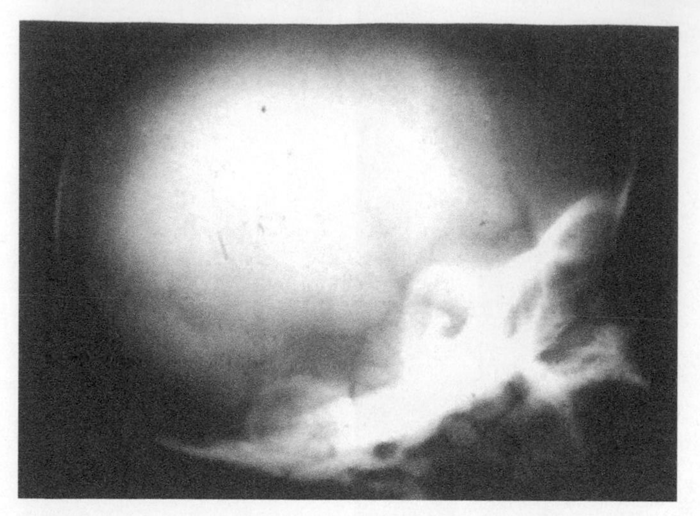

Another patient with type 2 autosomal dominant form, with increase in density of the skull base.

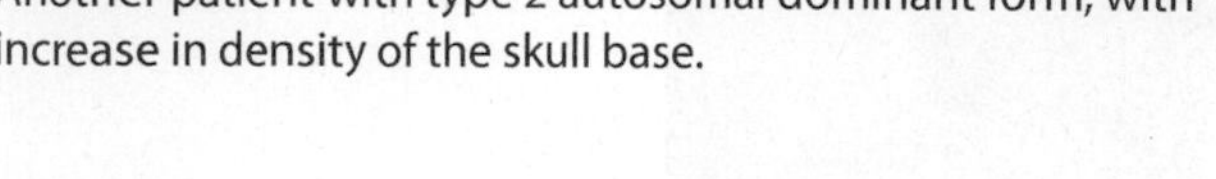

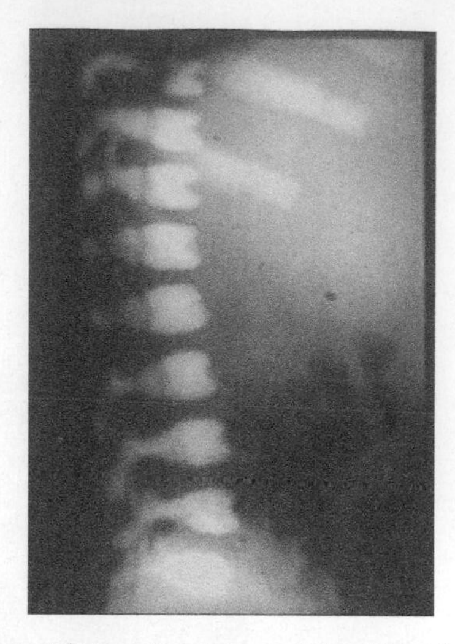

Another patient with type 2 autosomal dominant form, with increase in density of the spine and "sandwich" vertebrae. (All images courtesy of Dr. Akbar Bonakdarpour)

Answers

1. There is a generalized increase in bone density, with relative preservation of the cortices. There is an Erlenmeyer flask deformity. Although fractures are frequent, none are demonstrated here.
2. Lead toxicity, pyknodysostosis, Paget disease, osteoblastic metastasis, and osteopetrosis are all in the differential for osteosclerosis. Given the age of the patient, the most likely diagnosis is osteopetrosis.
3. Osteopetrosis is a result of a failure of osteoclasts to resorb bone.
4. The infantile autosomal recessive variant of osteopetrosis has a much higher morbidity and mortality.
5. The bones are dense in osteopetrosis, but weak. Therefore, fractures and fracture complications, such as delayed/nonunion as well as osteomyelitis, may occur. Encroachment on the medullary space may result in anemia. Other complications include nerve compression and abnormal dentition.

Pearls

- Osteopetrosis is a disease resulting from a failure of osteoclastic activity.
- There is an increase in bone density, however the bones are weaker and prone to fractures and complications of fractures.
- Two main forms exist: the more severe infantile autosomal recessive form and the milder adult autosomal dominant form.
- Adult forms may be diagnosed incidentally or with mild anemia.
- The bones are dense with medullary sclerosis and relative sparing of the cortices. Erlenmeyer flask deformity can be seen.
- Adult type 1 form shows uniform increase in bone density of the long bones, spine, and skull.
- Adult type 2 form shows the classic "bone-in-bone" appearance, with "sandwich vertebrae." The pelvis, spine, and skull base are often affected.

Suggested Readings

Ihde LL, Forrester DM, Gottsegen CJ, et al. Sclerosing bone dysplasias: review and differentiation from other causes of osteosclerosis. *Radiographics.* 2011;31(7):1865-1882.

Vanhoenacker FM, De Beuckeleer LH, Van Hul W, et al. Sclerosing bone dysplasias: genetic and radioclinical features. *Eur Radiol.* 2000;10(9):1423-1433.

Bilateral knee pain

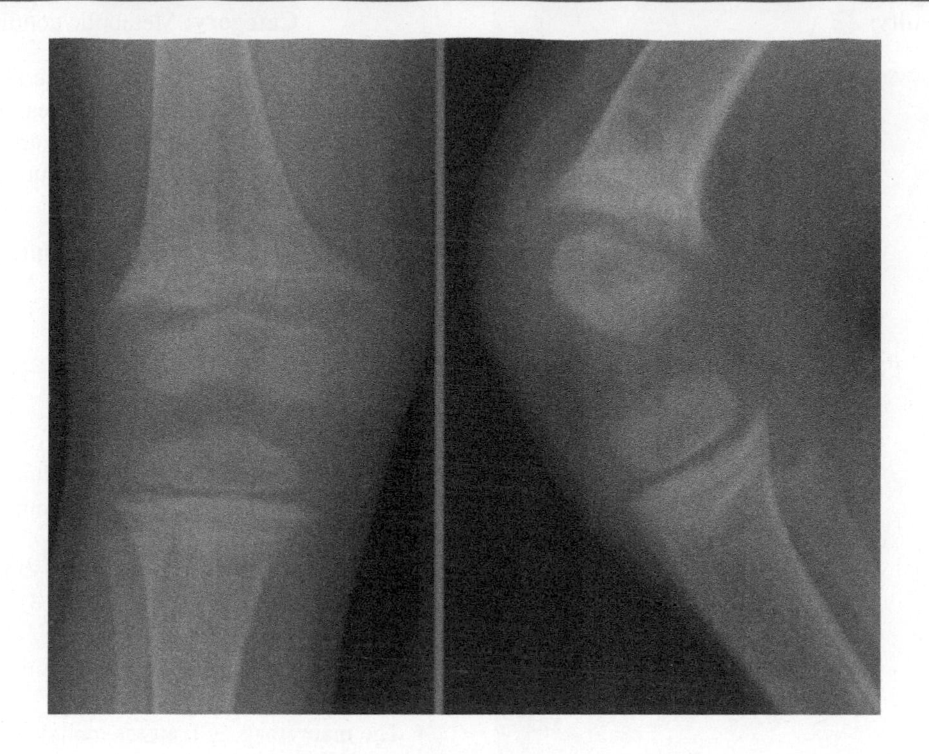

1. What are the imaging findings?

2. What is the differential diagnosis?

3. What is the diagnosis?

4. What are the other clinical and radiological features of this condition?

5. What are the main causes of this condition?

Rickets 1736

Case ranking/difficulty: 

Category: Metabolic conditions affecting bone

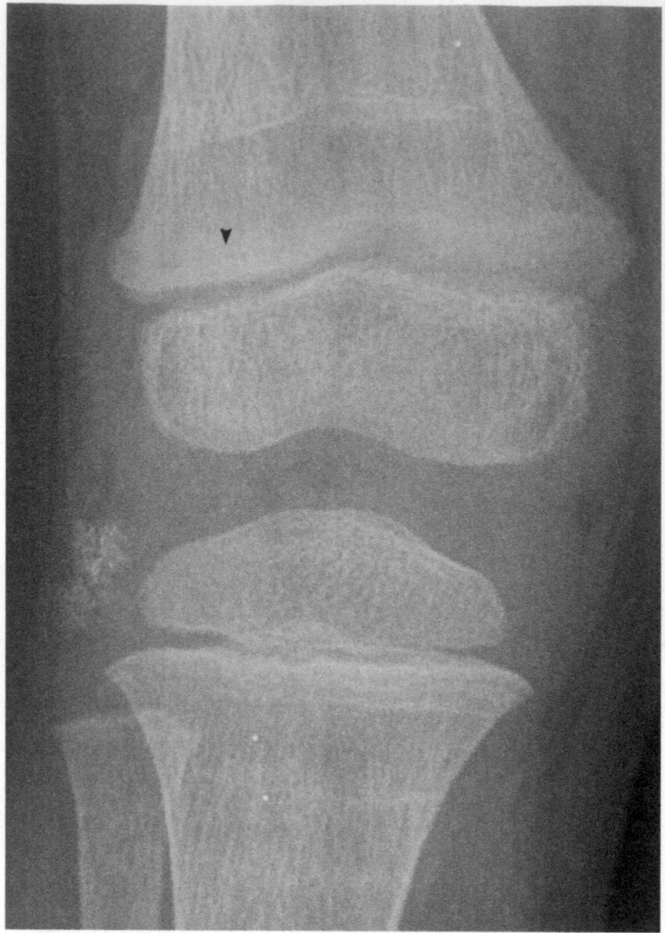

Post-treatment radiograph shows recovery with a somewhat dense metaphyseal band (*arrowhead*), a feature of treated rickets. (All images are courtesy of Dr. Akbar Bonakdarpour)

Answers

1. There is splaying, cupping and fraying of the metaphysis, and the growth plate is widened. The metaphysis is of reduced density and the cortex is indistinct.

2. The differential diagnosis includes scurvy, rickets, leukemia, and infection.

3. Mild bowing deformity of the knee with typical features of splaying, cupping, and fraying of the metaphysis and a widened growth plate, suggests the diagnosis of rickets.

4. In rickets, associated deformities of bones include bowing of long bones, triradiate pelvis, scoliosis, biconcave vertebrae, and basilar invagination. There can be a Harrison sulcus as a result of indrawing of the lower part of the chest wall. Flattening of the occiput and prominence of the frontal and parietal regions due to an accumulation of osteoid, leads to the craniotabes appearance of the skull.

5. Reduced dietary intake or increased loss because of malabsorption syndromes, diarrhea, or vomiting can lead to rickets. Breastfeeding children are also more likely to get rickets. Liver and renal failure are also important causes.

   Hypophosphatemia, either congenital or acquired, can result in rickets.

Pearls

- Rickets is caused by a deficiency of vitamin D, phosphorus, magnesium, or calcium. It is rare in developed countries and more common in developing countries.
- Rickets is classified as nutritional, vitamin D deficient, vitamin D resistant, and congenital.
- The main causes include decreased dietary intake, malabsorption, diarrhea, and vomiting. Liver and renal failure can also lead to rickets.
- The main imaging features include widening of the growth plate, fraying, splaying, and cupping of the metaphysis. The density of the metaphysis is reduced, and the cortex is indistinct because of accumulation of subperiosteal osteoid.
- There can be a "rickety rosary" appearance of the ribs, which may be a result of fracturing of the zone of provisional calcification during respiration, with or without a Harrison sulcus.
- Looser transformation zones are uncommon in children.
- Bone softening and accumulation of osteoid leads to associated deformities of bone, including bowing of long bones, triradiate pelvis, scoliosis, biconcave vertebrae, basilar invagination, and craniotabes.
- Healed rickets may result in dense metaphyseal bands.

Suggested Readings

Ecklund K, Doria AS, Jaramillo D. Rickets on MR images. *Pediatr Radiol.* 1999;29(9):673-675.

Nield LS, Mahajan P, Joshi A, Kamat D. Rickets: not a disease of the past. *Am Fam Physician.* 2006;74(4):619-626.

Chronic back pain

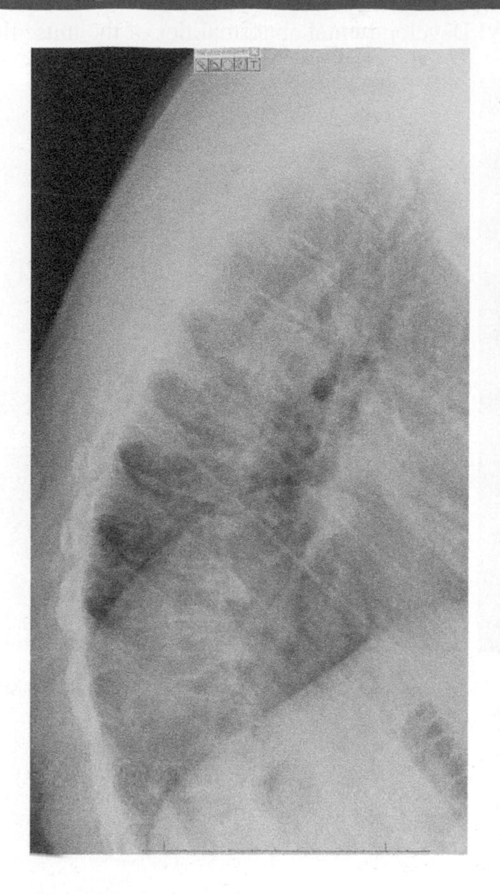

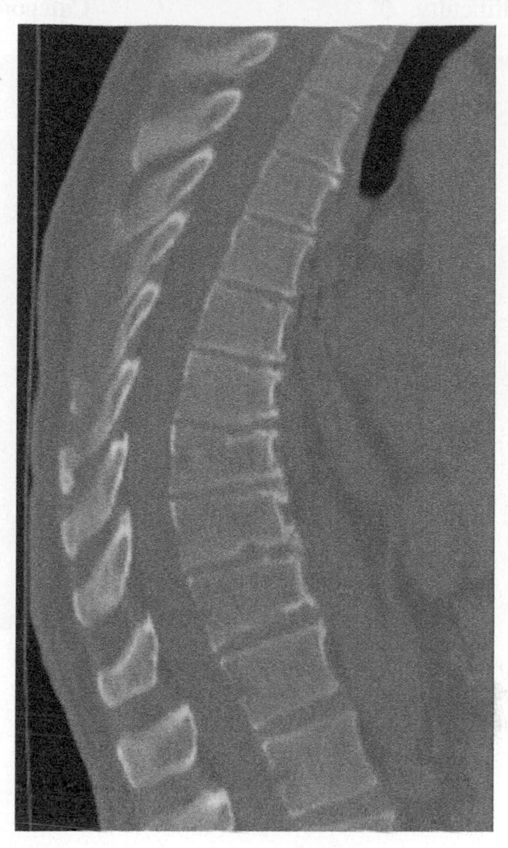

1. What are the radiograph and CT findings?

2. What is the differential diagnosis?

3. What is the most likely diagnosis?

4. How does the type 2 variant of this condition differ from type 1?

5. What are some of the associations of this entity?

Scheuermann disease 1452

Case ranking/difficulty:  **Category:** Developmental abnormalities of the musculoskeletal system

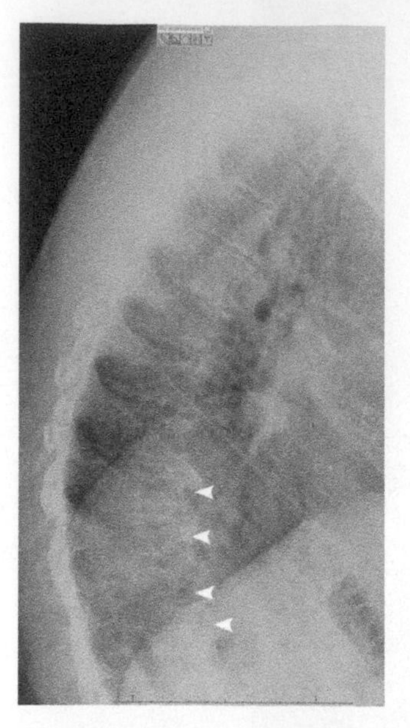

Lower thoracic kyphosis with multiple Schmorl nodes and increased AP diameter of the vertebrae.

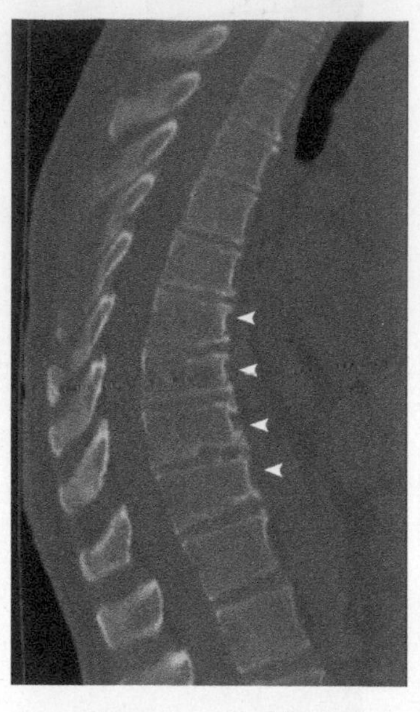

Four affected vertebral bodies from T8 to T11.

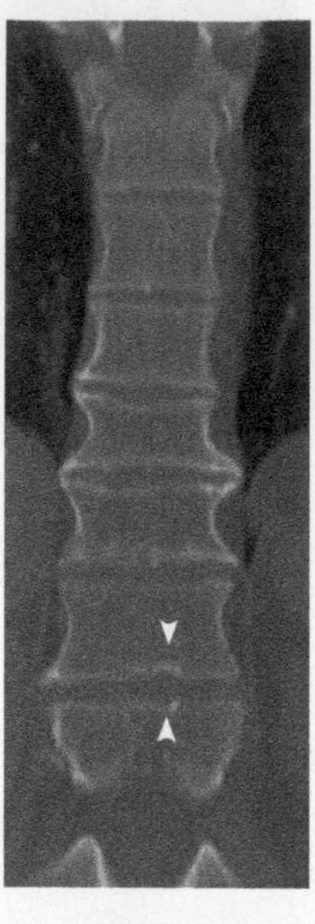

Multiple Schmorl nodes.

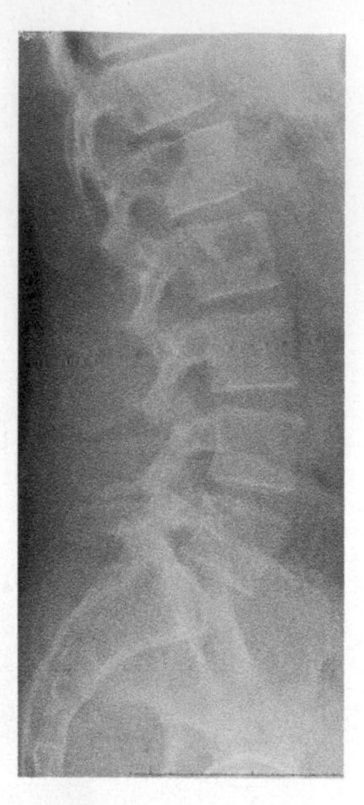

Lumbar spine is unaffected.

Answers

1. Lower thoracic kyphosis, multiple Schmorl nodes, increased diameter of the vertebral bodies with mild wedging, and involvement of 4 contiguous vertebrae.
2. Scheuermann disease, neurofibromatosis, postradiation scoliosis, and congenital kyphoscoliosis.
3. Given the imaging findings, the most likely diagnosis is Scheuermann disease.
4. Type 2 Scheuermann disease is characterized by disc space narrowing, anterior Schmorl nodes, involvement of less than 3 vertebral bodies, and normal vertebral body height and width.
5. Left-handedness, above average weight and height for age, family history, and spondylolysis or spondylolisthesis are associated with Scheuermann disease.

Pearls

- Scheuermann disease is an osteochondrosis of the secondary ossification centers of the spine.
- The lower thoracic and upper lumbar spine are most affected.
- AP and lateral standing radiographs are required.
- The classic or type 1 form is characterized by involvement of at least 3 contiguous vertebral bodies, wedging of greater than 5 degrees, kyphosis greater than 40 degrees, and multiple Schmorl nodes.
- Atypical or type 2 disease is characterized by involvement of only 1 or 2 bodies, anterior Schmorl nodes and disc space narrowing. The bodies are not wedged.
- MRI may be helpful in preoperative planning.

Suggested Readings

Gustavel M, Beals RK. Scheuermann's disease of the lumbar spine in identical twins. *AJR Am J Roentgenol.* 2002;179(4):1078-1079.

Wood KB, Melikian R, Villamil F. Adult Scheuermann kyphosis: evaluation, management, and new developments. *J Am Acad Orthop Surg.* 2012;20(2):113-121.

Chronic foot pain

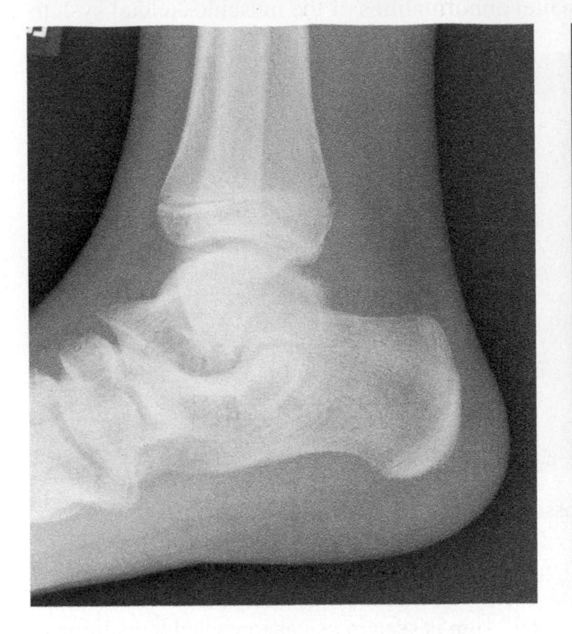

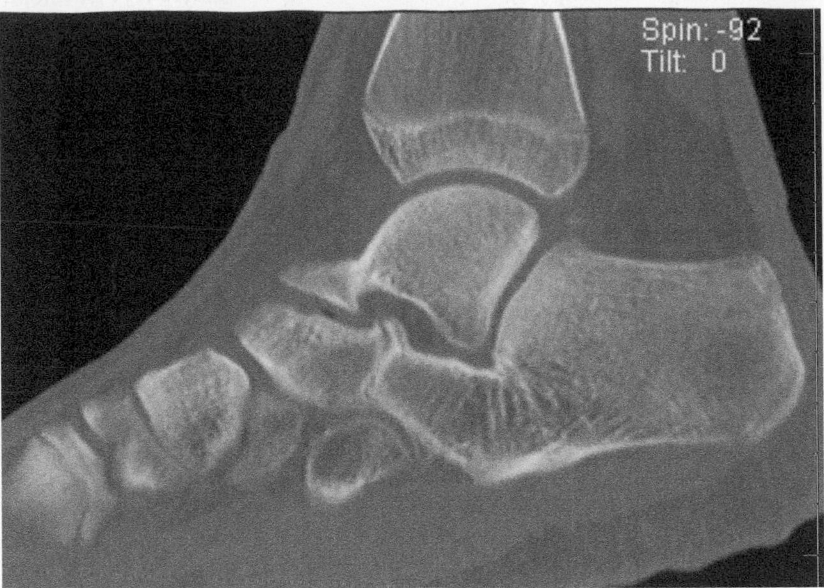

1. What are the plain radiograph findings?

2. What is the classic age of presentation of this finding?

3. What is the most common form of this entity?

4. What signs characterize this entity?

5. This entity is bilateral in what percentage of patients?

Nonosseous calcaneonavicular coalition 1320

Case ranking/difficulty: 

Category: Developmental abnormalities of the musculoskeletal system

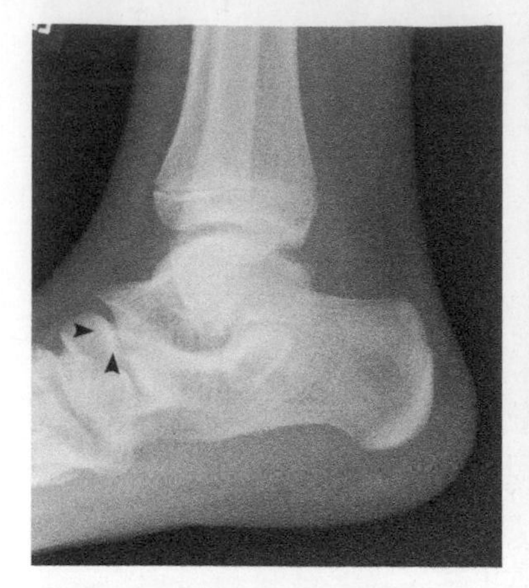

The anterior calcaneal process is broad and irregular, overlapping the navicular (anteater sign).

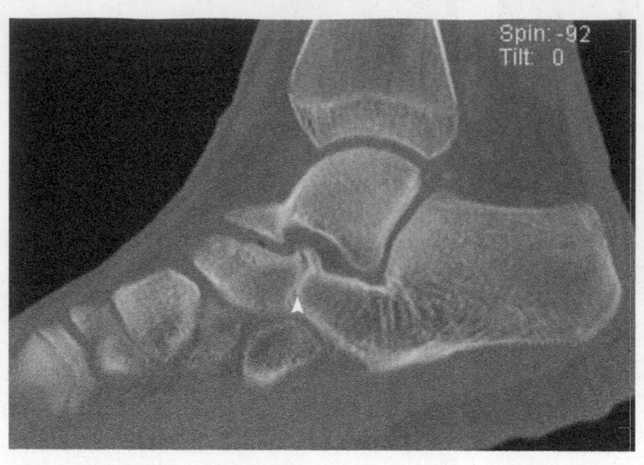

Sagittal reformatted image shows the nonosseous calcaneonavicular coalition.

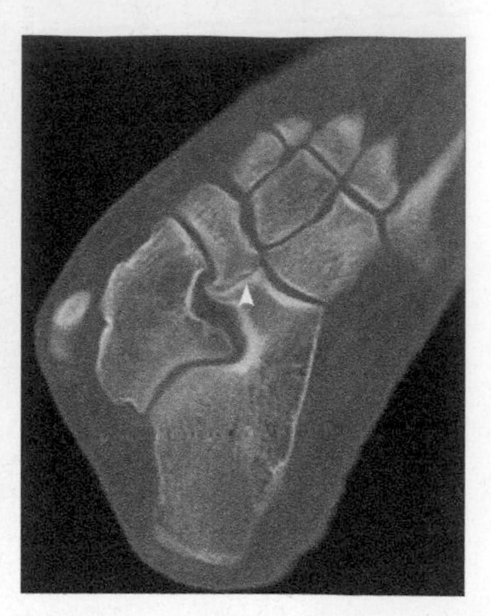

Oblique axial image shows the nonosseous coalition.

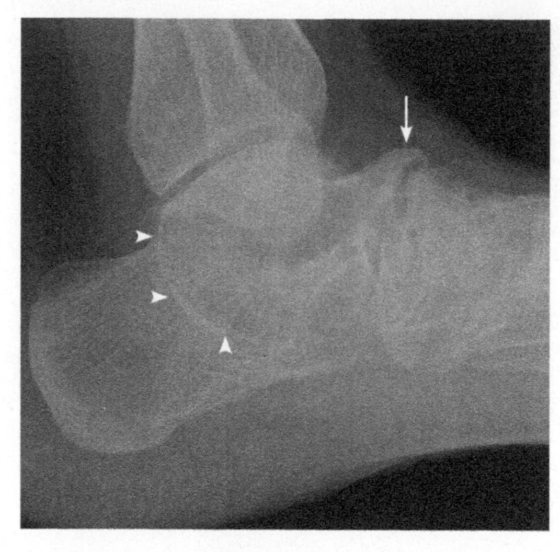

Continuous "C" sign (*arrowheads*) and talar beak (*arrow*) in another patient with a subtalar joint coalition.

Answers

1. The "anteater" sign is characteristic of a calcaneonavicular coalition. It is a broad irregular elongated anterior calcaneal process that overlaps the navicular on the lateral film.
2. Symptoms often correspond to ossification, either partial or complete. In calcaneonavicular coalition, this is at 8 to 12 years.
3. Calcaneonavicular coalitions are the most common coalitions.
4. The "anteater" sign is seen in calcaneonavicular coalitions.

   Talocalcaneal coalitions are characterized by a continuous "C" sign if osseous, and by a talar beak caused by abnormal traction on the talonavicular ligament.
5. Coalitions are typically bilateral in 40% to 60% of patients.

Pearls

- The most common coalition is a calcaneonavicular coalition.
- Coalitions may be osseous, fibrous, or cartilaginous.
- Classic sign for calcaneonavicular coalition is the "anteater" sign.
- This sign is a broad elongated anterior calcaneal process that overlaps the navicular on a lateral film.
- Classic age of presentation is 8 to 12 years for calcaneonavicular coalition.
- Coalitions are bilateral in 40% to 60%.
- Talocalcaneal coalitions demonstrate the continuous "C" sign, and a nonspecific talar "beak."

Suggested Readings

Nalaboff KM, Schweitzer ME. MRI of tarsal coalition: frequency, distribution, and innovative signs. *Bull NYU Hosp Jt Dis.* 2008;66(1):14-21.

Newman JS, Newberg AH. Congenital tarsal coalition: multimodality evaluation with emphasis on CT and MR imaging. *Radiographics.* 2000;20(2):321-332; quiz 526-527, 532.

Knee pain

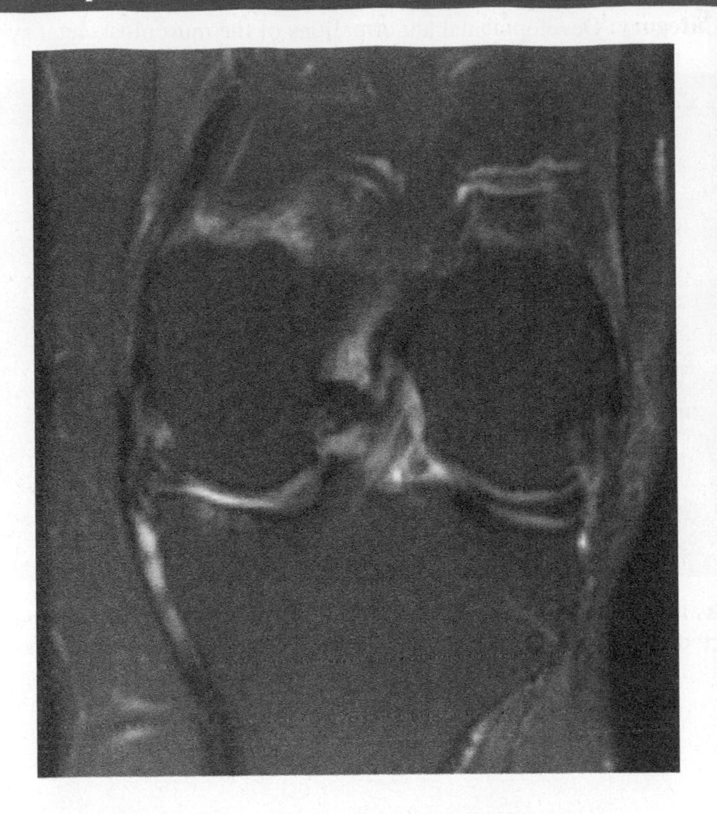

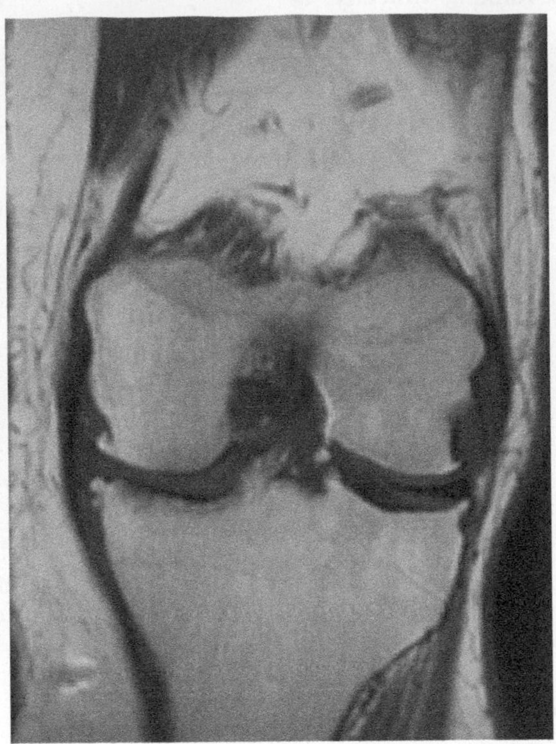

1. What is the abnormality on MRI?
2. What are the different varieties of this abnormality?
3. What is the abnormality seen in the Wrisberg variant?
4. What are the criteria used to diagnose complete and incomplete variants of this entity on MRI?
5. What is the management for this condition?

Discoid lateral meniscus 1410

Case ranking/difficulty: ✱ **Category:** Developmental abnormalities of the musculoskeletal system

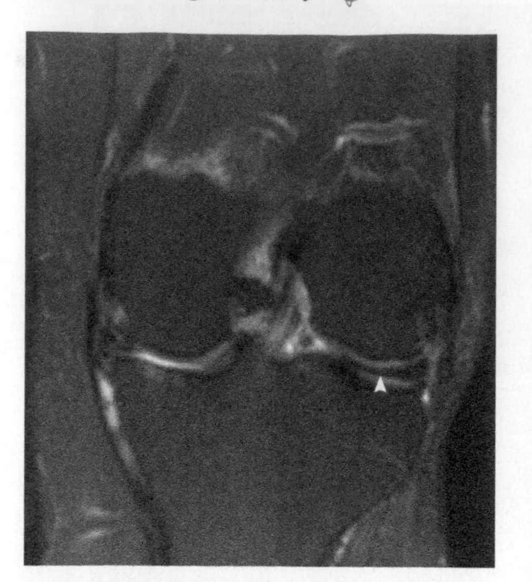

There is a slab-like appearance to the lateral meniscus (*arrowhead*). Medial osteoarthritis and tear of the medial meniscus body is also seen.

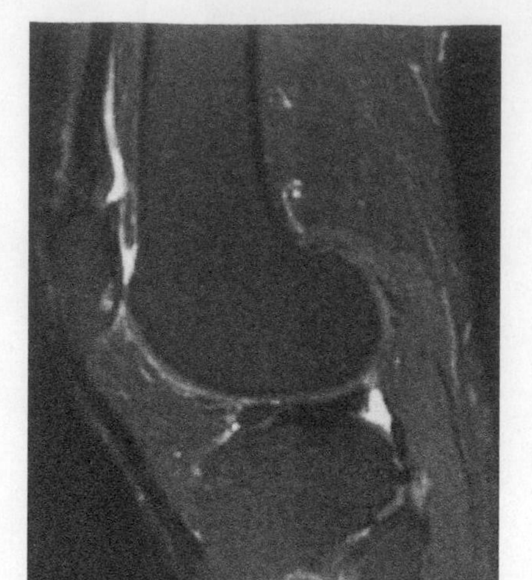

Meniscal tissue extends more medially than expected, or too many "bowties."

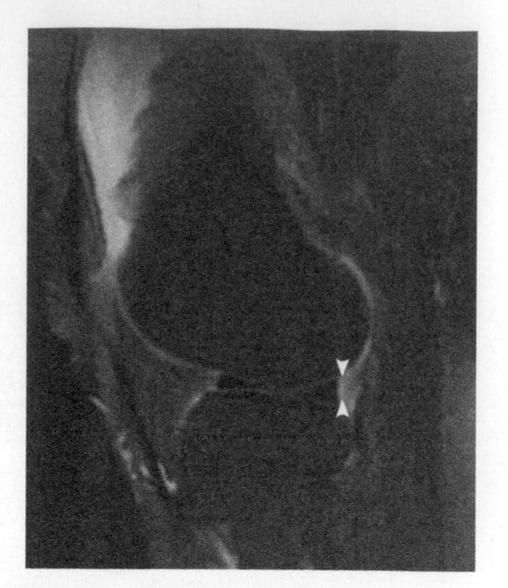

Another patient with Wrisberg variant of discoid lateral meniscus. Note absence of posterior attachments (*arrowheads*).

Answers

1. There is a slab-like lateral meniscus, consistent with an incomplete discoid lateral meniscus.
2. Watanabe classified discoid menisci into 3 types: complete, incomplete, and Wrisberg type.
3. A Wrisberg-type discoid lateral meniscus is characterized by an absent meniscotibial ligament and absent popliteomeniscal fascicles.
4. The criteria used to diagnose discoid menisci include more than 3 "bowties" on sagittal MR images, >20% ratio of meniscus to tibia on the coronal image, and a minimum meniscal diameter of 14 to 15 mm on a midcoronal image. Also used is 75% for the ratio of the sum of the width of the anterior and posterior horns to the meniscal diameter, on a sagittal slice that shows a maximum meniscal diameter.
5. Asymptomatic discoid menisci may be left alone. Treatment for symptomatic cases is to excise the meniscal tissue, leaving a rim measuring 6 to 7 mm circumferentially. Complete meniscectomy can be performed for a Wrisberg type.

Pearls

Discoid menisci are uncommon developmental variants that most commonly affect the lateral meniscus. Medial discoid menisci are rare.

They are frequently bilateral.

Three main types have been described by Watanabe:

- Type 1: A complete slab of meniscal tissue with complete tibial coverage.
- Type 2: An incomplete slab of meniscal tissue with 80% coverage of the lateral tibial plateau.
- Type 3: The Wrisberg variant, where the meniscus may have a normal morphology or is mildly hypertrophic but lacks its posterior attachments, that is, the meniscotibial ligament and meniscal fascicles, and is hypermobile.

MRI criteria for the more common complete and incomplete discoid menisci include more than 3 "bowties" on sagittal images and >20% coverage of the tibia on coronal images.

Treatment is with partial meniscal excision, with an attempt to maintain the morphology of a normal meniscus.

Suggested Readings

Rohren EM, Kosarek FJ, Helms CA. Discoid lateral meniscus and the frequency of meniscal tears. *Skeletal Radiol.* 2001;30(6):316-320.

Singh K, Helms CA, Jacobs MT, Higgins LD. MRI appearance of Wrisberg variant of discoid lateral meniscus. *AJR Am J Roentgenol.* 2006;187(2):384-387.

History of chronic neck pain

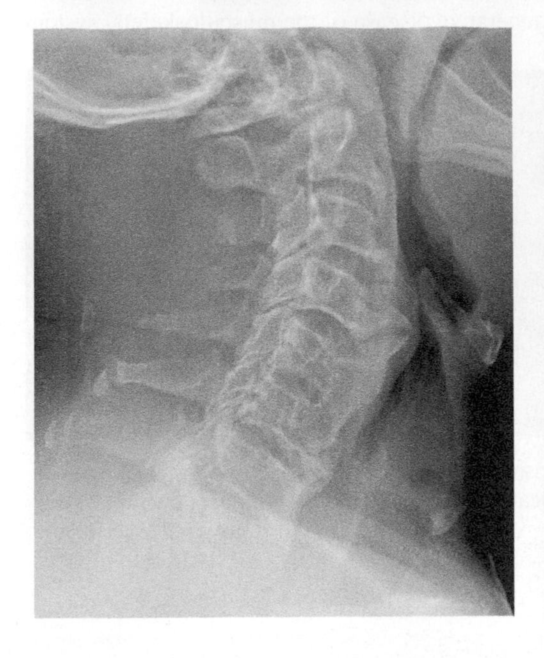

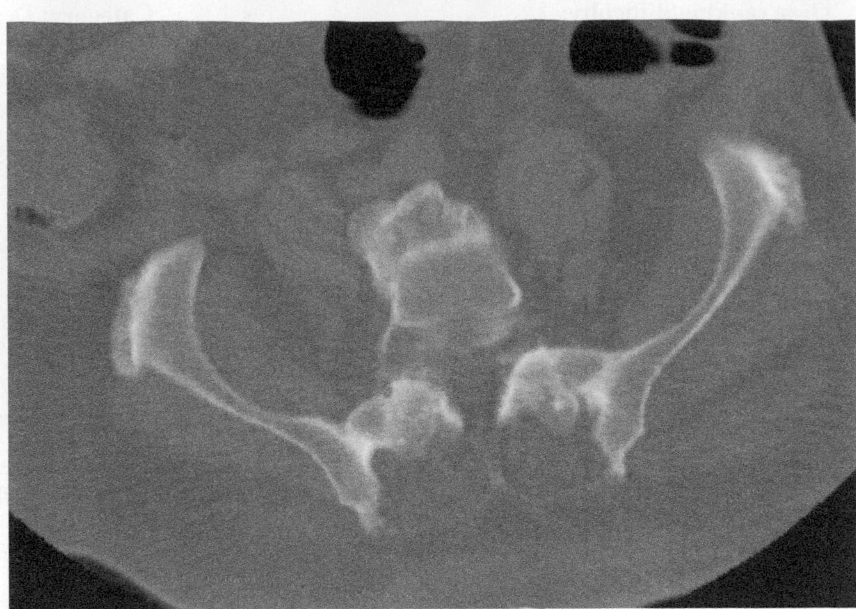

1. What are the radiograph findings?

2. What are included in the differential diagnosis?

3. What is the most commonly affected location in this disease?

4. What are important associations of this condition?

5. What is the management?

Diffuse idiopathic skeletal hyperostosis (DISH) 1343

Case ranking/difficulty: 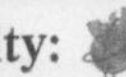

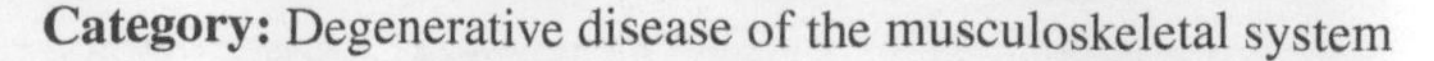

Category: Degenerative disease of the musculoskeletal system

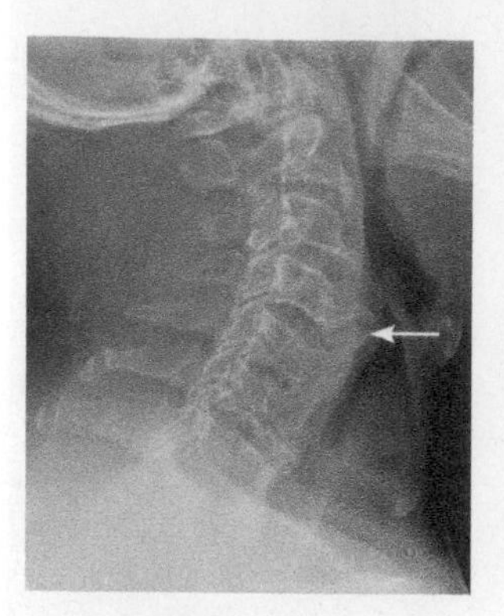

There is extensive anterior ossification, with preservation of the disk heights.

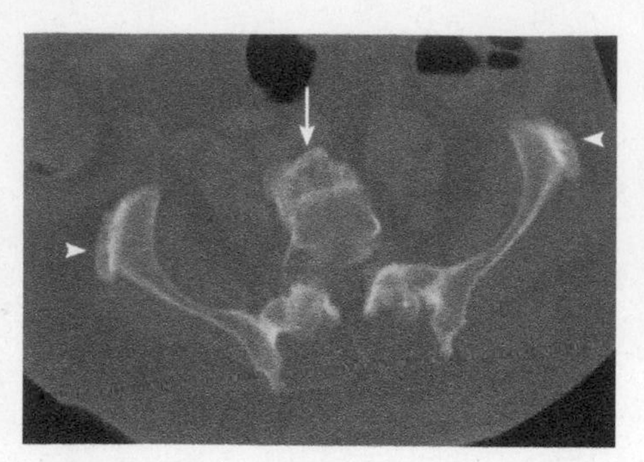

Extensive paraspinal ossification, and prominent enthesophytes at the iliac crests (*arrowheads*).

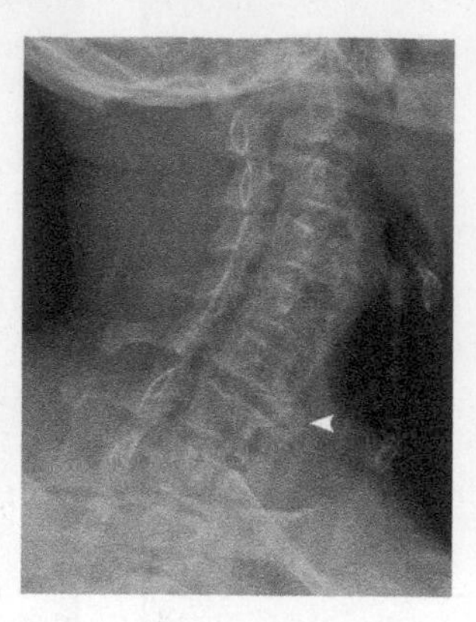

Extensive anterior ossification is again seen.

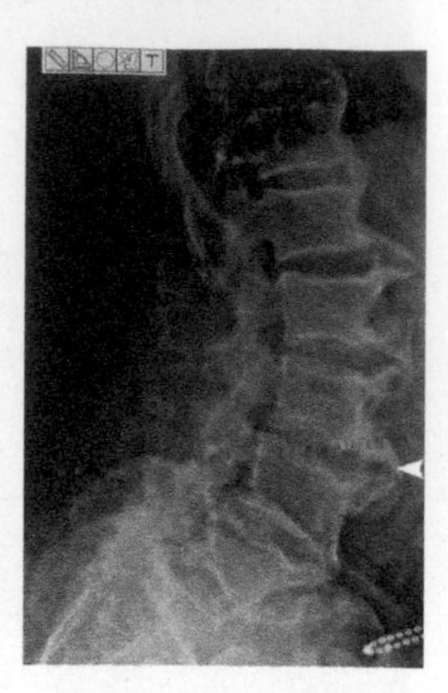

Lumbar spine shows similar flowing paraspinal ossification.

Answers

1. There is flowing paraspinal ossification involving more than 4 contiguous levels. A faint lucent line can usually be seen between the inferior vertebral bodies and the ossification in DISH but is not demonstrated in this case. There is enthesopathy at the C6 and C7 spinous processes and nuchal ligament ossification.

2. The flowing paraspinal nature of this ossification involving more than four contiguous levels is typical for DISH.

   Ankylosing spondylitis has smaller syndesmophytes with SI joint involvement, and degenerative disc disease would cause disc space narrowing. Fluorosis would cause increased bone density, and in acromegaly, the ossification does not have a flowing configuration and the disc heights may be increased.

3. DISH most commonly affects the thoracic spine, less commonly the cervical and lumbar spine and entheses.

4. Ossification of the posterior longitudinal ligament (OPLL), hyperostosis frontalis interna, ossification of the vertebral arch ligaments (OVAL), ossification of the stylohyoid ligament (Eagle syndrome), and heterotopic ossification are all recognized associations of DISH.

5. The vast majority of DISH cases are asymptomatic, and require no treatment. If there is pain and limitation of movement, then physical therapy and analgesia are indicated. In the rare cases of symptomatic compression of the esophagus, bronchus, IVC, or spinal cord, surgical decompression may be indicated.

Pearls

- DISH is most common in white men older than 50 years.
- It is characterized by flowing paraspinal ossification affecting at least four contiguous vertebral levels, with preserved discs and SI joints.
- The thoracic spine is most commonly affected, with the left side spared presumably by aortic pulsation.
- It is asymptomatic but may cause compression of the esophagus, bronchus, or IVC.
- It is associated with OPLL, OVAL, and hyperostosis frontalis interna.
- There is an increased risk of heterotopic ossification in the surgical bed, and perioperative radiation to the operative bed in individuals with DISH may be indicated in procedures such as a joint arthroplasty.

Suggested Readings

Resnick D, Guerra J, Robinson CA, Vint VC. Association of diffuse idiopathic skeletal hyperostosis (DISH) and calcification and ossification of the posterior longitudinal ligament. *AJR Am J Roentgenol.* 1978;131(6):1049–1053.

Taljanovic MS, Hunter TB, Wisneski RJ, et al. Imaging characteristics of diffuse idiopathic skeletal hyperostosis with an emphasis on acute spinal fractures: review. *AJR Am J Roentgenol.* 2009;193(3 Suppl):S10–S19, quiz S20–S24.

Incidental finding on CT head scan

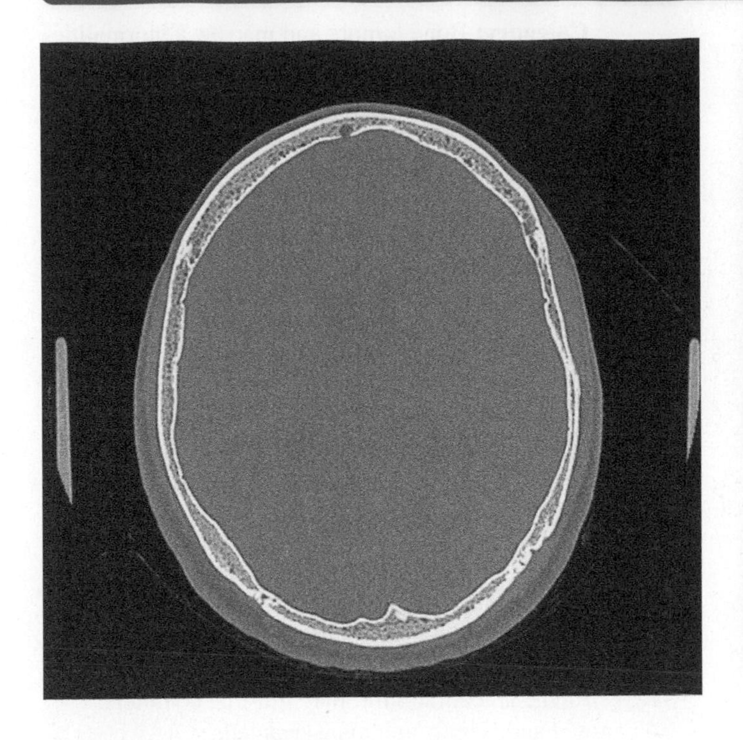

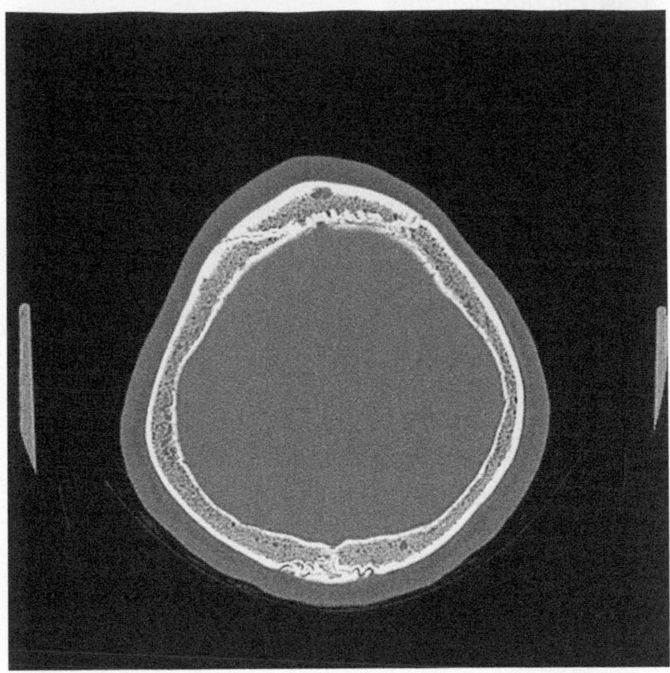

1. What is the differential diagnosis?
2. Where are these lesions commonly found?
3. What is the treatment for this entity?
4. What are the imaging features of this entity on MRI?
5. In which age group(s) is this entity more common?

Multiple lytic lesions of skull—pacchionian granulations 1836

Case ranking/difficulty:

Category: Bone tumors and marrow abnormalities

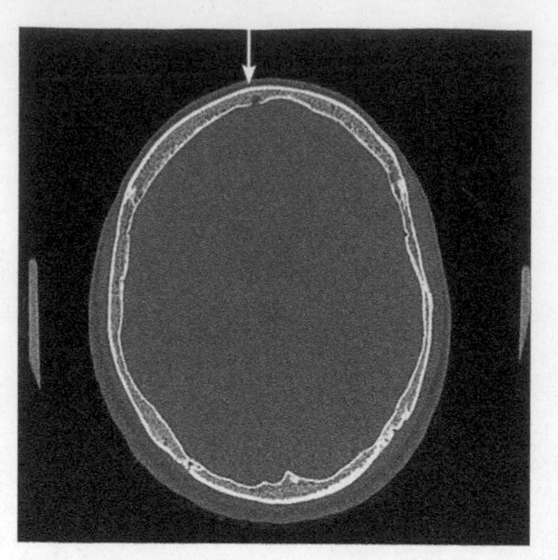

Lytic lesion in midline of frontal bone.

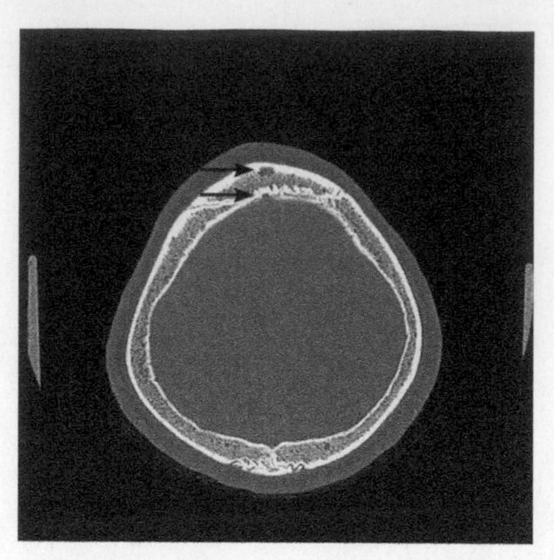

Two benign lytic lesions in midline of frontal bone consistent with arachnoid granulations.

Answers

1. The differential diagnoses of pacchionian granulations includes other causes of skull lytic lesions. However, the key distinguishing feature is the parasagittal location along the expected course of the superior sagittal sinus and accordingly arachnoid villi.
2. Pacchionian granulations are extrinsic erosions of the skull from hypertrophic arachnoid villi. They are not intrinsic lesions of bone. Consequently, they are found along the distribution of the arachnoid villi.
3. No treatment is required as arachnoid granulations are normal structures.
4. Pacchionian granulations have signal characteristics related to CSF (low T1, low FLAIR, high T2). There is free diffusion.
5. There is an increase in prevalence of arachnoid granulations with age, up to a peak in the seventh decade of life.

Pearls

- Pacchionian granulations are found in a parasagittal distribution along the course of the superior sagittal sinus and less frequently other dural venous sinuses.
- They must be considered in the differential diagnosis of parasagittal calvarial lytic lesions.
- As they are merely erosions of the skull from hypertrophic arachnoid villi, they must be confidently diagnosed and no treatment is warranted.
- Imaging characteristics are identical to CSF—that is, low T1, high STIR signal on MRI, and low attenuation on CT.
- The lesions increase in prevalence with age, being most common in the seventh decade of life. Accordingly, they should not generally be diagnosed in pediatric patients.

Suggested Readings

Schmalfuss IM, Camp M. Skull base: pseudolesion or true lesion? *Eur Radiol.* 2008;18(6):1232–1243.

VandeVyver V, Lemmerling M, De Foer B, Casselman J, Verstraete K. Arachnoid granulations of the posterior temporal bone wall: imaging appearance and differential diagnosis. *AJNR Am J Neuroradiol.* 2007;28(4):610–612.

Painful hip

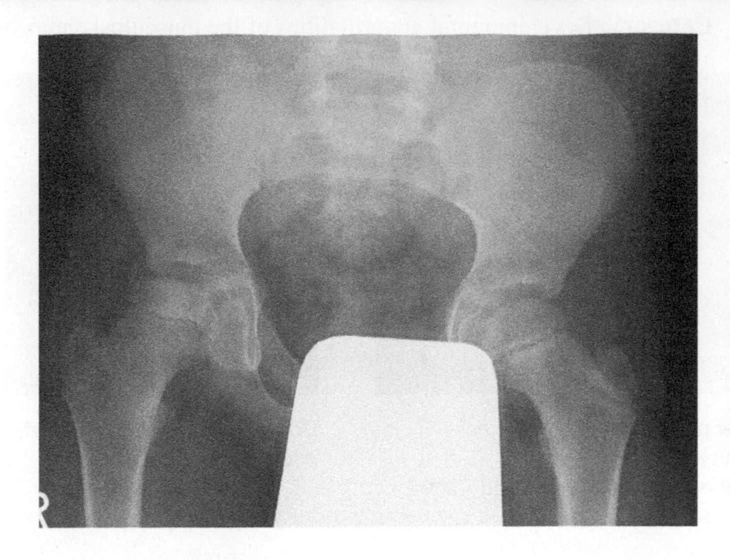

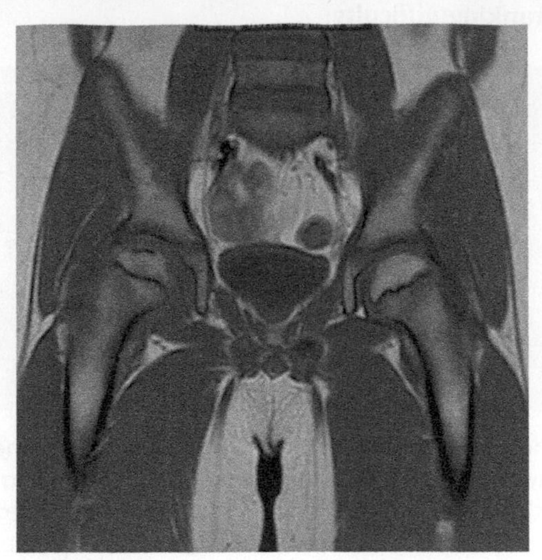

1. What are the radiographic findings?

2. What are the expected MRI findings?

3. What is the most likely diagnosis?

4. What is a double-line sign on MRI?

5. What are the patient demographics of this entity?

Legg-Calve-Perthes disease 1735

Case ranking/difficulty: **Category:** Developmental abnormalities of the musculoskeletal system

Frog lateral view shows the small physeal plate on right side (*arrowhead*), with a slightly sclerotic epiphysis.

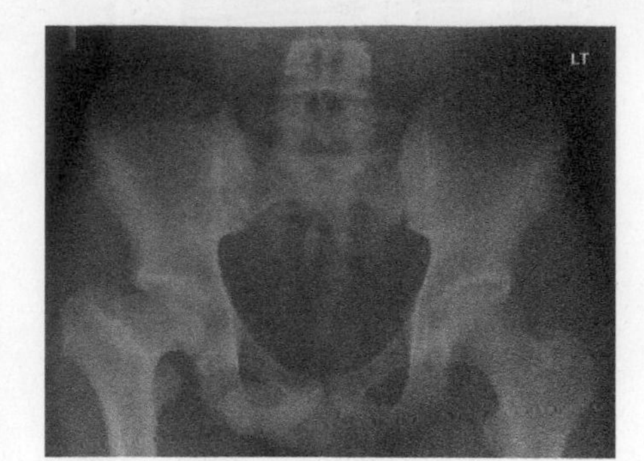

Another patient with coxa magna deformity of the right hip as a consequence of childhood Legg-Calve-Perthes disease.

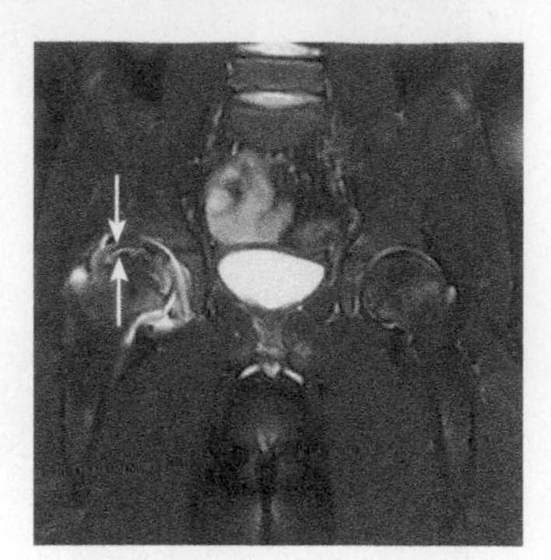

Double-line sign (*arrows*) with edema and effusion.

Answers

1. There is epiphyseal sclerosis, metaphyseal rarefaction, blurring of the physeal plate, reduced physeal plate height and a subchondral fracture.
2. Low T1 and high T2 marrow signal with a small subchondral fracture. There is also a "double-line sign" with outer low T1 and T2 signal, inner high T2 signal line, and a joint effusion.
3. Based on the clinical and radiologic features, the most likely diagnosis is Legg-Calve-Perthes disease.
4. An outer low signal intensity line of sclerosis and inner high signal intensity line because of granulation tissue on T2-weighted images is called the "double-line" sign. Some authors suggest it may also be partly a result of chemical shift artifact.
5. Legg-Calve-Perthes disease is most common among white male children, ages 4 to 12 years.

Pearls

- Legg-Calve-Perthes disease is idiopathic avascular necrosis of the femoral epiphysis, most commonly seen in boys 4 to 12 years of age.
- There are four stages of the disease: early, fragmentation, reparative, and healing.
- In the early stages, there is a reduction in the femoral epiphyseal size with sclerosis, joint effusion, ipsilateral reduced mineralization of bones, and blurring of the physeal plate.
- In the later stages, there is fragmentation of the femoral head, subchondral lucency and fracture. These changes are best seen on a lateral radiograph.
- The advanced reparative and healing stage of disease shows evidence of coxa plana or coxa magna on plain radiographs.
- T1 MRI shows a small femoral epiphysis with irregularity. STIR image of the hip will show an increased signal in the epiphysis with irregularity. There can be a "double-line" sign with a high signal line inside and a low signal line peripherally. Effusions may be present. In the later stages, the T2 signal may decrease.
- An "asterisk" sign may be present on CT and MRI, with thin sclerotic ray-like branching bands from a central dense band of thickened bony trabeculae, an early sign of this entity.
- MRI has the advantage of detecting early disease, assessing cartilaginous involvement and the degree of acetabular coverage.
- It is usually treated with traction, braces, and physiotherapy.

Suggested Readings

Dillman JR, Hernandez RJ. MRI of Legg-Calve-Perthes disease. *AJR Am J Roentgenol.* 2009;193(5):1394–1407.

Gross GW, Articolo GA, Bowen JR. Legg-Calve-Perthes disease: imaging evaluation and management. *Semin Musculoskelet Radiol.* 1999;3(4):379–391.

Hosalkar HS, Mulpuri K. Legg-Calvé-Perthes disease: where do we stand after 100 years? Editorial comment. *Clin Orthop Relat Res.* 2012;470(9):2345–2346.

Pain in left hip in a patient taking steroids

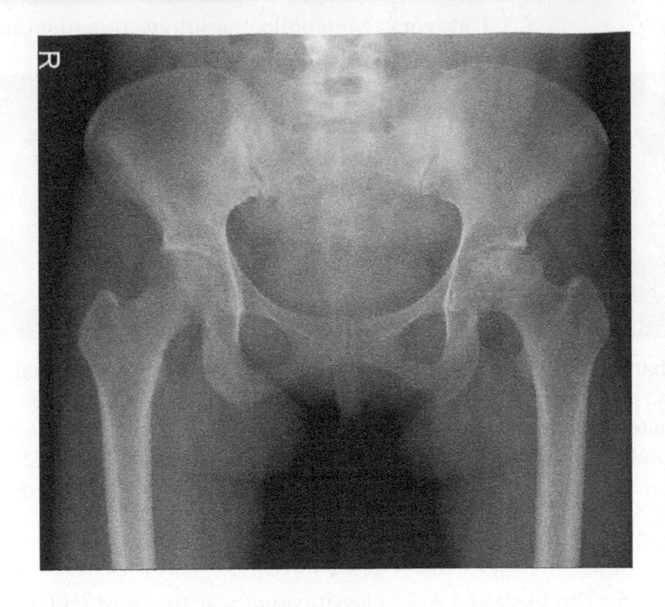

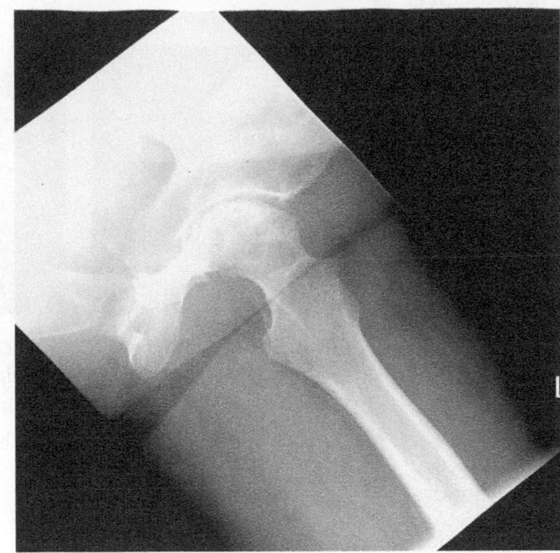

1. What is the most likely diagnosis?

2. What are recognized risk factors for this entity?

3. What are the characteristic radiographic and MRI features?

4. What is the imaging investigative modality of choice?

5. What are the names of staging systems to describe this entity?

Case ranking/difficulty: 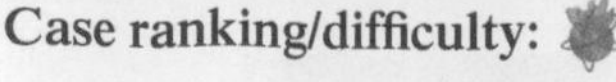

Category: Metabolic conditions affecting bone

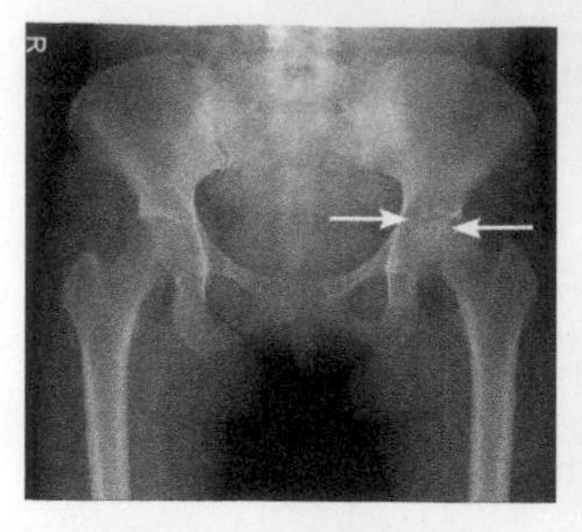

Established AVN of left femoral head with secondary osteoarthritis (stage 5). Crescentic lucencies are seen in weight-bearing surface consistent with subchondral fractures.

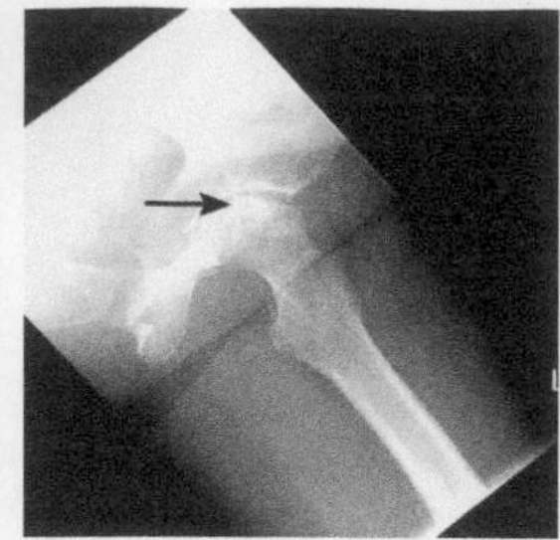

Contour abnormality, flattening, and loss of joint space (stage 5).

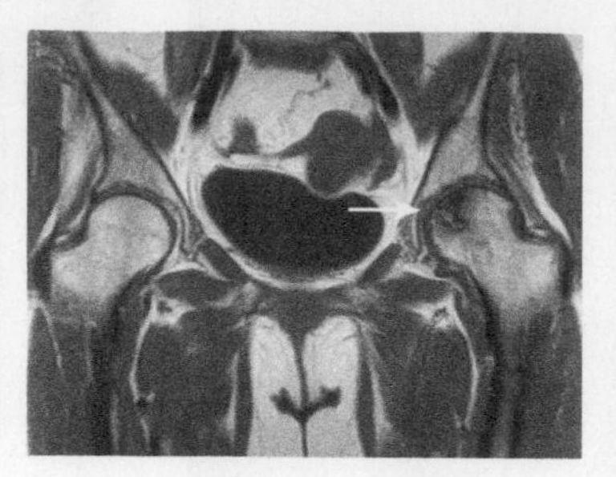

Early changes of left hip AVN showing crescentic low T1-marginated lesions prior to subchondral fracture.

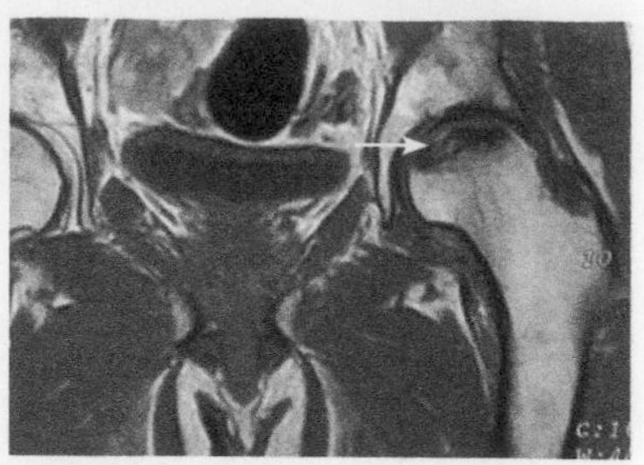

Established AVN with subchondral fracture and collapse of the weight-bearing surface of the femoral head, in conjunction with low T1 and T2 signal consistent with established, irreversible sclerosis.

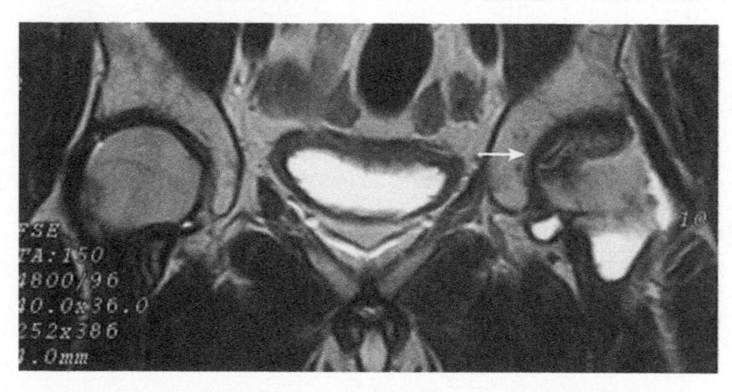

Established AVN with subchondral fracture and collapse of the weight-bearing surface of the femoral head, in conjunction with low T1 and T2 signal consistent with established, irreversible sclerosis.

Answers

1. Avascular necrosis (AVN) can be unilateral or bilateral; however in systemic disorders such as sickle cell disease, the changes are likely to be more symmetrical and there may be generalized sclerosis secondary to multiple medullary infarcts.
2. There are many risk factors for AVN, including trauma, steroids, alcohol, Caisson disease, SLE, and sickle cell disease.
3. AVN results in dead bone interspersed with poor new bone mineralization along dead trabeculae. The weakened bone matrix leads to multiple subchondral insufficiency fractures (crescentic lucencies) at weight-bearing surfaces, and ultimately flattening and deformity.

   The granulation tissue/sclerotic bone interface on MRI gives the "double-line" sign.
4. Although the diagnosis can be made on plain films, the earliest changes are detectable on MRI with loss of the normal marrow signal.
5. The Ficat and Arlet classification was the most widely used system based on radiographic findings alone. Steinberg's staging system includes MRI, scintigraphy, and clinical findings.

Pearls

- AVN is most common in the femoral head secondary to trauma, especially subcapital fractures.
- Other common causes include steroid treatment, alcohol, SLE, and sickle cell disease.
- Early diagnosis and treatment (removal of predisposing cause) is important to prevent complications, for example, deformity and osteoarthritis.
- MRI is the investigative modality of choice and detects marrow signal abnormality before the radiographic features of lucency, sclerosis, and subchondral fractures.
- A typical feature on MRI is the "double-line" sign, formed by the interface of inner (high signal intensity) granulation tissue with outer (low signal intensity) sclerotic bone.

Suggested Readings

Aaron RK, Voisinet A, Racine J, Ali Y, Feller ER. Corticosteroid-associated avascular necrosis: dose relationships and early diagnosis. *Ann N Y Acad Sci.* 2011;1240(1240):38–46.

Karantanas AH, Drakonaki EE. The role of MR imaging in avascular necrosis of the femoral head. *Semin Musculoskelet Radiol.* 2011;15(3):281–300.

Shigemura T, Nakamura J, Kishida S, et al. The incidence of alcohol-associated osteonecrosis of the knee is lower than the incidence of steroid-associated osteonecrosis of the knee: an MRI study. *Rheumatology (Oxford).* 2012;51(4):701–706.

Acute neurological symptoms with back pain—no history of fall or trauma

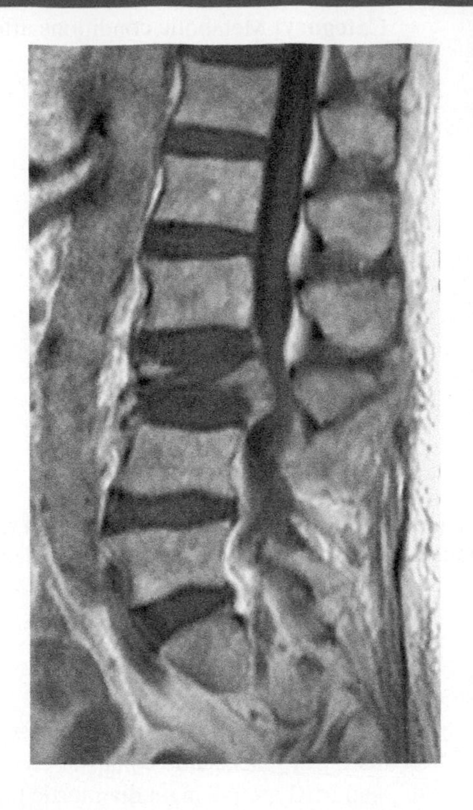

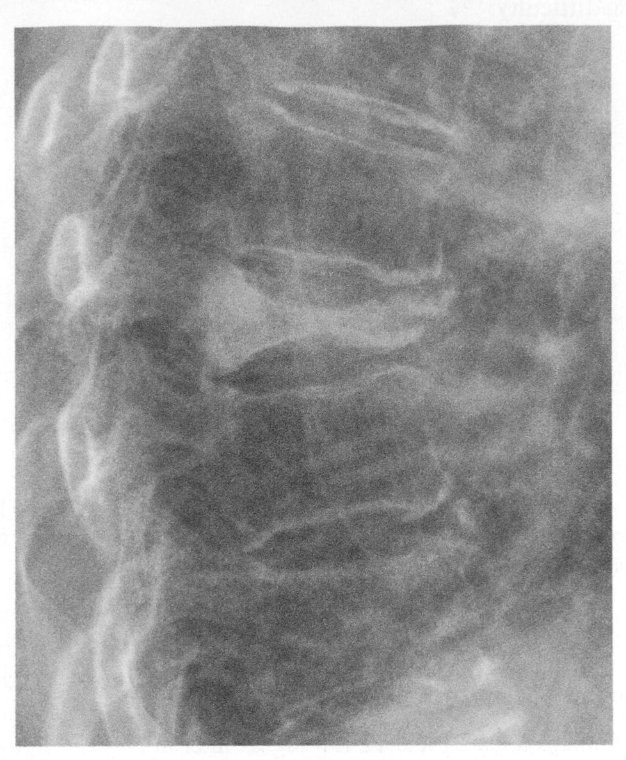

1. What are the radiographic findings?

2. What are the MRI findings?

3. What is the diagnosis?

4. What are the MR features favoring osteoporotic over metastatic vertebral collapse?

5. Contrast enhancement is useful in differentiating acute osteoporotic cord compression from metastatic cord compression. True or False?

Osteoporotic cauda equina compression 1007

Case ranking/difficulty: **Category:** Metabolic conditions affecting bone

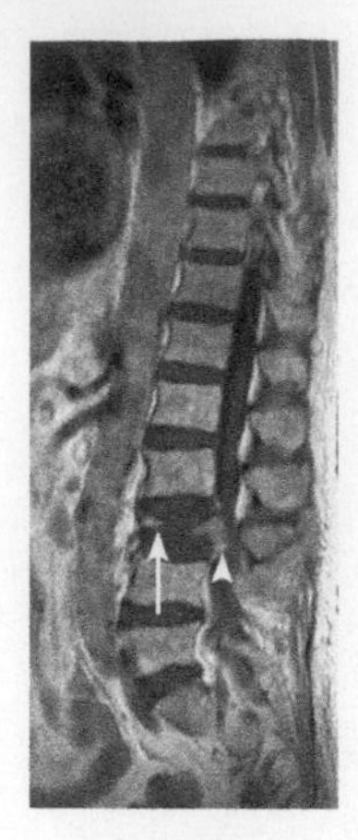

Osteoporotic cord compression with preserved fatty marrow posteriorly (*arrowhead*). The rest of the vertebral marrow signal is well preserved. Note low-signal-intensity band (*arrow*).

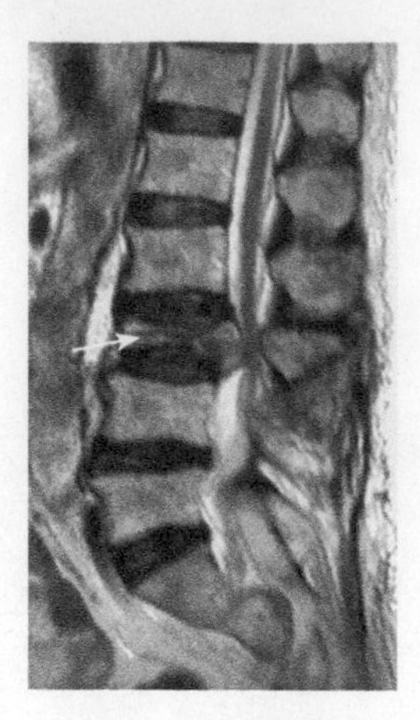

Low T1 band demonstrated with an *arrow*. Posterior retropulsed bone fragment with cauda equina compression is demonstrated.

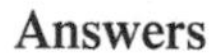

Answers

1. Severe anterior wedging of a midthoracic vertebra.
2. The MRI findings are a T1 and T2 low-signal-intensity band, retropulsion of a posterior bone fragment, and spared marrow signal within the affected vertebral body and other bodies. There is no posterior element involvement and no paraspinal mass.
3. The findings are suggestive of osteoporotic vertebral collapse.
4. Low-signal-intensity band on T1 and T2, areas of preserved bone marrow signal intensity in the affected and other vertebrae, multilevel collapse, no posterior element involvement, and no paraspinal mass. These MR features favor osteoporotic collapse.
5. True. Although it is controversial, some authors suggest heterogenous contrast enhancement in metastatic infiltration may be helpful in distinguishing this entity from cord compression secondary to osteoporotic collapse. An enhancing soft-tissue mass is also not seen in osteoporosis but can be seen in metastases.

Pearls

- Osteoporosis is a metabolic disorder affecting the modeling of bone, resulting in bone resorption. This leads to a reduction in bone mineral density.
- It is more common in females than in males, and one in three women older than the age of 65 years are affected.
- Osteoporosis is one of the major causes of nontraumatic vertebral collapse, and is important to differentiate from metastatic collapse.
- Plain film and MRI are the main diagnostic modalities.
- Plain film: Collapsed vertebra at one or multiple levels. Decreased density of bones with vertical striations, biconcave vertebrae, Schmorl nodes, and picture framing (prominence of the cortical outline as a result of disproportionate trabecula resorption and peripheral trabecula reinforcement).
- MRI: Low T1 and T2 signal-intensity bands, normal marrow signal intensity in other vertebrae and preserved marrow signal in the affected vertebra, posterior bone fragment retropulsion, absence of a paraspinal or epidural mass, and the presence of other compression fractures favors osteoporotic collapse over metastatic collapse.

Suggested Readings

Cuénod CA, Laredo JD, Chevret S, et al. Acute vertebral collapse due to osteoporosis or malignancy: appearance on unenhanced and gadolinium-enhanced MR images. *Radiology*. 1996;199(2):541–549.

Jung HS, Jee WH, McCauley TR, Ha KY, Choi KH. Discrimination of metastatic from acute osteoporotic compression spinal fractures with MR imaging. *Radiographics*. 2003;23(1):179–187.

Rumpel H, Chong Y, Porter DA, Chan LL. Benign versus metastatic vertebral compression fractures: combined diffusion-weighted MRI and MR spectroscopy aids differentiation. *Eur Radiol*. 2013;23(2):541–550.

Acute neurological symptoms with back pain—no history of trauma

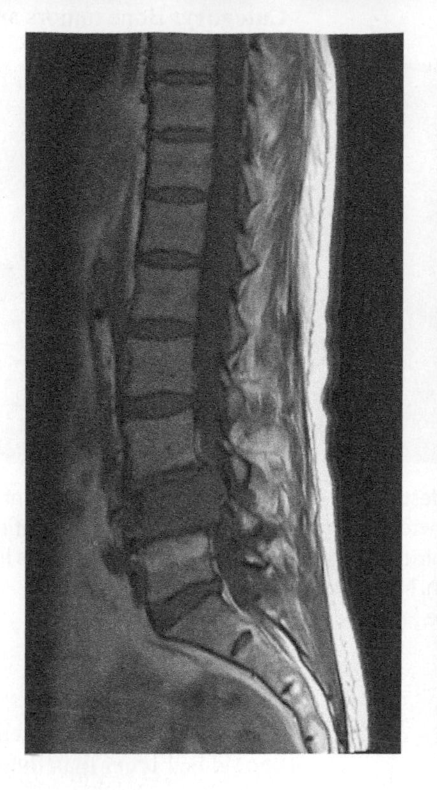

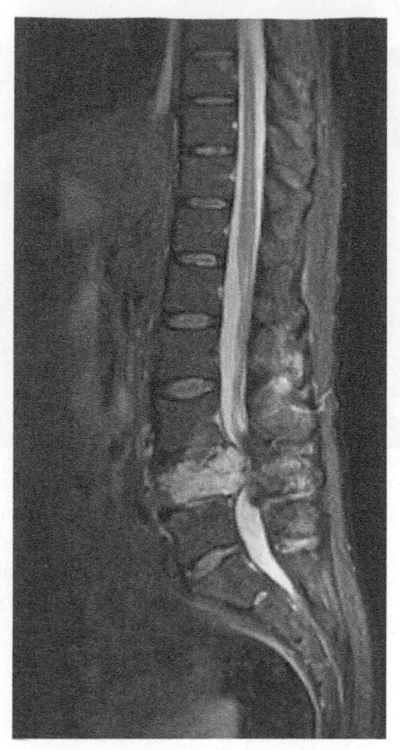

1. What are the MRI findings?

2. What are the differential diagnoses?

3. What are the specific distinguishing features of this entity on MRI?

4. T2-weighted images are best for evaluating marrow replacement. True or False?

5. What sequences are not useful in demonstrating this condition?

Metastatic cauda equina compression 1006

Case ranking/difficulty: 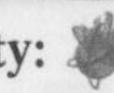 **Category:** Bone tumors and marrow abnormalities

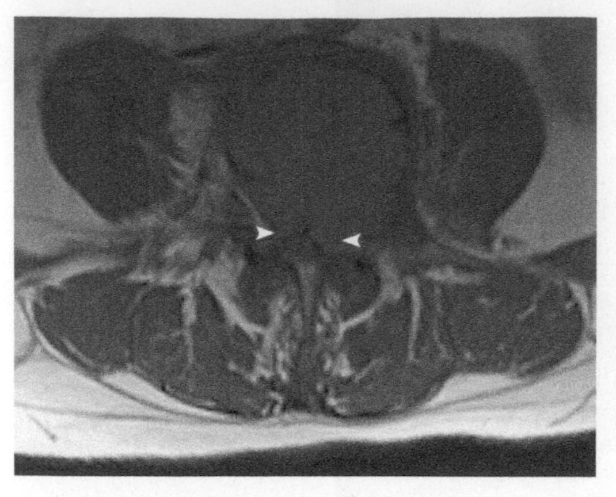

Axial image showing no room for CSF flow and the epidural fat completely compressed.

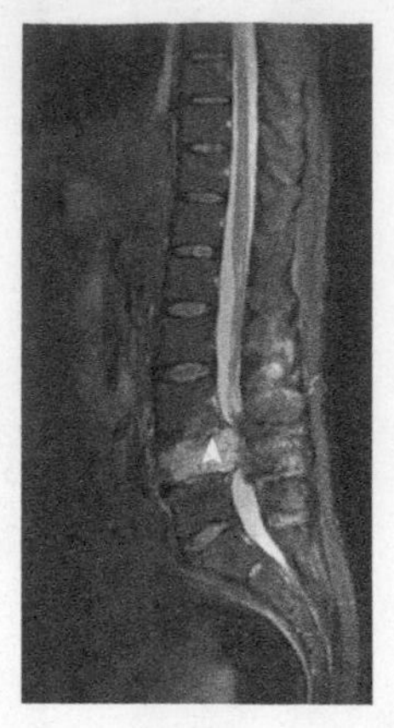

Metastatic destruction of the vertebral body with increased signal and diffuse posterior bulge, with cauda equina compression. Note subchondral low-intensity line (*arrowhead*).

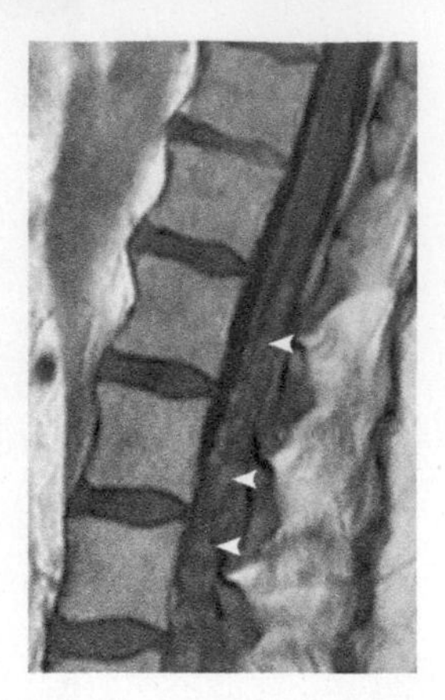

Contrast-enhanced image shows "sugar-coating" appearance of dural metastases in another patient.

Answers

1. T1 marrow replacement, vertebral collapse and diffuse posterior wall bulge, low signal intensity band, cauda equina compression, and single level involvement. Although a low-intensity band is seen in this case, it is more commonly seen in osteoporotic compression fractures.
2. The differential diagnosis includes osteoporotic fracture, metastatic collapse, infection, post-traumatic collapse, and chordoma.
3. MRI features suggesting metastatic compression include a diffuse posterior vertebral bulge, involvement of the posterior elements, paraspinal mass, epidural mass, other spinal involvement and "sugar coating" with contrast images (for dural metastases). T1-weighted images are useful to demonstrate multilevel marrow involvement.
4. False. T1 is the sequence of choice for evaluation of marrow replacement.
5. STIR and T2-weighted images can show increased signal in the infiltrated marrow but are nonspecific. Post-contrast images are useful to see dural metastases and paraspinal/epidural masses but are of uncertain usefulness in evaluating bony metastases. Gradient-echo and proton-density images are of little use.

Pearls

- Skeletal metastasis is the third most common site for metastases, and in the skeletal system the spinal column is the most common site.
- Abnormal marrow infiltration on T1 is an important indicator. T1 diffuse marrow infiltration should also be searched for, using the disc signal as a control (marrow signal should be higher than disc on the T1-weighted images).
- The following criteria on MRI favor metastatic collapse over osteoporotic collapse: diffuse posterior bulge, paraspinal or epidural mass, involvement of the posterior elements, and multiple level marrow involvement. A band of low T1 and T2 signal intensity is nonspecific but favors osteoporotic collapse.
- The use of contrast is of debatable usefulness in evaluating bony metastases. However "sugar coating" in the cases of dural metastases and of paraspinal or epidural masses are well demonstrated on post-contrast images.
- Urgent treatment is with cord decompression and spine stabilization. In palliative cases, vertebroplasty and kyphoplasty are offered for pain control.

Suggested Readings

Berwouts D, Remery M, Van Den Berghe T. Vertebral collapse caused by bone metastasis. *J Thorac Oncol.* 2011;6(4):823.

Jung HS, Jee WH, McCauley TR, Ha KY, Choi KH. Discrimination of metastatic from acute osteoporotic compression spinal fractures with MR imaging. *Radiographics.* 2003;23(1):179–187.

Lafforgue P, Bayle O, Massonnat J, et al. MRI in osteoporotic and metastatic vertebral compressions: apropos of 60 cases [in French]. *Ann Radiol (Paris).* 1991;34(3):157–166.

History given was child fell down

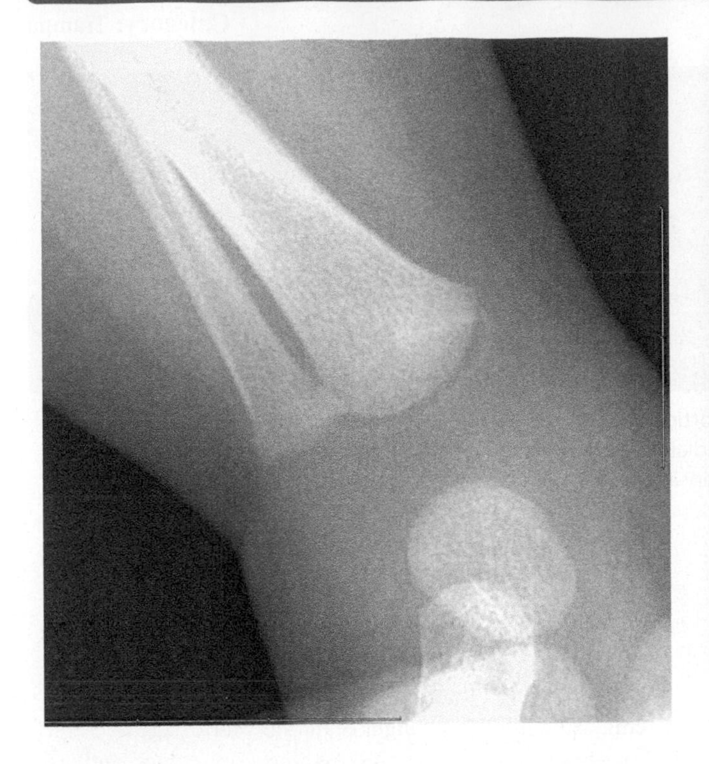

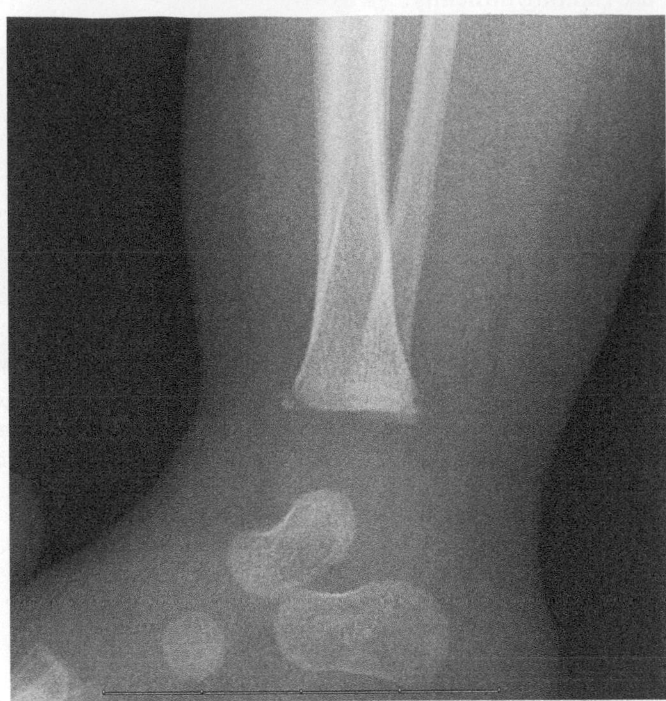

1. What names have been given to this entity?

2. What is the significance of the type of fracture depicted in this child's distal tibia?

3. What radiographic findings are the most specific for this entity?

4. What type of force is likely responsible for the distal tibial fracture depicted?

5. Which age group is at greatest risk for this entity?

Non-accidental trauma 2209

Case ranking/difficulty: 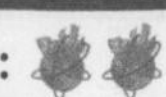

Category: Trauma

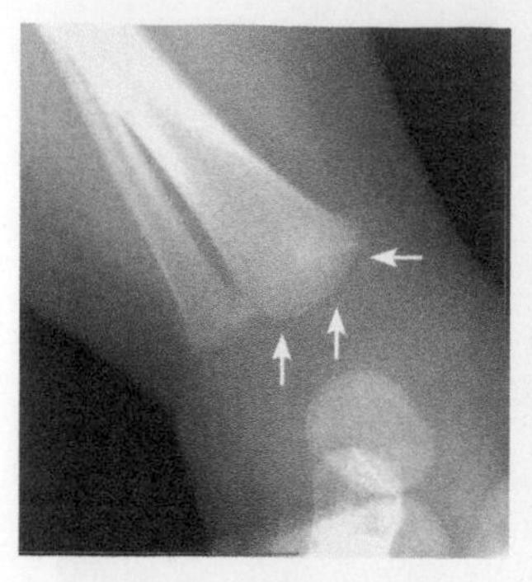

Radiograph demonstrates a fracture of the distal tibial metaphysis (*arrows*). The fracture has a "bucket-handle" appearance when imaged en face.

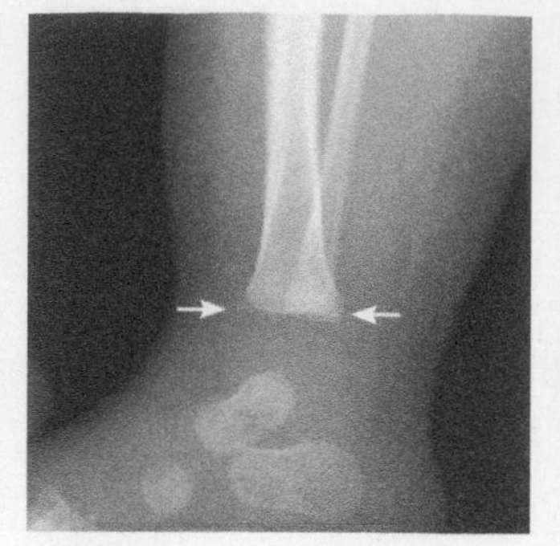

The fracture appears to involve the "corners" of the metaphysis (*arrows*) on the lateral projection.

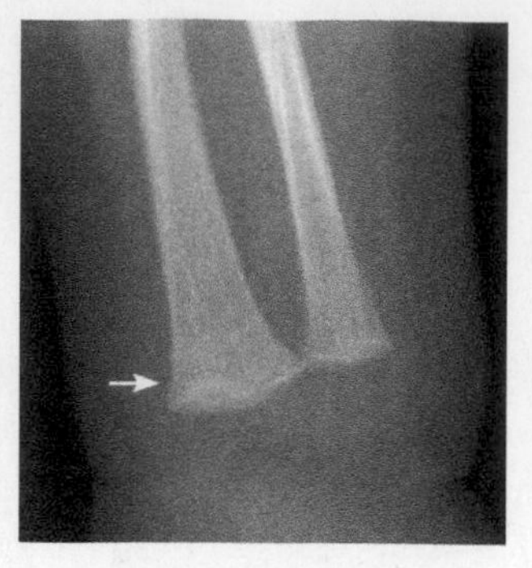

Cortical stepoff of the distal radial metaphysis (*arrow*) consistent with fracture.

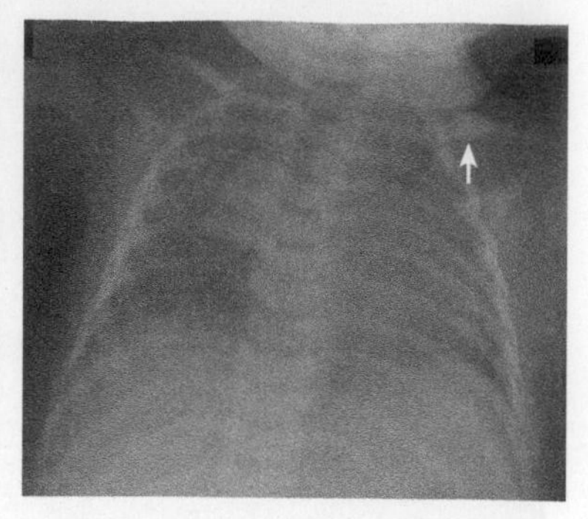

Healing fracture of the left clavicle (*arrow*).

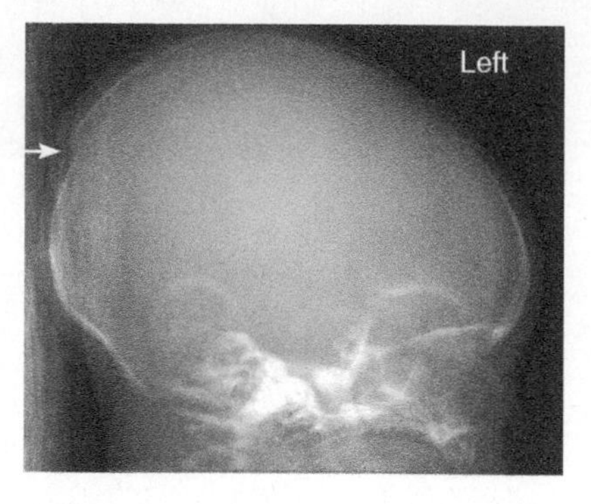

Lateral skull radiograph in a different patient (a 17-day-old girl) demonstrates a depressed skull fracture (*arrow*).

Answers

1. *Non-accidental trauma* and *non-accidental injury* are terms used today to describe what has previously been called child abuse, battered child syndrome, or shaken baby syndrome.

2. The radiographs depict a metaphyseal fracture. Metaphyseal fractures (also called *classic metaphyseal lesions* or *bucket-handle fractures*) are considered highly specific for non-accidental trauma.

3. Metaphyseal fractures and rib fractures are considered very specific for non-accidental trauma.

4. The metaphyseal fracture is thought to result from shear force caused by to-and-fro shaking of the extremities, as when an adult shakes an infant. A series of microfractures develops into a fracture line in the subepiphyseal region parallel to the physis.

5. Younger children are at higher risk. Children younger than one year of age accounted for 46% of fatalities caused by abuse or neglect, and children younger than age four years accounted for 81%.

Pearls

- In the United States in 2009, 476,000 children were physically abused.
- Non-accidental trauma is more common in younger children; children younger than one year of age account for 46% of fatalities caused by abuse or neglect, and children younger than age four years account for 81%.
- Skeletal injury is extremely common in non-accidental trauma.
- The radiographic finding of a metaphyseal corner fracture on the lateral film is highly specific for child abuse in children younger than two years of age. The appearance of this fracture en face is described as a "bucket-handle" fracture.
- Rib fractures, especially posterior rib or bilateral rib fractures, are also very specific for non-accidental trauma.
- Other specific findings include scapular fractures, sternal fractures, and vertebral spinous process fractures.
- Many other types of fracture occur commonly in both accidental and non-accidental trauma and are therefore not specific for non-accidental trauma.
- In general, when the provided history is inconsistent with the pattern or severity of injury, non-accidental trauma should be considered.
- Metabolic bone conditions such as osteogenesis imperfecta and rickets can mimic the skeletal findings in non-accidental trauma.

Suggested Readings

Dwek JR. The radiographic approach to child abuse. *Clin Orthop Relat Res*. 2011;469(3):776–789.

Lonergan GJ, Baker AM, Morey MK, Boos SC. From the archives of the AFIP. Child abuse: radiologic-pathologic correlation. *Radiographics*. 2003;23(4):811–845.

Motor vehicle accident

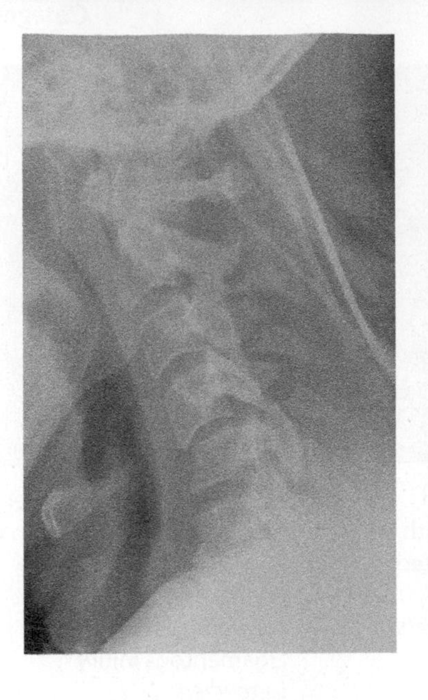

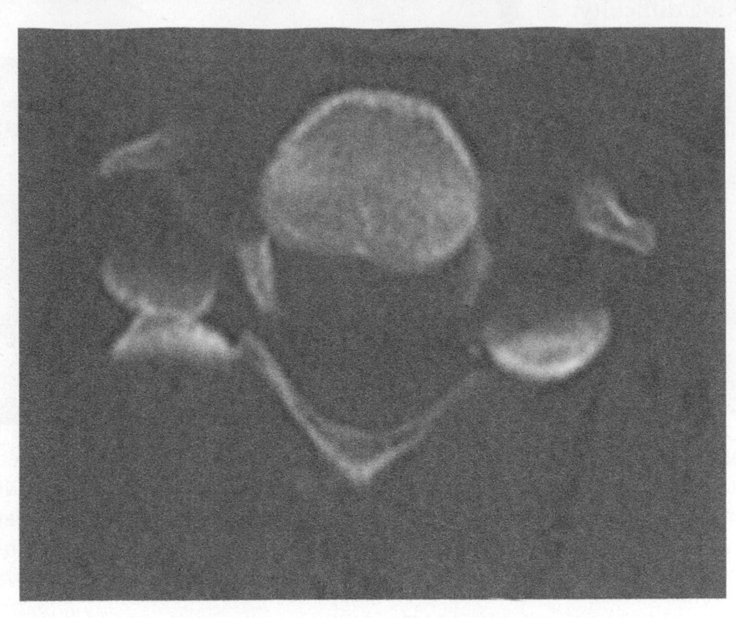

1. What are the imaging findings?
2. What is the mechanism of injury?
3. What injuries to the cervical spine are unstable?
4. In what injury is the hamburger sign seen?
5. What percentage of patients with bilateral injury have neurological compromise?

Jumped facet

2357

Case ranking/difficulty:

Category: Trauma

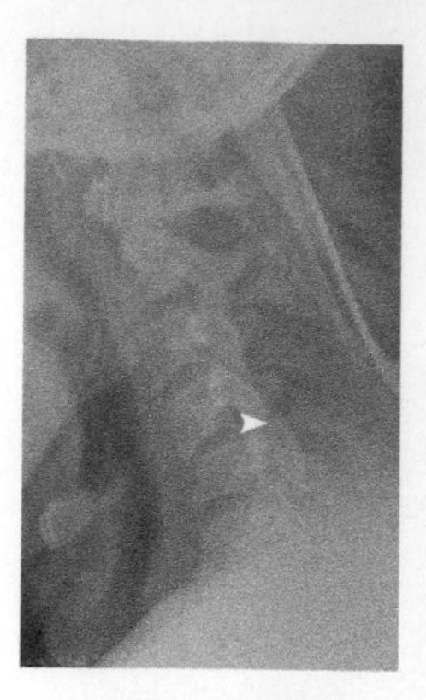

Anterolisthesis of C4 on C5, with a jumped facet (*arrowhead*) and multiple spinous process fractures.

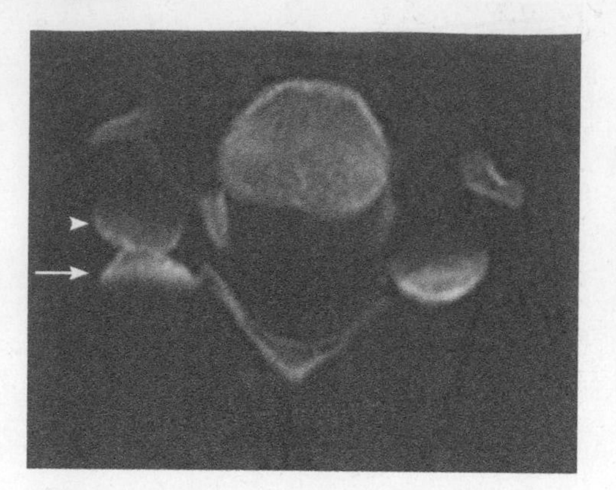

Right "hamburger" sign demonstrated. *Arrowhead* points to the inferior facet of the C4 vertebra, and the *arrow* points to the superior facet of C5.

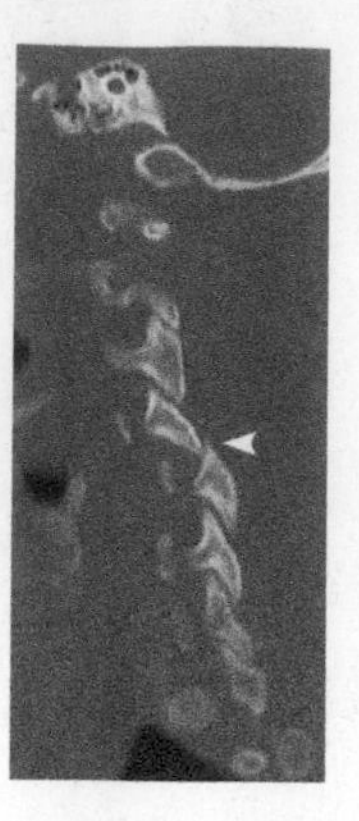

Jumped facet with an associated fracture (*arrowhead*).

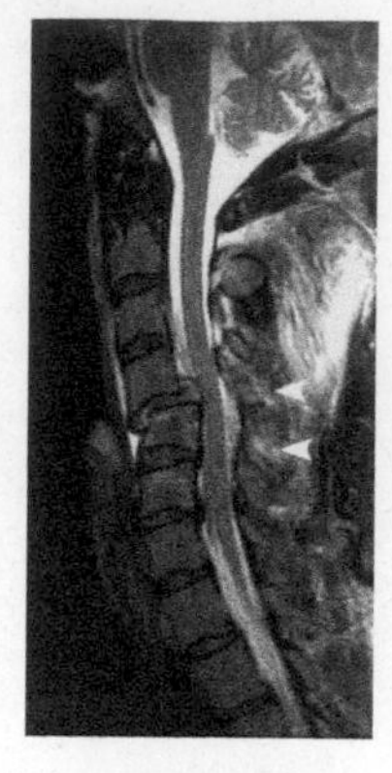

Uncovered disc with bulging, minimal cord edema and no cord transection. Ligamentous injury (*arrowheads*).

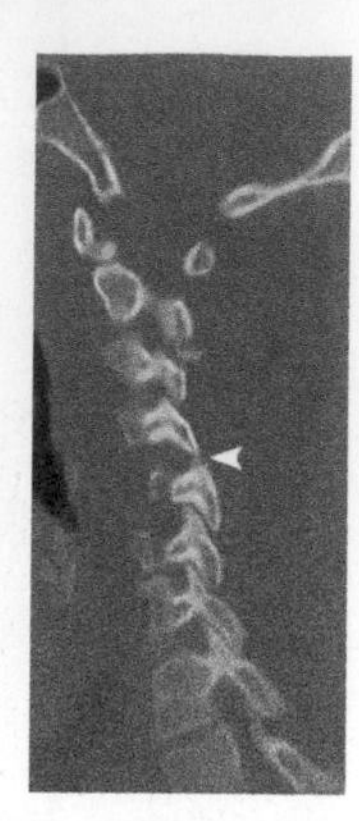

Perched facet on the left side.

Answers

1. There is a hyperflexion injury with a jumped facet, anterolisthesis of C4 on C5 and multiple spinous process fractures. The "hamburger" and "naked facet" signs are the same and are demonstrated here.
2. The mechanism for this injury is hyperflexion. A rotary component to the injury is contributory.
3. Flexion teardrop, Jefferson and Hangman fractures, type 2 dens fractures, and bilateral locked facets are unstable fractures. A unilateral locked facet with a fractured facet is also unstable. In addition, hyperextension dislocation is unstable.
4. A "hamburger" sign is seen in a jumped facet. On axial CT, the normal appearance of the facets is said to resemble a hamburger, with the superior articular facet of the vertebra below forming the top bun and the inferior facet of the vertebra above forming the bottom bun, and the space between the "meat." With a jumped facet, the bottom "bun" now lies anterior to the top "bun." This is known as the *hamburger* or *naked facet sign*.
5. Of patients with bilateral jumped facets, 75% have neurological compromise. The listhesis that occurs results in severe canal and foraminal stenosis, with cord compression or transection in severe cases.

Pearls

- A jumped facet is a result of a severe injury, usually MVA or a fall.
- The mechanism is hyperflexion rotation and is unstable when bilateral or associated with a facet fracture.
- In bilateral jumped facets, there is typically greater than 50% anterolisthesis and the subsequent spinal canal and neuroforaminal stenosis results in neurologic deficit in up to 75% of cases.
- Cord injury ranges from cord edema to cord transection.
- Associated fractures are common, including spinous process, facet, and a triangular corner fracture of the anterosuperior margin of the inferior involved vertebra.
- When the facets lie on to top of each other rather than overlapping, it is called a *perched facet*.
- The "hamburger" or "naked facet" sign is seen on axial CT images.
- Both CT and MRI are indicated: CT to define the fracture anatomy, and MRI to evaluate the cord, disc, and ligamentous structures.

Suggested Readings

Kornberg M. The computed tomographic appearance of a unilateral jumped cervical facet (the "false" facet joint sign). *Spine (Phila PA 1976).* 1986;11(10):1038–1040.

Sekula RF, Daffner RH, Quigley MR, et al. Exclusion of cervical spine instability in patients with blunt trauma with normal multidetector CT (MDCT) and radiography. *Br J Neurosurg.* 2008;22(5):669–674.

History of a motor vehicle accident

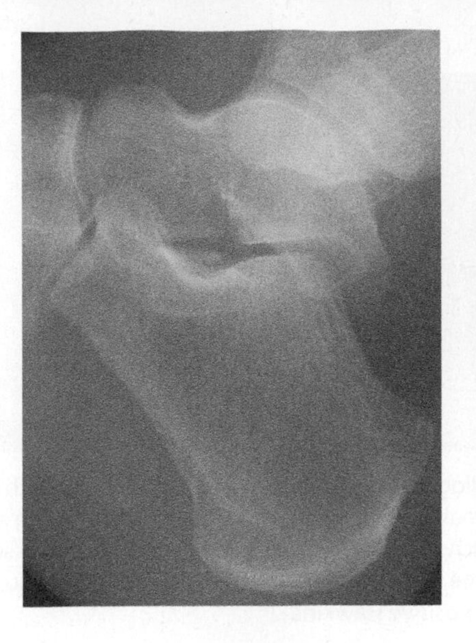

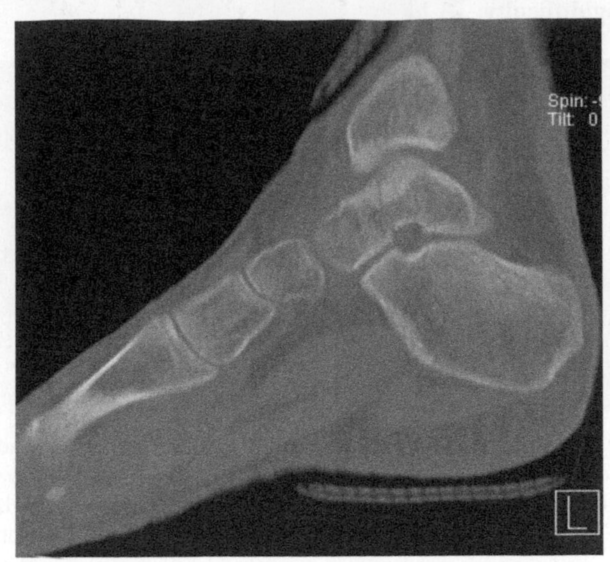

1. What are the imaging findings?

2. What other significant injuries would you be looking for?

3. What vessels provide the major arterial supply to the talar dome?

4. What is the Hawkins sign?

5. What is the significance of a positive Hawkins sign?

Talar neck fracture: Hawkins type 1 — 1462

Case ranking/difficulty: 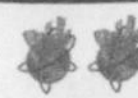

Category: Trauma

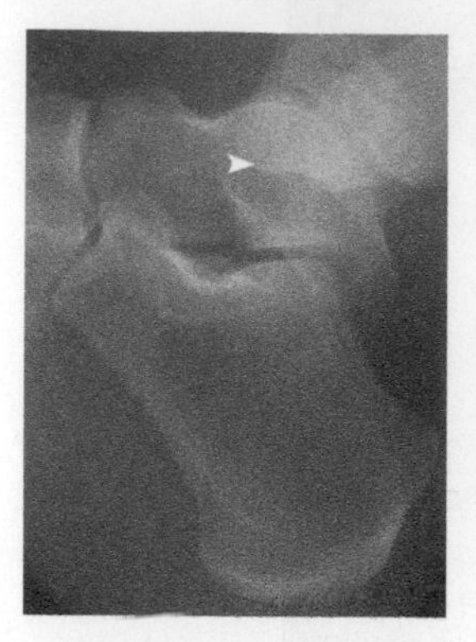

Minimally displaced talar neck fracture (*arrowhead*) and ankle effusion are seen.

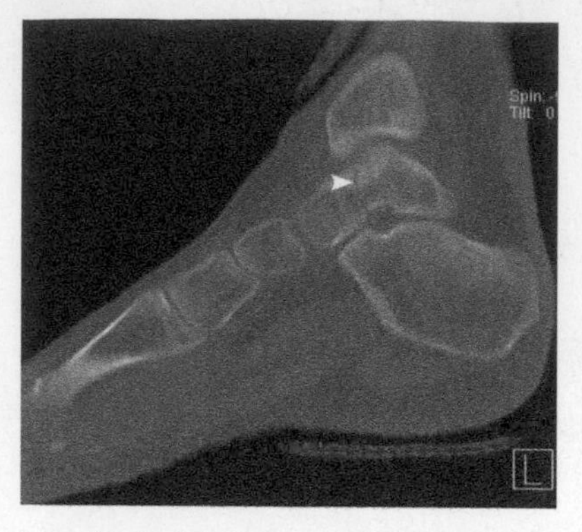

Nondisplaced fracture of the talar neck is seen.

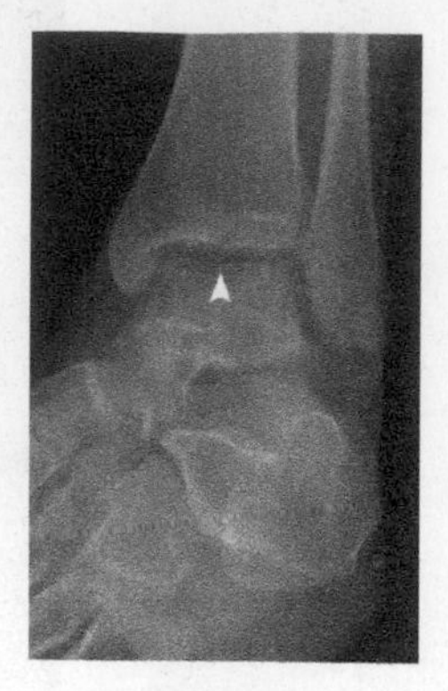

Radiographs 6 weeks later shows subchondral talar dome lucency, which is a positive Hawkins sign.

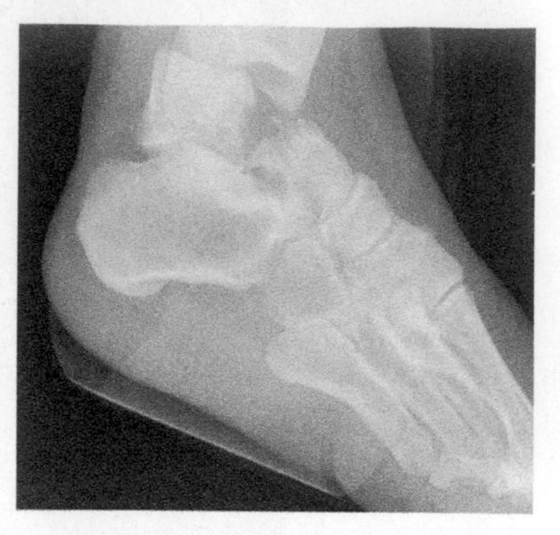

Another patient with Hawkins type 3 fracture, including a displaced talar neck fracture and associated subtalar and ankle joint subluxation.

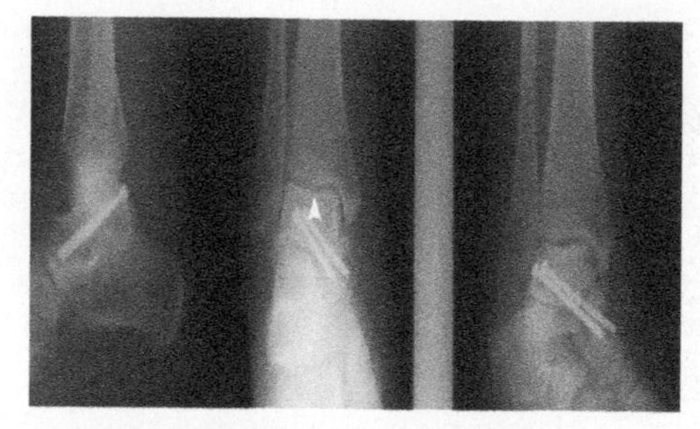

Same patient (Hawkins type 3) postsurgical screw fixation shows anatomic alignment of the fracture but with sclerosis of the talar dome (*arrowhead*), which is consistent with avascular necrosis.

Answers

1. There is a minimally displaced talar neck fracture with a small ankle effusion.
2. Dislocation/subluxation of the subtalar, tibiotalar, or talonavicular joints and significant fracture displacement.
3. The artery of the tarsal canal, which is a branch of the posterior tibial artery, is the major blood supply to the talar dome. The artery of the tarsal sinus, which is a branch of the peroneal artery, is the secondary blood supply.
4. Subchondral lucency in the talar dome occurring six to eight weeks after injury is called a *Hawkins sign*.
5. A positive Hawkins sign indicates a low risk for avascular necrosis of the talar dome. The band-like lucency that is seen in the dome is a result of preserved vascular perfusion, resulting in bone resorption.

Pearls

- Talar neck fractures are uncommon.
- Hawkins classified talar neck fractures into 4 types:
  - Type 1: Isolated nondisplaced talar neck fracture. Risk of AVN is 0–13%.
  - Type 2: Displaced talar neck fracture with subluxation/dislocation of the subtalar joint. Risk of AVN is 20–50%.
  - Type 3: Displaced talar neck fracture with dislocation of the subtalar and ankle joints. Risk of AVN is 69–100%.
  - Type 4: Displaced talar neck fractures with dislocation of the subtalar and ankle joints, as well as the talonavicular joint. Risk of AVN is 90–100%.
- The Hawkins sign is subchondral band-like lucency in the talar dome seen six to eight weeks after injury, and when present is a reliable indicator that avascular necrosis has not occurred and perfusion with hyperemia remains.
- If Hawkins sign is absent, there is a high risk for the development of avascular necrosis.

Suggested Readings

Donnelly EF. The Hawkins sign. *Radiology.* 1999;210(1): 195–196.

Hawkins LG. Fractures of the neck of the talus. *J Bone Joint Surg Am.* 1970;52(5):991–1002.

Fall from a tree

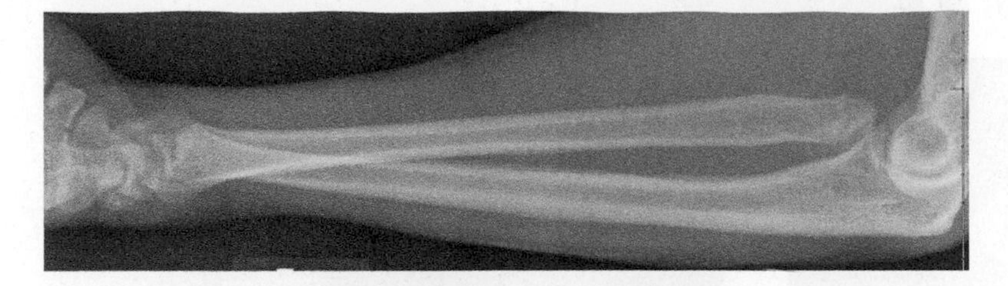

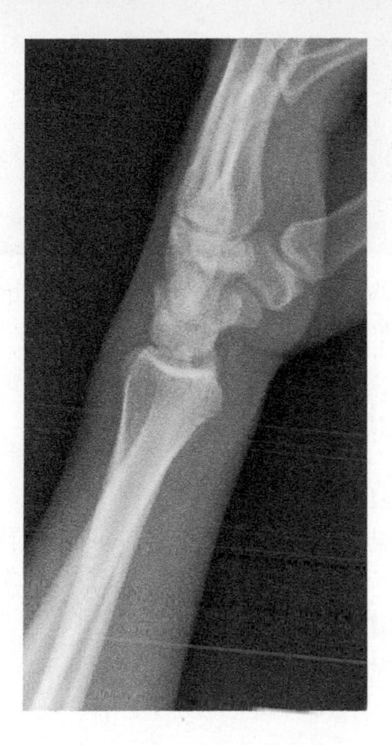

1. What are the imaging findings?

2. What is the accepted name for this injury?

3. What is the typical mechanism of injury?

4. What is a crisscross injury?

5. Are these injuries stable or unstable, and how are they treated?

Essex-Lopresti fracture–dislocation 2318

Case ranking/difficulty:

Category: Trauma

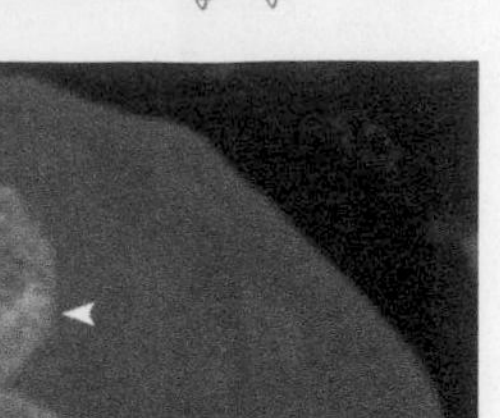

Volar dislocation of the distal ulna (*arrowhead*) at the DRUJ is well appreciated on CT.

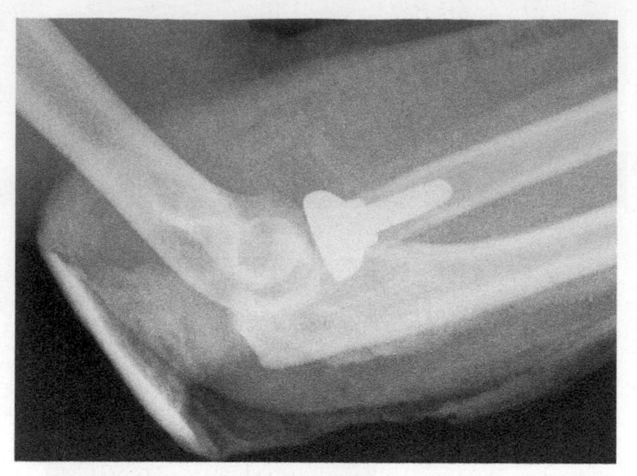

Treated with excision of the radial head and placement of a radial head prosthesis.

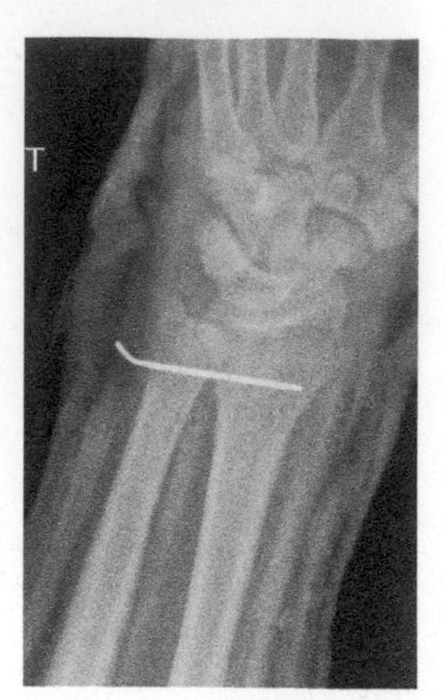

DRUJ dislocation was reduced and pinned.

Answers

1. There is a comminuted displaced radial head fracture, with volar dislocation of the ulna at the distal radio-ulnar joint (DRUJ).
2. The combination of a comminuted displaced radial head fracture and DRUJ dislocation is called an Essex-Lopresti fracture–dislocation.
3. Essex-Lopresti injuries are usually the result of a high velocity fall on the outstretched hand such as in parachuting, skiing, and falls from a height. Longitudinal migration of the radius occurs in the classic injury, with interosseous membrane disruption. Hyperpronation results in a dorsal dislocation of the distal ulna, hypersupination in a volar dislocation—these are the other variants.
4. The rare crisscross injury is a dislocation of the radial head at the elbow, and of the ulna at the DRUJ. The radial head dislocation is usually volar with a volar distal ulna dislocation.
5. The injury to the interosseous membrane that occurs in an Essex-Lopresti fracture–dislocation renders the injury unstable. Management is usually surgical: reduction of the radial head fracture and/or excision and prosthetic replacement of the radial head, with reduction and pinning of the DRUJ.

Pearls

- The Essex-Lopresti fracture–dislocation is a rare fracture–dislocation of the forearm.
- There is a displaced comminuted fracture of the radial head with dislocation of the ulna at the distal radioulnar joint (DRUJ).
- The DRUJ dislocation is volar in hypersupination injuries, and dorsal in hyperpronation injuries.
- The original fracture–dislocation described by Essex-Lopresti was a longitudinal migration of the radius.
- The rare "crisscross" injury is not a true Essex-Lopresti injury, and involves a volar radial head dislocation and volar dislocation of the ulna at the DRUJ.
- Essex-Lopresti injuries are inherently unstable, with injury to the interosseous membrane.
- There are two other forearm fracture–dislocations: Monteggia injuries, which are fractures of the proximal ulna with a radial head dislocation, and Galleazzi injuries, which are distal radial fractures with dislocation at the DRUJ.

Suggested Readings

Jungbluth P, Frangen TM, Arens S, Muhr G, Kälicke T. The undiagnosed Essex-Lopresti injury. *J Bone Joint Surg Br.* 2006;88(12):1629–1633.

Lendemans S, Taeger G, Nast-Kolb D. Dislocation fractures of the forearm. Galeazzi, Monteggia, and Essex-Lopresti injuries [in German]. *Unfallchirurg.* 2008;111(12): 1005–1014; quiz 1015–1016.

Patient fell while cleaning her garage

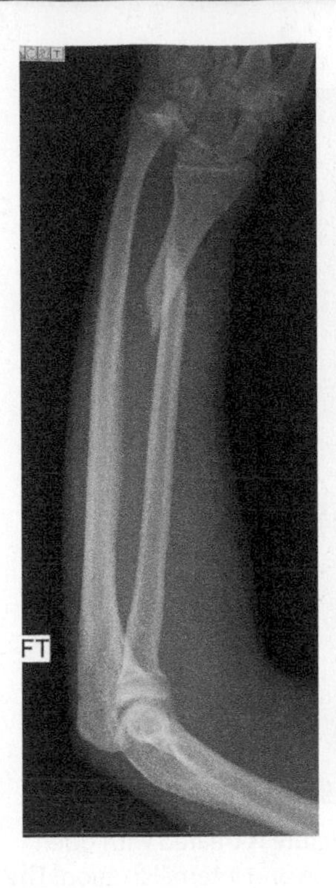
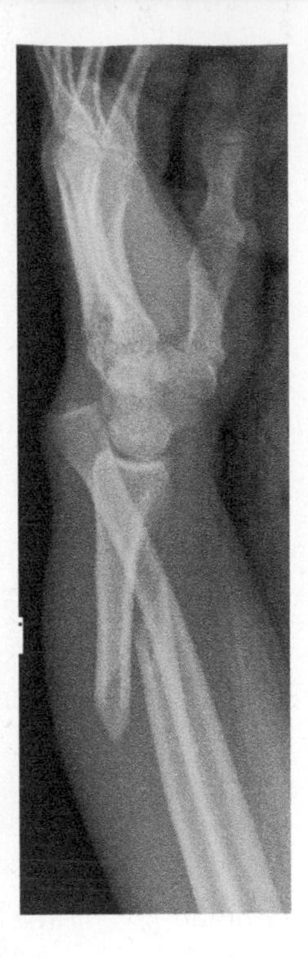

1. What are the radiograph findings?

2. What is the mechanism of injury?

3. The distal radius fracture is almost always located above what structure?

4. What is the treatment for this injury in an adult?

5. What is the injury pattern in an Essex-Lopresti injury of the forearm?

Galeazzi fracture–dislocation 1396

Case ranking/difficulty: 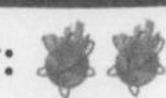

Category: Trauma

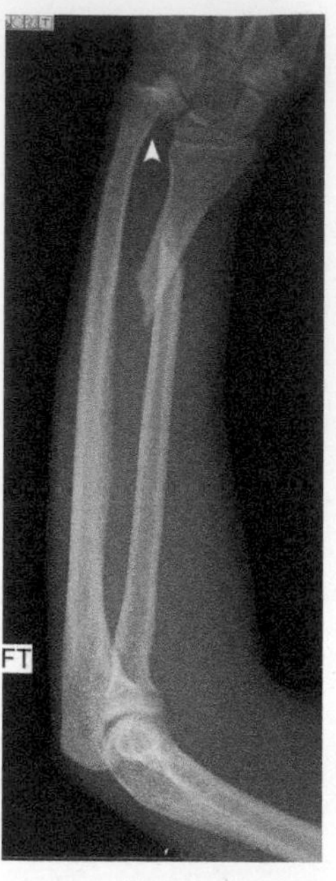

There is a displaced angulated fracture of the distal radius, with ulnar dislocation. An associated displaced ulnar styloid process fracture is seen (*arrowhead*).

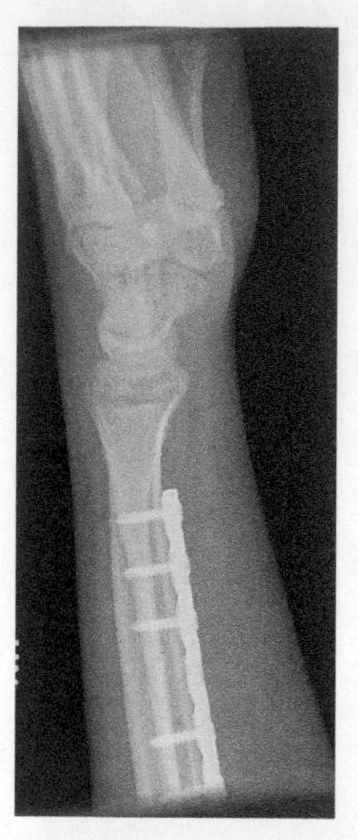

The fracture is treated with open reduction and internal fixation. The dislocation has been reduced.

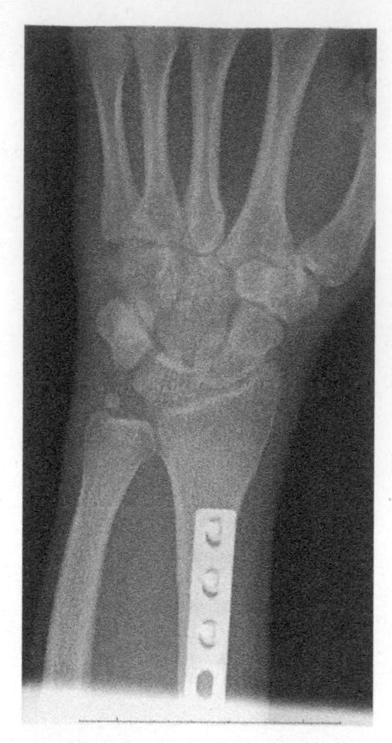

The radial height has been restored.

Answers

1. Displaced fracture of the distal radius, with dorsal dislocation of the distal ulna. This is a Galeazzi fracture–dislocation.
2. The typical mechanism is a fall on the outstretched hand while pronated. Direct trauma can sometimes result in this pattern.
3. The distal radius fracture is almost always located above the pronator quadratus muscle.
4. The management for a Galeazzi fracture–dislocation is open reduction and internal fixation in an adult. In a child, closed reduction and casting is performed.
5. An Essex-Lopresti forearm injury is a fracture of the radial head, accompanied by a dislocation of the distal ulna at the distal radioulnar joint. The interosseous membrane is injured.

Pearls

- Galeazzi fracture–dislocation occurs after a fall on the outstretched hand.
- The forearm is a "ring" structure, hence a distal radius fracture is accompanied by another injury.
- There is a displaced fracture of the distal radius with dorsal subluxation/dislocation of the distal ulna caused by ligamentous injury at the DRUJ.
- The fracture of the distal radius is almost always above the pronator quadratus muscle and is typically displaced and angulated.
- Volar subluxation can sometimes occur.
- In children, separation of the ulnar epiphysis may occur instead of ulnar dislocation.

Suggested Readings

Atesok KI, Jupiter JB, Weiss AP. Galeazzi fracture. *J Am Acad Orthop Surg.* 2011;19(10):623–633.

Carlsen BT, Dennison DG, Moran SL. Acute dislocations of the distal radioulnar joint and distal ulna fractures. *Hand Clin.* 2010;26(4):503–516.

Fall

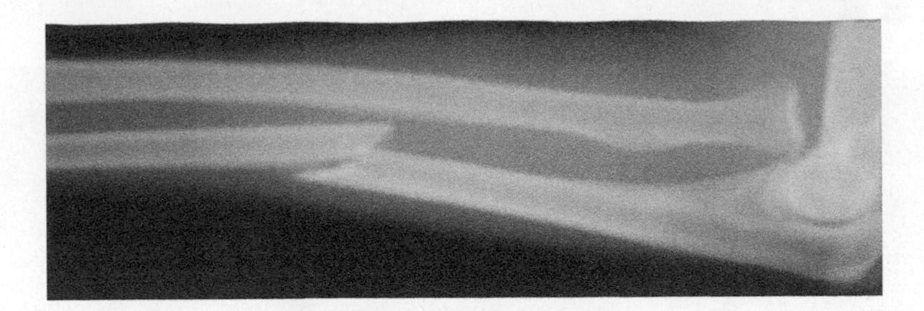

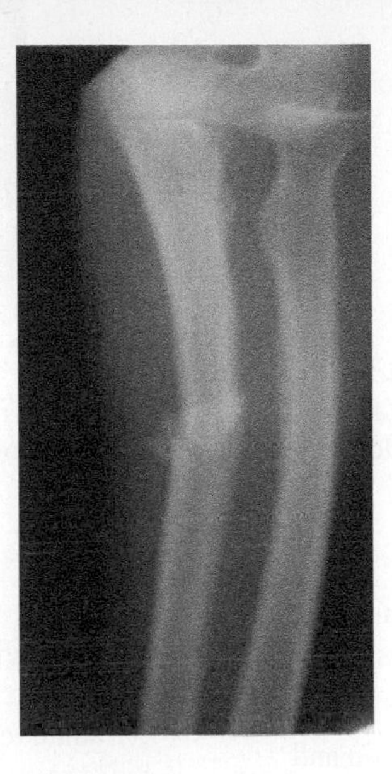

1. What are the radiograph findings?

2. What is the mechanism of injury?

3. What can be included in the differential, and what is the most likely diagnosis?

4. What are the different forms of this injury, and what is the most common form?

5. What are the major complications of this injury pattern?

Monteggia fracture–dislocation 1395

Case ranking/difficulty: ✱✱ **Category:** Trauma

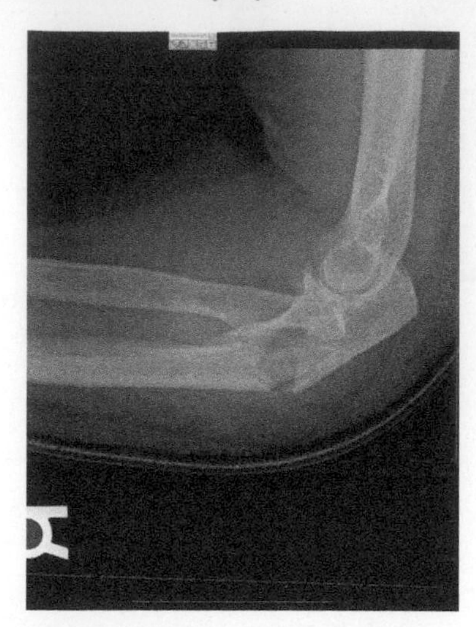

Companion case: proximal ulna fracture with a posteriorly directed fracture apex and posterior dislocation and fracture of the radial head. This a reverse Monteggia fracture (Bado type 2).

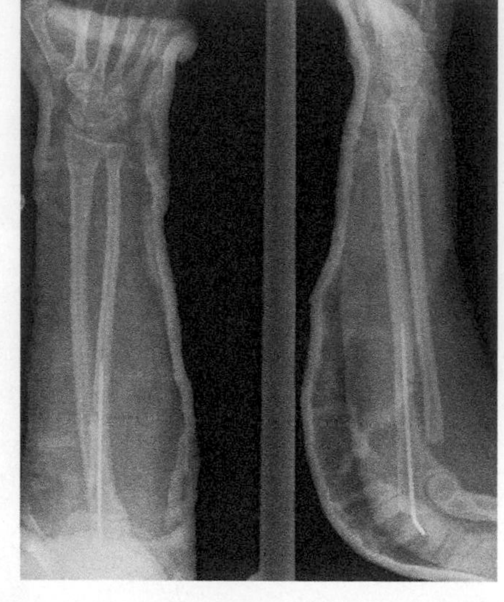

Another patient treated with rigid fixation of the ulna fracture and excision of the radial head.

Answers

1. Angulated fracture of the proximal ulna with anterior and radial dislocation of the radial head, consistent with a Monteggia fracture dislocation.
2. A fall on the outstretched hand in hyperpronation and direct trauma to the back of the elbow are the proposed mechanisms.
3. Essex-Lopresti injury, Galeazzi fracture–dislocation, and elbow dislocation are included in the differentials. A Monteggia fracture–dislocation is the diagnosis.
4. Bado described four forms, with type 1 being the most common.
   - Type 1: Fracture of the proximal ulna diaphysis with anterior radial head dislocation.
   - Type 2: Fracture of the proximal ulna diaphysis with posterior or posterolateral dislocation of the radial head.
   - Type 3: Fracture of the proximal ulna metaphysis with lateral or anterolateral radial head dislocation.
   - Type 4: Fracture of the proximal radius and ulna at the same level with anterior radial head dislocation. This is least common.
5. Complications include injury to the radial, median, and ulnar nerves, fracture nonunion and heterotopic ossification.

Pearls

- Monteggia fracture–dislocations occur after a fall on the outstretched hand when held in hyperpronation. Direct trauma to the back of the elbow is also implicated.
- There is a fracture of the proximal ulna and dislocation of the radial head.
- The apex of the ulna fracture is in the same direction as the radial head dislocation.
- Four types have been described by Bado.
- The most common form is a proximal ulna fracture, with an anterior apex angulation and an anterior dislocation of the radial head.
- The least common form consists of fractures of the proximal radius and ulna, with a radial head dislocation.

Suggested Readings

Beutel BG. Monteggia fractures in pediatric and adult populations. *Orthopedics.* 2012;35(2):138–144.

Sferopoulos NK. Monteggia type IV equivalent injury. *Open Orthop J.* 2011;5(5):198–200.

Acute right hip pain with no history of significant trauma

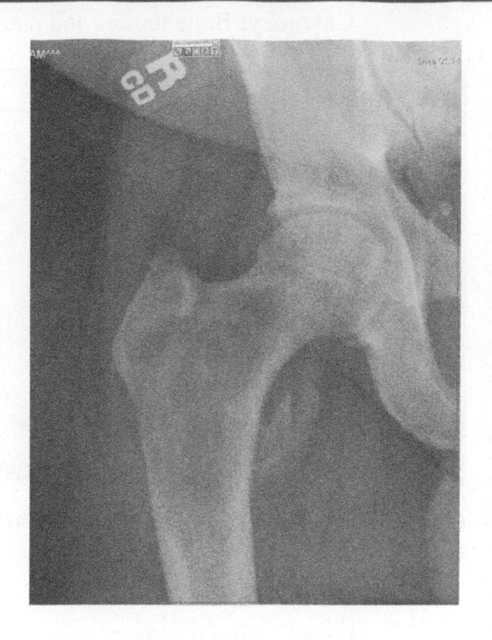

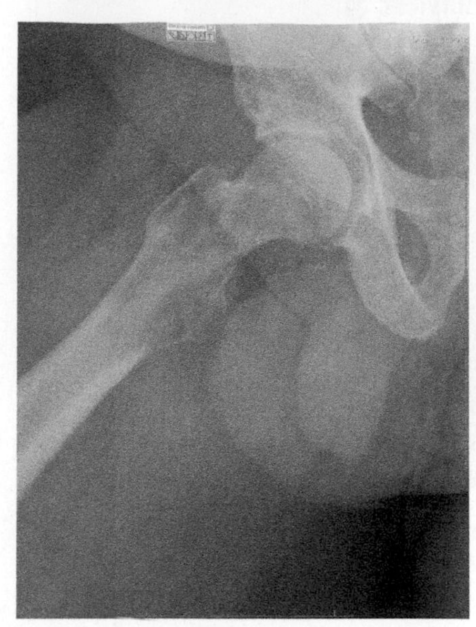

1. What are the radiological findings?

2. What are the usual etiologies for this appearance?

3. What are the next appropriate steps?

4. What is the main risk when this appearance is seen?

5. What is the management?

Lesser trochanter avulsion: metastatic disease 1363

Case ranking/difficulty: 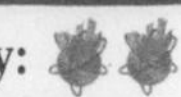

Category: Bone tumors and marrow abnormalities

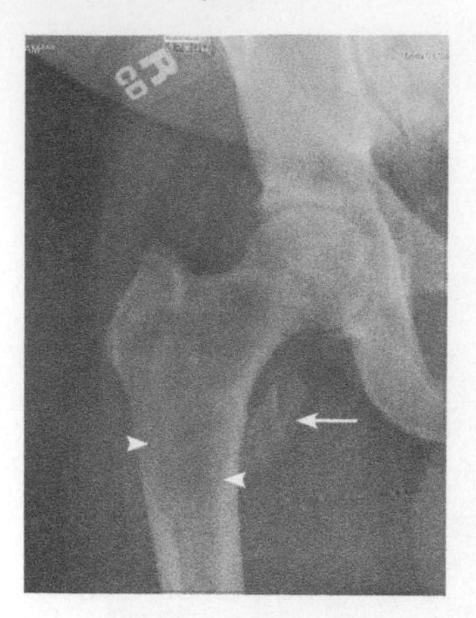

There is avulsion of the lesser trochanter (*arrow*). Focal osteolysis of the proximal femur with cortical thinning is noted (*arrowhead*).

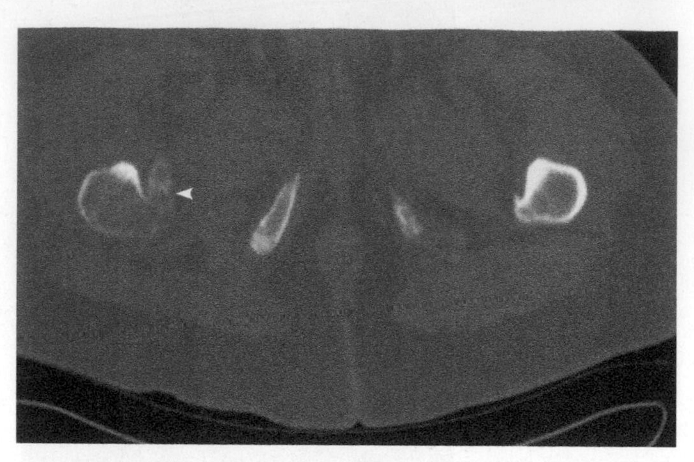

Osteolytic lesion with cortical destruction and lesser trochanter avulsion (*arrowhead*).

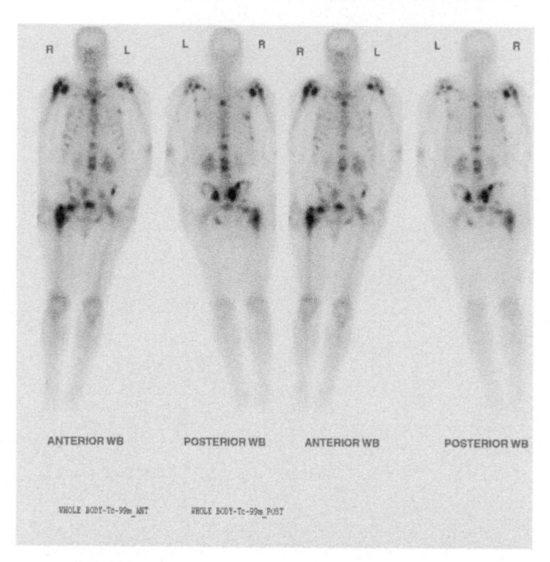

Diffuse metastatic foci are demonstrated.

Answers

1. There is an avulsion fracture of the lesser trochanter, with an osteolytic lesion in the proximal femur. There is cortical thinning.

2. In a patient older than age 40 years, lesser trochanter avulsion with minor or no trauma is highly suspicious for metastasis or primary bone tumor. In an adolescent, this may occur after strenuous hip flexion and is not pathologic.

3. Because this fracture is highly suspicious for underlying neoplasm, correlation for a history of neoplasm is warranted. If there is none, then further investigation with a bone scan is needed to evaluate for additional lesions. CT or MRI is indicated to assess the local extent of the lesion, and to determine the risk for pathologic fracture.

4. The main risk is an additional pathological fracture of the proximal femur.

5. Because of the high risk for pathologic fracture, prophylactic fixation of the femur is usually indicated.

Pearls

- Lesser trochanter avulsion in an adult after minor or no trauma should be considered to be a pathologic fracture until proven otherwise.
- The presence of this injury warrants further investigation with MRI and radionuclide bone scan.
- Lesser trochanter avulsions in adolescents may occur after strenuous hip flexion during sports, and are not pathologic.
- Prophylactic surgical fixation in adults is usually indicated to prevent pathologic fracture.
- Surgical management is not usually required in adolescents.

Suggested Readings

Khoury JG, Brandser EA, Found EM, Buckwalter JA. Non-traumatic lesser trochanter avulsion: a report of three cases. *Iowa Orthop J.* 1998;18(18):150–154.

Phillips CD, Pope TL, Jones JE, Keats TE, MacMillan RH. Nontraumatic avulsion of the lesser trochanter: a pathognomonic sign of metastatic disease? *Skeletal Radiol.* 1988;17(2):106–110.

History of a chronic disease, and sudden heel pain with no trauma

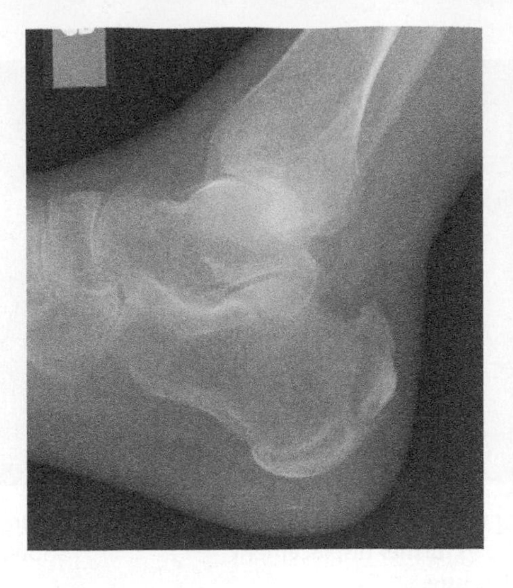
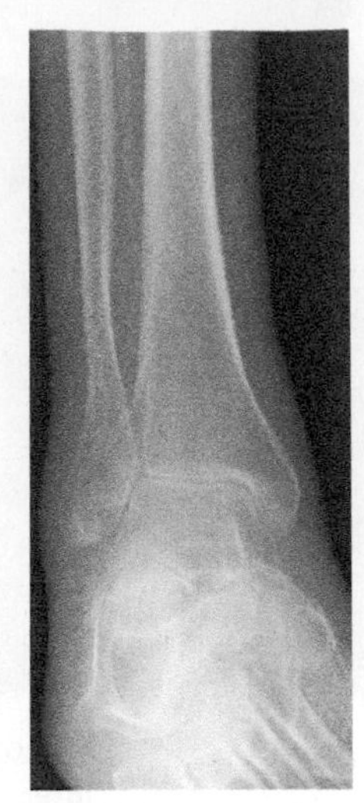

1. What are the pertinent radiograph findings?

2. What is the diagnosis?

3. What are predisposing factors for this entity?

4. What is the average time between the mean age of diabetes onset and the development of this fracture?

5. What is the definitive treatment?

Calcaneal insufficiency avulsion fracture 1532

Case ranking/difficulty: 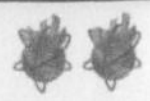

Category: Trauma

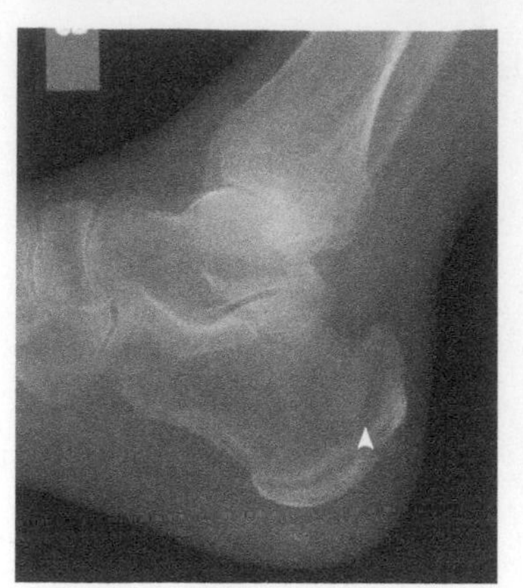

There is an acute, vertically oriented, and mildly displaced fracture of the posterior superior calcaneus. There is extensive vascular calcification.

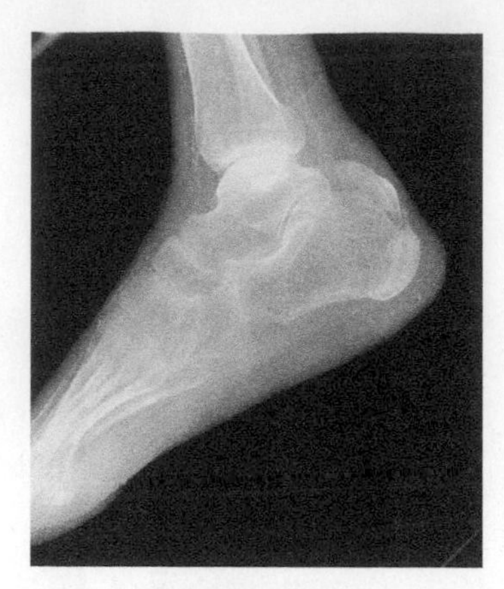

Radiograph taken three months later shows further displacement of the fracture.

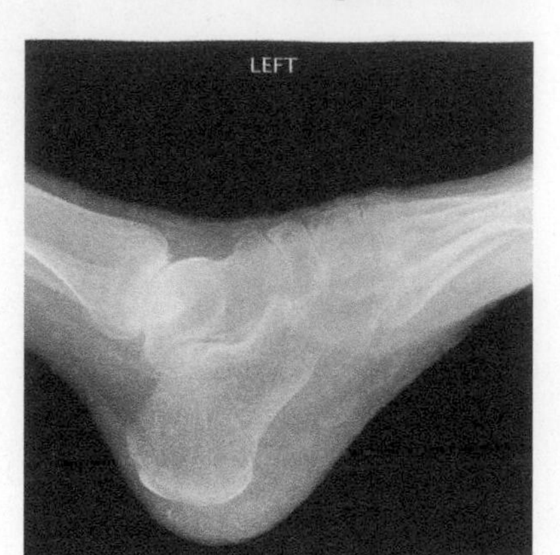

Lateral film of the contralateral side shows no fracture.

Answers

1. Vertically oriented, mildly displaced fracture of the posterior superior calcaneus, with vascular calcifications indicating the patient's diabetic status.
2. The diagnosis is a calcaneal insufficiency avulsion fracture (CIAF).
3. Diabetes mellitus, neuropathic foot, vascular insufficiency, soft-tissue infection, and osteoporosis are all contributory.
4. Average time from diabetes diagnosis to calcaneal avulsion fracture is 20 years.
5. Nondisplaced fractures can be treated conservatively and with good diabetes control, but the general tendency for this fracture to be displaced usually means surgical fixation is required.

Pearls

- Calcaneal insufficiency avulsion fractures (CIAFs) occur in patients with longstanding insulin-dependent diabetes.
- Typical time between the onset of diabetes and fracture is 20 years.
- Other conditions, such as peripheral vascular disease and hyperemia from soft-tissue infection, may also predispose to CIAF.
- The fractures are initially nondisplaced but rapidly progress to displacement.
- The fractures are vertically oriented at the posterior superior calcaneal tuberosity and often displaced by the pull of the Achilles tendon.
- MRI will detect changes of bone marrow edema and a fracture line before displacement occurs.
- Ultrasound can also show periosteal thickening and hyperemia on Doppler ultrasound in the early stages, before displacement occurs.

Suggested Readings

Arni D, Lambert V, Delmi M, Bianchi S. Insufficiency fracture of the calcaneum: Sonographic findings. *J Clin Ultrasound.* 2009;37(7):424–427.

Kathol MH, el-Khoury GY, Moore TE, Marsh JL. Calcaneal insufficiency avulsion fractures in patients with diabetes mellitus. *Radiology.* 1991;180(3):725–729.

History of anterior knee pain after running

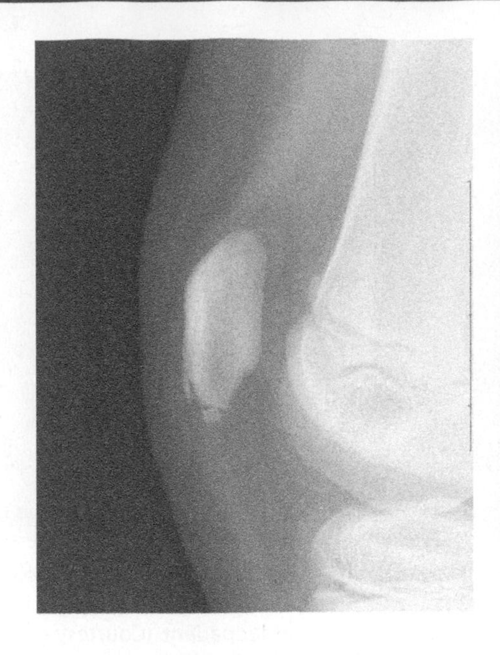

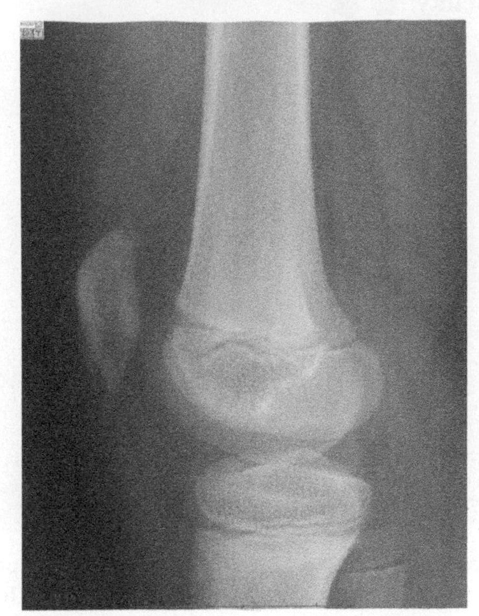

1. Which age group is commonly affected in this condition?

2. What is the proposed mechanism?

3. What are the typical radiological findings?

4. What is the significance of this injury?

5. What is the next most appropriate study?

Patella sleeve avulsion fracture 1345

Case ranking/difficulty: 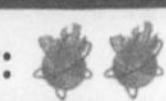 **Category:** Trauma

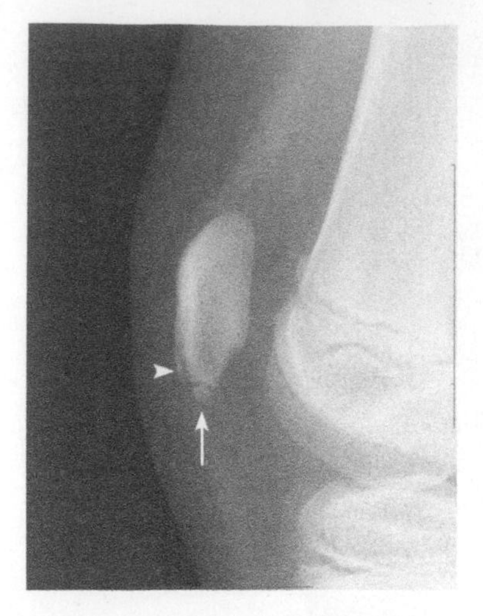

There is an avulsion fracture from the patella lower pole (*arrow*). Mild soft-tissue swelling is seen. Anterior patella density is an ossification center (*arrowhead*).

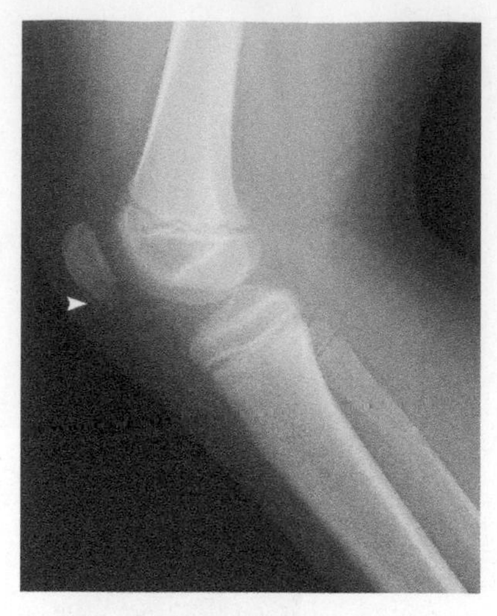

Another patient with a patella sleeve avulsion. (Courtesy of Children's Hospital of Philadelphia.)

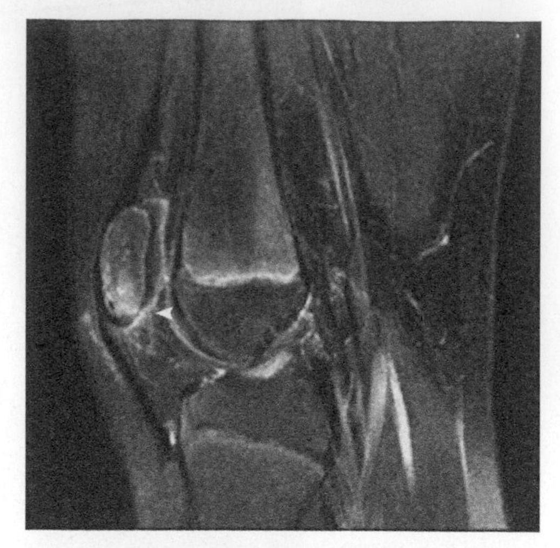

Osteochondral fracture well appreciated. The cartilaginous injury is minimal in this older patient. (Courtesy of Children's Hospital of Philadelphia.)

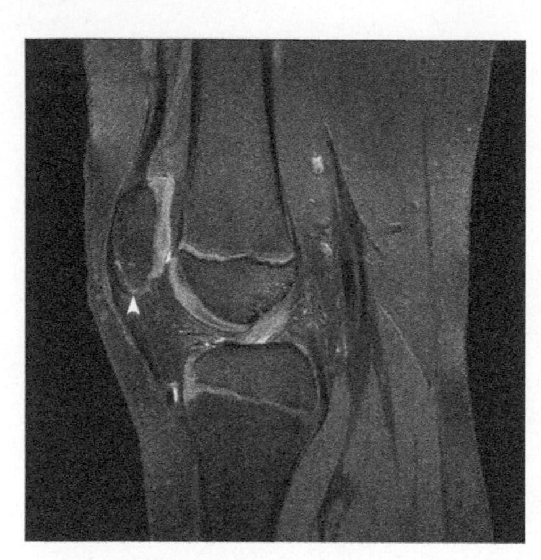

Osteochondral fracture. (Courtesy of Children's Hospital of Philadelphia.)

Answers

1. Patella sleeve avulsions are most common in the 8- to 12-years age group.

2. Patella sleeve avulsion results from a forced quadriceps contraction on a flexed knee. Sinding-Larsen-Johansson syndrome is an osteochondrosis of the lower pole of the patella affecting individuals aged 10 to 14 years.

3. Plain film radiographic findings of a patella sleeve avulsion include an avulsion fracture at the patella, soft-tissue swelling and joint effusion. Patella alta could be seen in some cases, if the patella tendon and its associated osseous fragment are completely avulsed.

4. The significance of a patella sleeve avulsion is that the cartilaginous and soft-tissue involvement is often disproportionate to the bony avulsion. Therefore, MRI is often necessary to assess the extensor mechanism and patella cartilage.

5. An MRI is often necessary to assess the extensor mechanism and patella cartilage, which may be injured in excess of the perceived osseous injury.

Pearls

- Lower pole patella avulsion fracture that occurs in young children.
- The size of the osseous fragment does not correlate with the severity of cartilage injury, as cartilage is a major component of a nonossified patella.
- MRI is usually indicated to evaluate the degree of cartilage injury.
- Results from forced contraction of the quadriceps on the flexed knee.
- Anterior patella ossification centers should not be confused with a patella sleeve avulsion.

Suggested Readings

Bates DG, Hresko MT, Jaramillo D. Patellar sleeve fracture: demonstration with MR imaging. *Radiology.* 1994;193(3):825–827.

Dupuis CS, Westra SJ, Makris J, Wallace EC. Injuries and conditions of the extensor mechanism of the pediatric knee. *Radiographics*. 2009;29(3):877–886.

Crush injury to knee while driving his golf cart

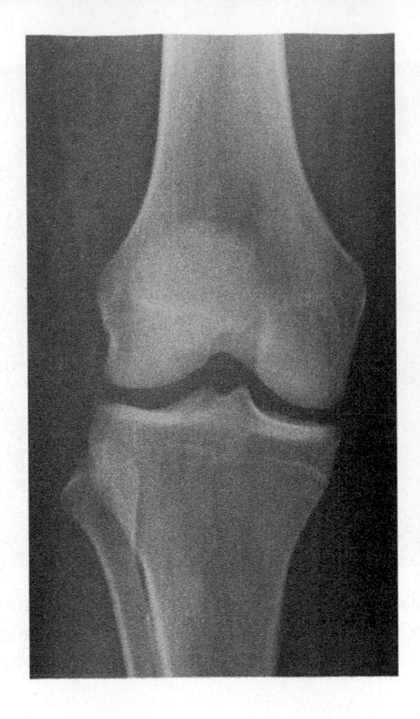

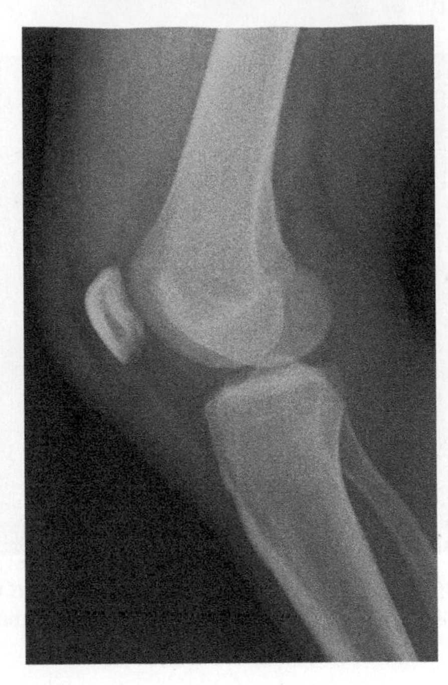

1. What is the abnormality seen on the AP and lateral plain films?

2. What is the next most appropriate imaging study?

3. This finding occurs in what clinical setting?

4. What patient population is most commonly affected?

5. What is the proposed mechanism?

Hoffa fracture 1315

Case ranking/difficulty: 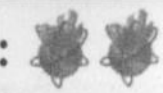

Category: Trauma

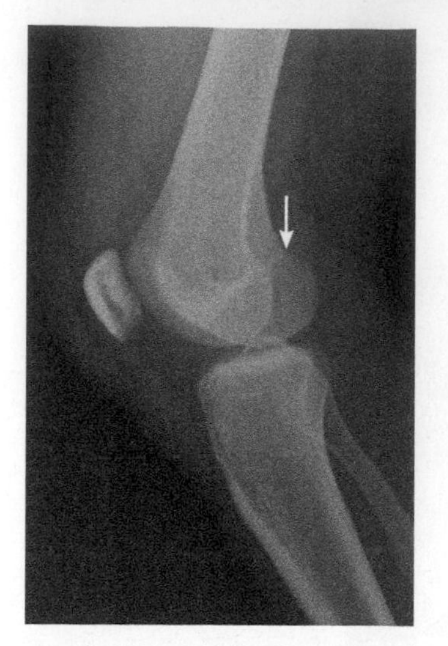

Very faint vertically oriented fracture line in the posterior medial femoral condyle.

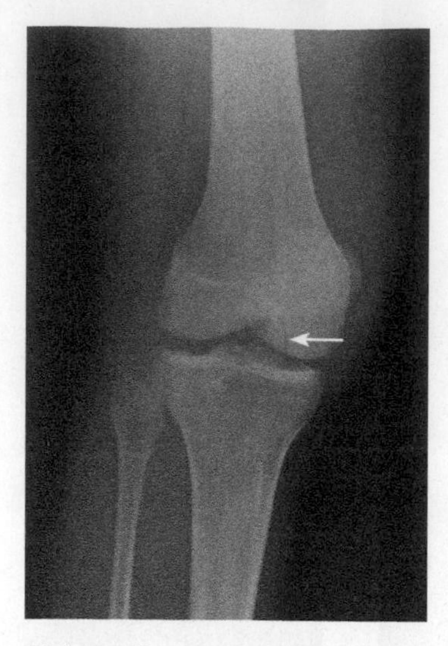

Oblique film clearly shows the fracture of the posterior medial femoral condyle.

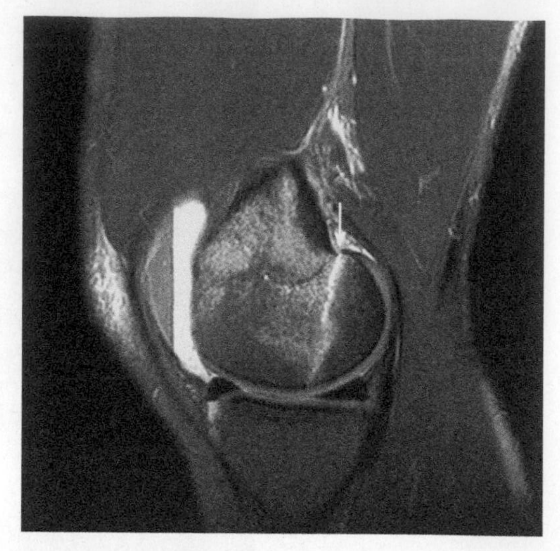

Coronally oriented posterior medial femoral condyle fracture, with associated bone marrow edema and lipohemarthrosis.

Answers

1. Faint visualization of a fracture in the posterior femoral condyle is seen only on the lateral film. A lipohemarthrosis is noted.
2. A trauma series of the knee should always include oblique films.
3. High-velocity injury.
4. Young active patients are the typical Hoffa fracture patient, as the injury is often associated with sports-related injuries and motor vehicle accidents.
5. Proposed mechanisms include axial loading with the knee in flexion and direct trauma possibly with an element of abduction.

Pearls

- A Hoffa fracture is a coronally oriented fracture in the posterior femoral condyle.
- The typical mechanism is axial loading in flexion.
- The lateral femoral condyle is affected more often than the medial.
- The injury occurs in the setting of high-velocity trauma.
- This fracture is often missed on standard AP and lateral film and is detected in only 69% of cases. Oblique views are useful.
- CT or MRI is usually required to confirm the diagnosis.

Suggested Readings

Dhillon MS, Mootha AK, Bali K, Prabhakar S, Dhatt SS, Kumar V. Coronal fractures of the medial femoral condyle: a series of 6 cases and review of literature. *Musculoskelet Surg*. 2012;96(1):49–54.

Thakar C. The Hoffa fracture—a fracture not to miss. *Emerg Med J*. 2010;27(5):391–392.

Pain in neck after diving into shallow pool

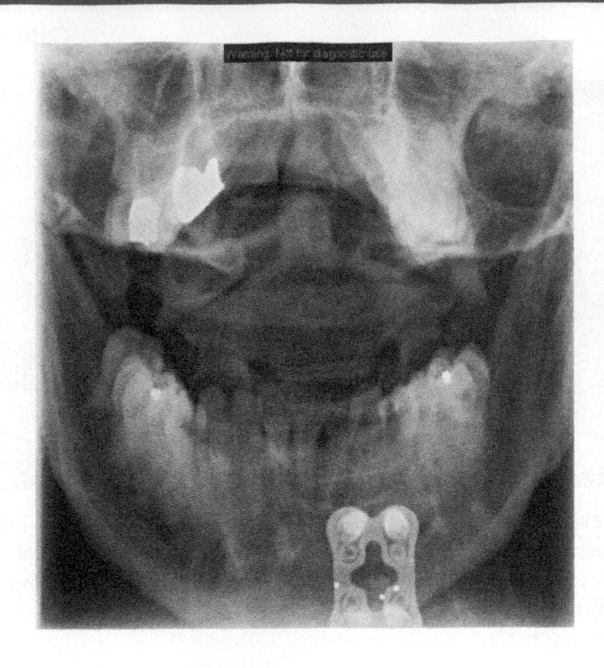

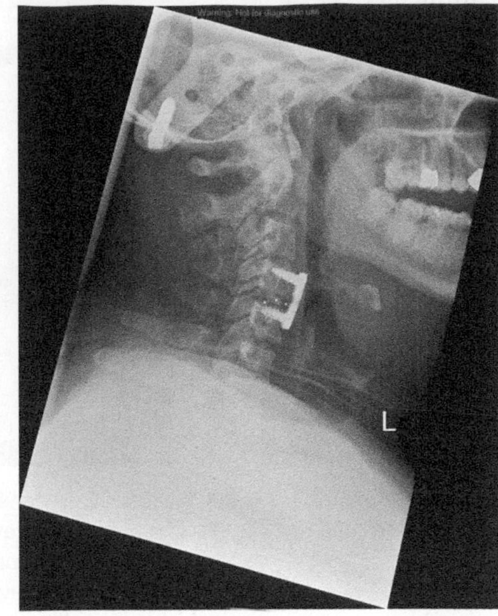

1. What is the mechanism of this injury?

2. What is used to determine the stability of the injury shown?

3. What ligament prevents posterior displacement of the odontoid peg?

4. What is the usual treatment for a stable burst fracture of C1?

5. What is the treatment required for the injury as shown?

Burst fracture of C1 (Jefferson) 527

Case ranking/difficulty: 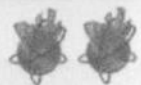

Category: Trauma

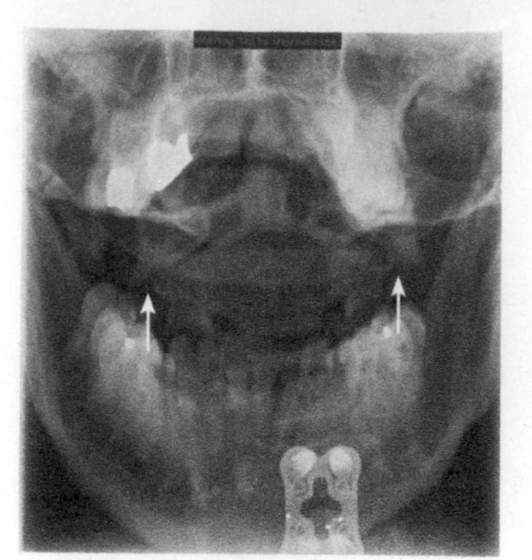

Open-mouth (peg) view showing separation of lateral masses of C1.

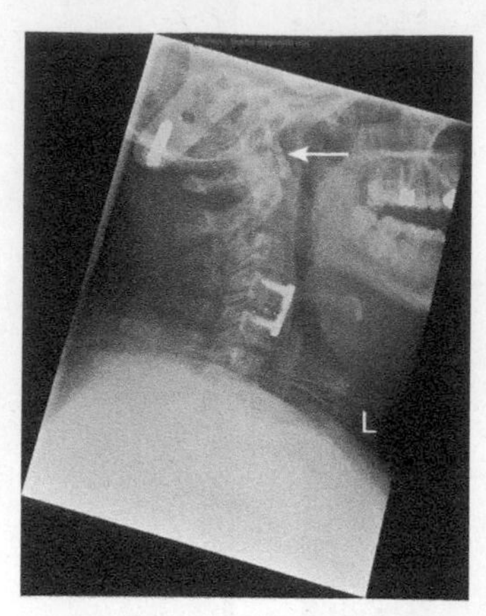

Lateral C-spine view shows C1 fracture with previous anterior cervical decompression and fusion. Note prevertebral soft-tissue swelling anterior to C1.

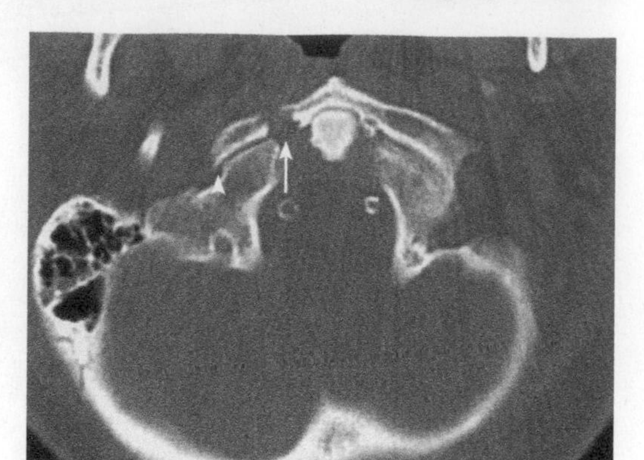

Fracture of right anterior arch of C1 demonstrated on axial CT (*arrow*). The right lateral mass of C1 has displaced laterally as a result (*arrowhead*).

Answers

1. Axial loading causes most burst fractures, especially C1 Jefferson fractures. The usual mechanism is sports-related injury or diving into a shallow swimming pool.
2. If the combined lateral mass displacement with respect to the articular surfaces of the axis is greater than 7 mm, the transverse ligament is considered to be ruptured, and the fracture is inherently unstable.
3. The transverse ligament of the atlas is the only structure that prevents posterior displacement of the odontoid peg. It is a very strong ligament; the integrity of which is vital to prevent cord injury. It is at risk of rupture with Jefferson fracture, especially when the lateral masses are involved.
4. The usual treatment for an undisplaced C1 fracture is a halo collar.
5. A displaced Jefferson fracture generally requires surgical stabilization of the cervical spine if the transverse ligament is ruptured, especially if associated with other cervical fractures. Many authorities will attempt nonoperative stabilization with a halo depending on the severity of the injury.

Pearls

- An axial-loading injury results in a burst fracture, which includes a Jefferson (C1) fracture.
- Stability is determined by the integrity of the transverse ligament.
- If the lateral masses of C1 are displaced by a total of 7 mm relative to C2, the transverse ligament is torn: the fracture is termed unstable and may require surgical fixation.
- MRI and CT are complementary investigations in cervical spine trauma to assess the cord and bony structures respectively.
- Initial assessment by plain films is adequate, if due care and attention is paid to the open-mouth odontoid peg view for displacement of the lateral masses of C1.
- Prevertebral soft-tissue swelling of greater than a third of the vertebral body from C1 to C3 in trauma cases should immediately trigger a CT examination to assess for an occult fracture.

Suggested Readings

Korinth MC, Kapser A, Weinzierl MR. Jefferson fracture in a child—illustrative case report. *Pediatr Neurosurg.* 2007;43(6):526–530.

Looby S, Flanders A. Spine trauma. *Radiol Clin North Am.* 2011;49(1):129–163.

Pratt H, Davies E, King L. Traumatic injuries of the C1/C2 complex: computed tomographic imaging appearances. *Curr Probl Diagn Radiol.* 2007;37(1):26–38.

Severe pain and swelling in knee after a skiing injury

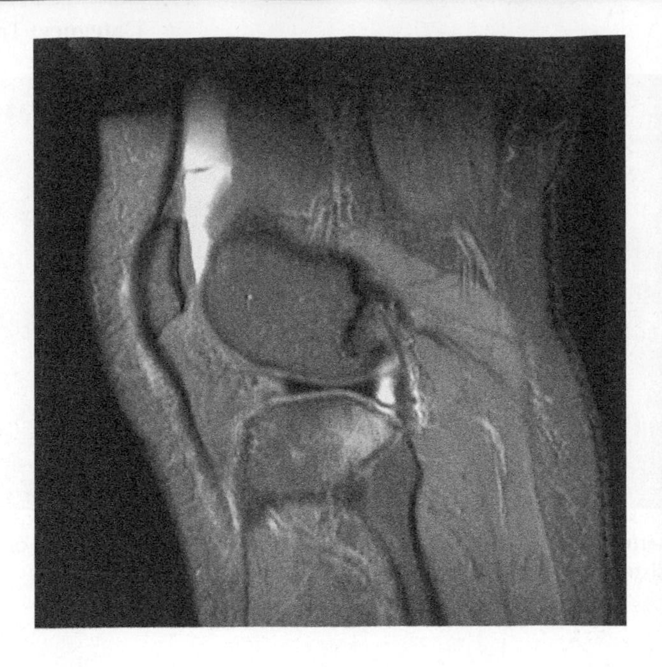

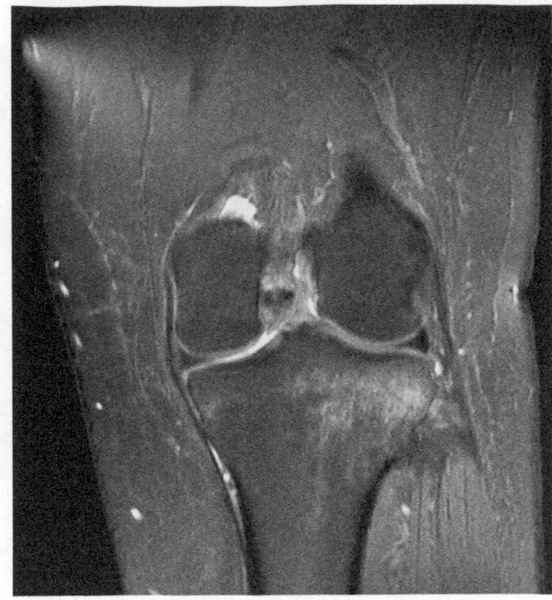

1. What is the mechanism of this injury?

2. Which soft-tissue structures are commonly damaged with this injury?

3. What is the management of this condition?

4. Which athletes are at risk of this injury?

5. What is the significance of anterior translation of the tibia on sagittal sequences?

Pivot-shift injury of knee 1702

Case ranking/difficulty: 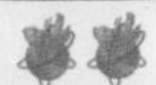

Category: Trauma

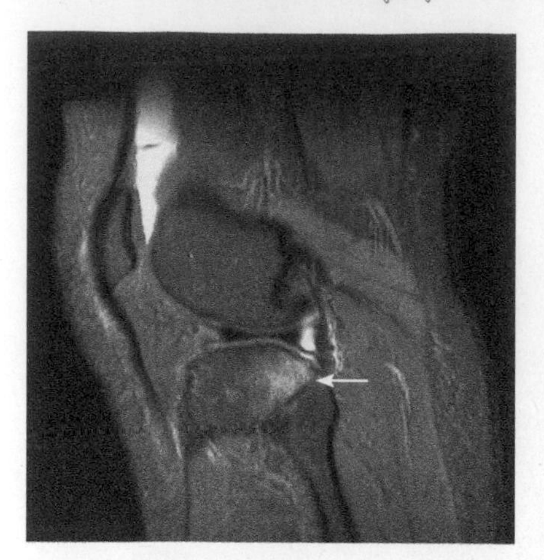

Marrow edema seen in posterior aspect of lateral tibial plateau is typical of a pivot-shift injury.

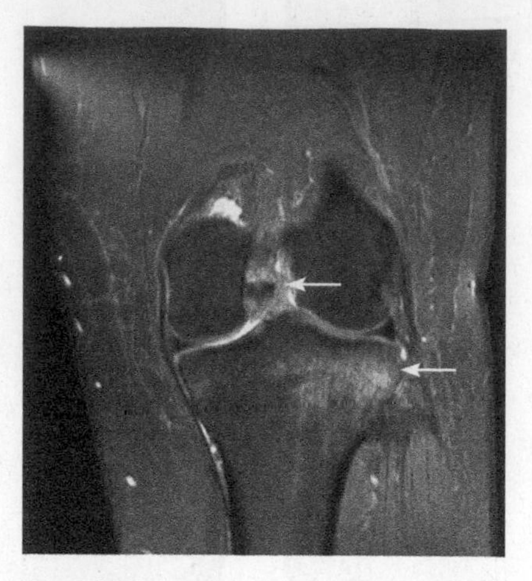

Tear of ACL and marrow edema in lateral tibial plateau consistent with a pivot-shift injury.

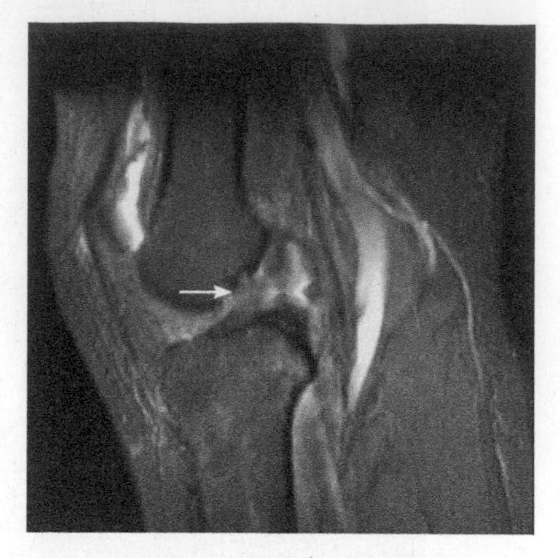

The ACL tear is well demonstrated on sagittal images.

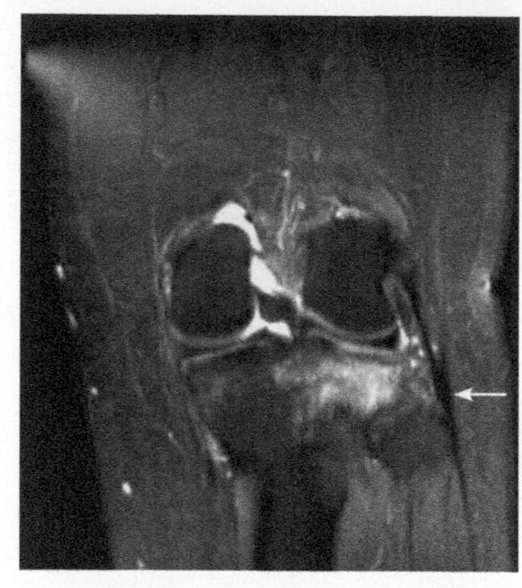

Although the posterolateral corner structures are intact in this patient, they must always be carefully evaluated in any pivot shift injury.

Answers

1. The pivot-shift mechanism is an extremely common mechanism of knee injury. It involves rapid deceleration with a rotational force.

2. Pivot shift injuries are associated with ACL, PCL, MCL, posterior horn of medial and lateral menisci, and posterolateral corner injuries.

3. The treatment depends on the structures damaged. If ACL/capsular/posterolateral corner structures are torn then repair is required. However an MRI is an essential investigation as it diagnoses the extent of internal derangement, if any, and may obviate the need for arthroscopy.

4. The pivot-shift injury requires a rapid deceleration and rotational force in a lower limb fixed to the ground. It cannot occur in a cyclist or swimmer as there is no excessive load to the ACL and no rotational component.

5. ACL rupture results in anterior translation of the tibia with respect to the femur.

Pearls

- The location of marrow edema in knee trauma provides important information as to the mechanism of injury.
- Pivot-shift knee injuries are associated with marrow edema in the posterior aspect of the lateral tibial plateau/fibular head and the lateral femoral condyle.
- A meticulous search for associated soft-tissue injuries should be performed, especially ACL, PCL, MCL, menisci, and posterolateral corner structures.

Suggested Readings

Fayad LM, Parellada JA, Parker L, Schweitzer ME. MR imaging of anterior cruciate ligament tears: is there a gender gap? *Skeletal Radiol*. 2003;32(11):639–646.

Sanders TG, Medynski MA, Feller JF, Lawhorn KW. Bone contusion patterns of the knee at MR imaging: footprint of the mechanism of injury. *Radiographics*. 2000;20 Spec No:S135–S151.

Yoo JH, Yang BK, Ryu HK. A case of fracture of posterior margin of lateral tibial plateau by pivot shift mechanism in chronic ACL insufficiency. *Arch Orthop Trauma Surg*. 2009;129(3):363–367.

Motor vehicle to bicycle injury

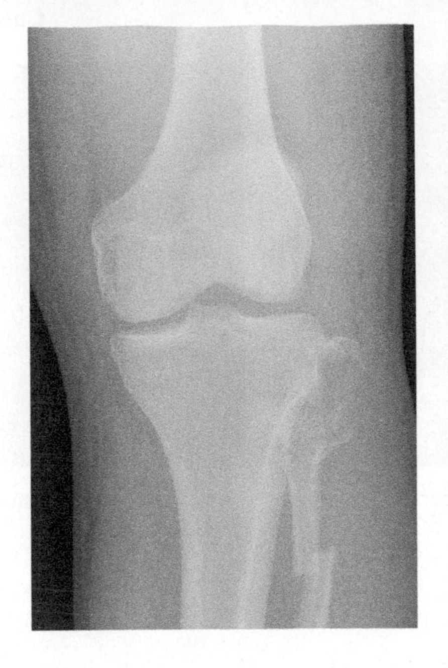

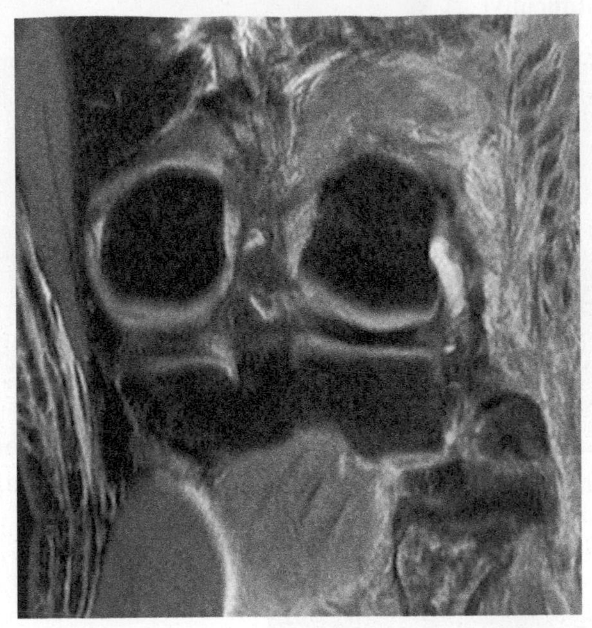

1. What are the MRI findings?

2. What is the diagnosis?

3. There is a paucity of joint fluid in posterolateral corner injury. True or False?

4. Arcuate fracture indicates a posterolateral corner injury. True or False?

5. What is the usual mechanism of injury?

Posterolateral corner injury 1289

Case ranking/difficulty: 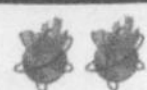

Category: Trauma

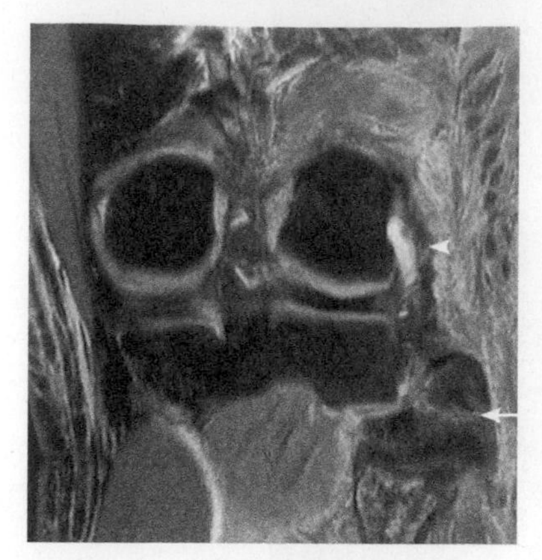

Fibular head fracture (*arrow*) and high-grade fibular collateral ligament injury (*arrowhead*).

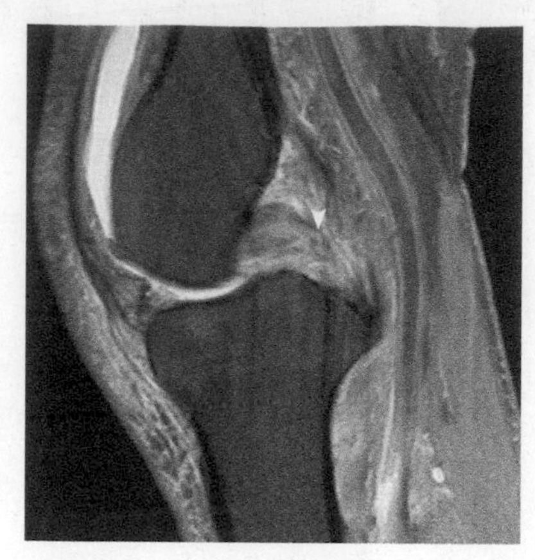

Posterior cruciate ligament tear.

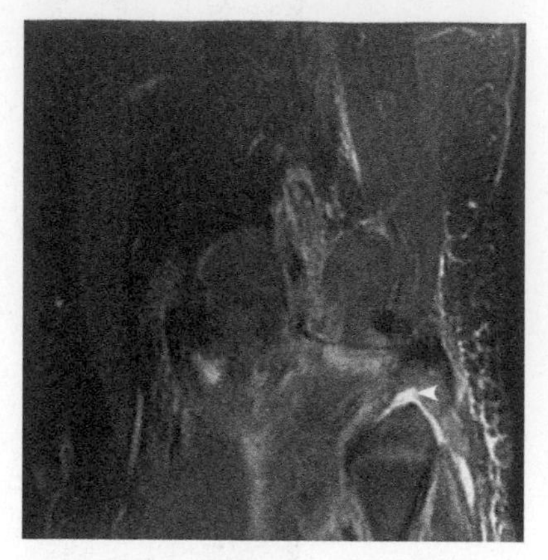

Conjoint tendon avulsion in another patient.

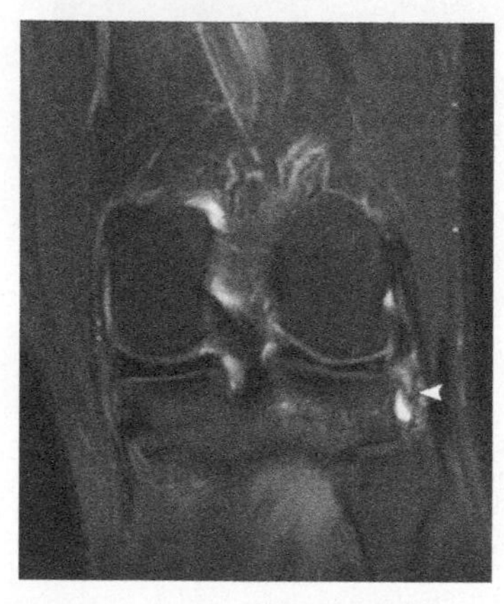

High-grade partial tear of the popliteofibular ligament in another patient.

Answers

1. Tears of the arcuate ligament, fabellofibular ligament and popliteofibular ligament are suspected because of the marked disproportionate posterolateral soft-tissue edema. There is definite lateral collateral ligament injury and associated posterior cruciate ligament tear.
2. Posterolateral corner injury.
3. Some studies have noted a paucity of joint fluid in posterolateral corner injury, consistent with joint capsule or arcuate ligament rupture and leakage of synovial fluid.
4. An arcuate fracture is an avulsion fracture of the fibular head, which suggests an underlying injury to the posterolateral corner structures particularly to the popliteofibular, fabellofibular, and arcuate ligaments.
5. Varus and external rotation injury, dashboard injury, external rotation and hyperextension injury.

Pearls

- The posterolateral corner includes many complex capsular and noncapsular structures.
- The components include the lateral gastrocnemius tendon, posterolateral joint capsule, fibular collateral ligament (FCL), popliteus tendon complex, arcuate ligament, popliteofibular ligament, and the fabellofibular ligament. The popliteofibular ligament is a particularly important stabilizer, along with the FCL and popliteus tendon.
- Isolated injuries are not unstable. Injury to two or more of the components are required for significant instability.
- A paucity of joint fluid is often seen in posterolateral corner injury, indicating arcuate ligament and/or capsular tears with synovial fluid leakage.
- Posterolateral corner injury is associated with ACL and PCL tears.
- The treatment usually includes surgical repair.
- If unrecognized, the resulting instability leads to early osteoarthritis of the knee and recurrent cruciate ligament tears, post reconstruction.

Suggested Readings

Apsingi S, Eachempati KK, Shah GK, Kumar S. Posterolateral corner injuries of the knee—a review. *J Indian Med Assoc.* 2011;109(6):400–403.

Huang GS, Yu JS, Munshi M, et al. Avulsion fracture of the head of the fibula (the "arcuate" sign): MR imaging findings predictive of injuries to the posterolateral ligaments and posterior cruciate ligament. *AJR Am J Roentgenol.* 2003;180(2):381–387.

Vinson EN, Major NM, Helms CA. The posterolateral corner of the knee. *AJR Am J Roentgenol.* 2008;190(2):449–458.

Acute knee injury with knee pain

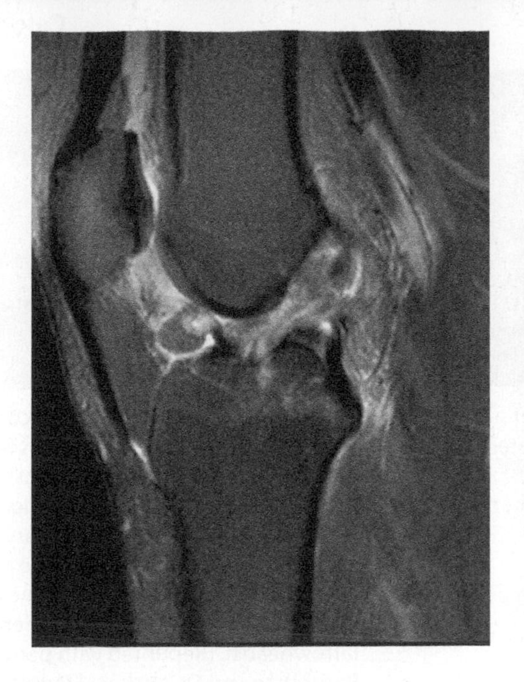

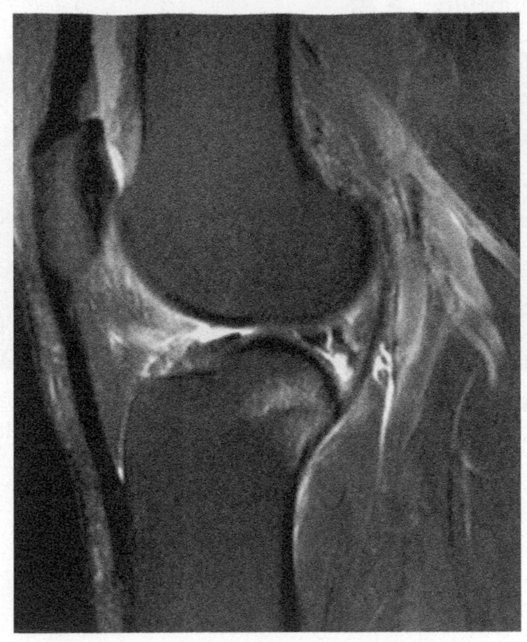

1. What are the MRI findings?

2. What is the differential diagnosis?

3. What is the significance of the meniscal abnormality?

4. What is the proposed mechanism for the meniscal abnormality?

5. What is the management?

Wrisberg rip tear lateral meniscus 1344

Case ranking/difficulty: 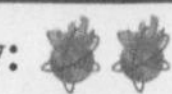 **Category:** Trauma

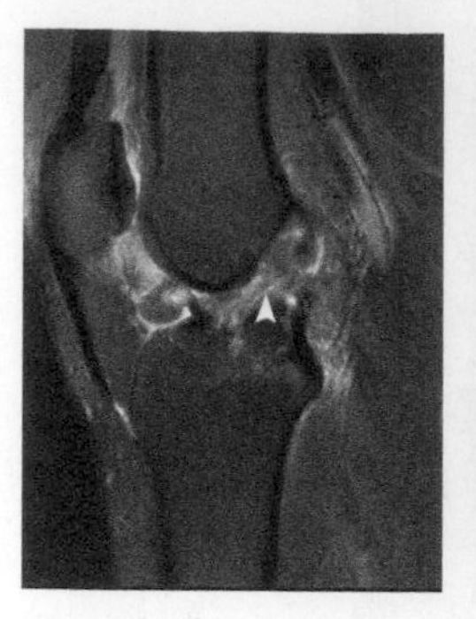

Complete tear of the ACL.

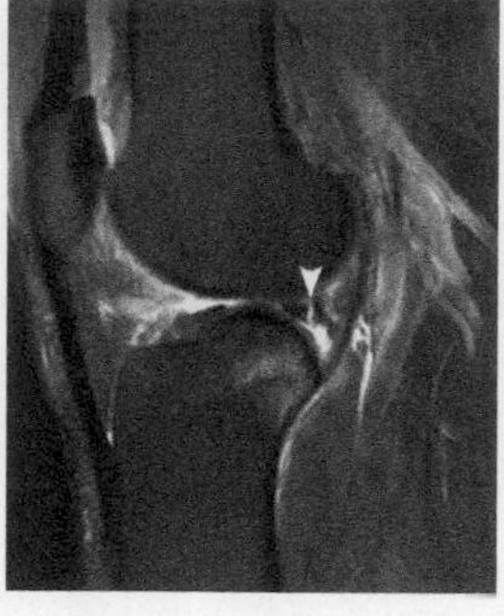

Longitudinal tear of the posterior horn lateral meniscus.

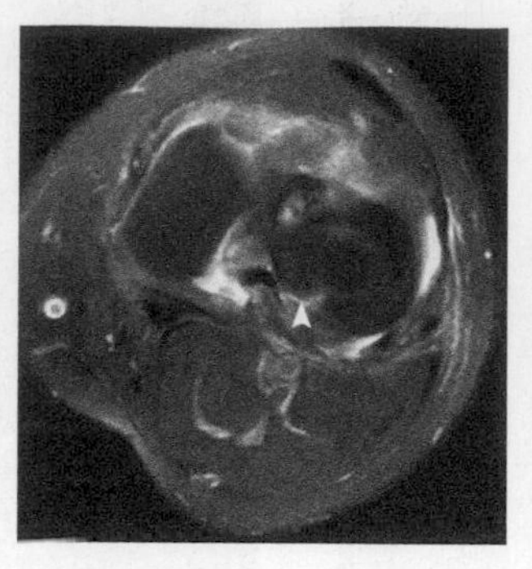

Longitudinal tear of the posterior horn lateral meniscus.

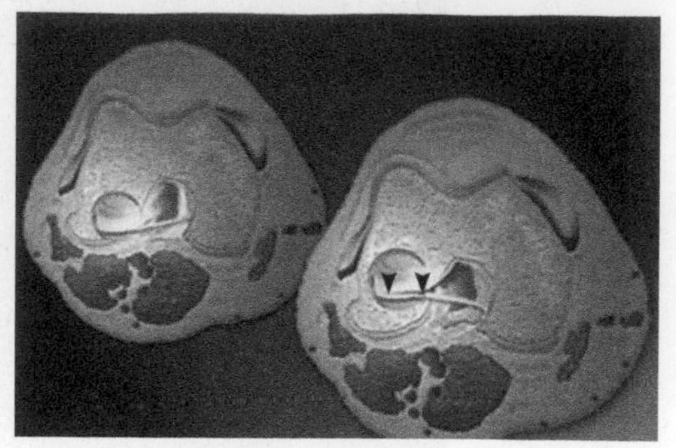

Illustration showing the oblique course of the ligament of Wrisberg as it courses from the medial femoral condyle to the posterior meniscal horn laterally. On the right, anterior translation of the tibia has occurred secondary to an ACL tear. As a result, traction upon the posterior horn of the lateral meniscus by the ligament of Wrisberg causes a longitudinal meniscal tear (arrowheads). (Reprinted with permission from Radsource and Dr. Michael Stadnick.)

Answers

1. There is a longitudinal tear of the posterior horn lateral meniscus, with a complete midportion ACL tear.
2. The fibers of the ACL are discontinuous, consistent with an ACL tear. A Wrisberg pseudotear, which is a simulated tear at the junction of the Wrisberg ligament attachment and the posterior horn lateral meniscus is possible, but the longitudinal signal in the lateral meniscus extends too far laterally. This is a true meniscal tear, the so-called Wrisberg "rip" tear.
3. The significance of a Wrisberg rip tear is that it always occurs with an ACL tear, and it is also a difficult tear to identify. Therefore, when an ACL tear is seen, close attention to the posterior horn lateral meniscus is warranted.
4. The longitudinal tear of the posterior horn of the lateral meniscus at the attachment of the Wrisberg ligament is likely caused by the anterior translation of the tibia relative to the femur that occurs in ACL tears. The tibial translation pulls on the Wrisberg attachment at the lateral meniscus while the femoral attachment remains fixed, resulting in a longitudinal split of the posterior horn lateral meniscus.
5. Meniscal repairs are best performed at the time of ACL reconstruction. Consequently, both the ACL reconstruction and meniscal repair are usually done at the same time.

Pearls

- A longitudinal tear of the posterior horn of the lateral meniscus, at the meniscal attachment of Wrisberg's ligament, has been termed a *Wrisberg "rip" tear*.
- It only occurs in association with an ACL tear.
- It should be considered a secondary sign of an ACL tear.
- Anterior translation of the tibia relative to the femur, as occurs in an ACL tear, puts traction on the Wrisberg ligament meniscal attachment, essentially splitting the posterior horn longitudinally.
- Treatment is usually surgical.

Suggested Readings

Awh MH, Stadnick M. Wrisberg pseudotear and Wrisberg rip. *MRI Web Clin*. October 2003.

De Smet AA, Mukherjee R. Clinical, MRI, and arthroscopic findings associated with failure to diagnose a lateral meniscal tear on knee MRI. *AJR Am J Roentgenol*. 2008;190(1):22–26.

Sudden blow to the medial aspect of patella during soccer

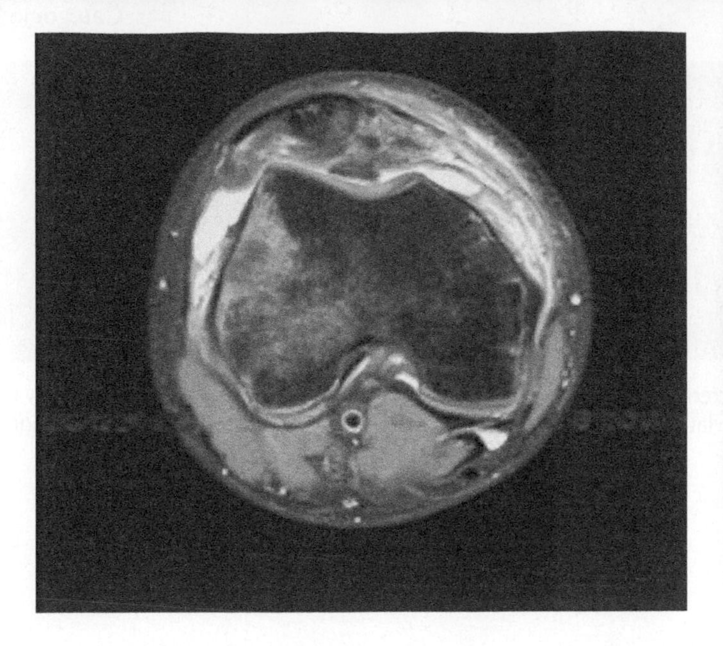

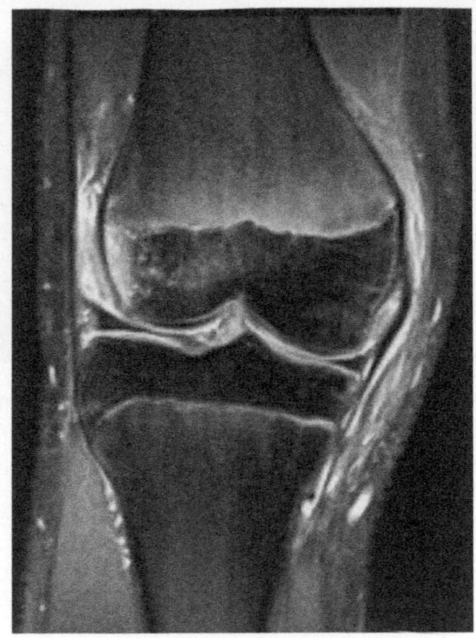

1. What sports are associated with this entity?

2. What ligament is almost always torn?

3. What are the predisposing factors?

4. Which imaging modality is best for dynamic assessment of patellar maltracking?

5. Which clinical examination is useful in confirming patellar subluxation?

Lateral patellar dislocation 478

Case ranking/difficulty: 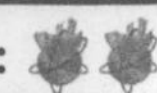

Category: Trauma

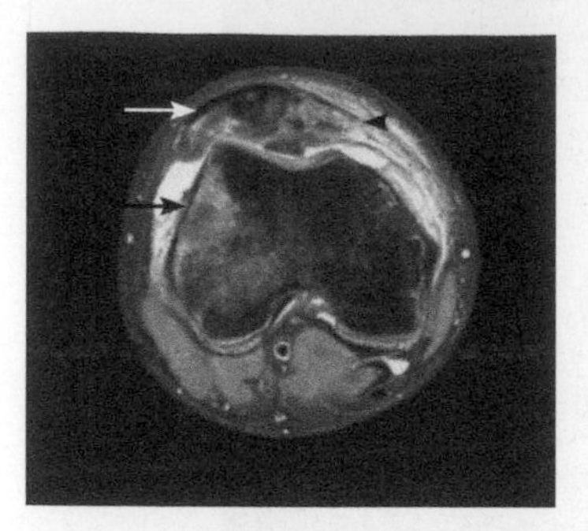

Marrow edema in lateral patellar facet and "kissing contusion" in lateral femoral condyle (*arrows*). The pattern here is a little atypical as more commonly there is edema within the medial patellar facet. Torn medial patellofemoral ligament (*arrowhead*).

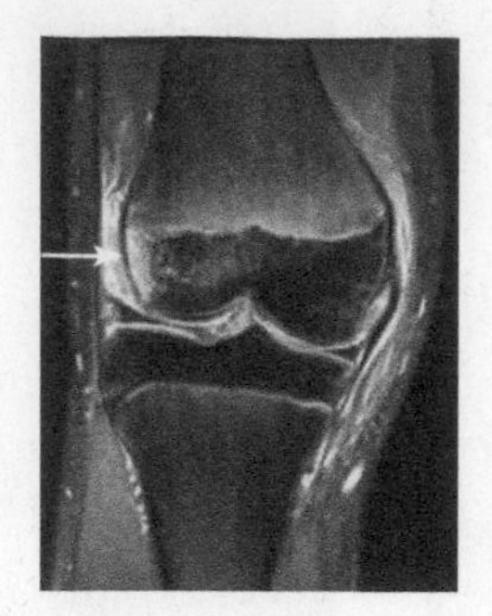

Characteristic pattern of marrow edema in lateral femoral condyle.

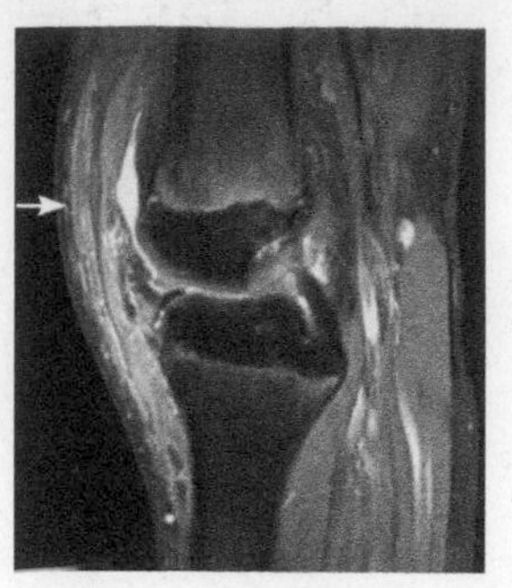

Large amount of prepatellar edema, and moderate suprapatellar effusion. Intact ACL, PCL, and menisci.

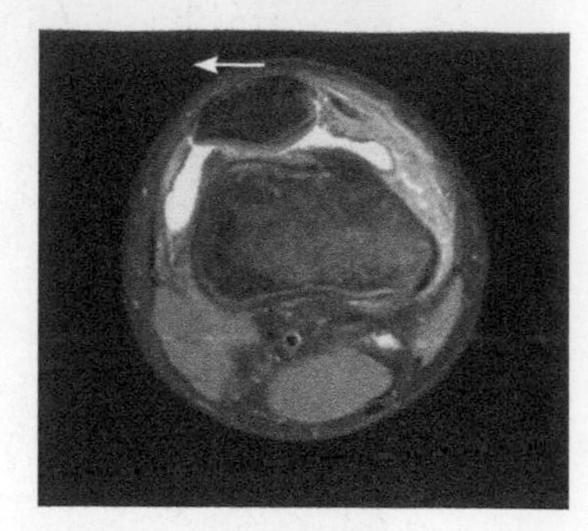

The patella lies laterally tilted and subluxed postdislocation.

Answers

1. Sudden movements against a contracted vastus medialis obliquus muscle can cause lateral dislocation of the patella in predisposed individuals with patellofemoral dysfunction. Sports in which this can occur include soccer, baseball, cricket, and tennis.

2. The medial patellofemoral ligament (medial retinaculum) is torn in 97% of cases of lateral patellar dislocation.

3. The predisposing conditions are those of patellofemoral dysfunction generally, for example, trochlear dysplasia, patella alta, lateralized tibial tubercle, and vastus medialis dysfunction.

4. Although CT and ultrasound have been used to assess patellar maltracking, the best modality is kinematic MRI using a fast gradient-recalled echo sequence.

   Lateral subluxation can be fully assessed with active contraction of the quadriceps using this technique.

5. The patellar apprehension test is sensitive for detecting patellar subluxation on clinical examination. It involves the examiner attempting to laterally sublux the patella while watching the patient's face. If the patient winces or contracts the quadriceps forcefully, the test is considered positive. The anterior drawer (Lachman) test is for ACL rupture. Apley grind test and the McMurray maneuver are for detecting meniscal tears.

Pearls

- A laterally subluxed patella with a large effusion/soft-tissue edema is suggestive of recent dislocation.
- A characteristic pattern of marrow edema in the medial patellar facet and lateral femoral condyle is highly suggestive of the diagnosis.
- Ninety-seven percent of injuries are associated with rupture of the medial patellofemoral ligament.
- The chondral surfaces of the patella and femoral trochlea should be evaluated for associated osteochondral defects, fractures, and stripping of the VM off the femur.
- Underlying causes of patellofemoral dysfunction should be sought, for example, patella alta, trochlear dysplasia, lateralized tibial tuberosity, patellar tilt, vastus medialis obliquus (VMO) tears, and weakness.
- Patella alta relates to the length of the patella hyaline cartilage with respect to the length of the patellar ligament and is most commonly assessed by the Insall-Salvati ratio.

Suggested Readings

Balcarek P, Ammon J, Frosch S, et al. Magnetic resonance imaging characteristics of the medial patellofemoral ligament lesion in acute lateral patellar dislocations considering trochlear dysplasia, patella alta, and tibial tuberosity-trochlear groove distance. *Arthroscopy.* 2010;26(7):926–935.

Peltola EK, Koskinen SK. Multidetector computed tomography evaluation of bony fragments and donor sites in acute patellar dislocation. *Acta Radiol.* 2011;52(1):86–90.

von Engelhardt LV, Raddatz M, Bouillon B, et al. How reliable is MRI in diagnosing cartilaginous lesions in patients with first and recurrent lateral patellar dislocations? *BMC Musculoskelet Disord.* 2010;11(11):149.

Sudden pain in the right foot

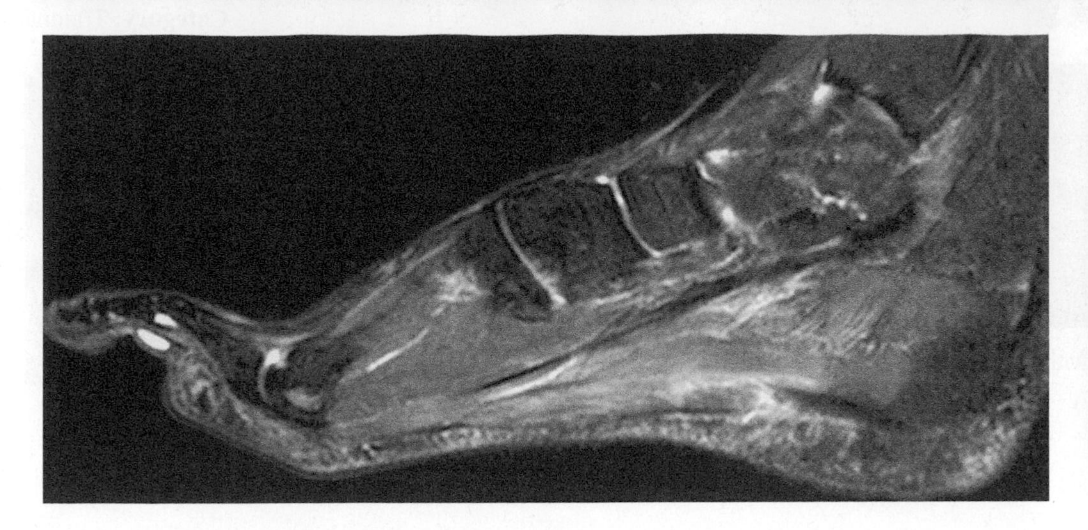

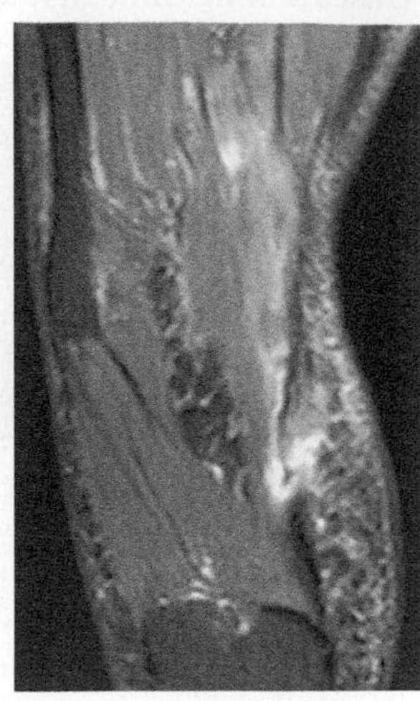

1. What are the MRI findings?

2. What is the differential diagnosis?

3. What is the diagnosis?

4. What are the different components of the affected structure?

5. What is the risk of rupture in patients who have had steroid injections?

Plantar fascia rupture 2262

Case ranking/difficulty: 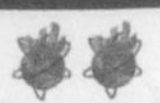 **Category:** Trauma

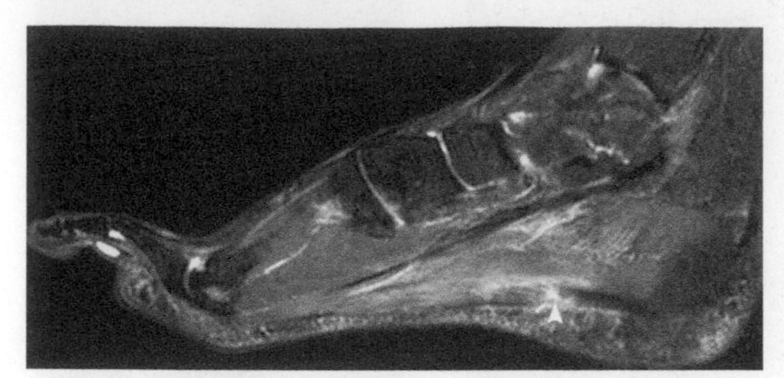

Discontinuity of plantar fascia with increased signal at the site of rupture.

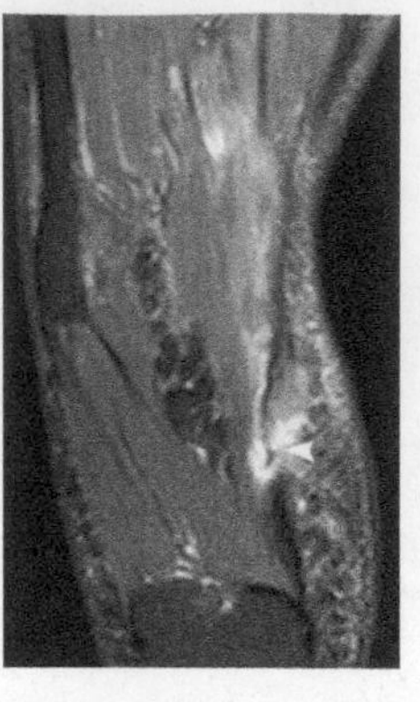

Fluid gap in the plantar fascia.

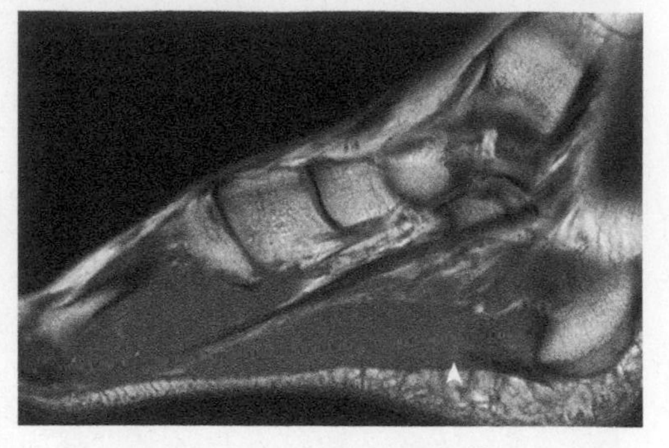

Complete rupture of the plantar fascia.

Answers

1. There is high T2 signal and low T1 signal with a fluid gap and edema in the plantar aponeurosis. This is consistent with a tear of the plantar fascia, with retraction.
2. The differential diagnosis includes rupture of the FHL or FDL tendons, plantar fascia tear, plantar fibromas, and plantar fasciitis.
3. The diagnosis is a full-thickness plantar fascia tear.
4. Medial, central, and lateral bands are the main components of the plantar fascia. The central band is the thickest and most important, and helps to maintain the plantar arch.
5. The risk of plantar fascia rupture after steroid injections is 10%.

Pearls

- Rupture of the planter fascia is very uncommon. It commonly occurs in athletic sports involving jumping and running, where there is sudden plantar flexion.
- Underlying plantar fascitis or recurrent steroid injections increases the chance of rupture. Plantar fasciitis can be caused by either repetitive trauma or inflammatory conditions, such as rheumatoid arthritis, Behçet disease, ankylosing spondylitis, or Reactive arthritis.
- Tears can be acute or chronic, and partial or complete.
- Ultrasound and MRI are the main imaging modalities. In the acute stage, there is a clear gap at the rupture site with hematoma and increased fluid collection on ultrasound. On MRI, low T1 and high T2/STIR signal intensity tear with fluid collection is seen. T1-weighted images helps to decide partial or complete tears. There is enhancement on post-contrast images.
- Chronic rupture shows scar tissue of low T1 and T2 signal intensity. In some cases of chronic rupture, along with fibrotic changes, there are cystic changes between the layers.
- Treatment is usually nonsurgical with ice, crutches, and anti-inflammatory drugs.
- Surgery is not routinely indicated.

Suggested Readings

Narváez JA, Narváez J, Ortega R, Aguilera C, Sánchez A, Andía E. Painful heel: MR imaging findings. *Radiographics.* 2000;20(2):333–352.

Theodorou DJ, Theodorou SJ, Farooki S, Kakitsubata Y, Resnick D. Disorders of the plantar aponeurosis: a spectrum of MR imaging findings. *AJR Am J Roentgenol.* 2001;176(1):97–104.

Theodorou DJ, Theodorou SJ, Kakitsubata Y, Lektrakul N, Gold GE, Roger B, Resnick D. Plantar fasciitis and fascial rupture: MR imaging findings in 26 patients supplemented with anatomic data in cadavers. *Radiographics.* 2000;20 Spec No:S181–S197.

Sudden pain in shoulder while waterskiing

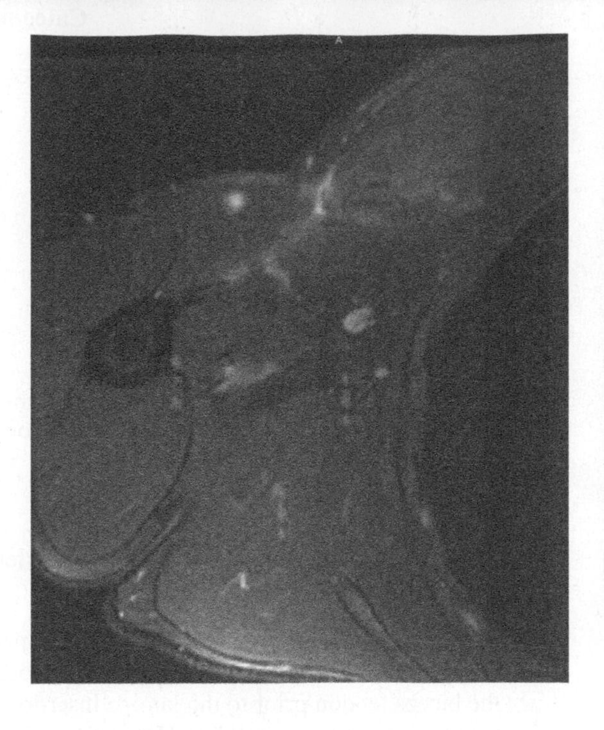

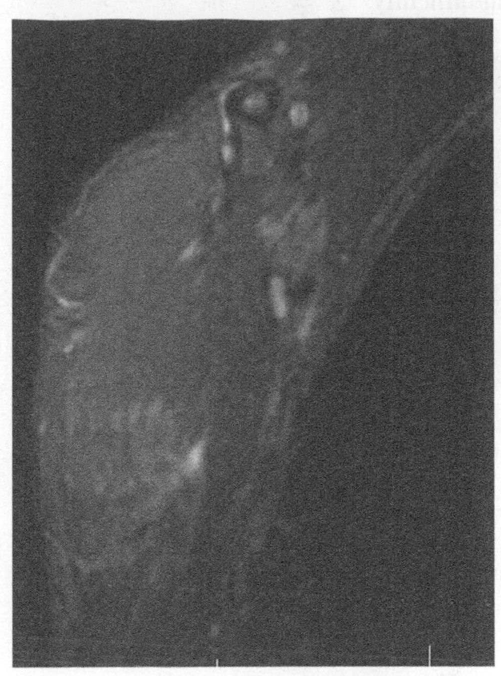

1. What are the MRI findings?

2. What are the origins of the affected structure?

3. Which laminae form the insertion of the affected structure, and where does it insert?

4. Regarding tears of this structure, most are insertional. True or False?

5. The affected structure contributes to the stability of the biceps tendon. True or False?

Pectoralis major tear 2305

Case ranking/difficulty: 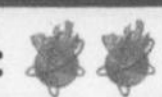

Category: Trauma

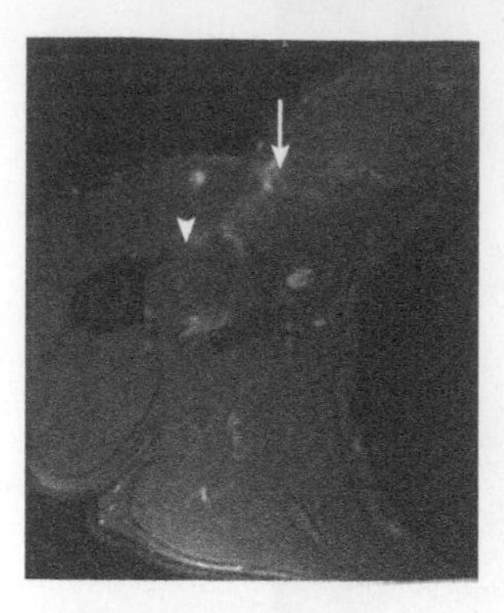

High-grade partial tear at the musculotendinous junction of the pectoralis major muscle, sternal head (*arrow*). The distal tendon (*arrowhead*) is intact.

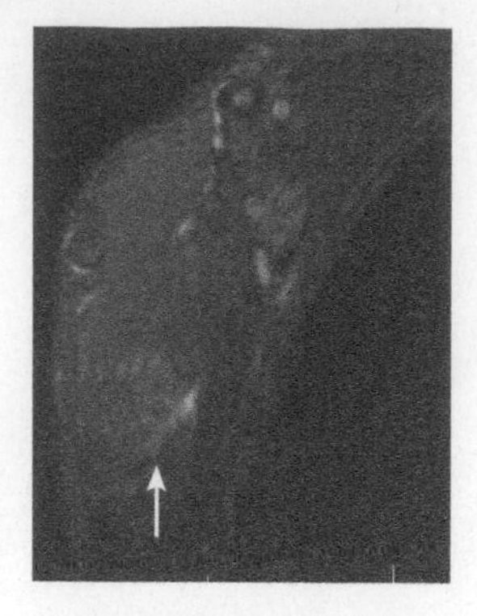

High-grade partial tear at the musculotendinous junction of the pectoralis major muscle, sternal head (*arrow*).

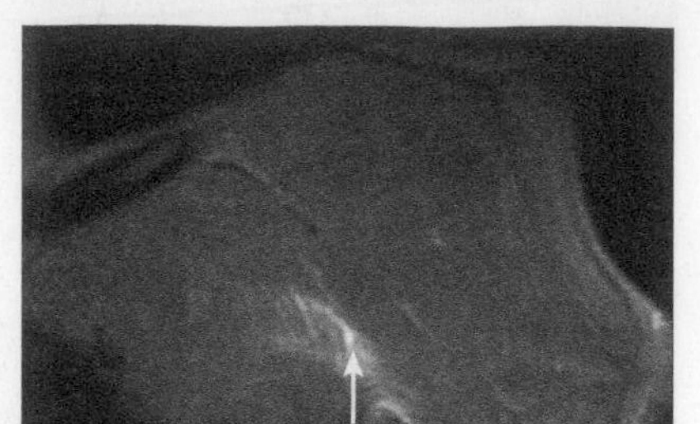

Another patient showing high grade partial tear at the sternal head musculotendinous junction, well appreciated on oblique coronal images.

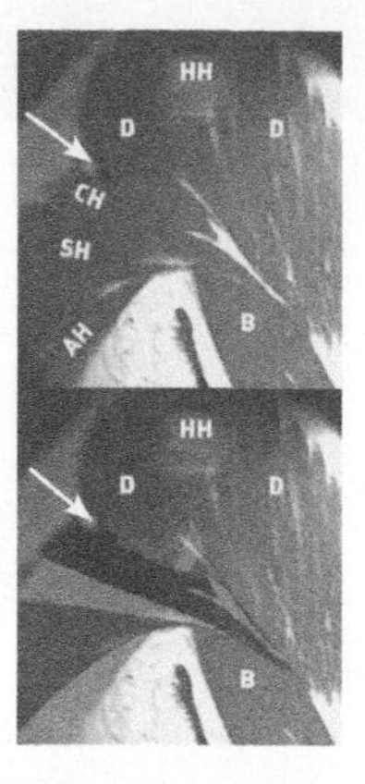

Normal pectoralis major anatomy. The cephalic vein within the deltopectoral groove (*arrow*) separates the deltoid muscle fibers and the clavicular head of the pectoralis major, an important anatomical landmark. CH, clavicular head; SH, sternal head; AH, Abdominal head. (Reprinted with permission from Radsource and Dr. Michael Stadnick.)

Answers

1. There is a high-grade partial tear at the sternal head of the pectoralis major muscle at the musculotendinous junction.
2. The pectoralis major muscle has three major origins: the clavicular, sternal, and abdominal heads. These heads arise from the clavicle, sternum, anterior ribs, and the external oblique fascia.
3. The pectoralis major tendon has two laminae, the sternal and clavicular laminae, which insert on the lateral intertubercular sulcus of the bicipital groove of the humerus.
4. False. Most pectoralis tears are at the musculotendinous junction of the sternal head, and are typically partial tears. Insertional tears are less common and tend to be complete tears.
5. True. The fibers of the sternal lamina of the pectoralis major tendon are partially attached to the long head of the biceps tendon prior to the lamina insertion, and help to stabilize the biceps tendon. Hence, insertional tears of the pectoralis major tendon can result in biceps tendon instability with mild subluxation.

Pearls

- The pectoralis major muscle origin has three heads: clavicular, sternal, and abdominal.
- The pectoralis major tendon has two laminae: the clavicular lamina and the sternal lamina.
- The sternal lamina courses upwards in a 180-degree fashion to insert proximal to the clavicular lamina.
- The abdominal fibers of the sternal lamina contribute to biceps tendon stability.
- Most tears are at the musculotendinous junction of the sternal head and are usually partial.
- Distal insertional tears are less common and are often complete tears.
- Oblique coronal MRI imaging is useful in evaluating the anatomy.

Suggested Readings

Connell DA, Potter HG, Sherman MF, Wickiewicz TL. Injuries of the pectoralis major muscle: evaluation with MR imaging. *Radiology.* 1999;210(3):785–791.

Lee J, Brookenthal KR, Ramsey ML, Kneeland JB, Herzog R. MR imaging assessment of the pectoralis major myotendinous unit: an MR imaging-anatomic correlative study with surgical correlation. *AJR Am J Roentgenol.* 2000;174(5):1371–1375.

Sudden popping sensation after lifting heavy object

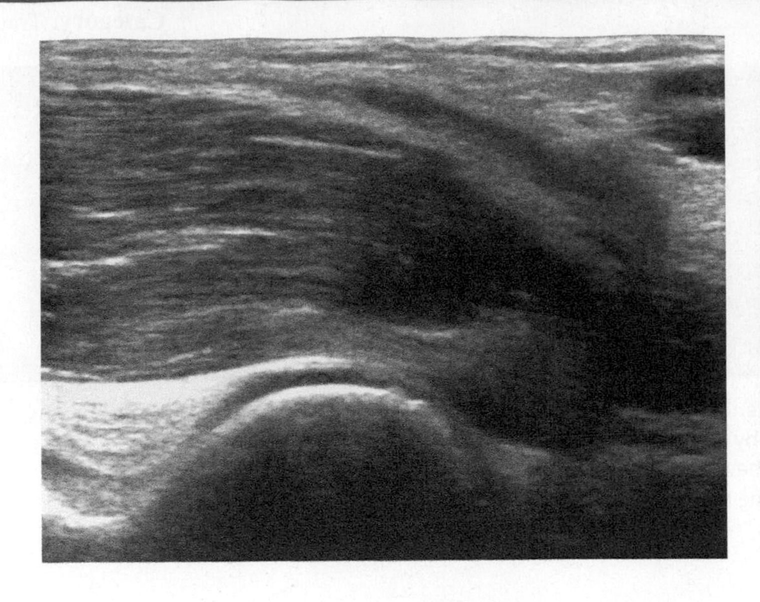

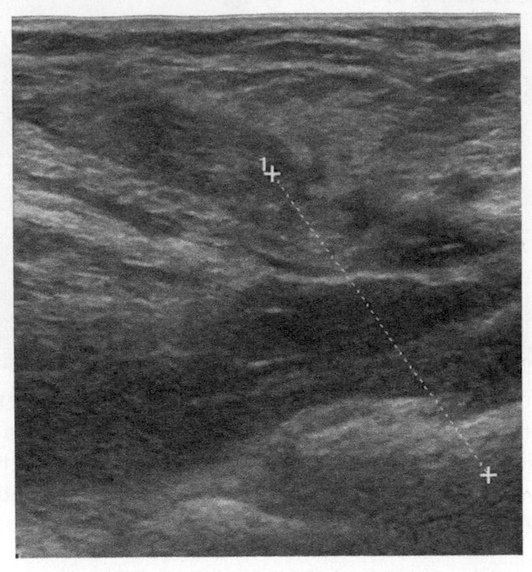

1. What are the ultrasound findings?
2. What is the diagnosis?
3. What are the expected MRI features of this condition, if it was partially injured?
4. What is the most common site of injury to this structure?
5. What MRI technique is useful in evaluating the distal biceps tendon?

Distal biceps tendon rupture 1444

Case ranking/difficulty: 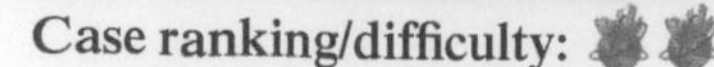

Category: Trauma

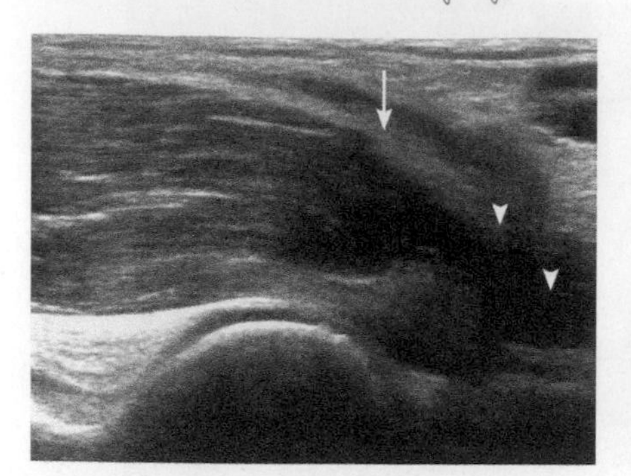

Ultrasound (longitudinal plane) image showing distal biceps rupture at the insertion on the radial tuberosity (*arrowheads*). Empty tendon sheath (*arrow*).

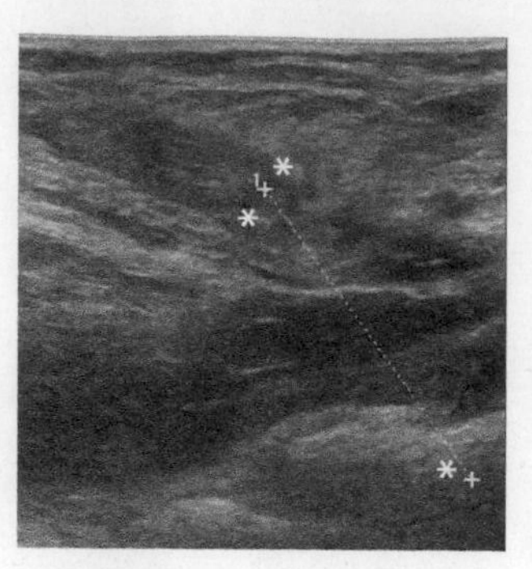

Degree of tendon retraction is outlined by the marker. *Asterisk* is the radius, *double asterisk* is the retracted tendon.

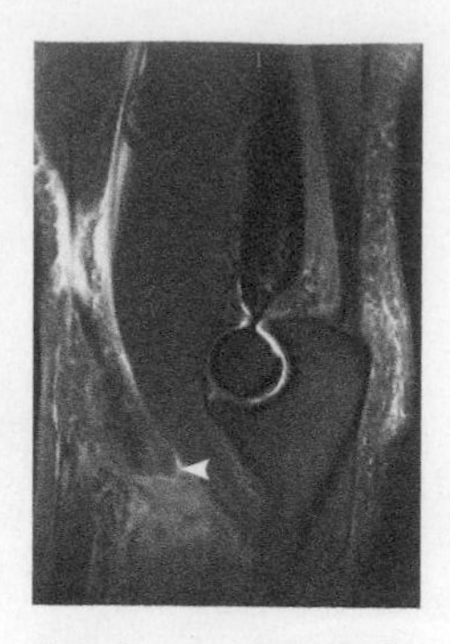

Another patient with a complete distal biceps tendon tear, and retraction (*arrowhead*).

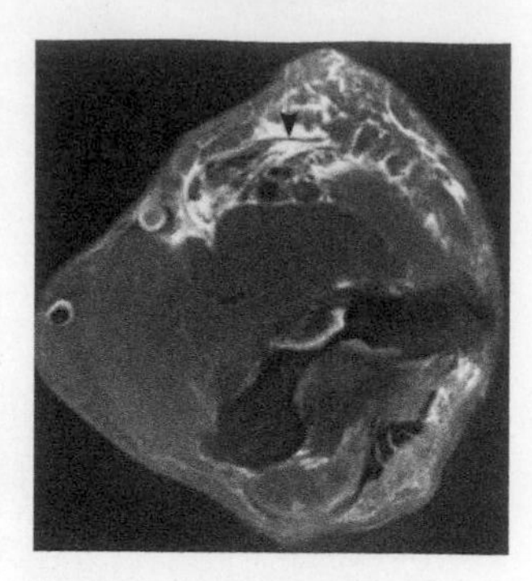

Intact lacertus fibrosus (*arrowhead*) prevents significant retraction.

Answers

1. There is a complete rupture of the distal biceps brachii tendon, with discontinuation of the distal biceps tendon and hematoma. There is also proximal retraction of the tendon.
2. Complete rupture of the distal biceps brachii tendon.
3. Tendinosis features, with partial discontinuity is typical. Distension of the bicipitoradial bursa and radial tuberosity marrow edema favor partial tear over tendinosis.
4. Three percent to 10% of biceps tears are distal tendon tears, and approximately 97% are proximal tears.
5. The flexed abducted and supinated (FABS) technique is useful in evaluating the distal biceps tendon.

Pearls

- Incidence is 1.2 per 100,000. Forty- to 60-year-old men are commonly affected.
- They are divided into acute or chronic, and partial or complete tears.
- Excessive load on the flexed and supinated forearm during weightlifting, football, and rugby is typical. Steroids also weakens the tendon, and the tendon can rupture without trauma.
- X-ray can sometimes show soft-tissue deformity, otherwise it is normal.
- Ultrasound shows a partial or complete tear. There is a lack of continuity of the tendon on full-thickness tears, and in partial tears there is a wavy discontinuation of the biceps tendon fibers. Hematoma is variably seen, depending upon the time of injury.
- On MRI, T2-weighted images shows edema within the biceps tendon, tendon rupture with discontinuity, and proximal retraction on fluid sensitivity sequences. An intact lacertus fibrosus prevents significant retraction of the tendon.
- Partial-thickness tears are generally treated conservatively, and full-thickness acute tears are treated surgically.

Suggested Readings

Le Huec JC, Moinard M, Liquois F, Zipoli B, Chauveaux D, Le Rebeller A. Distal rupture of the tendon of biceps brachii. Evaluation by MRI and the results of repair. *J Bone Joint Surg Br.* 1996;78(5):767–770.

Marnitz T, Spiegel D, Hug K, et al. MR imaging findings in flexed abducted supinated (FABS) position and clinical presentation following refixation of distal biceps tendon rupture using bioabsorbable suture anchors. *Rofo.* 2012;184(5):432–436.

Sudden pain at the back of thigh while running

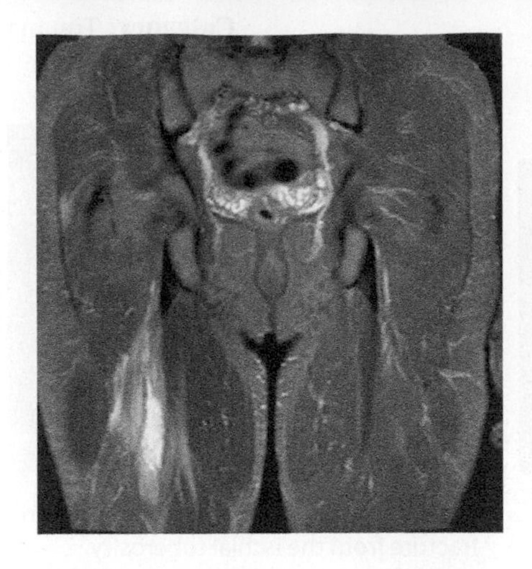

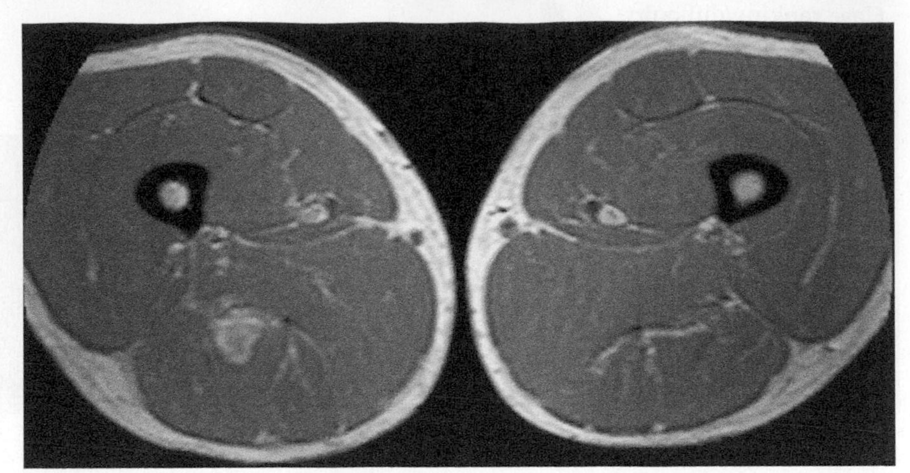

1. What are the MRI findings?

2. What are the main components of the hamstring muscle complex?

3. Where is avulsion injury of this complex most common?

4. Muscle strain of this structure is most often seen in which anatomical location?

5. What other important findings should be sought after when evaluating this injury?

Hamstring tear 1861

Case ranking/difficulty: **Category:** Trauma

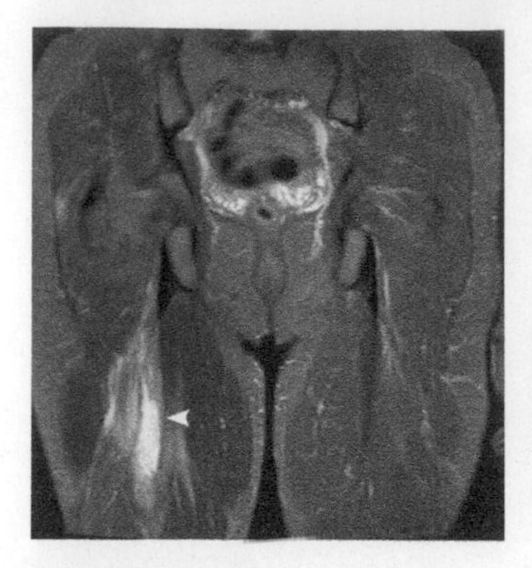

High signal with discontinuity in the hamstring, consistent with a high-grade partial tear of the biceps femoris musculotendinous junction.

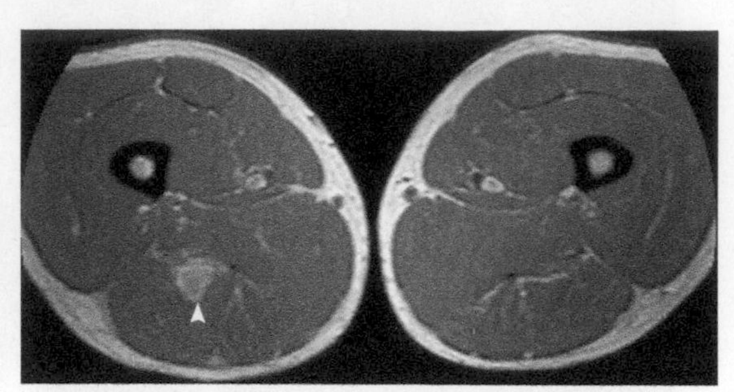

Intermediate/high T1 signal hematoma with discontinuity, consistent with hamstring muscle complex (HMC) group high-grade partial tear.

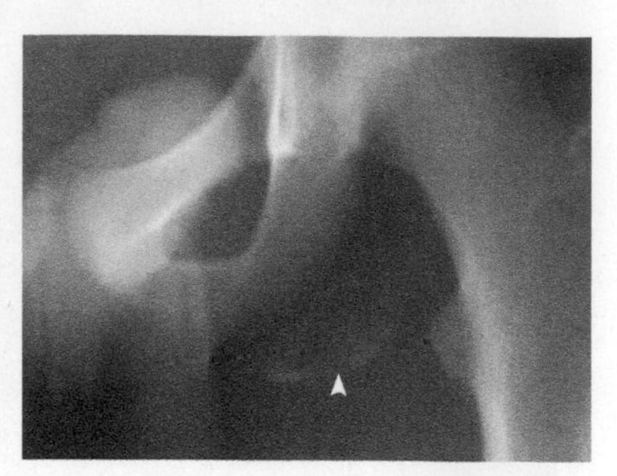

Another patient with hamstring avulsion fracture from the ischial tuberosity.

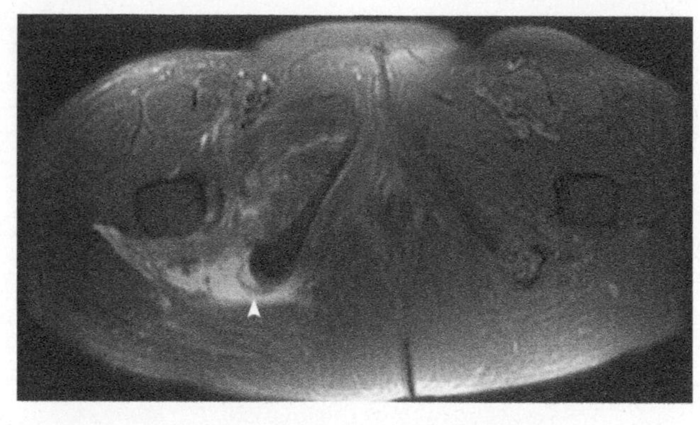

Hamstring avulsion from the ischial tuberosity in another patient.

Answers

1. MRI shows intermediate to high T1 and high STIR signal in the biceps femoris, with high-grade partial tear and hematoma formation at the musculotendinous junction. There is no avulsion at the ischial tuberosity.
2. The hamstring complex is comprised of the biceps femoris, semimembranosus and semitendinosus. There is some debate amongst anatomists regarding the inclusion of the adductor magnus in this group.
3. Avulsion of the hamstring muscle complex (HMC) is common at the ischial tuberosity, and mainly of the conjoint semitendinosus-biceps tendon.
4. HMC strain or partial tear is most common at the musculotendinous junction of the hamstring group.
5. As the management of the patient is determined by many different factors, it is important to observe the status of the tendon and surrounding soft tissues. Enthesopathy, chronic tear, scarring, bone bruising, and hematoma should be mentioned in the report.

   Usually avulsion of the tendon requires surgical repair, and strain requires conservative management.

Pearls

- HMC injury could be either avulsion injuries or muscle tear/strain. Avulsion injuries could be partial or complete, osseous or muscular alone. In adolescents, it is often osseous because of the unfused apophysis at the ischial tuberosity site.
- MRI accurately shows the avulsion and hematoma in acute cases, especially in fluid-sensitive coronal and axial STIR sequences.
- Ultrasound is also helpful in the early stages because of its sensitivity in detecting a fluid gap.
- HMC strain occurs mainly at the musculotendinous junction, where there is a 10- to 12-cm zone of transition that is relatively hypovascular.

Suggested Readings

De Smet AA, Best TM. MR imaging of the distribution and location of acute hamstring injuries in athletes. *AJR Am J Roentgenol.* 2000;174(2):393–399.

Koulouris G, Connell D. Hamstring muscle complex: an imaging review. *Radiographics.* 2005;25(3):571–586.

Sudden onset of calf pain while exercising

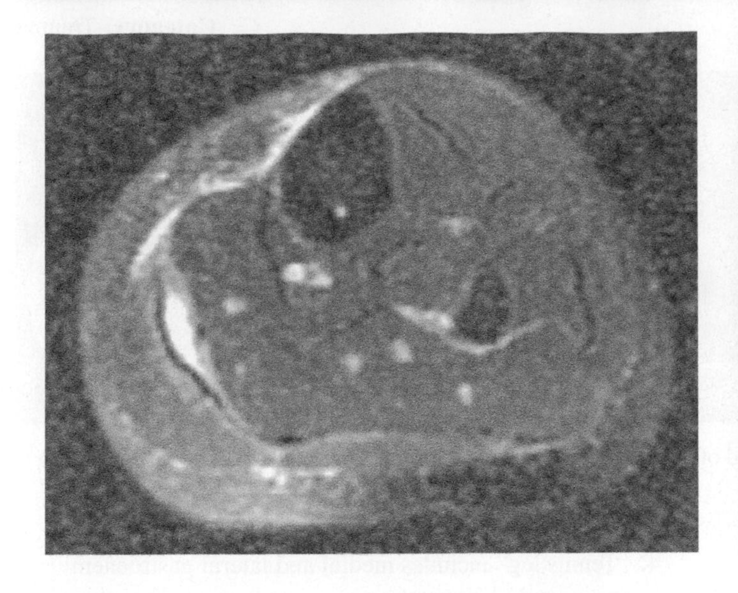

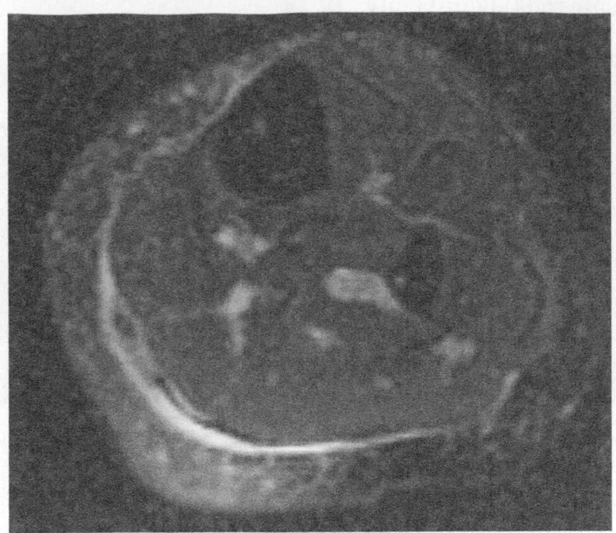

1. What are the MRI findings?

2. Given the clinical picture and MRI findings, what are the most likely differentials?

3. The plantaris muscle is absent in what percentage of the population?

4. What constitutes the clinical entity of a tennis leg?

5. What is the management?

Plantaris tear

1392

Case ranking/difficulty: 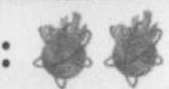

Category: Trauma

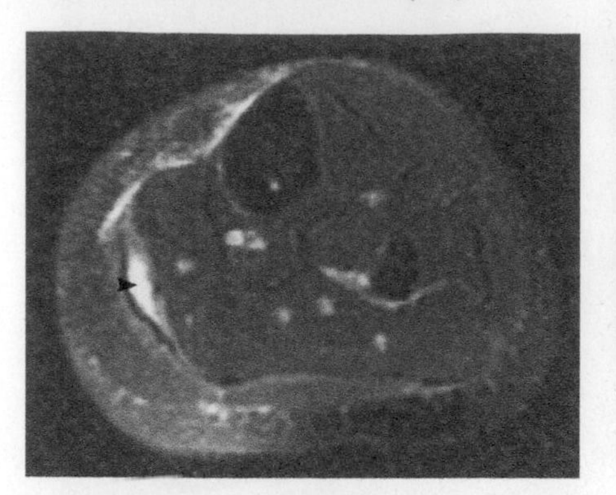

There is a lentiform fluid collection between the medial gastrocnemius and soleus muscles.

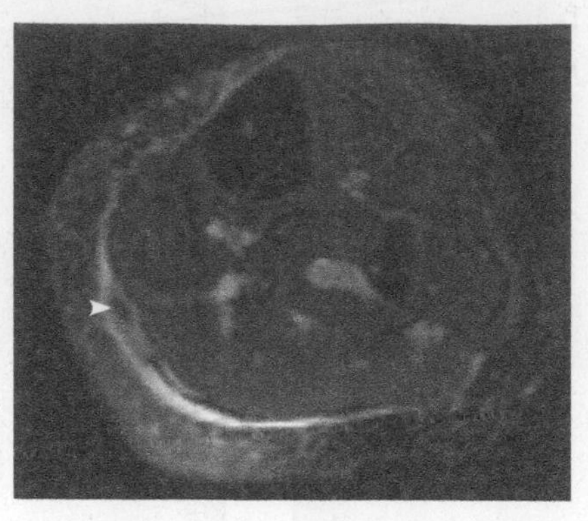

The retracted end of the tendon is seen more distally.

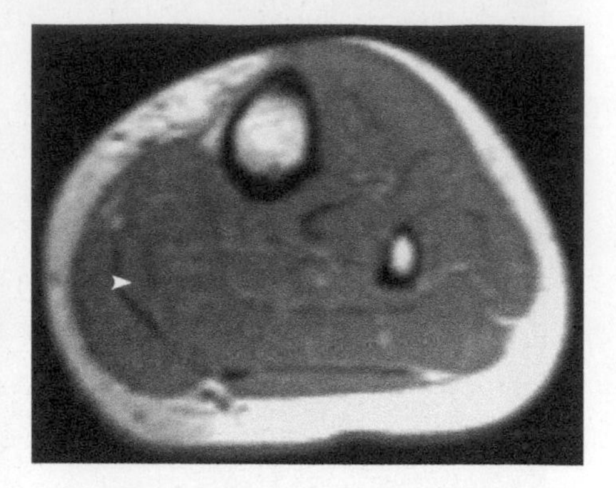

The lentiform fluid collection is isointense to skeletal muscle.

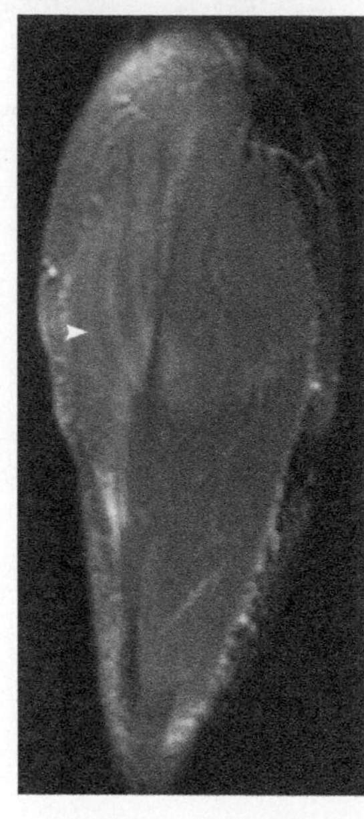

Medial gastrocnemius edema is seen. This may represent associated muscular strain.

Answers

1. There is a lentiform fluid collection between the medial gastrocnemius and soleus muscles. There is also mild strain of the medial gastrocnemius muscle.
2. A ruptured popliteal cyst or DVT can present with acute calf pain. However, the presence of a fluid collection between the medial gastrocnemius and the soleus is typically seen in a ruptured popliteal cyst, medial gastrocnemius injury or a plantaris tear. Because of the location and history, a plantaris tendon tear is most likely.
3. The plantaris is absent in 7% to 10% of individuals.
4. "Tennis leg" includes medial and lateral gastrocnemius strain, and plantaris rupture, as well as a soleus strain.
5. The treatment for plantaris tears is overwhelmingly conservative with rest, elevation and NSAIDs. A fasciotomy may be performed if there is a compartment syndrome.

Pearls

- The plantaris muscle has a short muscle and a long tendon.
- It originates in the posterior lateral femoral condyle and inserts in the posterior superior medial calcaneus.
- It is absent in 7% to 10% of the population.
- Tears typically occur at the musculotendinous junction.
- Like the gastrocnemius muscle, the plantaris crosses two joints and is therefore prone to injury.
- MRI shows an oval fluid collection between the soleus and medial gastrocnemius muscles. Associated strains of these muscles are common. Injuries to these three muscles have been termed *tennis leg*.
- A retracted tendon is important to identify, to differentiate it from other etiologies.

Suggested Readings

Delgado GJ, Chung CB, Lektrakul N, et al. Tennis leg: clinical US study of 141 patients and anatomic investigation of four cadavers with MR imaging and US. *Radiology.* 2002;224(1):112–119.

Helms CA, Fritz RC, Garvin GJ. Plantaris muscle injury: evaluation with MR imaging. *Radiology.* 1995;195(1):201–203.

History of injury to the knee

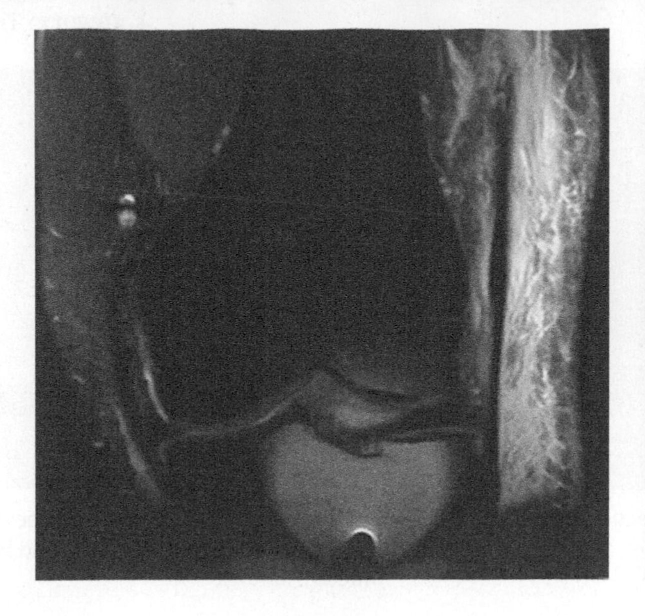

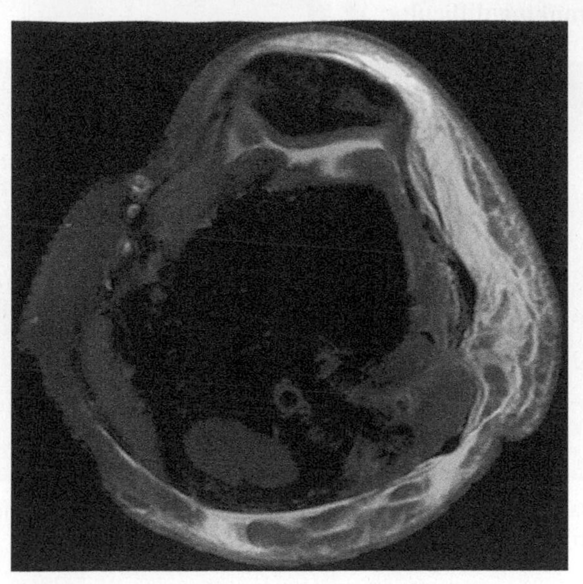

1. What are the MRI findings?

2. What is the diagnosis?

3. What are the MRI findings dependent on?

4. What are the main differential diagnoses?

5. What are the treatment options?

Morel-Lavallee lesion 1005

Case ranking/difficulty: 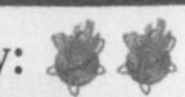

Category: Trauma

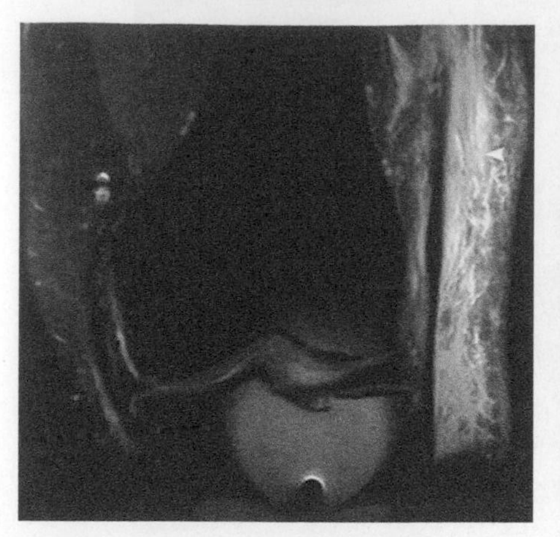

Perifascial fluid collection, which is high signal on T2-weighted images.

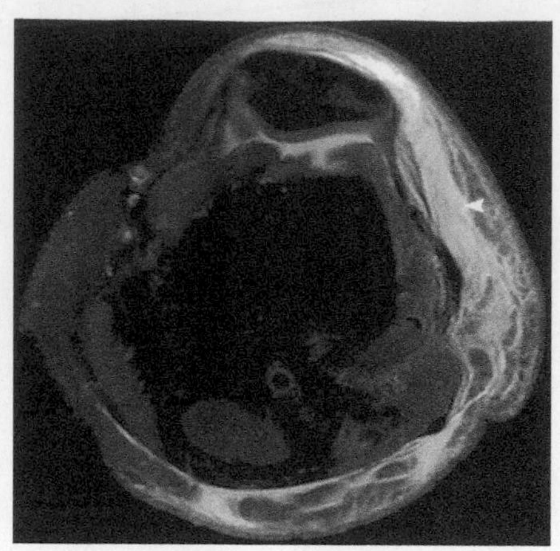

Perifascial fluid collection.

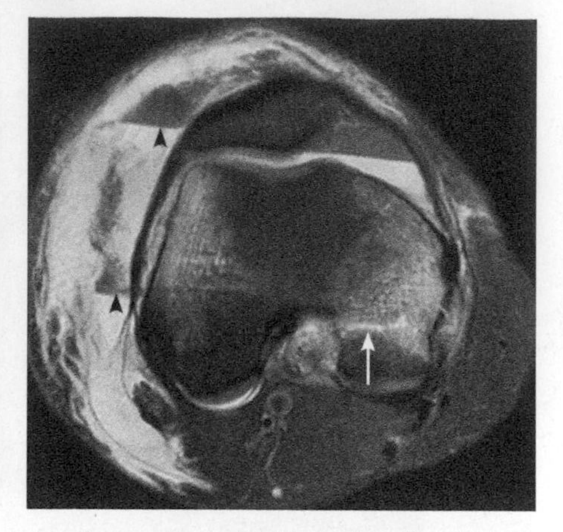

Another patient with Morel-Lavallee lesions (*arrowheads*), lipohemarthrosis, and Hoffa fracture (*arrow*).

Answers

1. There is a fluid collection with a pseudocapsule in the perifascial layer, which is comprised of hemolymph. Different constituents such as lymph, fat and blood may make the diagnosis difficult.
2. Morel-Lavallee lesion. This occurs secondary to a shearing degloving blunt injury with tangential forces, leading to a hemolymphatic collection in between the skin and subcutaneous tissues and the fascial layer.
3. Relative proportion of blood, lymph and fat, as well as the fibrous pseudocapsule determine the MRI characteristics of the lesion.
4. The main differential diagnoses are soft-tissue neoplasm, bursitis, ganglion, hematoma, and knee joint effusion.
5. Tight bandage as a conservative measure.

   Surgical drainage can be performed, and exploration and removal of capsule is suggested to avoid the chance of recurrence.

Pearls

- Morel-Lavallee lesions are a consequence of a blunt shearing degloving injury, leading to separation of the hypodermis and subcutaneous tissues from the fascial layer, and therefore to an accumulation of hemolymphatic collection with a pseudocapsule.
- Ultrasound and MRI are the investigative modalities of choice. These demonstrate the anatomical space clearly, with a collection in the perifascial plane containing blood and lymph products. The signal characteristics depend on the maturity of the blood products. This may create a diagnostic challenge.
- Most common sites are the lateral aspect of the thigh, buttock, back, and around the knee.
- Treatment options range from a conservative tight bandage to surgical drainage and removal of the capsule, to avoid recurrence.

Suggested Readings

Borrero CG, Maxwell N, Kavanagh E. MRI findings of prepatellar Morel-Lavallée effusions. *Skeletal Radiol.* 2008;37(5):451–455.

Köhler D, Pohlemann T. Operative treatment of the peripelvic Morel-Lavallée lesion [in German]. *Oper Orthop Traumatol.* 2011;23(1):15–20.

van Gennip S, van Bokhoven SC, van den Eede E. Pain at the knee: the Morel-Lavallée lesion, a case series. *Clin J Sport Med.* 2012;22(2):163–166.

Chronic ankle pain, getting worse

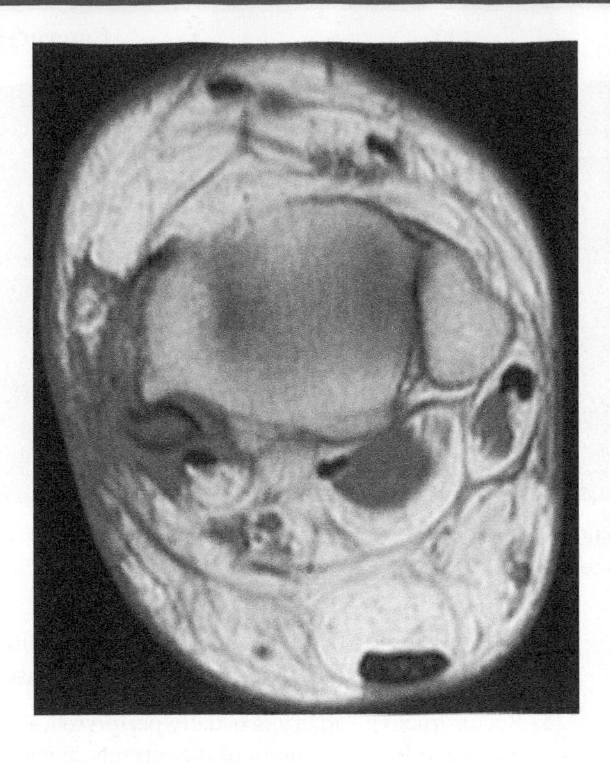

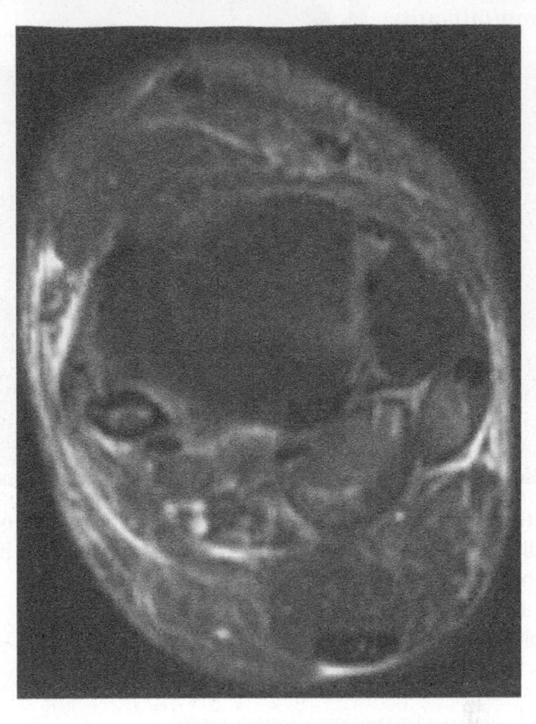

1. What are the MRI findings?

2. What contributes to these findings?

3. Why is there a propensity for this tendon to tear in this location?

4. What are typical insertion sites for the posterior tibial tendon?

5. What is the management for this condition?

Posterior tibial tendon subluxation 1473

Case ranking/difficulty: 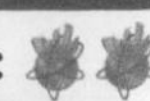

Category: Trauma

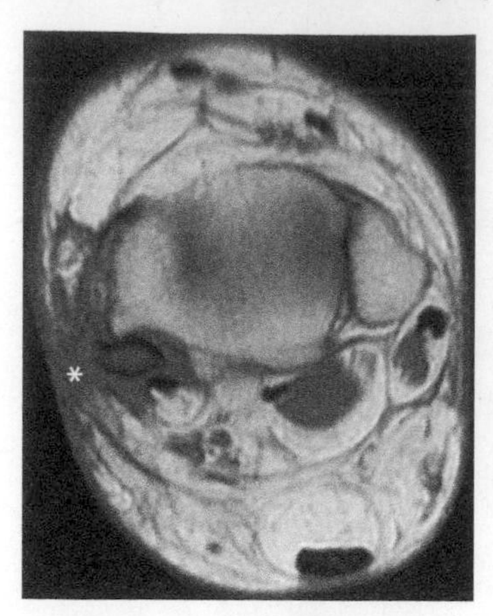

The posterior tibial tendon is subluxed medially and is tendinotic and partially torn. There is mild tenosynovitis and a large posterior medial malleolus spur. The flexor retinaculum is torn (*asterisk*).

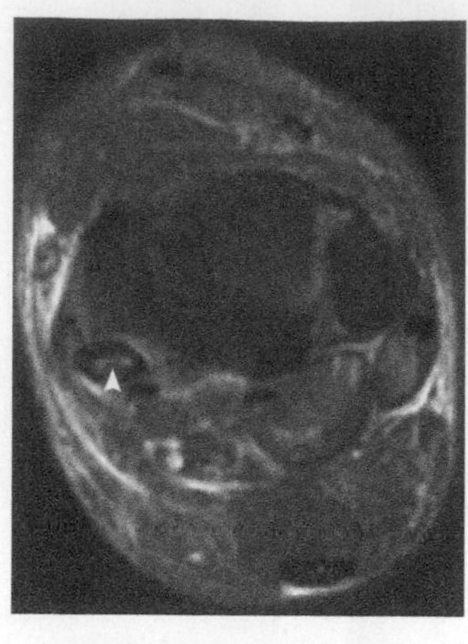

A split tear of the posterior tibial tendon (PTT) is seen.

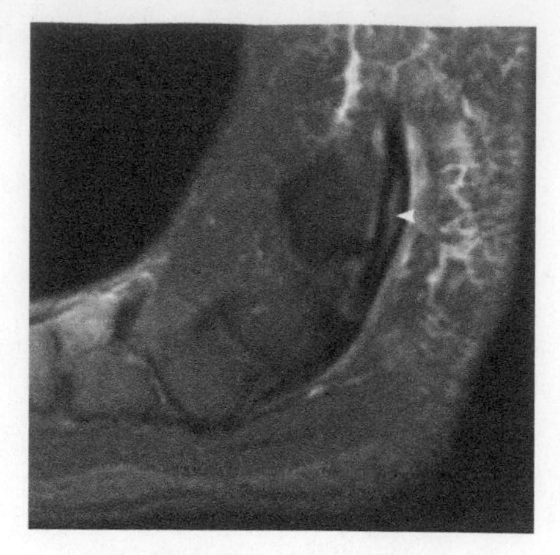

Split tear is well demonstrated.

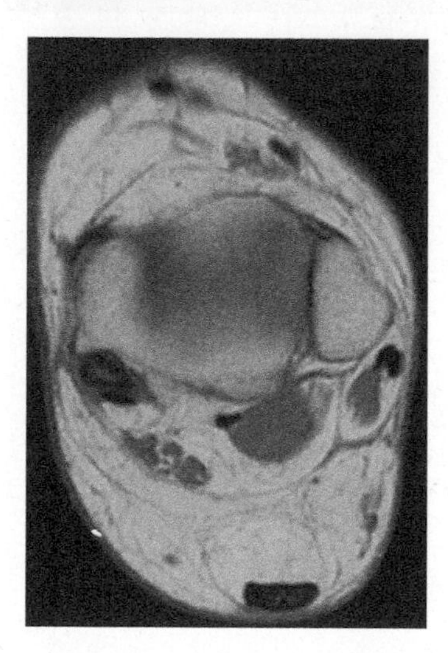

Study 7 months prior shows the tendinotic PTT but no subluxation, and the retinaculum was intact.

Answers

1. The flexor retinaculum is disrupted, with a split tear of the posterior tibial tendon (PTT), tenosynovitis, and medial subluxation. A medial malleolus spur is seen, which contributes to the mechanical attrition.
2. A divided or torn retinaculum, shallow retromalleolar sulcus, trauma, and steroid injections are contributory.
3. The PTT has a watershed area of hypovascularity in the retromalleolar sulcus, and is prone to mechanical attrition.
4. The PTT inserts on the medial navicular, cuneiforms, and the second, third, and fourth metatarsal bases.
5. Reconstructive surgery is usually performed, which may involve groove deepening of the retromalleolar sulcus. If the PTT is torn, repair of the tendon may be indicated.

Pearls

- The PTT inserts on the medial navicular and distally at the cuneiforms and the second through fifth metatarsal bases.
- The flexor retinaculum keeps the PTT located in the retromalleolar sulcus.
- In the retromalleolar sulcus, the PTT is prone to injury because of mechanical attrition and the relative hypovascularity of the tendon in this location (watershed zone).
- In a traumatic event, the flexor retinaculum tears and the tendon can sublux or dislocate.
- A shallow retromalleolar sulcus can contribute to subluxation.
- Associated tendinosis or tearing of the PTT may result from recurrent subluxation.

Suggested Readings

Bencardino J, Rosenberg ZS, Beltran J, et al. MR imaging of dislocation of the posterior tibial tendon. *AJR Am J Roentgenol.* 1997;169(4):1109–1112.

Rosenberg ZS, Beltran J, Bencardino JT. From the RSNA Refresher Courses. Radiological Society of North America. MR imaging of the ankle and foot. *Radiographics.* 2000;20 Spec No:S153–S179.

Chronic lateral ankle pain

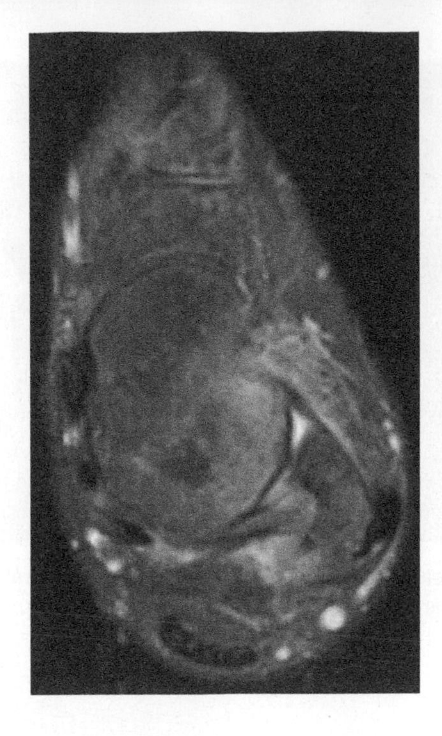
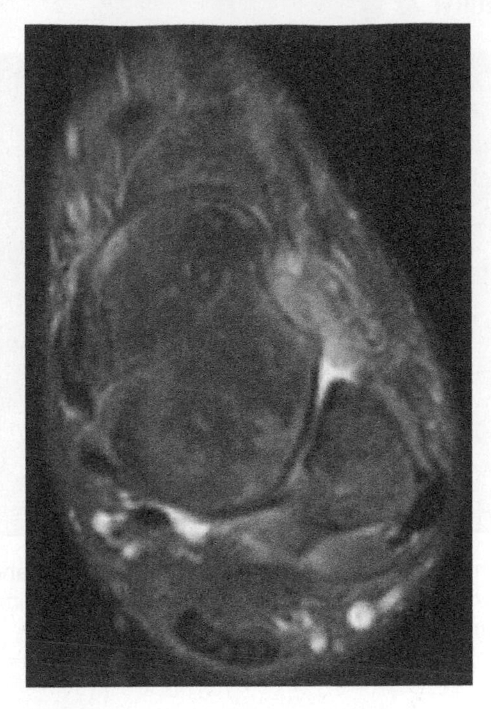

1. What are the MRI findings?

2. What is the proposed mechanism of injury?

3. What are injuries often associated with the primary abnormality?

4. What is the most common form of this injury?

5. What is the treatment?

Peroneal tendon subluxation 1377

Case ranking/difficulty: 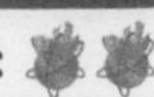 **Category:** Trauma

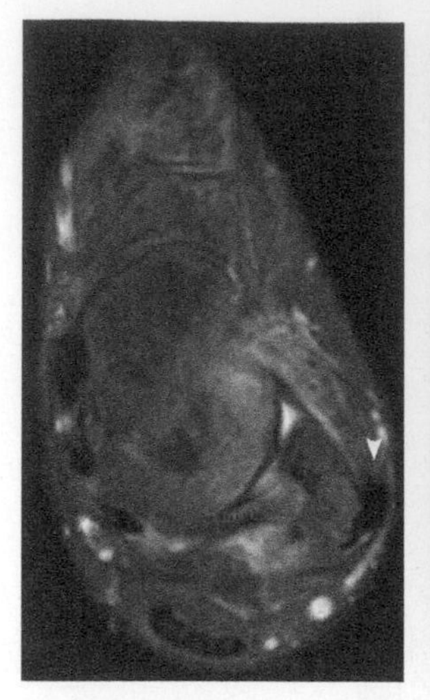

Lateral subluxation of the peroneal tendons is seen. The peroneal retinaculum is torn (*arrowhead*).

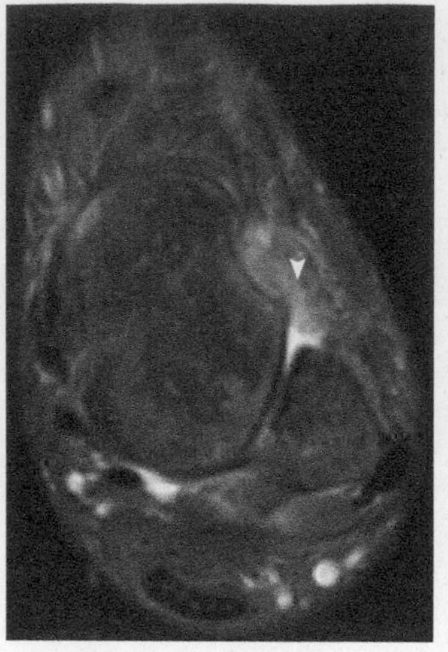

Partial tearing of the talar attachment of the anterior talofibular ligament (*arrowhead*) and lateral peroneal subluxation.

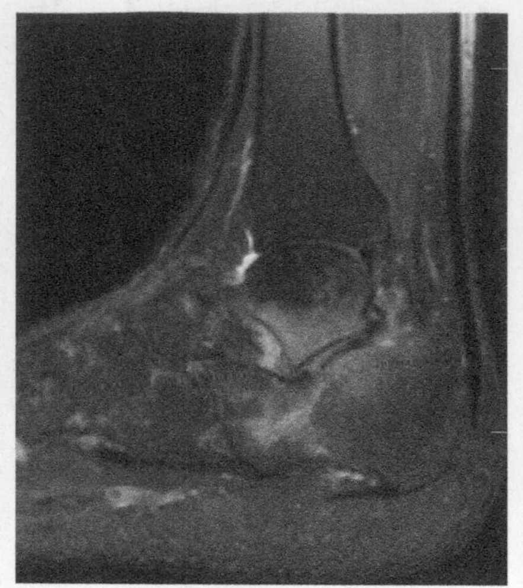

Calcaneal fracture and talus contusion with marrow edema are also seen.

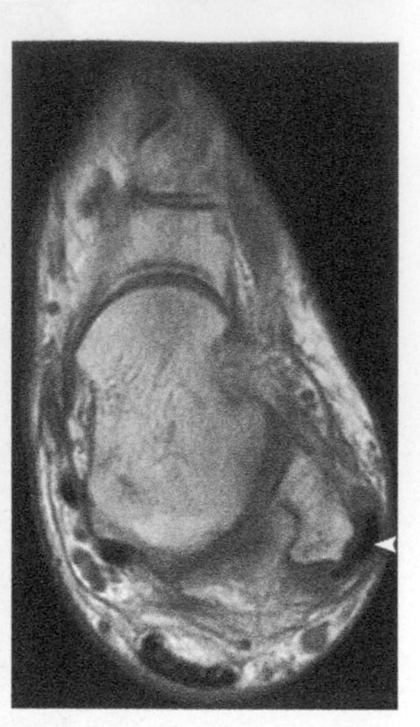

Lateral peroneal subluxation is seen.

Answers

1. The peroneal tendons are subluxed laterally, and the superior peroneal retinaculum is torn and stripped from the fibula along with the fibula periosteum. There is an associated partial tear of the anterior talofibular ligament, and talus edema.
2. The proposed mechanism for traumatic peroneal subluxation is forced dorsiflexion, as in a skiing injury. Inversion may be contributory.
3. Lateral ligament and peroneal tendon tear or tenosynovitis, are commonly associated injuries. Lateral fibula cortex avulsion fracture can occur.
4. The most common form of superior peroneal retinaculum injury is stripping of the retinaculum along with the fibula periosteum at the fibula attachment but without tear.
5. Closed reduction and casting for six weeks is the initial management. Instability is common, however, and surgical repair of the retinaculum with or without deepening of the peroneal groove is usually required.

Pearls

- Peroneal tendon subluxation occurs after significant dorsiflexion injury. Inversion may be contributory.
- The most common injury is stripping of the fibular attachment of the retinaculum along with the fibula periosteum, but the retinaculum itself remains intact.
- A tiny avulsion fracture from the lateral fibula cortex may be seen in more severe injuries.
- Associated peroneal tendon tear or tenosynovitis is common, as well as lateral ligament injury.
- A shallow or convex peroneal groove may be contributory.
- Surgery is typically required.

Suggested Readings

Schweitzer ME, Eid ME, Deely D, Wapner K, Hecht P. Using MR imaging to differentiate peroneal splits from other peroneal disorders. *AJR Am J Roentgenol.* 1997;168(1):129–133.

Tjin A Ton ER, Schweitzer ME, Karasick D. MR imaging of peroneal tendon disorders. *AJR Am J Roentgenol.* 1997;168(1):135–140.

History of dislocated thumb 4 days prior; difficulty grasping

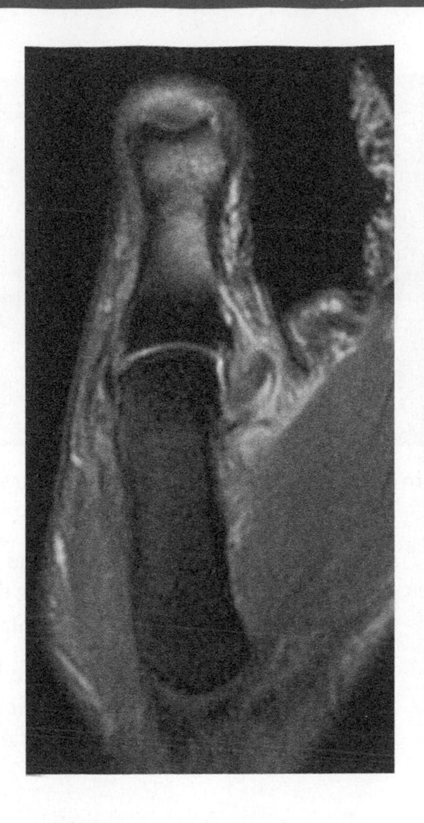

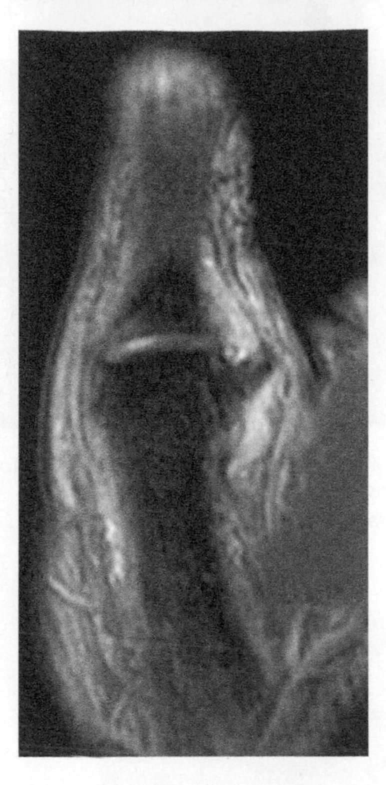

1. What are the MRI findings?

2. What is the name given to this finding?

3. What percentage of patients with a complete UCL tear develop this lesion?

4. What is the mechanism of injury?

5. What is the treatment?

Stener lesion 1415

Case ranking/difficulty: 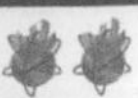

Category: Trauma

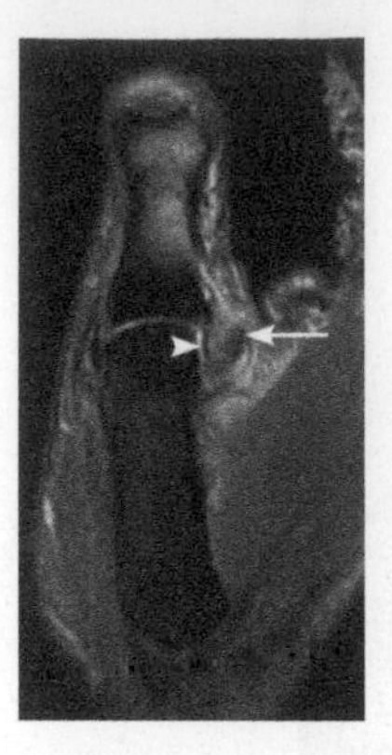

Torn retracted ulnar collateral ligament (*arrow*), with the adductor aponeurosis (*arrowhead*) interposed between the retracted ligament and the osseous structures.

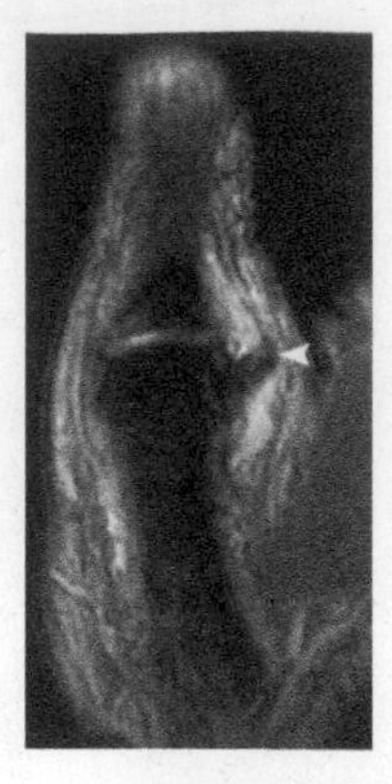

Torn retracted UCL.

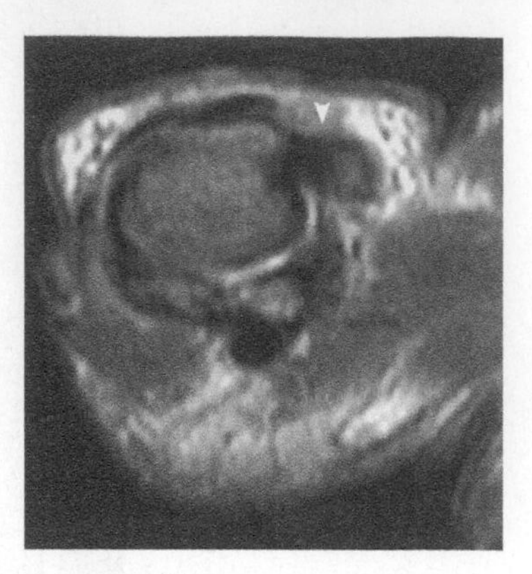

Torn retracted UCL.

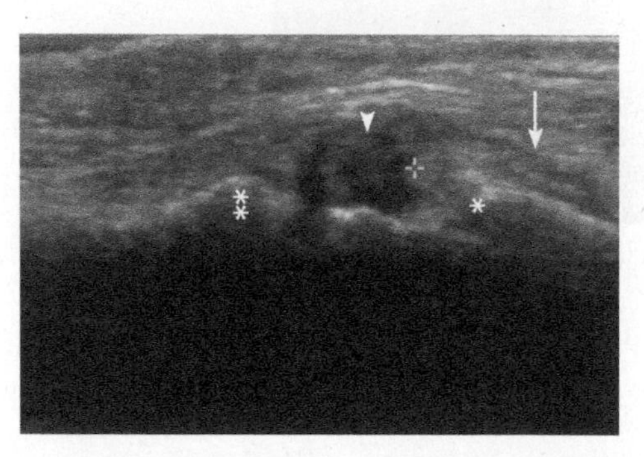

Hypoechoic tear of the UCL distally with a coiled retracted ligament (*arrowhead*) in another patient with an isolated UCL tear. *Asterisk* represents the metacarpal head, *double asterisk* represents the proximal phalanx, and the *arrow* represents the adductor aponeurosis with no interposition.

Answers

1. The UCL is torn at its phalangeal attachment and retracted proximally, with the adductor aponeurosis now deep to the retracted ligament giving a "yo-yo on a string" appearance.

2. The particular finding of adductor aponeurosis interposition in a torn retracted UCL is called a *Stener lesion*.

3. More than 80% of patients with a complete UCL tear develop a Stener lesion.

4. A hyperabduction injury is the classic mechanism, with sudden valgus stress on a taut ligament. A fall on the outstretched hand is also common.

5. Although isolated, incomplete UCL injuries are treated with a thumb spica, a Stener lesion needs to be treated surgically within three weeks of the injury.

Pearls

- A Stener lesion occurs with forced hyperabduction at the thumb MCP.
- It was originally described in Scottish gamekeepers, but is more common now in skiers.
- The torn retracted UCL lies external to the adductor pollicis aponeurosis, which prevents adequate repair and healing.
- The combination of the retracted ligament and aponeurosis interposition gives a "yo-yo on a string" appearance, with the aponeurosis the string and the retracted ligament the ball.
- Treatment is surgical.

Suggested Readings

Haramati N, Hiller N, Dowdle J, et al. MRI of the Stener lesion. *Skeletal Radiol.* 1995;24(7):515–518.

Lohman M, Vasenius J, Kivisaari A, Kivisaari L. MR imaging in chronic rupture of the ulnar collateral ligament of the thumb. *Acta Radiol.* 2001;42(1):10–14.

Snapping of ring finger flexor tendon with pain

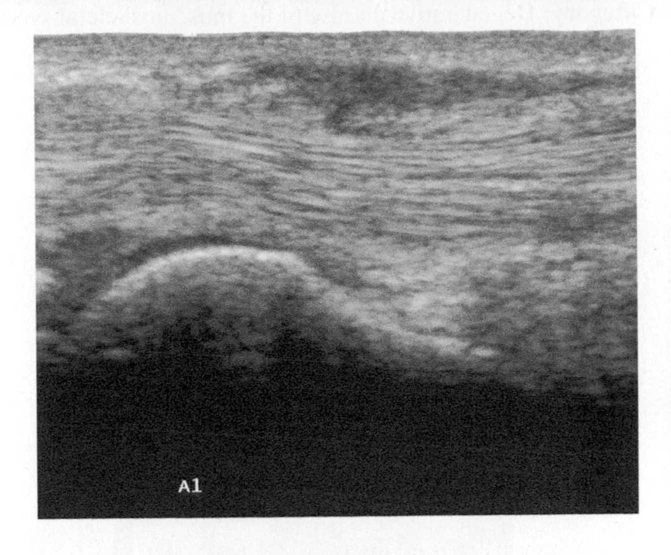

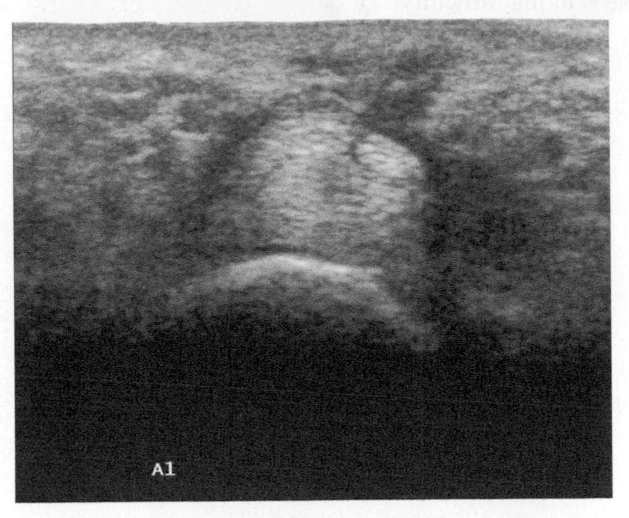

1. Which structure is pathologically thickened in this condition?
2. Which digit is most commonly implicated?
3. What are the possible treatments?
4. What are the imaging features of this entity?
5. What are the predisposing factors?

Trigger finger

Case ranking/difficulty: 

Category: Degenerative disease of the musculoskeletal system

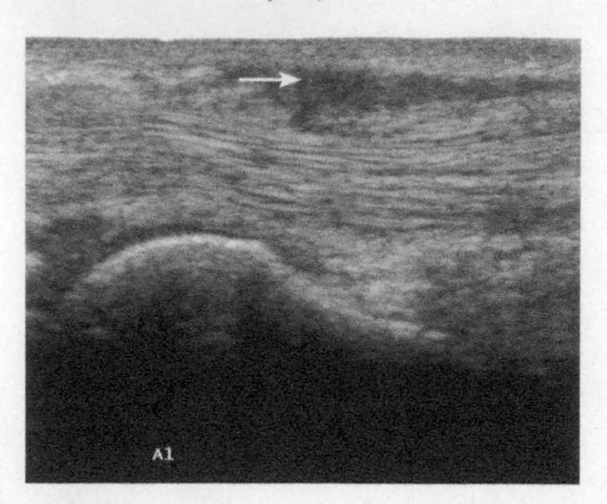

Nodular thickening of A1 pulley proximal to MCP joint.

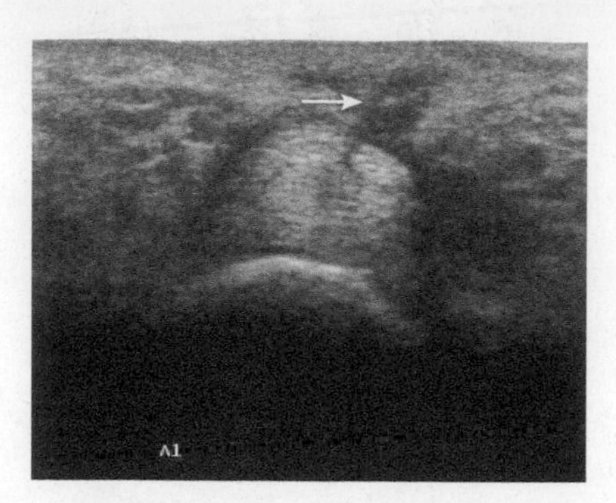

Nodular thickening of A1 pulley on axial images.

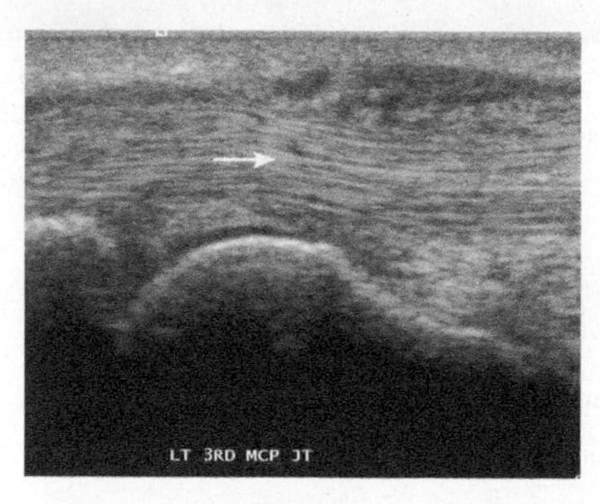

The underlying flexor tendon fibers are entirely normal, demonstrating high reflectivity and a striated appearance.

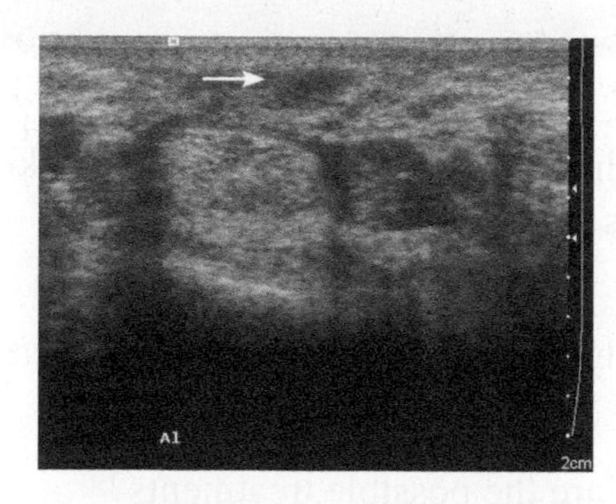

Further demonstration of nodular thickening of pulley.

Answers

1. Annular and cruciform pulleys are connective tissue condensations that enable the smooth functioning of the flexor tendons that they encase. The A1 pulley is implicated in trigger finger.
2. Most cases involve the ring finger.
3. Percutaneous release and steroid injection can both be performed using ultrasound guidance. Dry needling and autologous blood injection are tendon therapies for resistant tendinopathies: for example, Achilles, patellar tendons.
4. Trigger finger is caused by nodular thickening of the A1 pulley in most cases. On ultrasound this is hypoechoic, and on MRI it appears as uniformly low T1 and T2 signal.
5. People who are prone to repetitive finger movements, for example, piano players, typists and athletes, are at greater risk of trigger finger. Rheumatoid arthritis and diabetes are also predisposing factors. In particular, rheumatoid can cause tendinopathies and tenosynovitis which can further lead to constriction at sites of tendon movement.

Pearls

- Trigger finger can be diagnosed clinically and radiologically.
- The abnormality is usually related to abnormal thickening or nodularity of the A1 flexor tendon pulley.
- Ultrasound is the imaging modality of choice as it allows dynamic assessment and can guide percutaneous therapy.
- Treatments include corticosteroid injection, percutaneous release with a cutting needle, and surgical release.

Suggested Readings

Guerini H, Pessis E, Theumann N, et al. Sonographic appearance of trigger fingers. *J Ultrasound Med.* 2008;27(10):1407–1413.

Gyuricza C, Umoh E, Wolfe SW. Multiple pulley rupture following corticosteroid injection for trigger digit: case report. *J Hand Surg Am.* 2009;34(8):1444–1448.

Rajeswaran G, Lee JC, Eckersley R, Katsarma E, Healy JC. Ultrasound-guided percutaneous release of the annular pulley in trigger digit. *Eur Radiol.* 2009;19(9):2232–2237.

Forced ulnar deviation of wrist

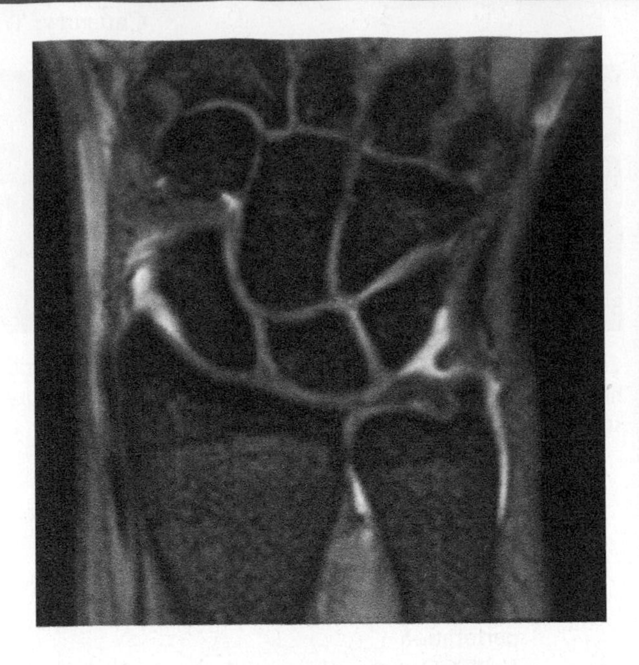

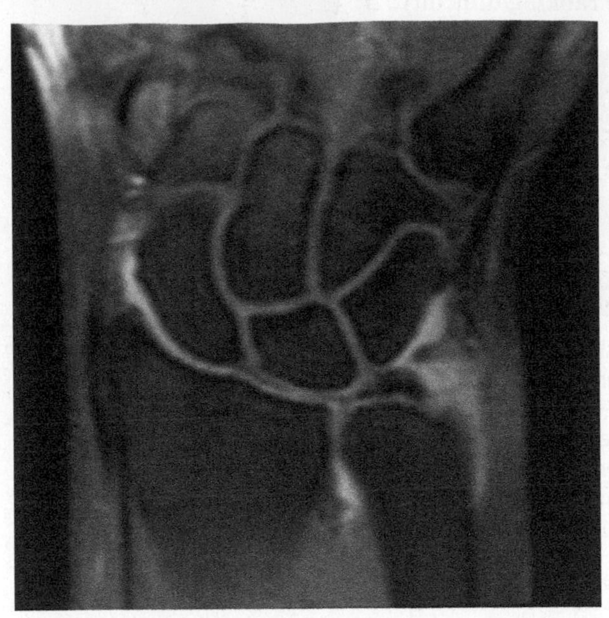

1. What features are associated with this entity?
2. Which modality is appropriate for evaluating this entity?
3. Which tendon is intimately associated with the involved structure?
4. What part of the involved structure has the best blood supply?
5. What is the name of the commonly used classification for injuries to this structure?

Triangular fibrocartilage tear 336

Case ranking/difficulty: 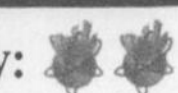

Category: Trauma

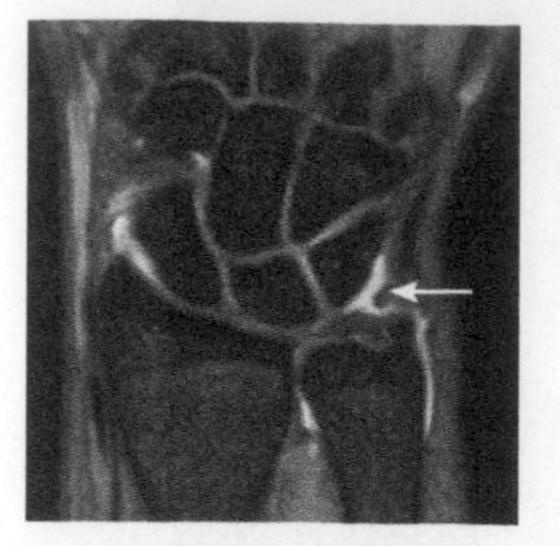

Ulnar-sided triangular fibrocartilaginous complex (TFCC) tear and contrast within distal radioulnar joint and along the medial ulna, demonstrated after intra-articular gadolinium injection.

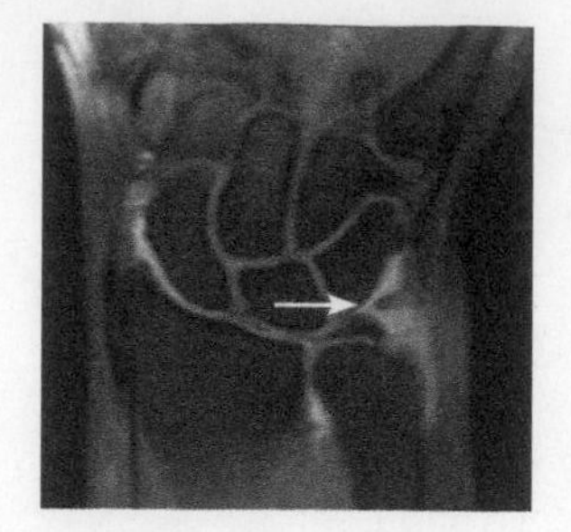

TFCC tear is shown.

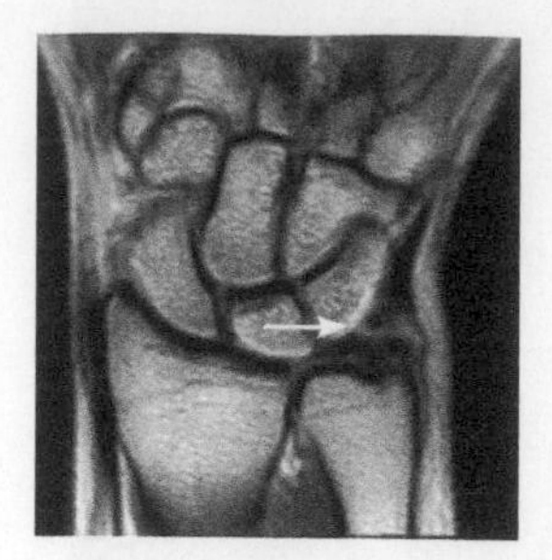

Contrast-enhanced T1 with high-signal gadolinium seen outlining a TFCC tear.

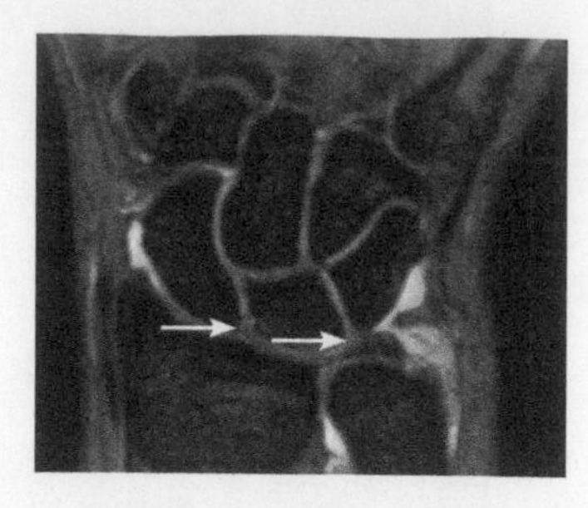

The scapholunate and lunotriquetral ligaments are intact. The injury is chiefly related to the TFCC.

Answers

1. Positive ulnar variance is associated with ulnar impaction, leading to degeneration and central perforation of the triangular fibrocartilaginous complex (TFCC). These central tears are increasingly common with advancing age and often asymptomatic.

2. Contrast arthrography and MR/CT arthrography are sensitive and reliable for diagnosing TFCC tears. Alternatively, direct wrist arthroscopy can be performed, although this carries unnecessary patient risk, especially in those patients in whom no intervention is required.

3. The extensor carpi ulnaris tendon is broadly attached to the TFCC and uses it as a pulley. Consequently, damage to the TFCC can increase moment through the ECU tendon by 30%, causing tendonitis and eventually rupture.

4. There is a rich blood supply to the outer third of the TFCC. This is entirely analogous to the "red zone" of the knee menisci. Consequently, repair of central tears are relatively unsuccessful, and these lesions are best managed with conservative treatment or debridement if symptomatic.

5. The Palmer classification is commonly used for grading TFCC tears, distinguishing traumatic from degenerative tears:

   - Class 1: Traumatic
     - A: central perforation
     - B: ulnar avulsion with or without distal ulnar fracture
     - C: distal avulsion
     - D: radial avulsion with or without sigmoid notch fracture
   - Class 2: Degenerative (ulnocarpal abutment syndrome)
     - A: TFCC wear
     - B: TFCC wear with lunate and/or ulnar chondromalacia
     - C: TFCC perforation with lunate and/or ulnar chondromalacia
     - D: TFCC perforation with lunate and/or ulnar chondromalacia and lunotriquetral ligament perforation
     - E: TFCC perforation with lunate and/or ulnar chondromalacia, lunotriquetral ligament perforation, and ulnocarpal arthritis

Pearls

- TFCC tears are broadly classified into traumatic (class I) and degenerative (class II) etiologies.
- Acute tears are associated with distal radius fractures (falling on an outstretched hand), or forced ulnar deviation.
- Degenerative tears are associated with ulnocarpal abutment resulting from positive ulnar variance.
- Contrast or CT/MRI arthrography are mandatory imaging studies in evaluating tears reliably. Contrast communicating between the radiocarpal and distal radioulnar joint is diagnostic of a TFCC tear.
- Peripheral blood supply is excellent, analogous to the "red zone" of the knee menisci. These tears usually heal successfully after surgical repair.

Suggested Readings

Joshy S, Ghosh S, Lee K, Deshmukh SC. Accuracy of direct magnetic resonance arthrography in the diagnosis of triangular fibrocartilage complex tears of the wrist. *Int Orthop.* 2008;32(2):251–253.

Maizlin ZV, Brown JA, Clement JJ, et al. MR arthrography of the wrist: controversies and concepts. *Hand (N Y).* 2009;4(1):66–73.

Severe pain on abduction of shoulder

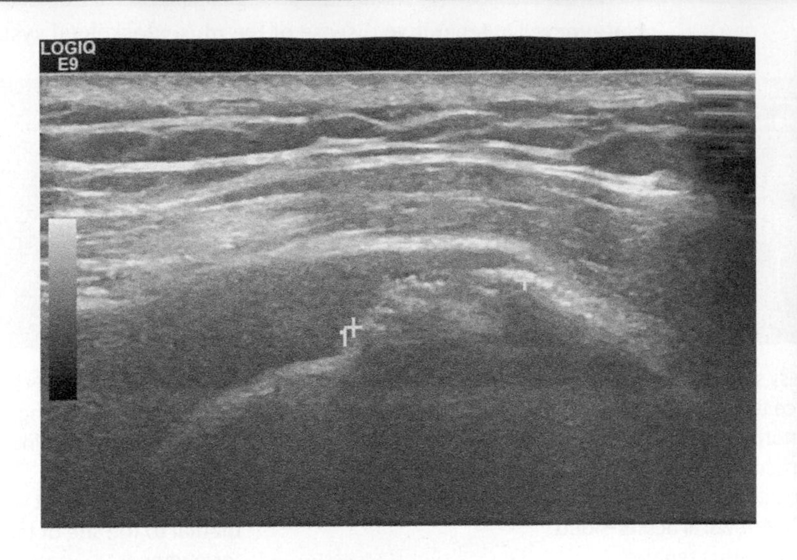

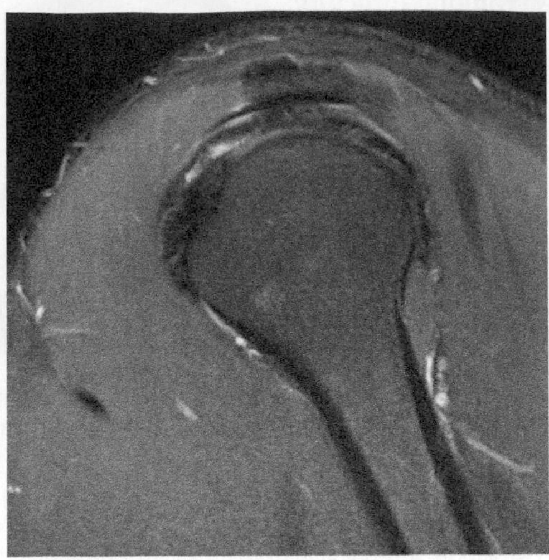

1. What is the differential diagnosis?

2. What is the innervation of the affected structure?

3. What are the imaging modalities of choice for this entity?

4. What is the etiology of the pathology shown?

5. What is the appropriate management for this entity?

PASTA (partial articular supraspinatus tendon avulsion) lesion 2250

Case ranking/difficulty: 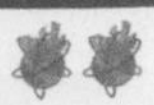

Category: Degenerative disease of the musculoskeletal system

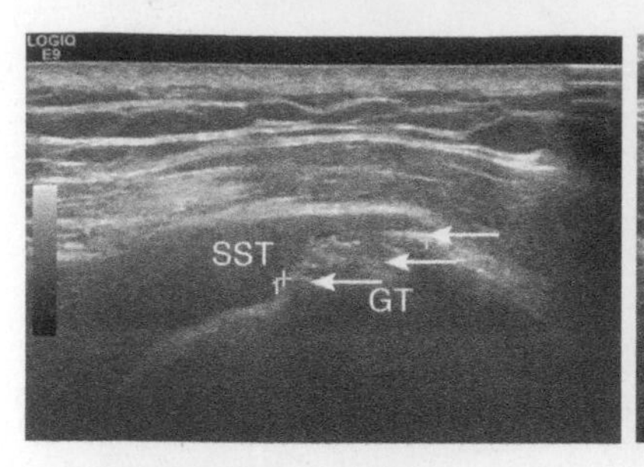

Partial-thickness supraspinatus articular surface tear demonstrated by loss of the normal contour and thickness of articular surface of tendon with cortical irregularity at the greater tuberosity (GT). *Arrows*, articular-sided tear; *SST*, supraspinatus tendon.

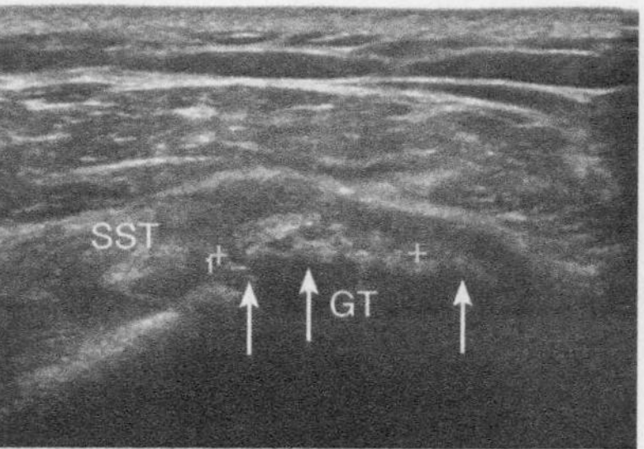

Partial-thickness supraspinatus articular surface tear demonstrated by loss of the normal contour and thickness of articular surface of tendon with cortical irregularity at the greater tuberosity (GT). *Arrows*, articular-sided tear; *SST*, supraspinatus tendon.

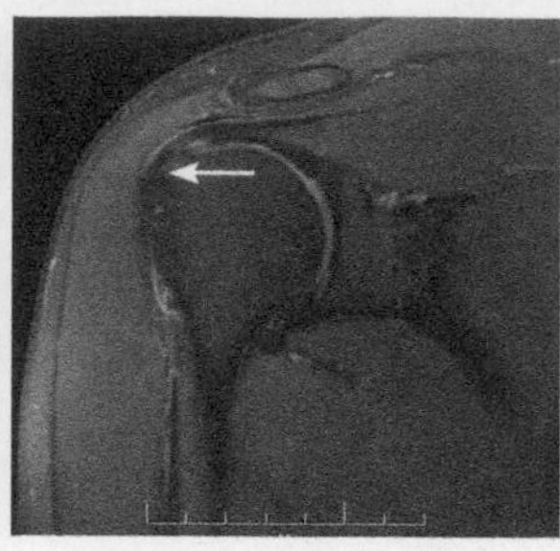

Coronal T2 fat-saturated image demonstrating articular surface tear of supraspinatus insertion.

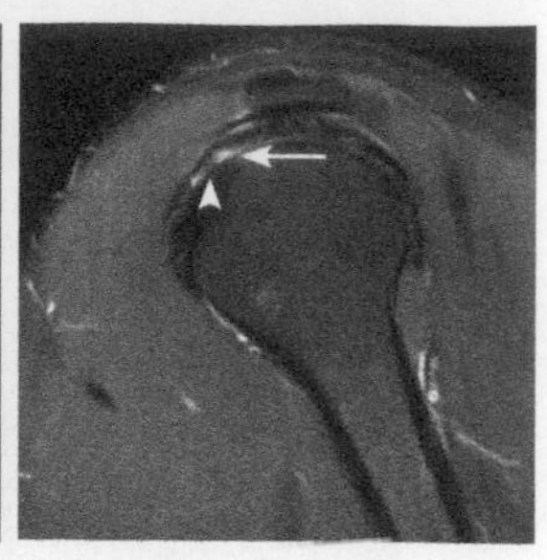

Articular-sided tear is seen at the anterior leading edge of the supraspinatus tendon (*arrow*). The biceps tendon is just medial to the site of tear (*arrowhead*).

Answers

1. The main differential diagnosis for this appearance is between a fracture of the greater tuberosity and a PASTA (partial articular supraspinatus tendon avulsion) lesion. A plain radiograph and history is useful to differentiate between the two. The bursal surface of the tendon is smooth: hence, it is not a full-thickness tear.

2. The suprascapular nerve (C5 and C6 roots) innervates both the supra- and infraspinatus muscles. The nerve supplies the infraspinatus muscle after passing over the spinoglenoid notch. The axillary nerve supplies deltoid, teres minor and the shoulder joint capsule.

3. Ultrasound is the imaging modality of choice for the rotator cuff in the United Kingdom, and MRI is preferred in the United States. Precise measurements can be obtained, dynamic assessment can be done and therapy can be delivered (eg, subacromial injection) via ultrasound guidance.

4. Either degeneration or an acute injury, for example, a fall, may cause a PASTA lesion. Calcific tendinosis per se would not give this pattern of tendon tear.

5. Partial-thickness tears may be managed conservatively with rest, physiotherapy, NSAIDs, and occasional subacromial injections for pain relief. More aggressive arthroscopic or open surgical repair depends on the patient's activity profile, age, premorbid conditions, and choice. In selected patients, surgical repair may be beneficial in restoring the patient to a near-normal standard of function.

Pearls

- PASTA lesions are also known as (articular) "rim-rent" tears and are partial-thickness tears of the articular surface of the supraspinatus (or infraspinatus) tendon footplate.
- The term *rim-rent* may sometimes refer to an articular or bursal-sided tear of either supraspinatus or infraspinatus. Therefore, care must be exercised in terminology when communicating findings to clinicians. However, a PASTA lesion is by definition an articular-sided partial tear.
- Cortical irregularity at the greater tuberosity with loss of the distal tendon thickness on the articular surface on ultrasound should prompt the radiologist to consider the diagnosis of a PASTA lesion.
- The crucial distinction between this type of tear and a full-thickness tear is that the bursal surface of the tendon is completely intact.
- An MRI is of equivalent sensitivity to ultrasound in diagnosing a PASTA lesion.
- Management depends on patient premorbid function and symptoms. It includes rest, NSAIDs, cortisone injections, physical therapy, and arthroscopic repair.

Suggested Readings

Sperling JW, Dahm DL. Double suture technique to delineate PASTA lesions. *Arthroscopy*. 2006;22(6):681.1–2.

Vinson EN, Helms CA, Higgins LD. Rim-rent tear of the rotator cuff: a common and easily overlooked partial tear. *AJR Am J Roentgenol.* 2007;189(4):943–946.

Waibl B, Buess E. Partial-thickness articular surface supraspinatus tears: a new transtendon suture technique. *Arthroscopy*. 2005;21(3):376–381.

Medial joint line pain, previous history of acute twisting knee injury (images from two patients)

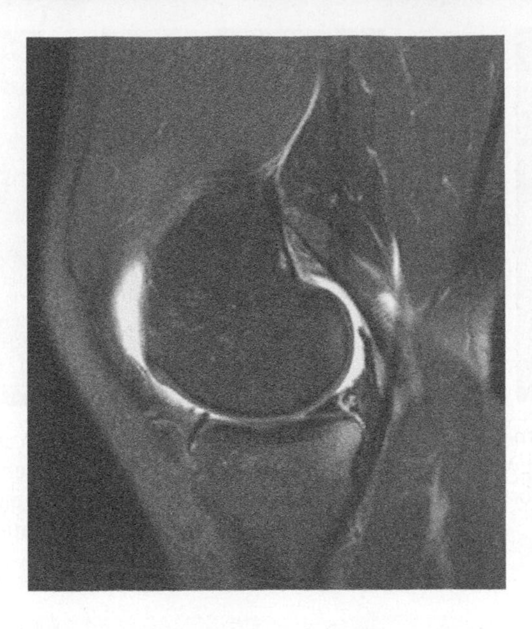

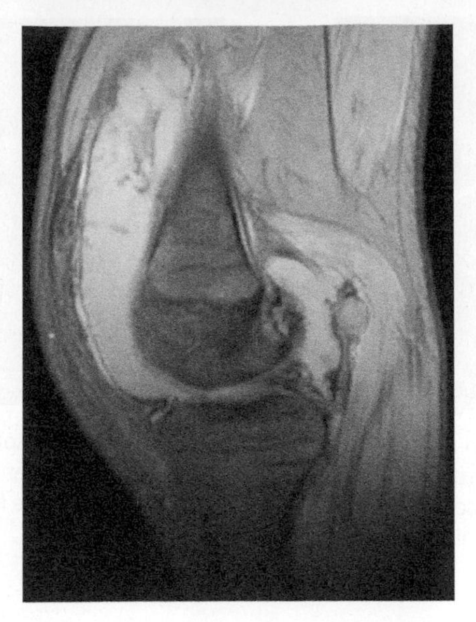

1. What is the differential diagnosis in these 2 patients?

2. What ligaments attach the root of the meniscus to the joint capsule?

3. What test on clinical examination may be positive with this entity?

4. What is the most favorable location for a meniscal tear?

5. What other finding on coronal imaging may be suggestive of this diagnosis?

Meniscocapsular separation 1648

Case ranking/difficulty:

Category: Trauma

Fluid tracks through the posterior capsular attachment of the medial meniscus consistent with meniscocapsular separation.

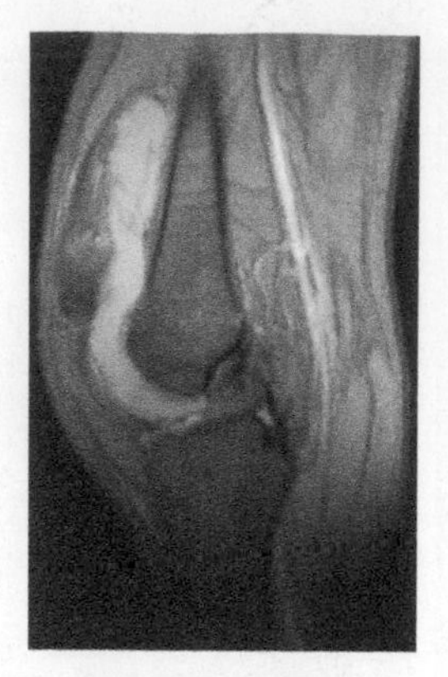

The ACL is also completely torn in the second patient, consistent with a pivot-shift injury and a large force.

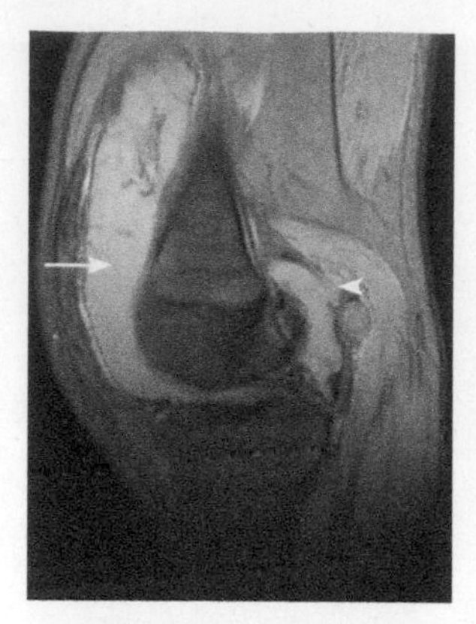

There is a massive effusion (*arrow*) and associated capsular tear (*arrowhead*) posteriorly in the second patient with meniscocapsular separation.

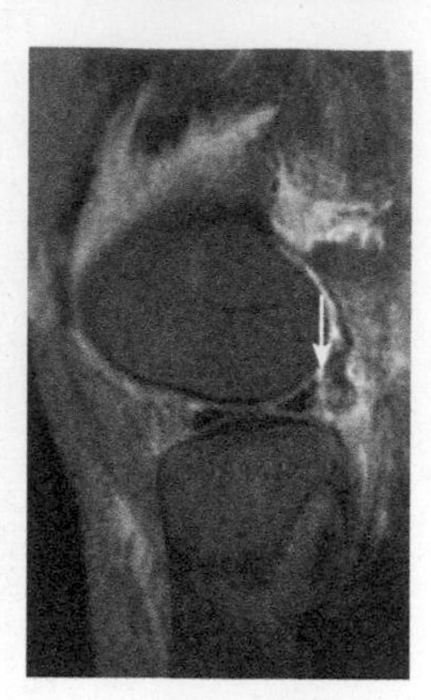

A case of lateral meniscocapsular separation in a third patient.

Answers

1. There is excess fluid between the posterior horn of the medial meniscus and the capsule. The meniscofemoral ligament is not visualized in continuity. The likely diagnosis is meniscocapsular separation. There may be an associated capsular injury. A peripheral longitudinal tear at the posterior horn/root junction may have similar appearances, although the tear in this case would be through the meniscal substance rather than capsular attachments.

2. The meniscofemoral and meniscotibial ligaments are condensations of the joint capsule; they attach the meniscus to the capsule peripherally.

3. McMurray and Apley tests assess the integrity of the menisci.

4. Peripheral (red-zone) tears are in the well vascularized portion of the meniscus. They tend to heal better with conservative management and have a better chance of full recovery post surgery.

5. On coronal imaging, meniscocapsular separation may be suggested by fluid tracking deep to the MCL.

Pearls

- Meniscocapsular separation should be considered and actively excluded when the clinical history and examination are suggestive of a meniscal tear, although a meniscal tear is not immediately apparent.
- Imaging findings are of detachment of the meniscus from the capsular attachments (meniscofemoral and/or meniscotibial ligaments) on sagittal and coronal images, localized effusion between the posterior edge of the meniscus and the capsule, and a change in the contour of the posterior horn.
- As they are peripheral (red-zone) injuries, they are well vascularized and tend to heal well if surgical repair is performed.
- Incomplete meniscocapsular separation is suggested by the presence of edema within the meniscofemoral and meniscotibial ligaments.
- Associated injuries are common—look for prior ACL, MCL, and LCL injuries.
- Distinction should be made between a peripheral meniscal tear and a true meniscocapsular injury by the presence or absence of meniscal tissue peripheral to the tear line.

Suggested Readings

De Maeseneer M, Shahabpour M, Vanderdood K, Van Roy F, Osteaux M. Medial meniscocapsular separation: MR imaging criteria and diagnostic pitfalls. *Eur J Radiol.* 2002;41(3):242–252.

Hetsroni I, Lillemoe K, Marx RG. Small medial meniscocapsular separations: a potential cause of chronic medial-side knee pain. *Arthroscopy.* 2011;27(11):1536–1542.

Pain in elbow several days after elbow joint dislocation

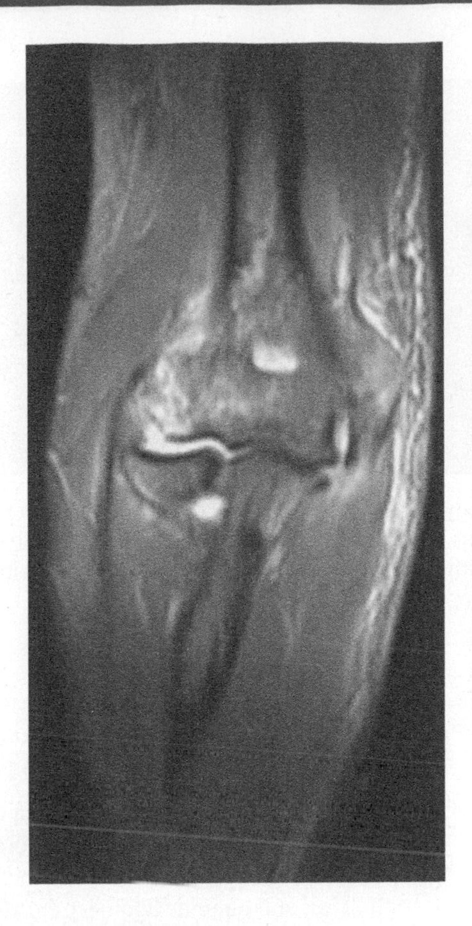

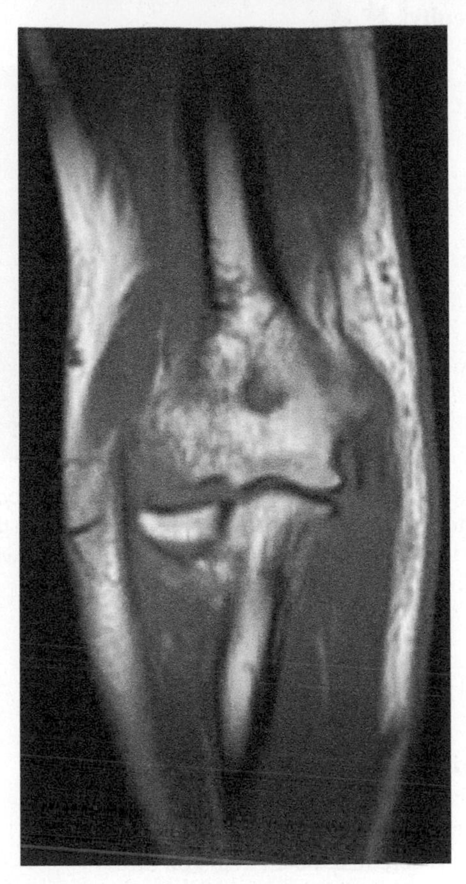

1. What is the mechanism of injury?
2. What are the abnormal structures in this entity?
3. Which neurovascular structures may be at risk at the time of the initial injury?
4. What clinical symptoms may arise from olecranon loose bodies?
5. What is the optimal time of repair of the damaged structure?

Lateral ulnar collateral ligament (LUCL) injury of elbow 2232

Case ranking/difficulty: 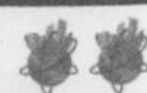

Category: Trauma

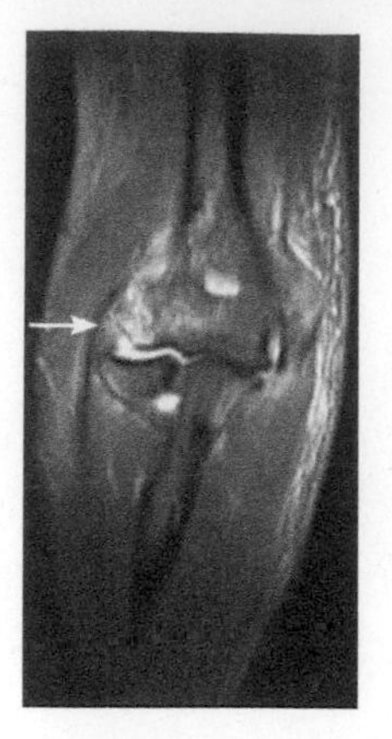

Marrow edema in capitellum secondary to avulsion injury of lateral ulnar collateral ligament (LUCL).

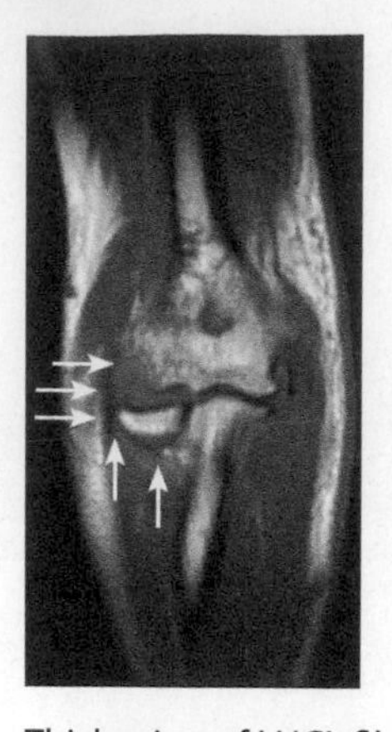

Thickening of LUCL fibres and marrow edema at insertion onto capitellum consistent with an avulsion injury (LUCL annotated with *arrows*).

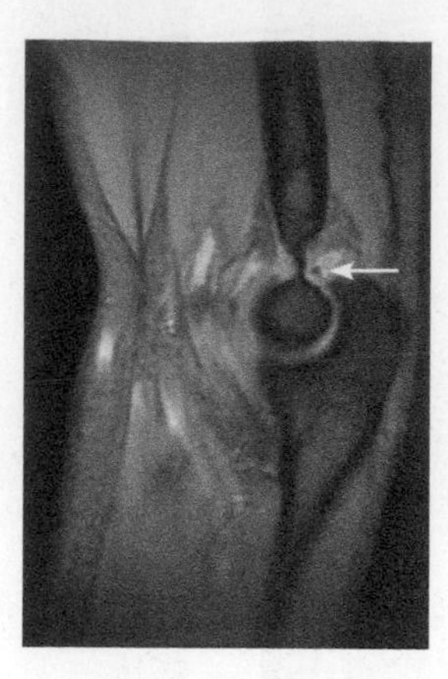

Tiny loose body is seen adjacent to the olecranon consistent with a capsular avulsion.

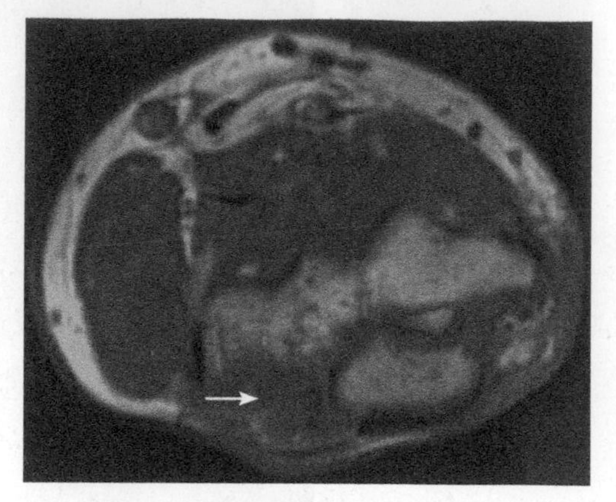

Axial T1 images show low signal within the capitellum consistent with marrow edema at the site of the avulsion injury.

Answers

1. Posterior elbow dislocation commonly results in tearing of the lateral collateral ligament complex, including the radial collateral ligament and lateral ulnar collateral ligament (LUCL). There may be an avulsion of the capitellum where the lateral ligaments attach.
2. Posterior dislocation of the elbow results in damage to the radial-sided ligamentous structures primarily, for example, radial collateral ligament and LUCL. These may need operative repair to prevent potential chronic elbow instability. The capitellum may be involved as a result of an avulsion injury of these ligaments.

   Coronoid and olecranon fractures may also be seen because of direct impaction but are not present in this particular case.
3. The brachial artery, median nerve, and ulnar nerve are all at risk of damage from elbow dislocations. Confirmation of the brachial artery pulse and intact motor/sensory function distally is important when examining the patient.
4. Olecranon loose bodies may result from posterior elbow dislocations. They can be a continued source of problems with symptoms of locking, pain worsening when the elbow is extended and loss of control when throwing.
5. Repair of the lateral ulnar collateral ligament should ideally be performed within two weeks. After this time, better results may be achieved with autologous tendon reconstruction of the ligament.

Pearls

- An elbow dislocation is usually posterior and has a constellation of common injuries: coronoid, olecranon, radial head fractures, radial collateral, lateral ulnar collateral, and annular ligament injuries are common. Ulnar collateral ligament injuries may also occur.
- A lateral ulnar collateral injury may be associated with a capitellar fracture and result in chronic posterior rotatory instability.
- Loose bodies should be carefully evaluated and an attempt should be made to decide if they are adherent to inflamed capsule or genuinely free-floating.
- MRI is the investigation of choice after elbow dislocation, as careful assessment of ligamentous integrity is essential.
- If there is diagnostic difficulty, an MR arthrogram may be performed using dilute gadolinium injected via the radiocapitellar joint.

Suggested Readings

Rhyou IH, Kim YS. New mechanism of the posterior elbow dislocation. *Knee Surg Sports Traumatol Arthrosc.* 2012;20(12):2535–2541.

Takigawa N, Ryu J, Kish VL, Kinoshita M, Abe M. Functional anatomy of the lateral collateral ligament complex of the elbow: morphology and strain. *J Hand Surg Br.* 2005;30(2):143–147.

Hyperextension injury to the little finger

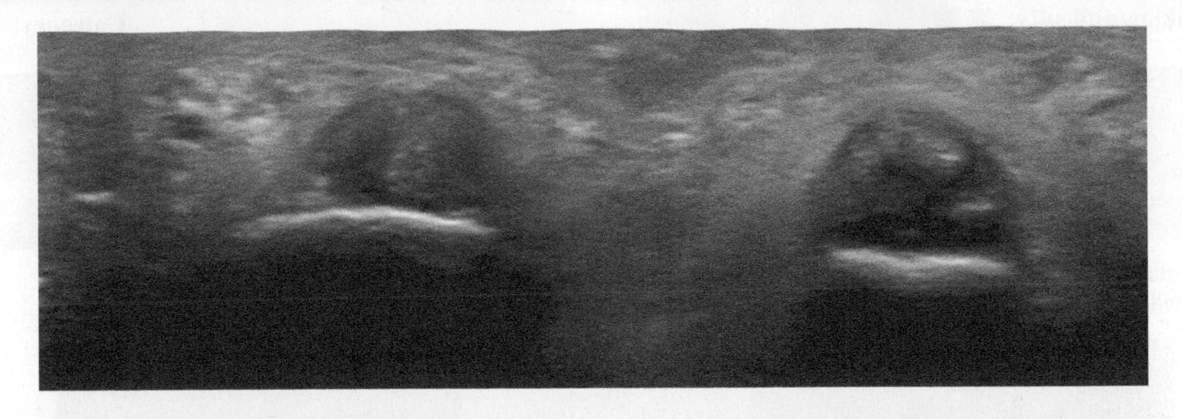

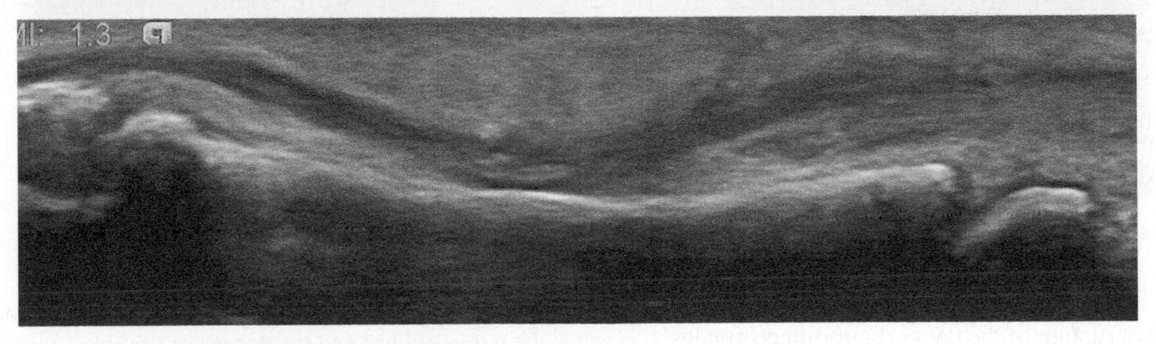

1. What are the ultrasound findings?

2. What are the anatomical attachments of the flexor tendons to the volar aspect of the phalanx?

3. What are the described types of flexor tendon injuries?

4. What are zones of the hands when describing this injury?

5. What is the mechanism of injury?

Jersey finger—flexor digitorum profundus tendon rupture 1399

Case ranking/difficulty: 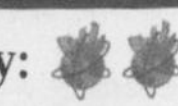

Category: Trauma

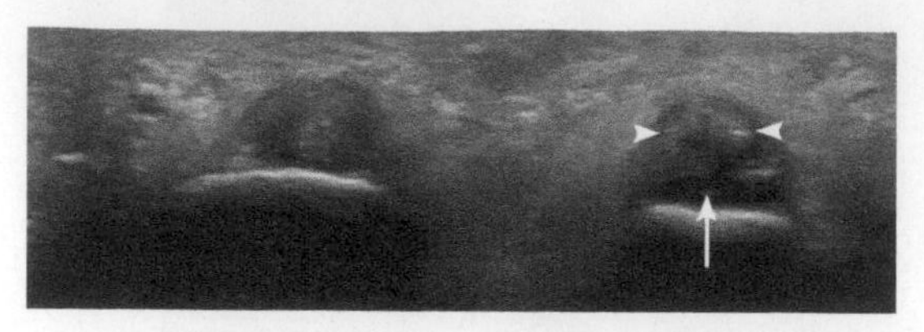

Missing central FDP tendon (*arrow*). Two slips of FDS are demonstrated (*arrowheads*).

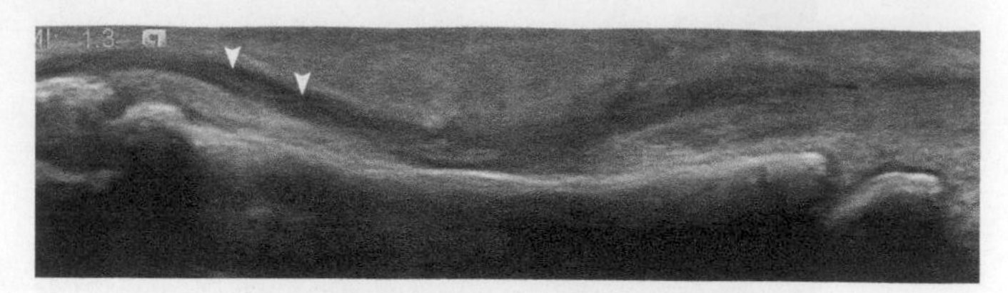

Empty FDP tendon sheath (*arrowheads*).

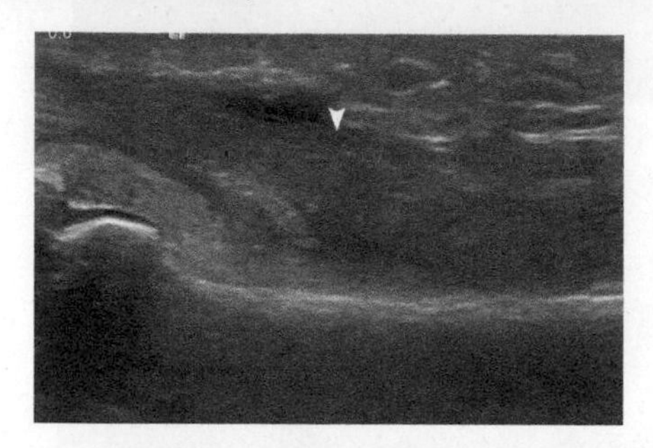

Curled and retracted FDP tendon (*arrowhead*).

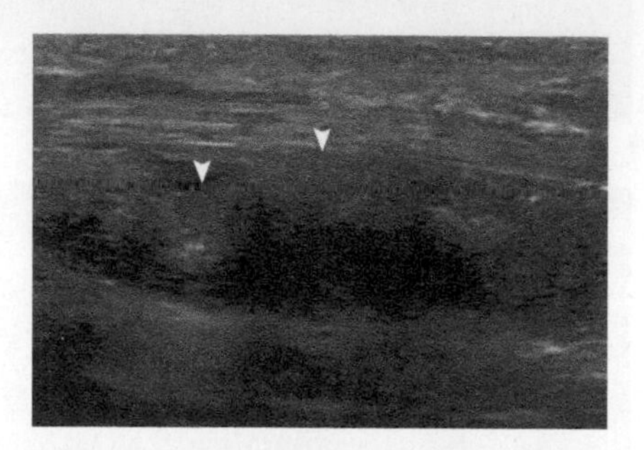

Arrowhead showing retracted tendon.

Answers

1. There is a rupture of the flexor digitorum profundus (FDP) tendon with retraction.
2. Vincula longa and vincula brevia are thin, vascularized, synovial bands that contribute to the stability of the tendon.
3. There are 4 types:
   - Type 1: Retraction of tendon up to the palm, treatment no later than 7 days after injury.
   - Type 2: Retraction to the PIP joint. Small fleck of calcification is often noted, vincula longa prevents necrosis as a result of preserved vascularity.
   - Type 3: Retraction to the base of the distal phalanx with a fracture fragment, not passing beyond the DIPJ or A4 pulley.
   - Type 4: Type 3 with avulsion of FDP from the fracture fragment and proximal retraction to the palm.
4. There are also described zones of tendon retraction: zone I is up to the PIP joint; zone II to the MCP joint; zone III up to the wrist; zone IV is at the wrist; and zone V is proximal to the wrist. The zones are different for the thumb.
5. Hyperextension of a flexed finger is the mechanism of injury in a Jersey finger.

Pearls

- FDP tendon rupture is also called *Jersey finger*. The mechanism is usually a forced extension of the flexed finger.
- Ultrasound is the investigative modality of choice. MRI is supplementary.
- It is important to know the anatomy and describe the tendon rupture and the degree of proximal retraction, as well as any bony avulsion, and also to describe the zonal location of the retracted tendon.
- The classification of FDP injury by Leddy and Packer is useful in the management plan:
  - Type 1: Retraction of tendon up to the palm, treatment is required no later than 7 days after injury.
  - Type 2: Retraction to the level of the PIP joint. The intact vincula longa prevents necrosis because of preserved vascularity.
  - Type 3: Retraction to the base of the distal phalanx with a fracture fragment, not passing beyond the distal interphalangeal joint or A4 pulley as the large bone fragment is "caught" in the tendon sheath. Treatment options depend on the time of presentation and the location of the retracted tendon.
  - Type 4: Tendon separates from the bony fragment and retracts to the palm.
- Surgical repair and tendon transfer are carried out. Postoperative physiotherapy plays an important role.

Suggested Readings

Clavero JA, Alomar X, Monill JM, et al. MR imaging of ligament and tendon injuries of the fingers. *Radiographics*. 2002;22(2):237–256.

Drapé JL, Tardif-Chastenet de Gery S, Silbermann-Hoffman O, et al. Closed ruptures of the flexor digitorum tendons: MRI evaluation. *Skeletal Radiol*. 1998;27(11):617–624.

Severe pain in great toe during football practice

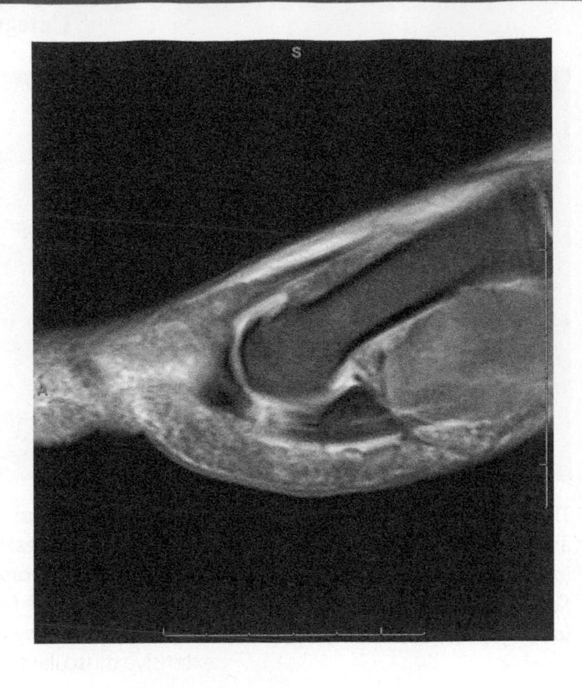

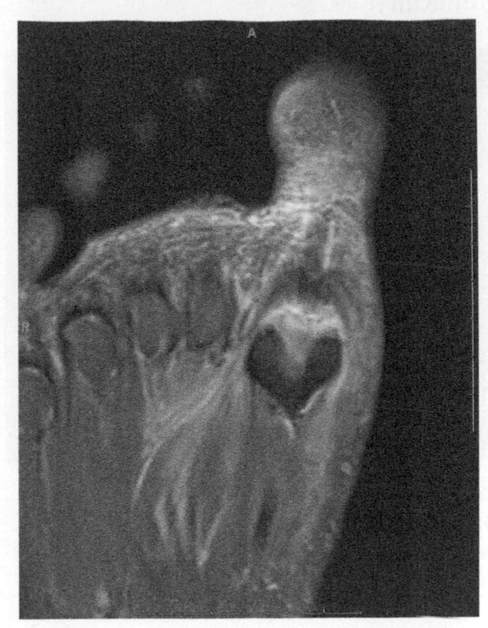

1. What are the MRI findings?

2. What is the most likely diagnosis?

3. What are the components of the great toe capsuloligamentous complex?

4. On MRI, there is a normal recess at the attachment of the plantar plate to the proximal phalanx. True or False?

5. What are the indications for surgery in these patients?

Turf toe 1411

Case ranking/difficulty: 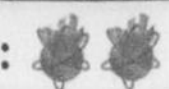 **Category:** Trauma

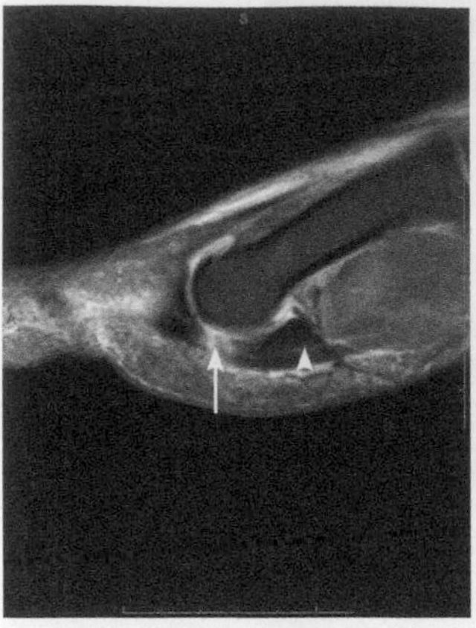

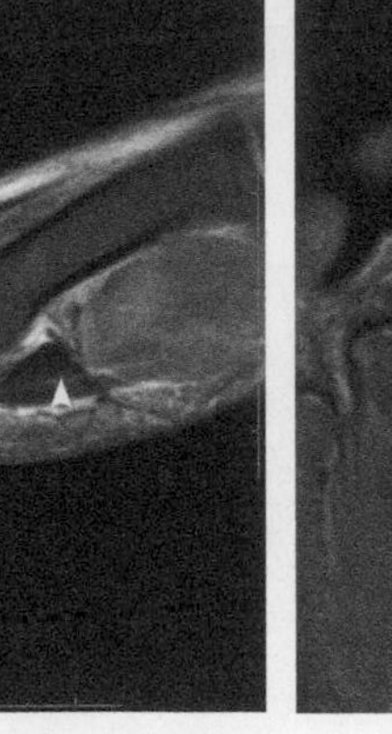

Tear of the plantar plate (*arrow*) with proximal migration of the sesamoids (*arrowhead*).

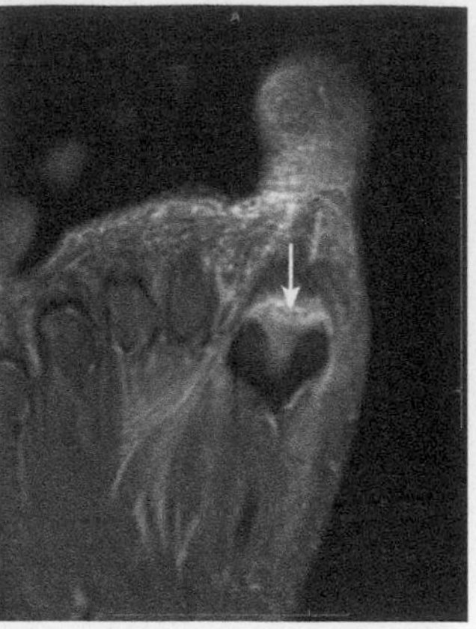

There is disruption of the plantar plate (*arrow*).

There is partial tear of the abductor hallucis tendon (*arrow*). Tenosynovitis of the flexor hallucis longus tendon (*arrowhead*) is noted.

There is disruption of the sesamoid-phalangeal ligaments (*arrows*), which is worse medially. Tenosynovitis of the flexor hallucis longus tendon (*arrowhead*) and extensive muscular edema is noted.

Answers

1. There is proximal migration of the sesamoids with tearing of the plantar plate, the sesamoid–phalangeal ligaments, and the abductor hallucis tendon. In addition, there is tenosynovitis of the flexor hallucis longus tendon.
2. The clinical history and MRI findings are consistent with turf toe.
3. Plantar plate, intersesamoid, and sesamoid–phalangeal ligaments, as well as the accessory sesamoid ligaments and abductor/adductor hallucis tendons.
4. There is a normal recess centrally at the attachment of the plantar plate to the base of the proximal phalanx. It is central, smooth, regular, and incomplete, unlike a tear of the plantar plate.
5. Extensive injury in a professional athlete or in a patient refractory to conservative management may require surgical intervention. Surgery should be performed as early as possible, as scarring in the operative bed often makes surgical intervention difficult.

Pearls

- Turf toe is an injury to the capsuloligamentous structures of the great toe.
- Radiographs may show widening of the intersesamoid space or proximal migration of the sesamoids. Fractures of the sesamoids may also occur.
- MRI can show the extent of injury to the plantar plate, associated ligaments, and tendons. Sesamoid displacement and fracture/contusion is also well demonstrated.
- A normal recess at the plantar plate phalangeal attachment distally can be seen, which is important to differentiate from a tear.
- Injury to the intersesamoid ligament will result in widening of the intersesamoid distance.
- Injury to the sesamoid–phalangeal ligaments will result in proximal migration of the sesamoids.

Suggested Readings

Crain JM, Phancao JP, Stidham K. MR imaging of turf toe. *Magn Reson Imaging Clin N Am.* 2008;16(1):93–103, vi.

Yao L, Do HM, Cracchiolo A, Farahani K. Plantar plate of the foot: findings on conventional arthrography and MR imaging. *AJR Am J Roentgenol.* 1994;163(3):641–644.

Severe pain on abduction of the thumb

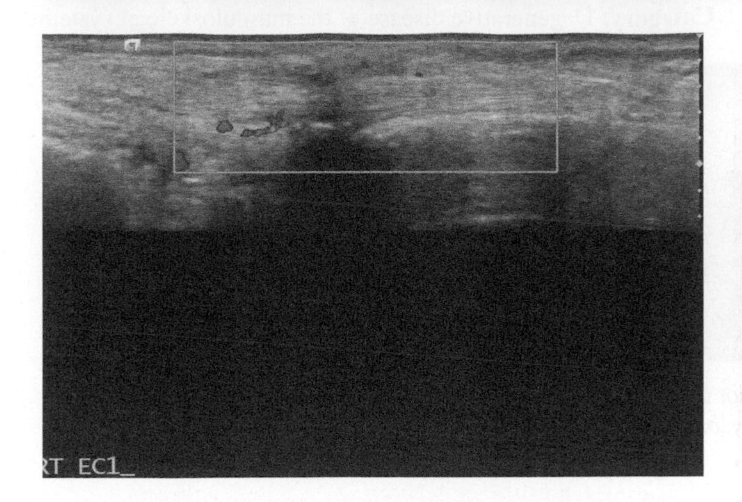

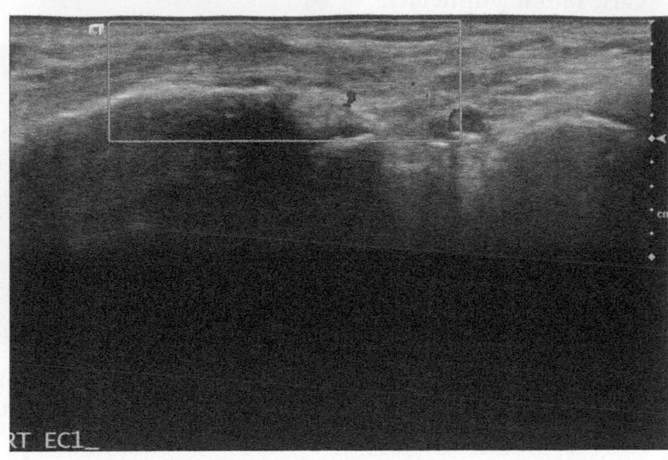

1. What is the differential diagnosis of this condition?
2. What is the abnormal structure shown?
3. What are the imaging modalities of choice for this condition?
4. What are the possible treatments for this condition?
5. What clinical test can confirm the presence of this condition?

De Quervain tenosynovitis 1649

Case ranking/difficulty: 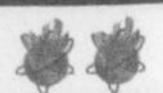

Category: Degenerative disease of the musculoskeletal system

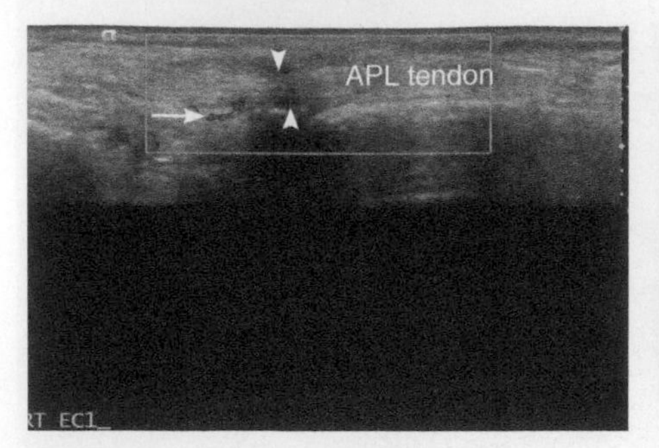

Fluid in first extensor sheath (*arrowhead*) with neovascularity (*arrow*).

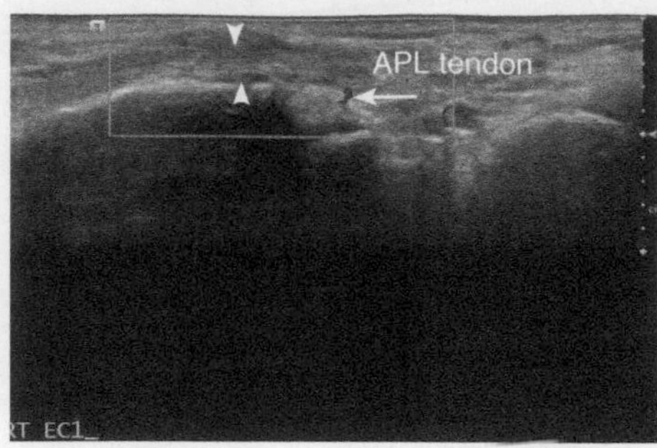

Fluid in first extensor sheath (*arrowhead*) with neovascularity (*arrow*).

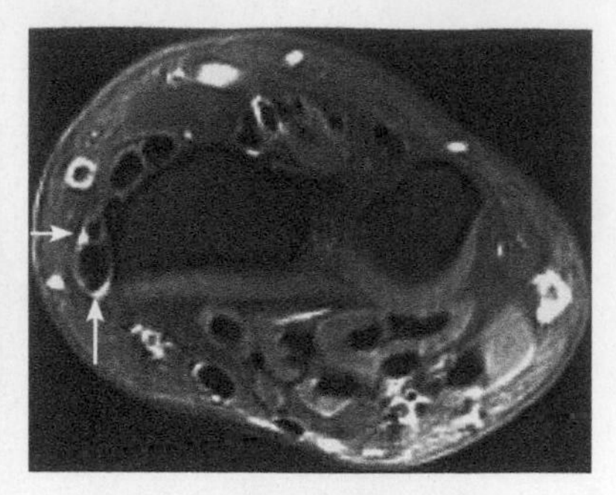

An effusion in the first extensor compartment is typical of De Quervain tenosynovitis.

Answers

1. De Quervain tenosynovitis can be related to overuse, inflammatory conditions, for example, rheumatoid arthritis, or infection.
2. The common synovial sheath containing the abductor pollicis longus and extensor pollicis brevis tendons is by convention labelled as the first compartment.
3. MRI and ultrasound are both suitable for diagnosis of De Quervain's tenosynovitis. Ultrasound has the advantage of guiding percutaneous injection therapy.
4. Treatment includes rest, splinting, NSAIDs, percutaneous steroid injection and extensor compartment release.
5. The Finkelstein test involves ulnar deviation with a flexed thumb. It is almost invariably positive with De Quervain tenosynovitis.

Pearls

- De Quervain tenosynovitis is a common condition, usually secondary to repetitive frictional forces.
- It involves the abductor pollicis longus (APL) and extensor pollicis brevis (EPB) tendons as they pass over the radial styloid.
- Patients with inflammatory arthritis, especially rheumatoid, may also present with this condition in addition to involvement of other tendon compartments, for example, extensor compartment 6 (ECU).
- Ultrasound is the examination of choice, as it enables percutaneous corticosteroid injection to be performed at the time of scanning.
- MRI will show fluid within the first extensor synovial sheath, although the underlying tendons are usually normal.
- Axial and coronal T1/STIR images are ideal for evaluation.
- The Finkelstein test can be performed prior to the ultrasound examination to add to diagnostic confidence. It is almost always positive in affected individuals.

Suggested Readings

Abrisham SJ, Karbasi MH, Zare J, Behnamfar Z, Tafti AD, Shishesaz B. De Quervain tenosynovitis: clinical outcomes of surgical treatment with longitudinal and transverse incision. *Oman Med J.* 2011;26(2):91–93.

Choi SJ, Ahn JH, Lee YJ, et al. de Quervain disease: US identification of anatomic variations in the first extensor compartment with an emphasis on subcompartmentalization. *Radiology.* 2011;260(2): 480–486.

Pagonis T, Ditsios K, Toli P, Givissis P, Christodoulou A. Improved corticosteroid treatment of recalcitrant de Quervain tenosynovitis with a novel 4-point injection technique. *Am J Sports Med.* 2011;39(2):398–403.

Anterior knee pain for 2 years

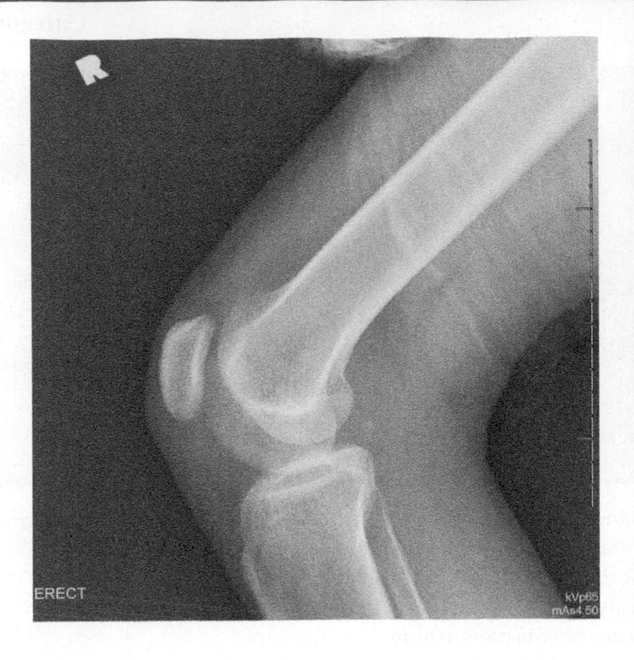

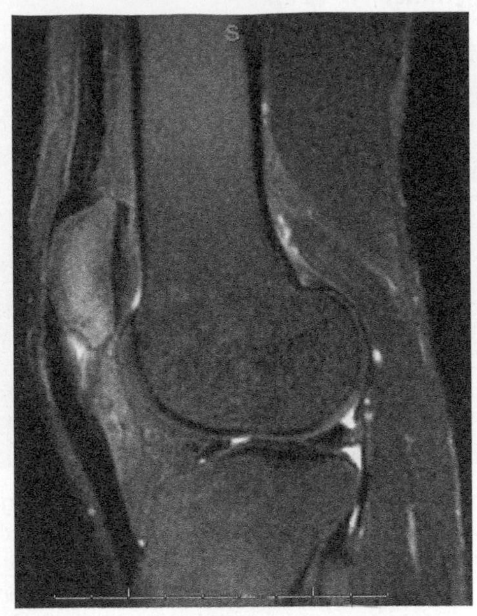

1. What are the MRI findings?

2. What is the etiology?

3. What is the differential diagnosis for the entity depicted?

4. Is this entity more common in men or women?

5. This entity is most prevalent among athletes in which sports?

Jumper's knee

1557

Case ranking/difficulty:

Category: Trauma

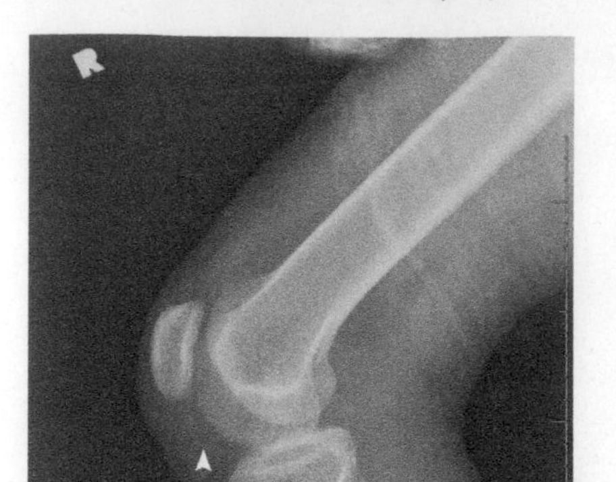

No osseous abnormality is present, but mild edema is demonstrated in the superior portion of the Hoffa fat pad (*arrowhead*).

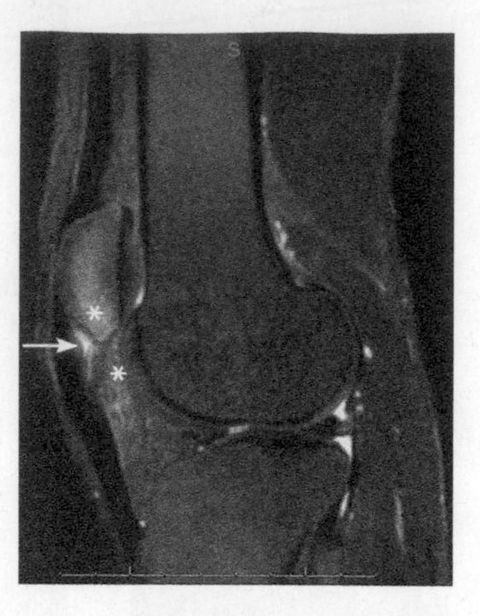

Thickening and increased signal intensity in the proximal patellar tendon consistent with tendinosis, as well as a focal area of fluid signal intensity consistent with partial tear (*arrow*). Marrow edema pattern is present in the inferior pole of the patella (*superior asterisk*), and edema is present in the superior aspect of the Hoffa fat (*inferior asterisk*).

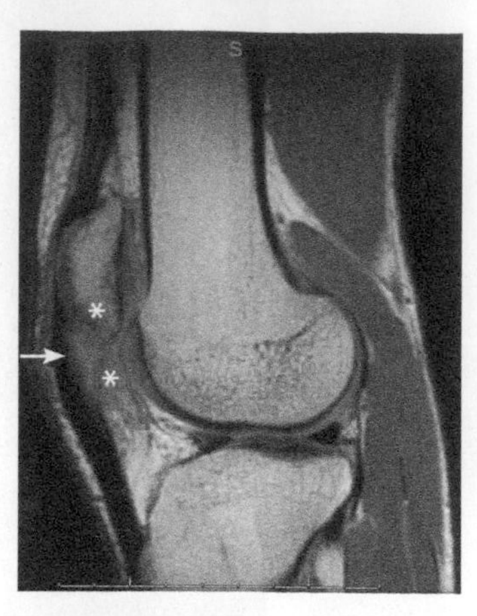

Similar findings in another patient

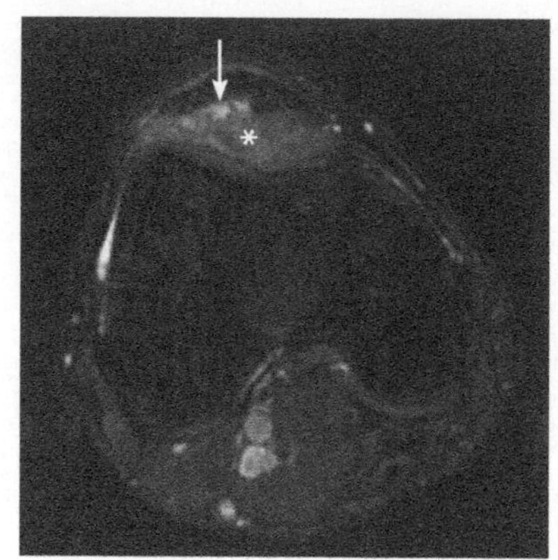

Partial tendon tear (*arrow*). Edema is present in the superior aspect of the Hoffa fat (*asterisk*).

Answers

1. Proximal patellar tendinosis and edema in the superior aspect of the Hoffa fat.
2. Jumper's knee is an overuse condition caused by repetitive activity, most commonly jumping sports.
3. The clinical differential diagnosis may include patellar tracking disorder, infrapatellar bursitis, and impingement as a result of a patellar plica.
4. The gender ratio for jumper's knee is 1:0.6 (men-to-women).
5. It is most prevalent in jumping sports such as volleyball and basketball.

Pearls

- Jumper's knee, or proximal patellar tendinosis, is a common overuse condition of the knee that typically afflicts jumping athletes.
- It is most common among basketball and volleyball players.
- Patients typically present with gradual onset of anterior knee pain related to activity.
- On physical examination, tenderness is localized to the inferior pole of the patella and proximal patellar tendon.
- MRI demonstrates thickening and increased signal of the proximal patellar tendon near the patellar attachment. Associated edema in the Hoffa fat pad and the lower pole of the patella is common.
- Partial-thickness tearing of the patellar tendon may be present, characteristically in the posterior central aspect of the tendon proximally.

Suggested Readings

Lian OB, Engebretsen L, Bahr R. Prevalence of jumper's knee among elite athletes from different sports: a cross-sectional study. *Am J Sports Med.* 2005;33(4):561–567.

Zwerver J, Bredeweg SW, van den Akker-Scheek I. Prevalence of jumper's knee among nonelite athletes from different sports: a cross-sectional survey. *Am J Sports Med.* 2011;39(9):1984–1988.

Athlete with right-sided groin pain that is worse with activity

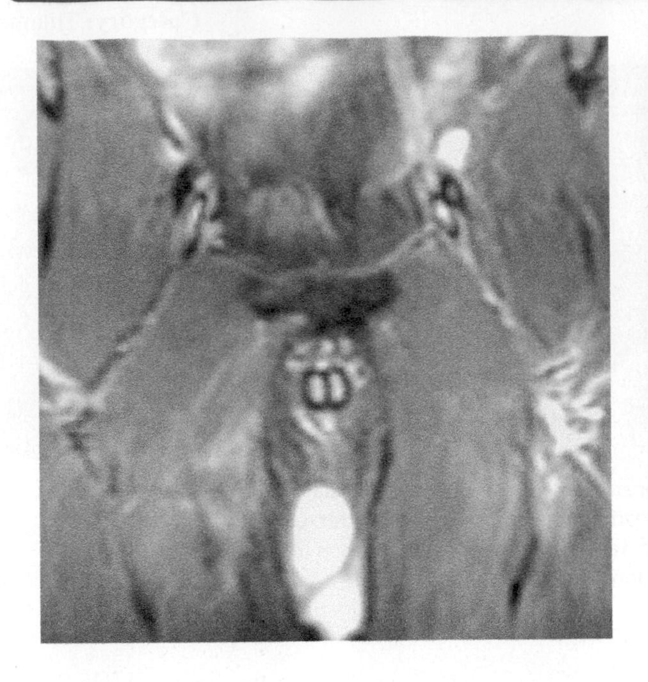

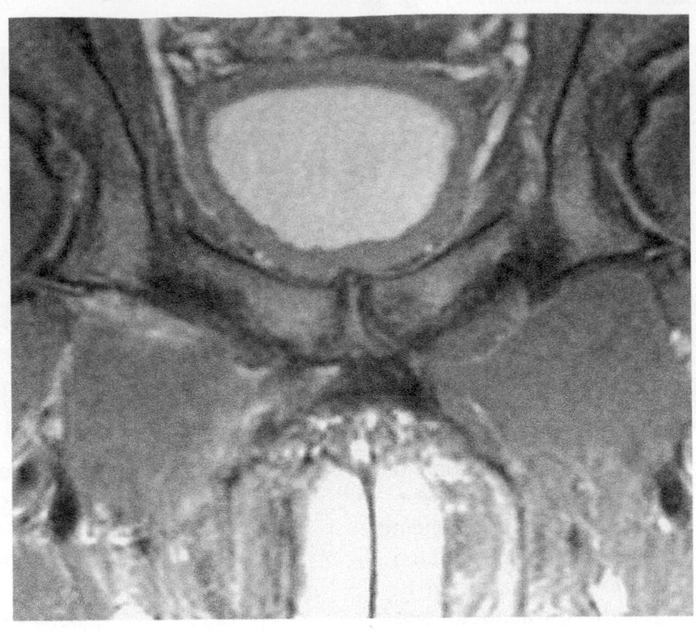

1. What muscles attach at or near the pubic symphysis?
2. What structures are commonly abnormal in this entity?
3. In this entity, the hernia is usually located where?
4. What is the clinical differential diagnosis?
5. What other names have been given to groin pain in athletes?

Athletic pubalgia 1455

Case ranking/difficulty: 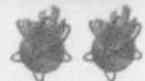

Category: Trauma

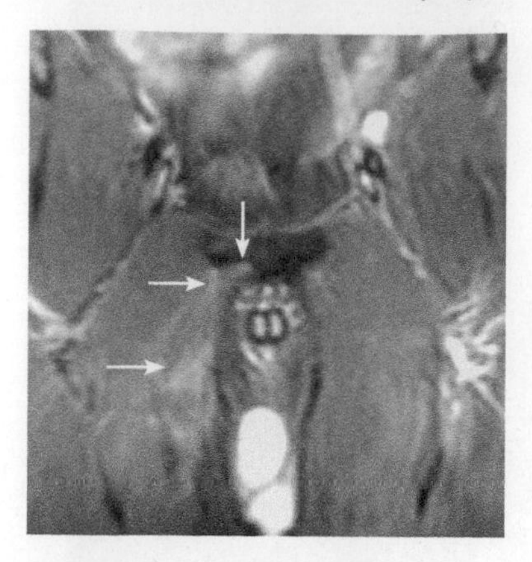

A tear of the right rectus abdominis–adductor aponeurosis is present (*superior, vertical arrow*) extending into the adductor longus tendon (*middle arrow*). Edema pattern is present within the adductor muscles (*inferior arrow*).

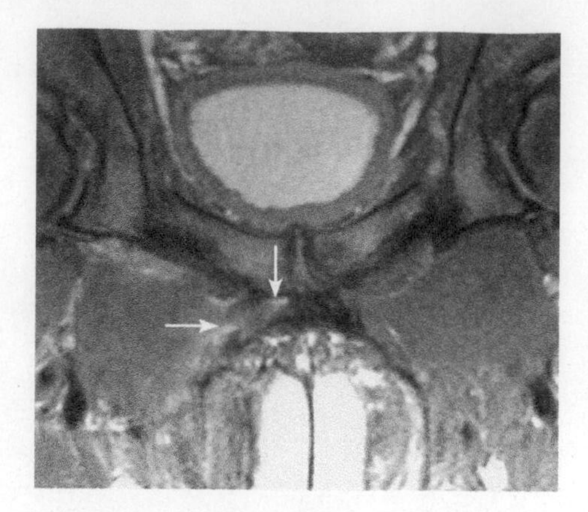

Oblique coronal image demonstrates tear of the right rectus abdominis–adductor aponeurosis (*superior arrow*) extending into the adductor longus tendon (*inferior arrow*).

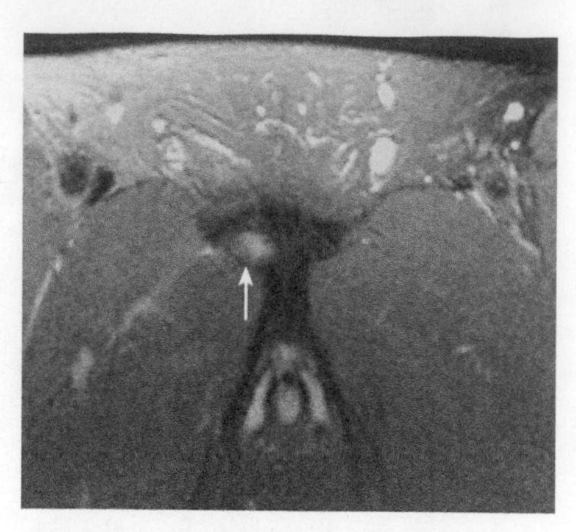

Oblique axial image shows a tear of the right rectus abdominis–adductor aponeurosis (*arrow*).

Answers

1. Muscles that attach at or near the pubic symphysis include the rectus abdominis and the thigh adductor group muscles, which include the pectineus, adductor longus, adductor brevis, gracilis, and adductor magnus. The rectus abdominis muscles attach at the superior aspect of the pubic symphysis. The pectineus originates from the superior pubic ramus. The adductor longus originates from the pubic body just below the pubic crest. The adductor brevis originates from the anterior surface of the pubic body and inferior ramus. The gracilis originates from the ischiopubic ramus. The adductor magnus originates from the ischial tuberosity and ischiopubic ramus. The sartorius muscle originates at and inferior to the anterior superior iliac spine, not near the pubic symphysis.
2. The rectus abdominis and adductor tendons (including pectineus, adductor longus, and adductor brevis) are usually involved in athletic pubalgia.
3. Although athletic pubalgia is sometimes termed "sports hernia," this is actually a misnomer. Usually no hernia is present in these patients.
4. Acetabular labral tear, stress fracture, inguinal hernia, femoroacetabular impingement, and snapping hip syndrome are in the clinical differential.
5. Sports hernia, sportsman's hernia, footballer's groin, hockey groin, and Gilmore's groin are all terms that have been used to describe athletic pubalgia.

Pearls

- Athletic pubalgia refers to activity-related groin pain in athletes.
- It usually afflicts high-performance athletes at the collegiate or professional level.
- It more commonly occurs in players of soccer, hockey, football, and Australian-rules football.
- On MRI, abnormalities are typically located near the pubic symphysis and include bone marrow edema pattern at the pubic symphysis, thigh adductor tendon injury, and rectus abdominis insertional injury.
- Tears may occur in the rectus abdominis-adductor aponeurosis, which is a fibrous plate that overlies the pubic symphysis anteriorly.
- Bone marrow edema pattern may occur in isolation, or in association with the tendon/aponeurosis tears.

Suggested Readings

Mullens FE, Zoga AC, Morrison WB, Meyers WC. Review of MRI Technique and imaging findings in athletic pubalgia and the "sports hernia". *Eur J Radiol.* 2012;81(12):3780–3792.

Zoga AC, Kavanagh EC, Omar IM, et al. Athletic pubalgia and the "sports hernia": MR imaging findings. *Radiology.* 2008;247(3):797–807.

Medial knee pain for 4 years

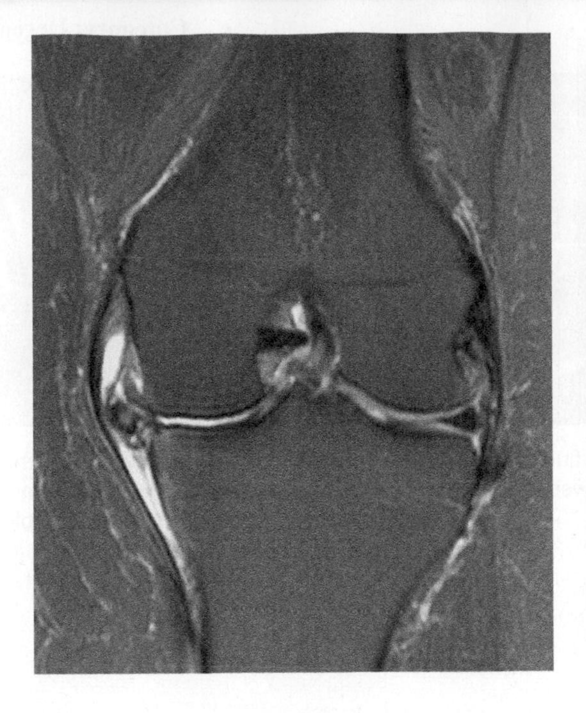

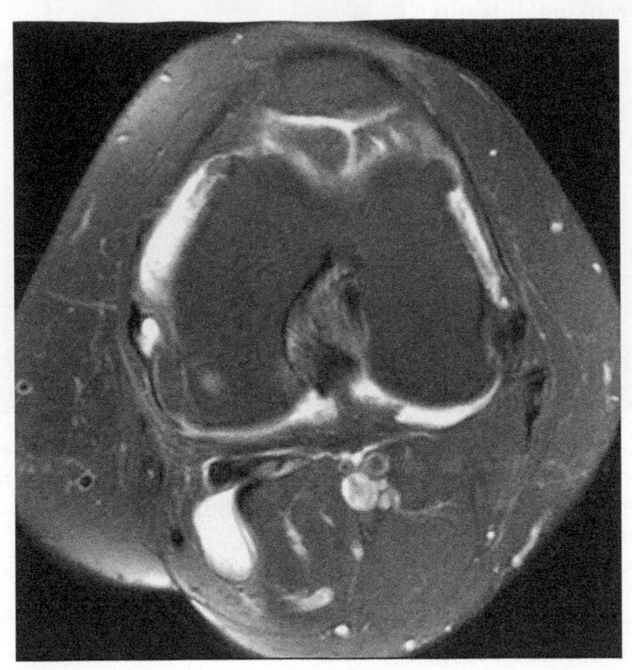

1. What are the pertinent imaging findings?

2. What are included in the differential for a cystic lesion at the medial knee?

3. What forms the medial supporting structures of the knee?

4. What are the components of the MCL?

5. What is the appropriate treatment for this condition?

Medial collateral ligament bursitis 1326

Case ranking/difficulty: ✱✱ **Category:** Degenerative

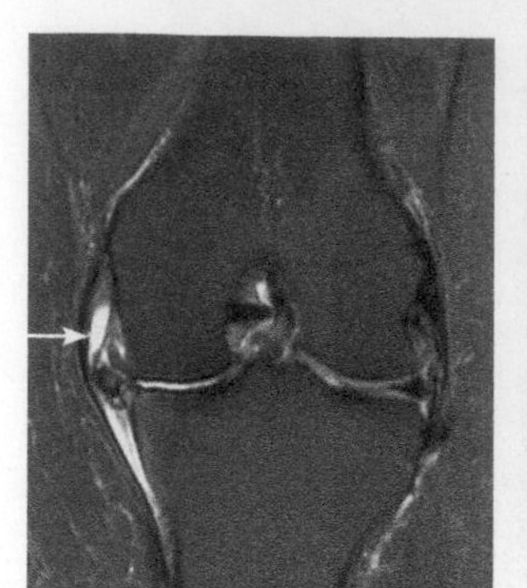

Cystic fluid collection between the 2 layers of the MCL (*arrow*), extending above and below the joint line. Degenerative tear of the medial meniscus, meniscal extrusion, and medial compartment osteoarthritis are also seen.

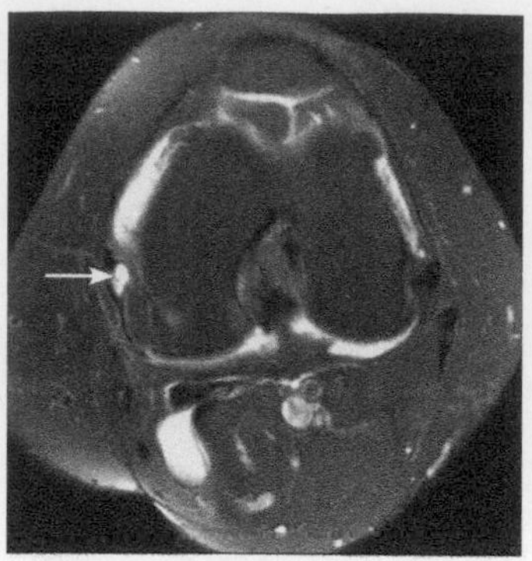

The fluid collection lies between the 2 layers of the MCL. Popliteal cyst is incidentally noted.

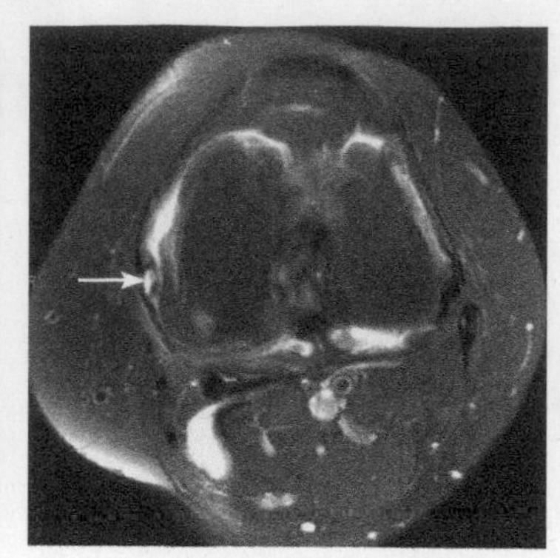

The fluid collection is again seen between the 2 layers of the MCL.

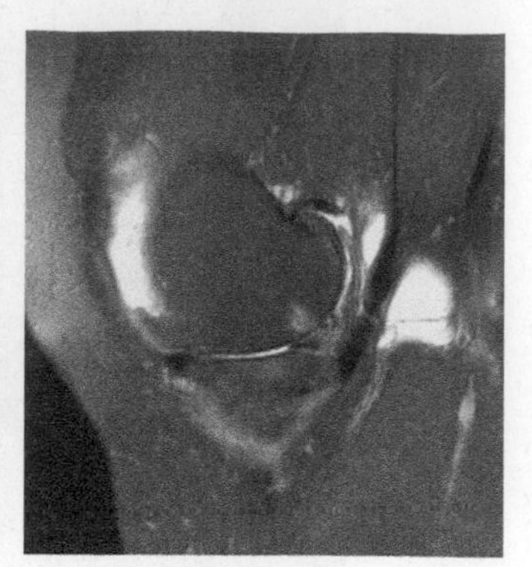

Degenerative medial meniscus tear, medial compartment osteoarthritis, and popliteal cyst are other demonstrated findings in this patient.

Answers

1. There is a cystic lesion between the 2 layers of the MCL consistent with MCL bursitis. There is a degenerative tear of the medial meniscus, and the meniscal body is medially extruded. There is also medial compartment osteoarthritis.

2. Cystic lesions around the medial knee include MCL bursitis, pes anserine bursitis, tibial collateral ligament-semimembranosus bursitis, parameniscal cyst, ganglion and synovial cysts, and a Baker cyst. Rarely, a sarcoma may appear purely cystic.

3. The medial supporting structures are formed by 3 layers. The most superficial layer (layer 1) is formed by the crural fascia, and the sartorius muscle lies within the posterior aspect of this fascia. The middle layer (layer 2) is the superficial MCL and the deep layer (layer 3) is the deep MCL. Layers 1 and 2 fuse anteriorly, and layers 2 and 3 fuse posteriorly.

4. The MCL has a superficial and a deep layer, the latter formed by the deep meniscofemoral and the deep meniscotibial (coronary) ligament as well as the joint capsule.

5. Conservative management with NSAIDs or cyst injection/aspiration is all that is required in the majority of cases. With failure of conservative management, surgical debridement is required and is curative.

Pearls

- Well-defined cystic lesion located between the superficial and deep layers of the MCL.
- Contributory factors include trauma, osteophytic spurs, genu valgus, rheumatoid arthritis, flatfoot deformity, and friction to the medial knee.
- The lesion typically extends above the joint line, unlike pes anserine and tibial collateral ligament-semimembranosus bursitis, which are usually located below the joint line.
- Parameniscal cyst is another cystic lesion that is in the differential for medial cystic lesions located above the joint line.

Suggested Readings

De Maeseneer M, Shahabpour M, Pouders C. MRI spectrum of medial collateral ligament injuries and pitfalls in diagnosis. *JBR-BTR.* 2010;93(2):97–103.

De Maeseneer M, Shahabpour M, Van Roy F, et al. MR imaging of the medial collateral ligament bursa: findings in patients and anatomic data derived from cadavers. *AJR Am J Roentgenol.* 2001;177(4):911–917.

28-year-old female runner with knee pain for months

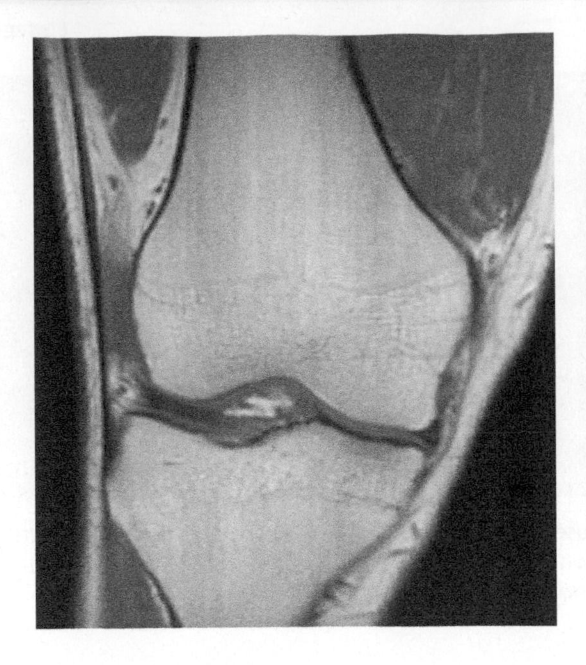

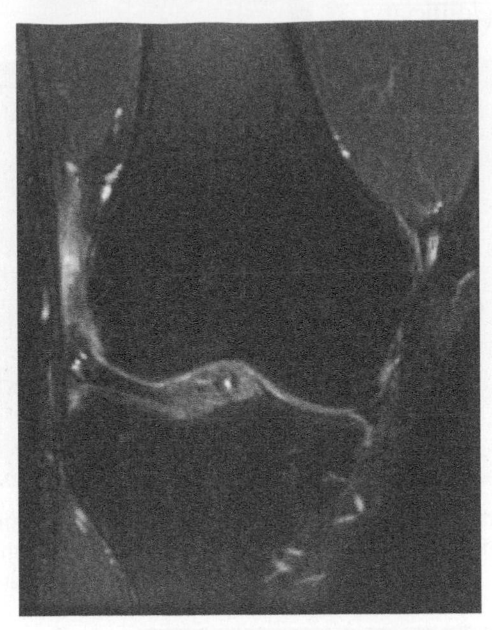

1. What are the MRI findings?

2. What additional findings may be seen in these patients?

3. Which patients are at risk?

4. What is in the differential diagnosis?

5. What is the treatment?

Case ranking/difficulty: 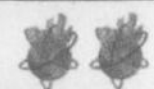

Category: Trauma

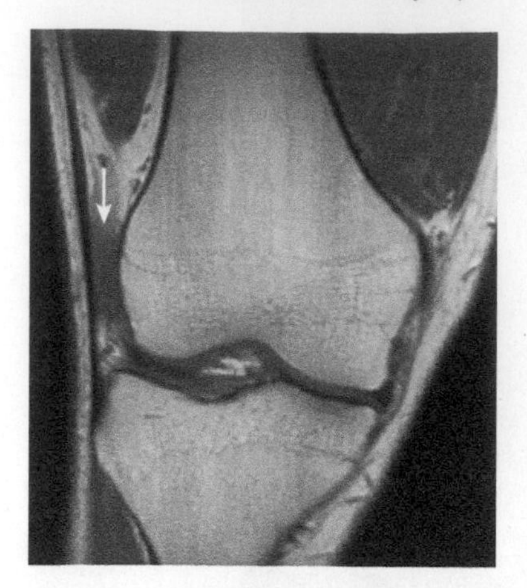

There is inflammatory stranding deep to the iliotibial band (ITB).

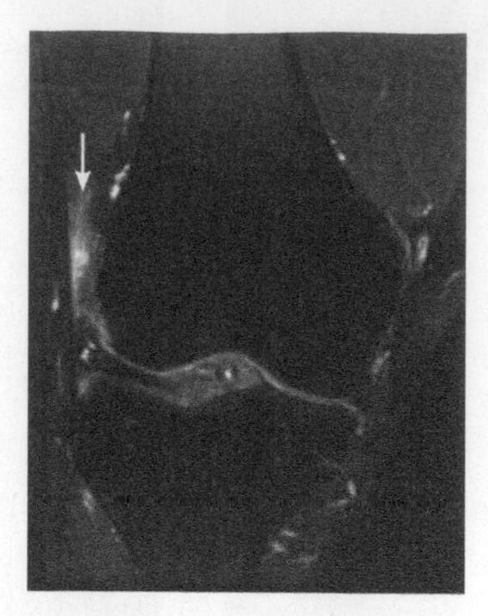

There is diffuse edema deep to the ITB without edema in the ITB, or external to it.

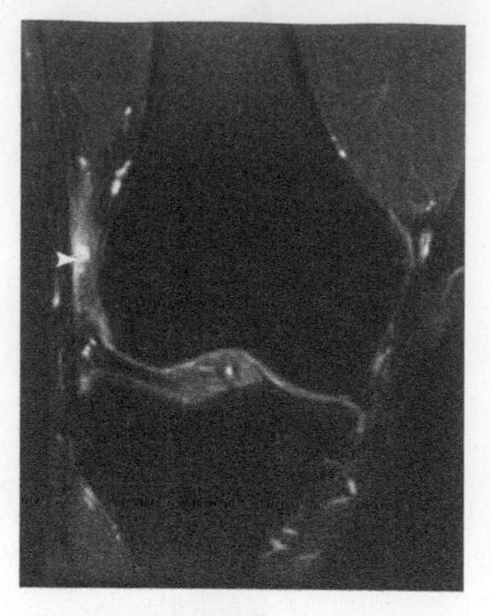

Early adventitial bursa formation is seen (*arrowhead*).

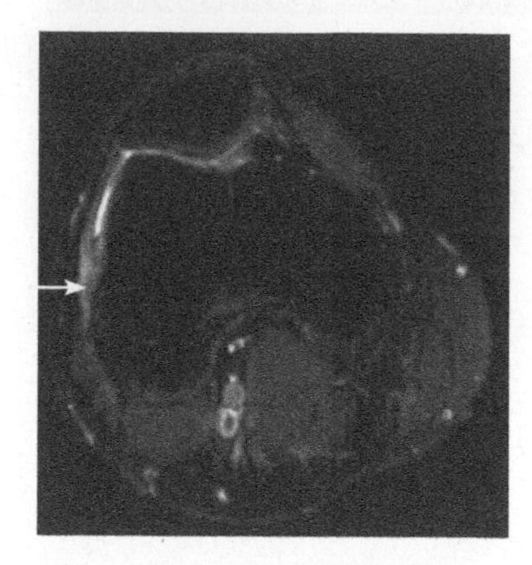

Edema deep to the ITB is seen.

Answers

1. There is poorly defined edema deep to the iliotibial band (ITB) with an otherwise normal ITB, consistent with iliotibial band friction syndrome.

2. Cystic adventitial bursae may form deep to the ITB. Early bursa formation is seen in this case. In chronic cases, the ITB may be thickened with superficial edema. An ITB tear is extremely rare.

3. ITB friction syndrome is classically seen in runners. Predisposing factors include genu varum, hyperpronation, prominent lateral epicondyle, and a congenitally wide ITB.

4. The clinical differential for lateral knee pain would include a lateral meniscus tear, and lateral collateral ligament injury. These are easily excluded on MRI. On MRI, the cystic adventitial bursae that may form in the region of inflammation may be confused with a lateral recess of the suprapatella bursa.

5. Management is typically lifestyle modification, with NSAIDs and rest. Steroid injections can be performed as indicated in more difficult cases. Surgical release of the posterior ITB fibers may be performed, but is rarely indicated.

Pearls

- ITB friction syndrome is an overuse syndrome classically seen in runners.
- Genu varum, a prominent lateral epicondyle, and hyperpronation may contribute to ITB syndrome.
- There is poorly defined edema deep to the ITB in the adjacent fat, located at or posterior to the lateral femoral condyle.
- Cystic adventitial bursae may develop secondary to repetitive trauma.
- This bursa is differentiated from the lateral recess of the knee joint by its location at and posterior to the lateral femoral epicondyle on axial images. The recess is anterior.
- The ITB may eventually become thickened in chronic cases, with edema superficial to the ITB.

Suggested Readings

Muhle C, Ahn JM, Yeh L, et al. Iliotibial band friction syndrome: MR imaging findings in 16 patients and MR arthrographic study of six cadaveric knees. *Radiology.* 1999;212(1):103–110.

Murphy BJ, Hechtman KS, Uribe JW, Selesnick H, Smith RL, Zlatkin MB. Iliotibial band friction syndrome: MR imaging findings. *Radiology.* 1992;185(2):569–571.

Pain and limitation of movement—history of previous arthroscopic surgery

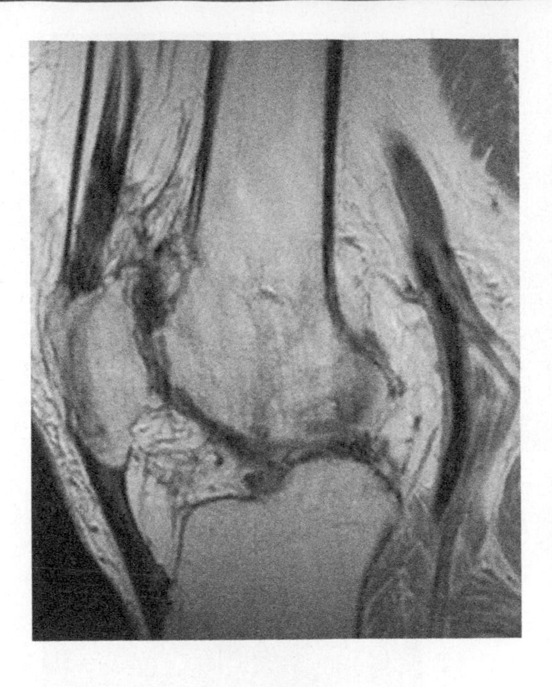

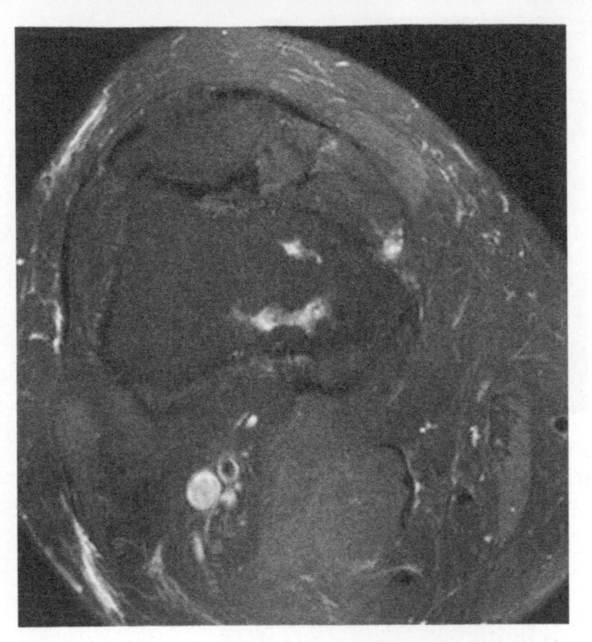

1. What are the MRI findings?

2. What is the differential diagnosis?

3. What is a cyclops lesion?

4. What increases the severity of generalized arthrofibrosis?

5. What is the management for this condition?

Arthrofibrosis of the knee 1429

Case ranking/difficulty: 

Category: Degenerative disease of the musculoskeletal system

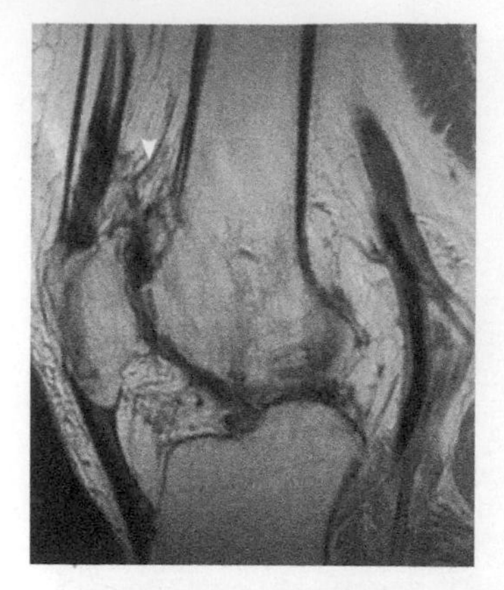

There is extensive scarring in the Hoffa fat pad and in the suprapatellar fat. There is almost no joint fluid.

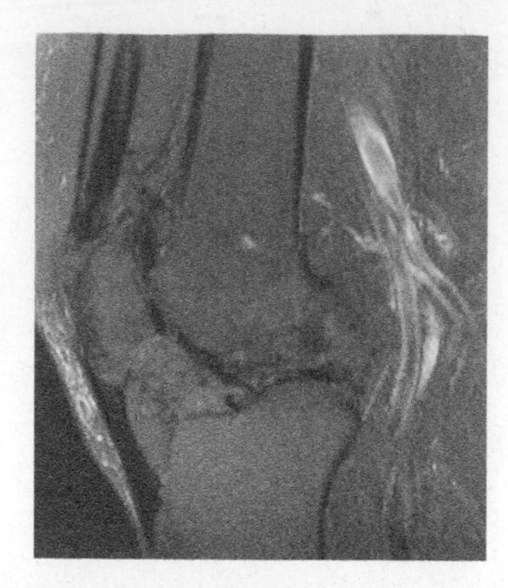

Similar findings as in figure on the left.

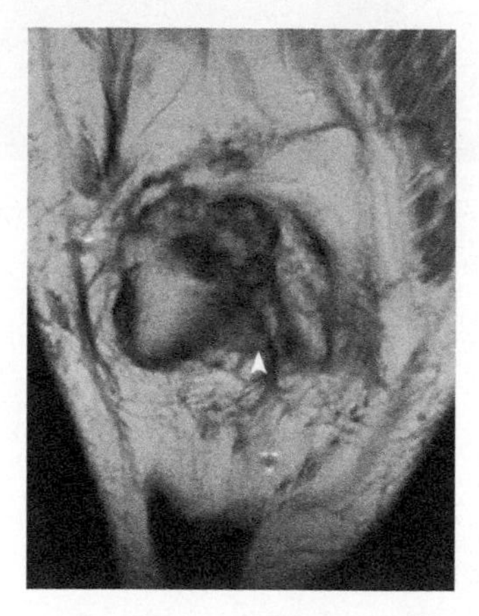

Extensive scarring in the joint is again seen.

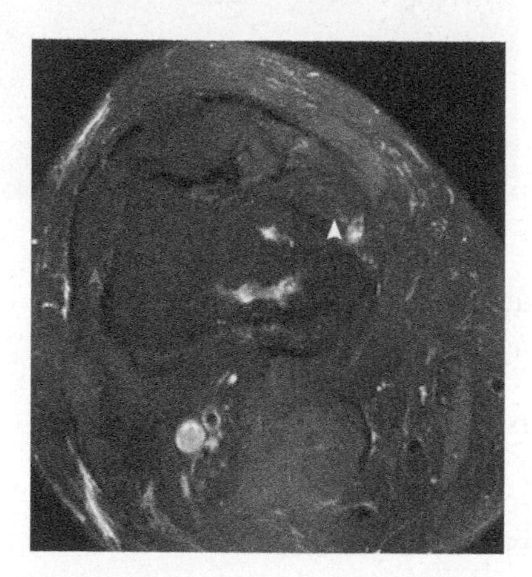

Axial image shows the absence of joint fluid and compensatory hypertrophy of the intra-articular fat (*arrowhead*).

Answers

1. There is a paucity of joint fluid with scarring in a Hoffa fat pad. The intra-articular fat is hypertrophic.
2. PVNS and hemophilia would show normal or increased joint fluid. The history of prior surgery, extensive scarring and the paucity of joint fluid suggest generalized arthrofibrosis as the diagnosis.
3. A cyclops lesion is a localized form of arthrofibrosis at the base of the ACL following an ACL reconstruction. It may be localized postoperative scarring, or scarring around the entrapped native ACL fibers.
4. There is a genetic predisposition for arthrofibrosis. However, the severity of knee injury and the extent of related surgery, as well as the length of immobilization, are risk factors.
5. The management is initially physical therapy, followed by manipulation under anesthesia. If these fail, then surgical removal of scar is performed.

Pearls

- Arthrofibrosis of the knee occurs after open or arthroscopic surgical procedures.
- Generalized arthrofibrosis results in low T1 and T2 scar tissue forming along the arthroscopic tract, or diffusely in the joint capsule.
- There is often a paucity of joint fluid.
- MRI is useful in delineating the location of scar tissue, and guides the surgeon for operative planning.
- Treatment is with physical therapy, manipulation under anesthesia, or surgical resection of scar.

Suggested Readings

Chen MR, Dragoo JL. Arthroscopic releases for arthrofibrosis of the knee. *J Am Acad Orthop Surg.* 2011;19(11):709–716.

Recht MP, Kramer J. MR imaging of the postoperative knee: a pictorial essay. *Radiographics.* 2003;22(4):765–774.

Chronic knee pain

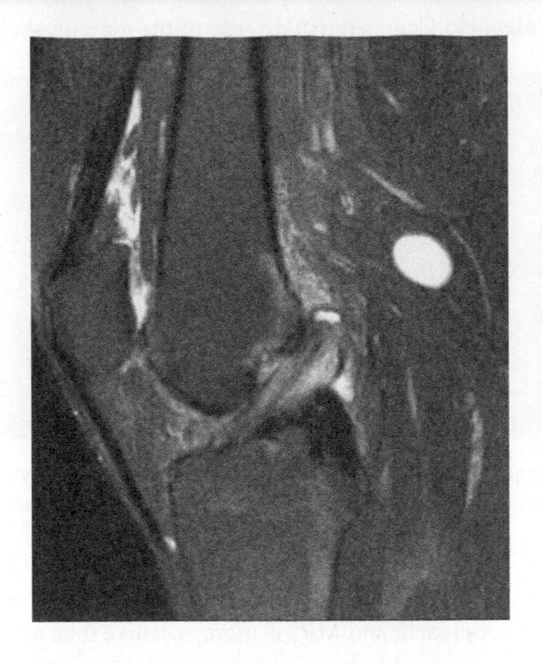

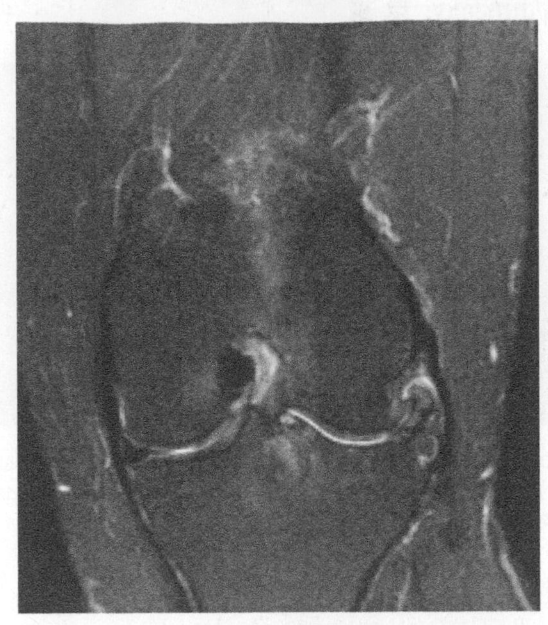

1. What MRI findings are demonstrated?
2. What are the proposed etiologies?
3. What is the mean age of this condition?
4. On arthroscopy, what is the best approach and what are the findings?
5. What is the management for this condition?

Mucoid degeneration of the anterior cruciate ligament 1324

Case ranking/difficulty: 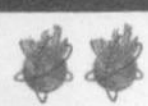

Category: Degenerative disease of the musculoskeletal system

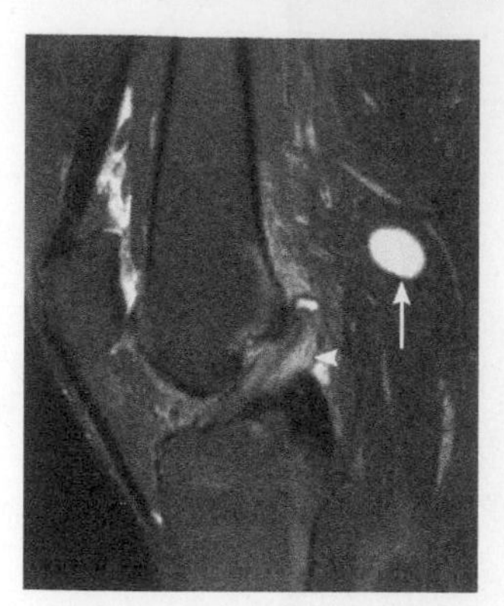

Marked enlargement of the ACL with increased signal (*arrowhead*). Incidental popliteal venous varix is noted (*arrow*).

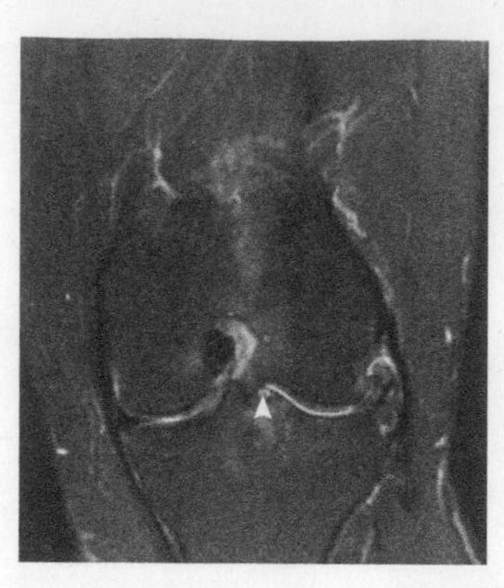

Enlarged ACL with increased signal and proximal tibia cysts (*arrowhead*).

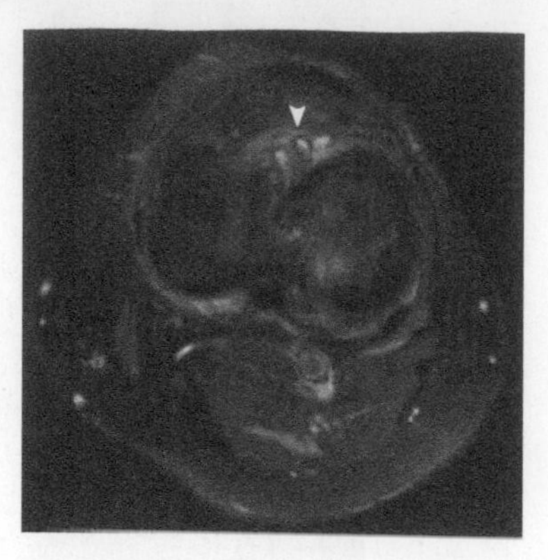

Intra-articular ganglion cysts are seen anterior to the ACL footprint.

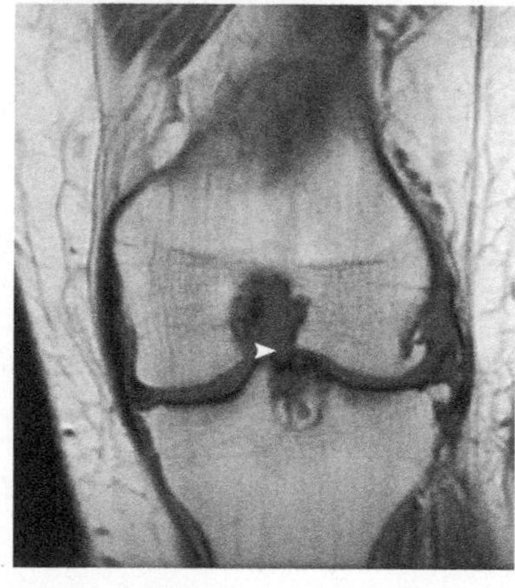

Poor definition of the ACL fibers with loss of the normal fat at the base of the ACL.

Answers

1. The ACL is enlarged with increased T2 signal but with preserved fibers. Associated cysts in the proximal tibia and intra-articular ganglion cysts are frequent associations, and are demonstrated in this case.

2. Senescent degeneration, as well as congenital or acquired synovial entrapment between the ACL fibers, are the proposed etiologies of ACL mucoid degeneration.

   Minor or nonspecific trauma also has been implicated.

3. The mean age for ACL mucoid degeneration alone is 43 years. The mean age for coincident ACL ganglia and mucoid degeneration is 45 years. The mean age for ACL ganglion cysts alone is 39 years.

4. Changes of ACL mucoid degeneration are best assessed on arthroscopy with a posterior approach, and mucoid material can be expressed on probing. The ligament can appear normal on arthroscopy especially with an anterior approach, and MRI is more sensitive than arthroscopy.

5. If discovered incidentally on MRI and the patient is asymptomatic, no treatment is required.

   When symptomatic, management is initially conservative with NSAIDs. Failure of conservative management may require excision of the ACL.

Pearls

- In mucoid degeneration, the ACL is enlarged and has increased T2 signal.
- The fibers are usually not well seen on T1-weighted images, but are seen to be intact on the T2-weighted images.
- There is loss of the normal fat at the base of the ACL on T1-weighted images.
- There are often associated cysts in the proximal tibia, and intra-articular ganglion cysts.
- Mucoid degeneration often leads to ganglion cyst formation in the ACL.
- Arthroscopy may not show the changes, especially with an anterior approach.

Suggested Readings

Bergin D, Morrison WB, Carrino JA, Nallamshetty SN, Bartolozzi AR. Anterior cruciate ligament ganglia and mucoid degeneration: coexistence and clinical correlation. *AJR Am J Roentgenol.* 2004;182(5):1283–1287.

Recht MP, Applegate G, Kaplan P, et al. The MR appearance of cruciate ganglion cysts: a report of 16 cases. *Skeletal Radiol.* 1994;23(8):597–600.

Anterior knee pain

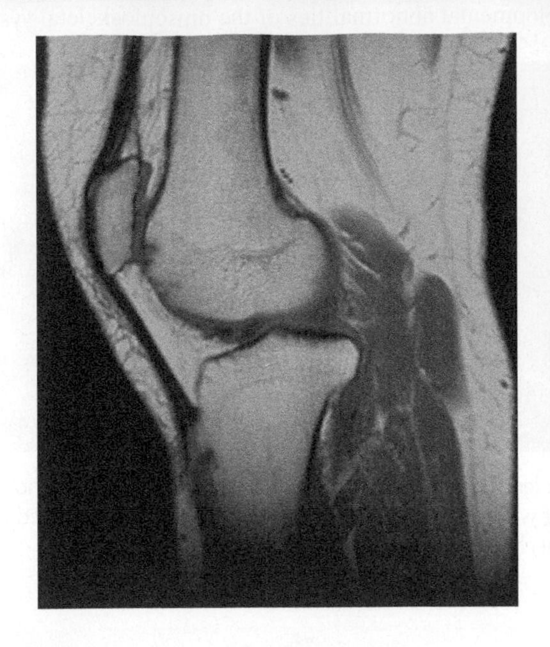

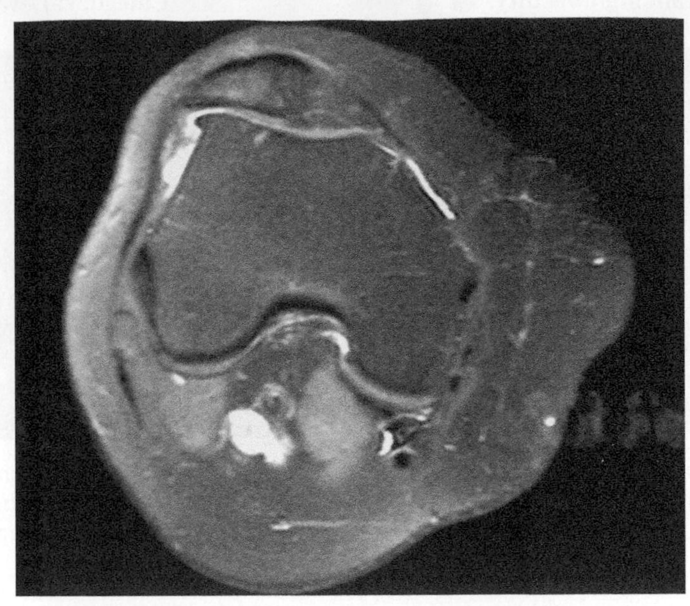

1. What is the differential diagnosis of anterior knee pain?

2. What are the imaging features of this condition?

3. What are the possible surgical treatments?

4. What are the features of transient patellar dislocation?

5. What is considered to be a normal femoral trochlear sulcus angle?

Patellofemoral dysfunction 1720

Case ranking/difficulty: 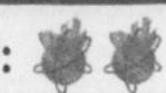 **Category:** Developmental abnormalities of the musculoskeletal system

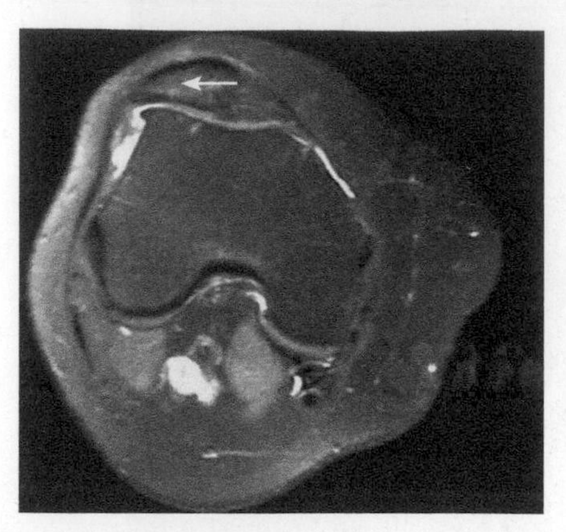

Lateral patellar translation in conjunction with shallow femoral trochlea.

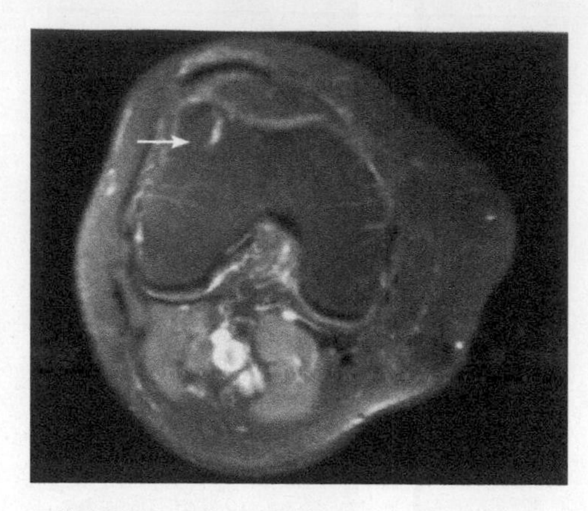

Full-thickness chondral loss in femoral trochlea with subchondral stress changes consistent with patellofemoral chondropathy.

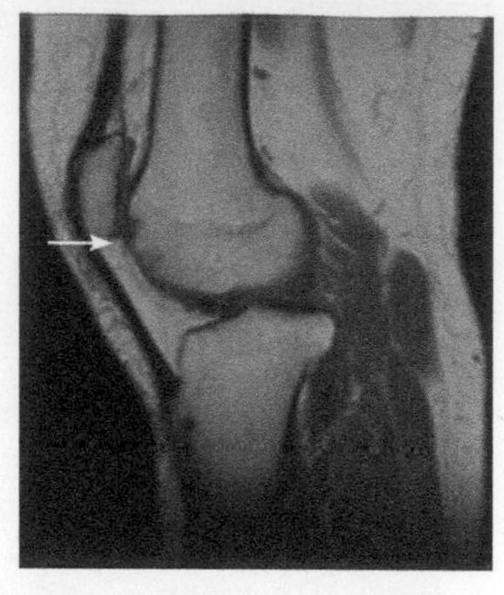

Severe femoral trochlea subchondral changes are well demonstrated on T1 images.

Answers

1. Anterior knee pain results from abnormalities of the extensor mechanism or patellofemoral joint.

   Common causes of anterior knee pain include quadriceps tendonitis, patellar maltracking abnormalities, including patella alta (high-riding patella), lateral patellar subluxation, previous patellar dislocation, femoral trochlear dysplasia, and chondromalacia patellae.

   Sinding-Larsen-Johansson syndrome (distal patella apophysitis) is a cause of anterior knee pain in adolescents. It is similar to Osgood-Schlatter syndrome, although the latter is traction apophysitis of the tibial tuberosity.

2. A torn medial patellar retinaculum is diagnostic of previous transient patellar dislocation, which is usually related to a predisposing factor for patellofemoral dysfunction, for example, femoral trochlear dysplasia, or lateralized patellar tendon.

3. The Elmslie-Trillat-Maquet procedure involves medialization of the tibial tuberosity.

4. Lateral patellar dislocation is a common injury in certain sports, for example, cricketers. If imaged acutely, there will be marrow edema in a characteristic distribution of medial patellar facet and lateral femoral trochlea. The underlying cause is often patella alta or femoral trochlear dysplasia, which predisposes to dislocation.

5. A normal trochlear sulcus angle is 140 degrees ±2 degrees.

Pearls

- Patellofemoral dysfunction is an important cause of anterior knee pain.
- Assessment of cartilage integrity and osteochondral defects is essential.
- Evaluation of underlying causes should be sought and commented on in the radiological report, for example, patella alta, patellar tilt, shallow femoral trochlear groove, lateralized patellar tendon, and signs of previous lateral patellar dislocation. MRI T2 fat-saturated images (or equivalent) in the axial plane are the most useful imaging sequences for assessing the patellofemoral compartment. Additional information can be obtained from T1/STIR sagittal images, for example patellar tendon length.

Suggested Readings

Mulford JS, Wakeley CJ, Eldridge JD. Assessment and management of chronic patellofemoral instability. *J Bone Joint Surg Br.* 2007;89(6):709–716.

Pal S, Besier TF, Draper CE, et al. Patellar tilt correlates with vastus lateralis: vastus medialis activation ratio in maltracking patellofemoral pain patients. *J Orthop Res.* 2012;30(6):927–933.

Stefanik JJ, Guermazi A, Zhu Y, et al. Quadriceps weakness, patella alta, and structural features of patellofemoral osteoarthritis. *Arthritis Care Res (Hoboken).* 2011;63(10):1391–1397.

Ulnar-sided wrist pain

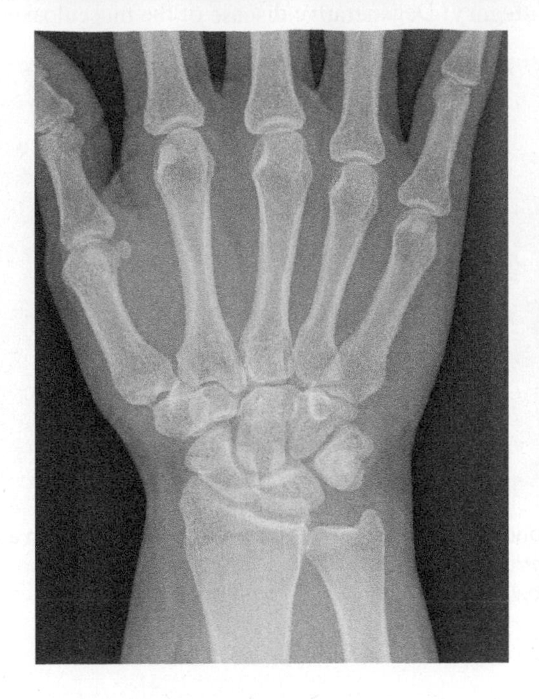

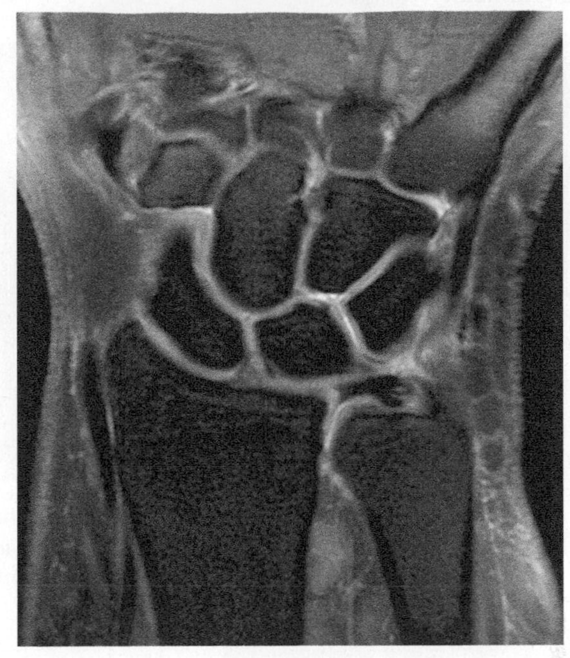

1. What are the MRI findings?
2. What are the expected imaging findings on a CT arthrogram?
3. What are the different morphologic types of the involved bone?
4. What is the proposed mechanism of injury?
5. What percentage of individuals have this syndrome?

Hamate-lunate impaction syndrome 1599

Case ranking/difficulty: 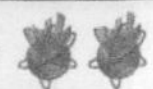 **Category:** Degenerative disease of the musculoskeletal system

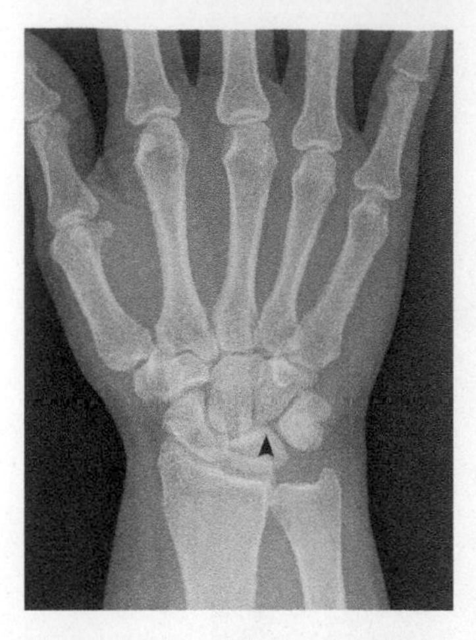

Type II lunate with an extra facet articulating with the hamate (*arrowhead*).

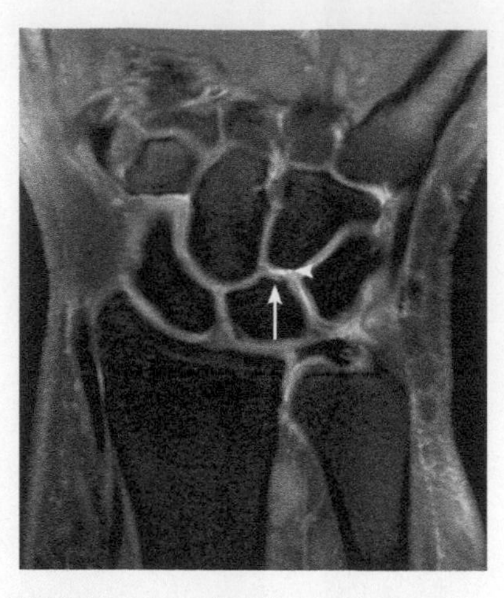

Type II lunate with chondrolysis at the hamate-lunate joint (*arrowhead*), and extra lunate facet (*arrow*).

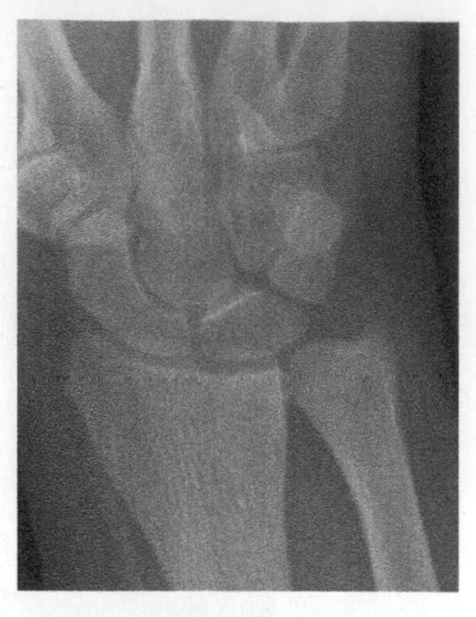

Another patient with a type 1 lunate; single facet articulating with the capitate.

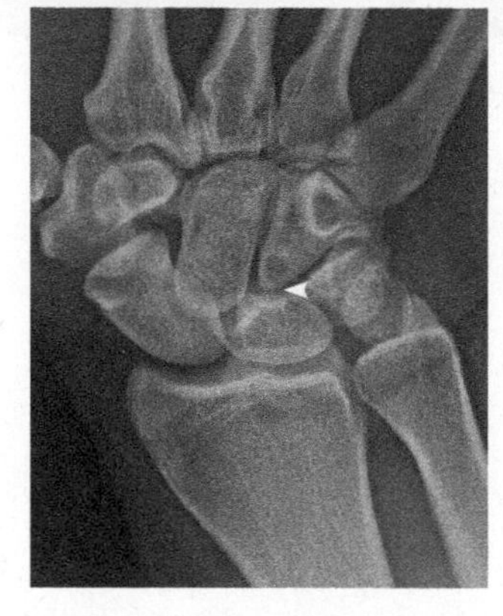

Type 2 lunate in another patient with hamate-lunate arthritis (*arrowhead*) at the second facet and cystic change.

Answers

1. There is a type II lunate with chondrolysis of the hamate-lunate joint.
2. Type II lunate with chondrolysis at the hamate-lunate joint, especially involving the hamate cartilage. Degenerative changes in the hamate-lunate joint with subchondral sclerosis, reduction in joint space, and sometimes osteophytes and subchondral cysts are seen.
3. Type I: The lunate has no articulation with the hamate.

   Type II: The lunate has an extra medial facet that articulates with the hamate.
4. Abnormal loading of the hamate-lunate joint in ulnar deviation leads to degenerative changes.
5. Fifty percent of lunates are type II, and 25% of these individuals develop hamate-lunate impaction syndrome.

Pearls

- Hamate-lunate syndrome is associated with a type II lunate.
- A type II lunate is a type of lunate where there is an additional medial facet articulating with the hamate. A type I lunate does not have such an articulation.
- Fifty percent of lunates are type II, and of these individuals, 25% develop hamate-lunate impaction syndrome.
- In a type II lunate, there is abnormal biomechanics of the wrist, especially during the ulnar deviation of the wrist. This leads to chondromalacic and degenerative changes of the hamate-lunate joint.
- MRI demonstrates an abnormal articulation of the lunate and subchondral bone marrow edema of the hamate and lunate. On cartilage sensitive images, there is chondrolysis, especially on the hamate side of the articulation, with subchondral cysts and subchondral sclerosis.

Suggested Readings

Cerezal L, del Piñal F, Abascal F, García-Valtuille R, Pereda T, Canga A. Imaging findings in ulnar-sided wrist impaction syndromes. *Radiographics*. 2002;22(1): 105–121.

Watanabe A, Souza F, Vezeridis PS, Blazar P, Yoshioka H. Ulnar-sided wrist pain. II. Clinical imaging and treatment. *Skeletal Radiol*. 2010;39(9):837–857.

Chronic left wrist pain

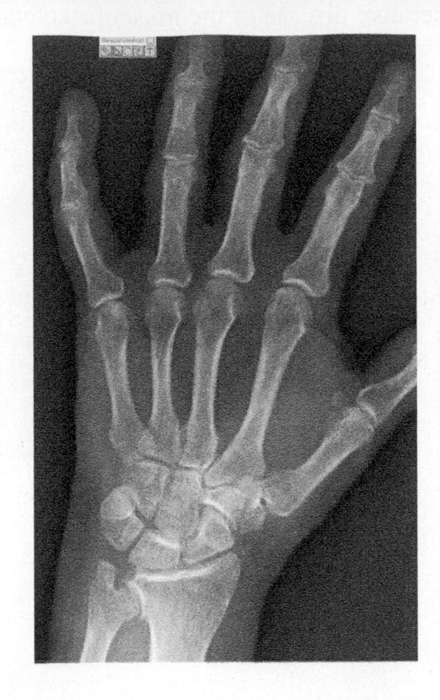

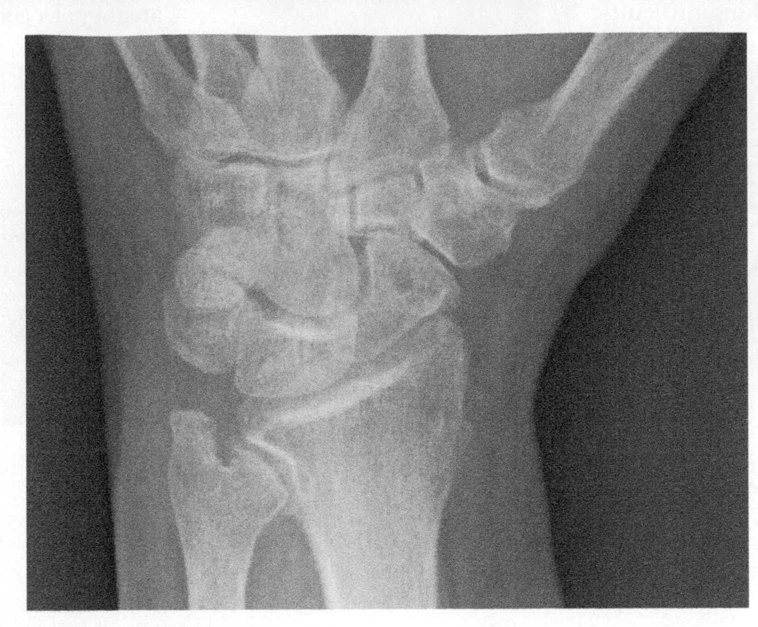

1. What are the radiograph findings?

2. What is the diagnosis?

3. What are the predisposing factors for this condition?

4. What is the pathophysiology of the condition?

5. What tests can be performed to diagnose this condition in the early stages, before erosive changes occur?

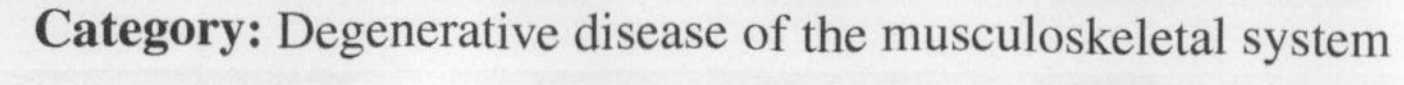

Ulnar impingement syndrome 1441

Case ranking/difficulty: 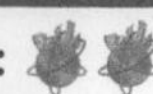

Category: Degenerative disease of the musculoskeletal system

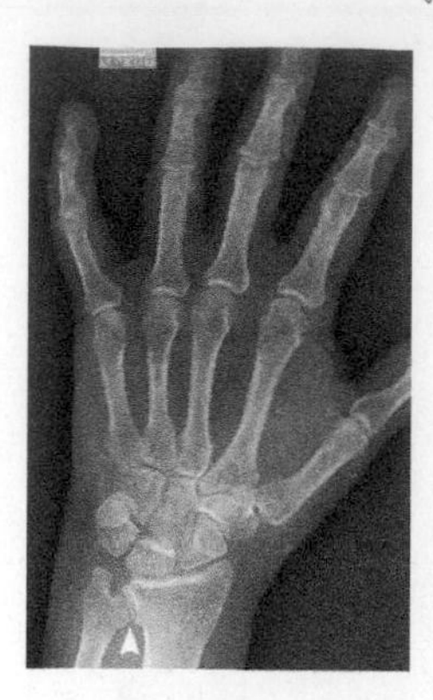

There is a short ulna, with radioulnar convergence and osteoarthritic changes at the distal radioulnar joint.

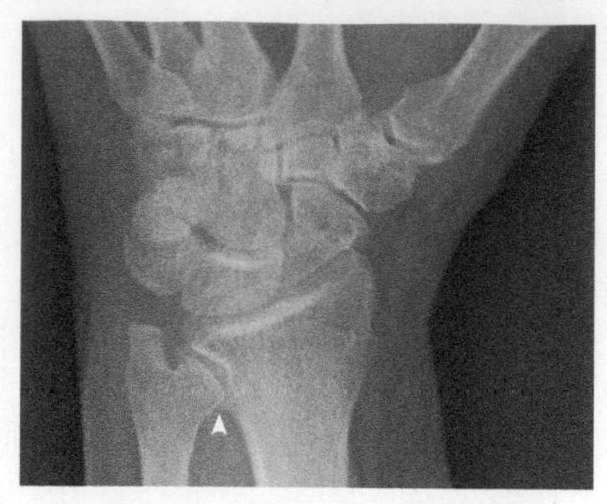

Radioulnar convergence with impingement.

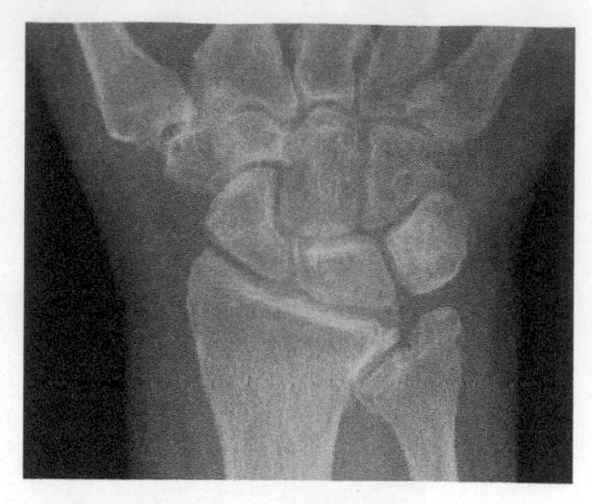

The changes are bilateral.

Answers

1. There is a short ulna, with ulnar convergence on the distal radius. The sigmoid notch is scalloped and sclerotic.
2. The findings of a short ulna with a sclerotic and scalloped sigmoid notch is consistent with ulnar impingement syndrome.
3. A congenital short ulna, and surgical resection of the distal ulna for a malunited Colles fracture, Madelung deformity, or rheumatoid arthritis are causes of ulnar impingement syndrome.
4. A short ulna will result in unopposed action of the abductor pollicis longus, extensor pollicis brevis, and pronator quadratus. This will lead to ulnar convergence of the ulna on the radius.
5. Although clinical testing may be suggestive, MRI is much more sensitive in detecting the changes. The stress view described by Lees and Scheker also has been reported to be useful.

Pearls

- Ulnar impingement results from a congenitally short ulna, or shortening caused by surgical correction of a malunited Colles fracture, Madelung deformity, or rheumatoid arthritis.
- There is pain on pronation and supination.
- Radioulnar convergence results in sclerosis, erosions osteophytes, and scalloping at the distal radioulnar articulation.
- Sclerosis precedes the development of erosions.
- Stress views or MRI will detect early changes.
- Treatment is with aggressive ulnar shortening or ulnar head prosthesis in the acquired form, and distractive ulnar lengthening in the congenital form.

Suggested Readings

Cerezal L, del Piñal F, Abascal F, García-Valtuille R, Pereda T, Canga A. Imaging findings in ulnar-sided wrist impaction syndromes. *Radiographics*. 2002;22(1):105–121.

Coggins CA. Imaging of ulnar-sided wrist pain. *Clin Sports Med.* 2006;25(3):505–526, vii.

Longstanding painful wrist

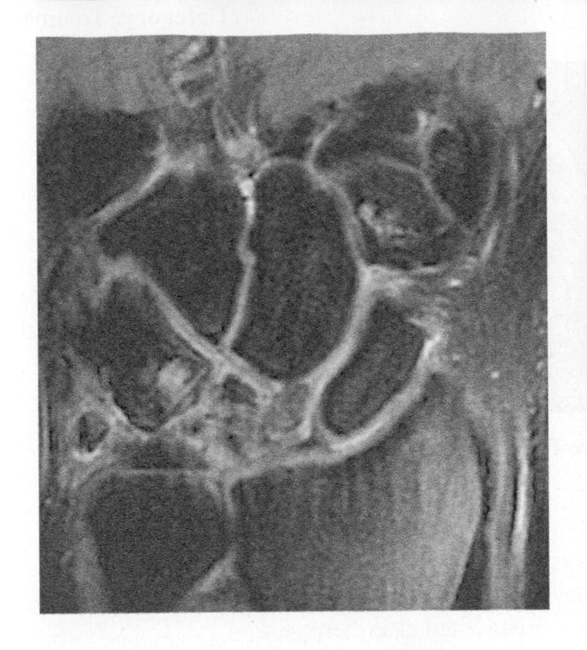

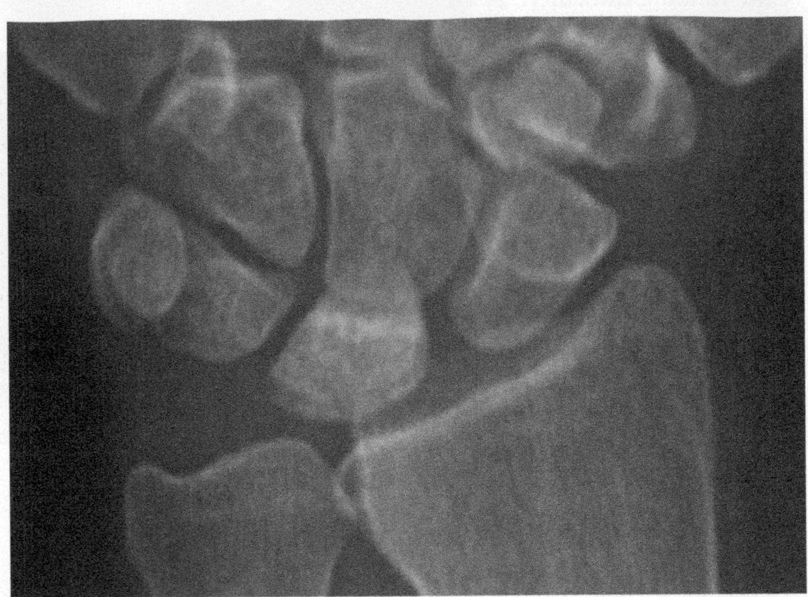

1. What are the radiographic findings?

2. What are the MRI findings?

3. What is the diagnosis?

4. What is the classification based on radiographs?

5. What is the proposed MRI classification of this entity?

Kienböck disease 1555

Case ranking/difficulty: 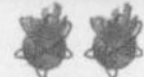

Category: Trauma

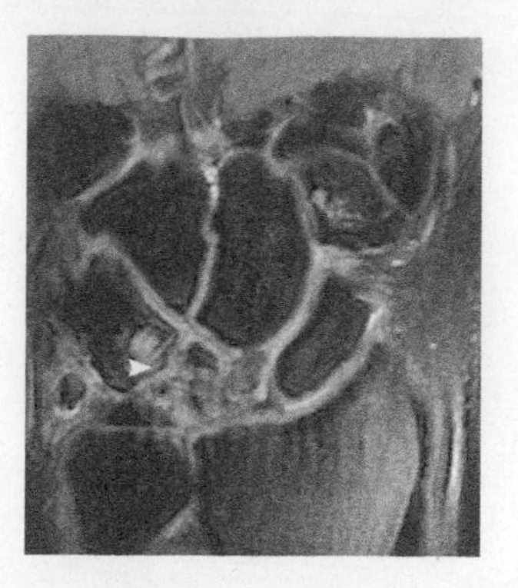

MRI better demonstrates the lunate collapse, with increased T2 signal in the lunate and degenerative changes in the lunotriquetral joint (*arrowhead*).

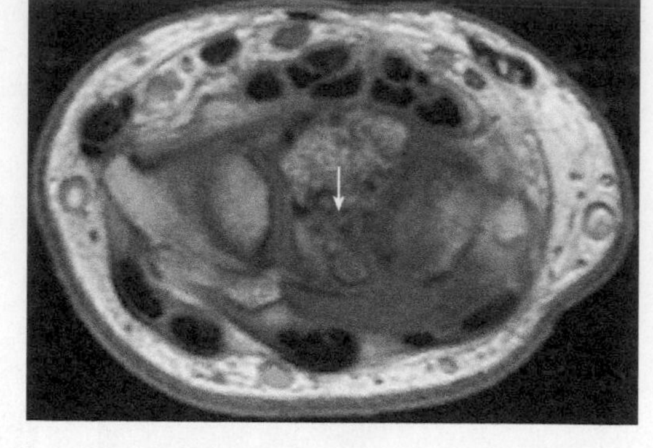

Low T1 signal and fragmentation of the lunate.

Answers

1. There is a sclerosis of the lunate without definite collapse. There is no associated negative ulnar variance.
2. Bone marrow edema in the lunate is demonstrated with high T2 and low T1 signal. There is cystic change and fragmentation of the lunate. Degenerative changes of the triquetrum with cysts are also noted. This is likely stage IV collapse based on MRI criteria.
3. The MRI findings are compatible with advanced Kienböck disease.
4. The Lichtman classification is described below:
    - Stage 1: Normal, linear or compression fracture
    - Stage 2: Sclerotic changes of the lunate
    - Stage 3A: Collapse of lunate without fixed scaphoid rotation
    - Stage 3B: Lunate collapse with fixed scaphoid rotation
    - Stage 4: Stage 3 with degenerative changes of the carpus
5. The proposed MRI classification for lunate osteonecrosis is described below:
    - Stage 0: Low T1 fracture line, no diffuse marrow signal change
    - Stage 1: Diffuse low T1 and high T2/STIR signal
    - Stage 2: Sclerosis of lunate
    - Stage 3: Progressive collapse of the lunate, associated with scapholunate ligament tear
    - Stage 4: All of the above with degenerative changes

Pearls

- Osteonecrosis of the lunate is called Kienböck disease.
- Negative ulnar variance is present in 75% of cases. This predisposes the lunate to more shear and compressive forces, as the lunate is subject to load normally distributed elsewhere.
- Repetitive trauma or acute injury along with its unfavorable anatomical blood supply, leads to devascularization of the lunate and subsequent avascular necrosis.
- X-ray shows sclerosis with eventual collapse of the lunate.
- In advanced cases, there is proximal carpal row collapse with SLAC wrist, as the capitate migrates proximally into the space created by the lunate.
- CT findings are similar to plain film findings.
- MRI shows low T1 and high T2/STIR signal intensity within the lunate. Low T2 signal is seen in the later stages. There may be fragmentation and collapse of the lunate. In advanced cases, there is collapse of the proximal row, chondrolysis, and degenerative changes.
- The early stages are treated with conservative measures, immobilization and revascularization surgeries. In later stages with degenerative changes, proximal row carpectomy or wrist arthrodesis are surgical options. Surgical core decompression of the lunate has also been described.

Suggested Readings

Bain GI, Durrant AW. Arthroscopic assessment of avascular necrosis. *Hand Clin.* 2011;27(3):323–329.

Ogawa T, Nishiura Y, Hara Y, Okamoto Y, Ochiai N. Correlation of histopathology with magnetic resonance imaging in Kienböck disease. *J Hand Surg Am.* 2012;37(1):83–89.

Schmitt R, Fellner F, Obletter N, Fiedler E, Bautz W. Diagnosis and staging of lunate necrosis. A current review [in German]. *Handchir Mikrochir Plast Chir.* 1998;30(3):142–150.

Patient with chronic ankle pain and limitation of motion

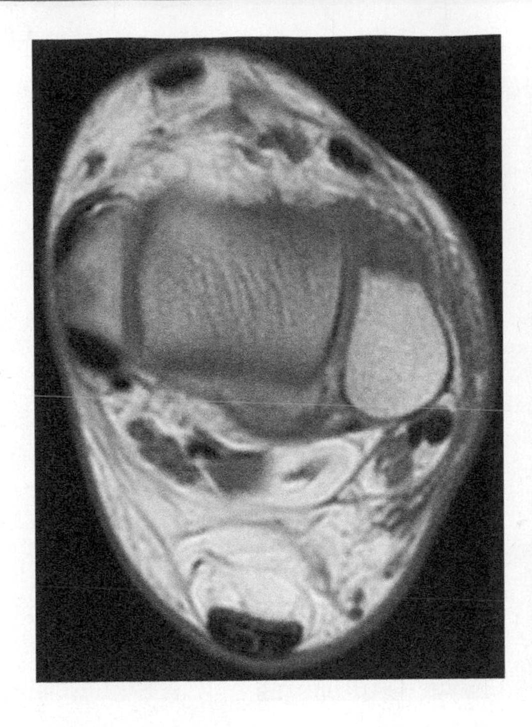

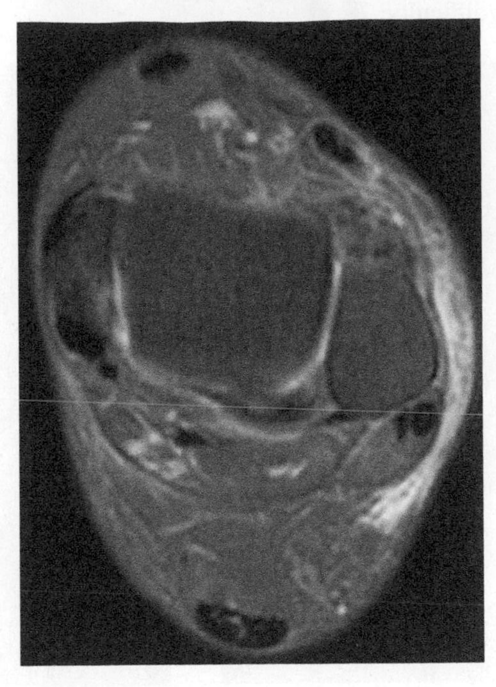

1. What is the abnormality seen on MRI?

2. What are important causes for this syndrome?

3. What is the typical mechanism of injury?

4. What is the least common type of ankle impingement?

5. What are the most appropriate imaging modalities when ankle impingement is suspected?

Anterolateral impingement — 1318

Case ranking/difficulty: 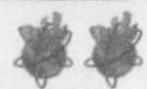

Category: Trauma

Marked T1 hypointensity, thickening, and heterogeneity in the expected position of the anterior tibiofibular ligament (*arrow*). A normal ligament was not identified.

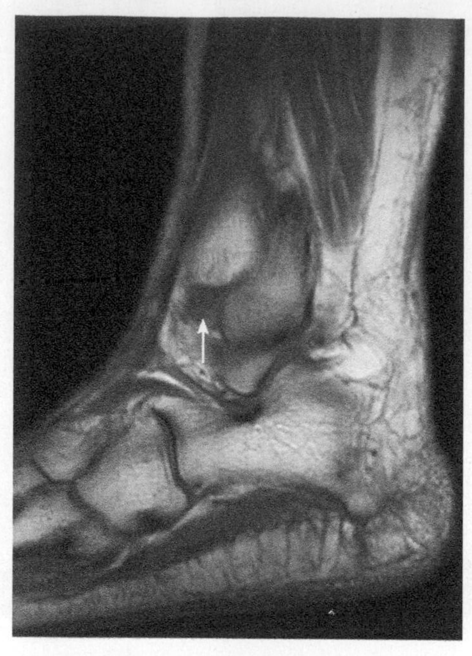

Sagittal image shows the scar tissue in the anterolateral gutter.

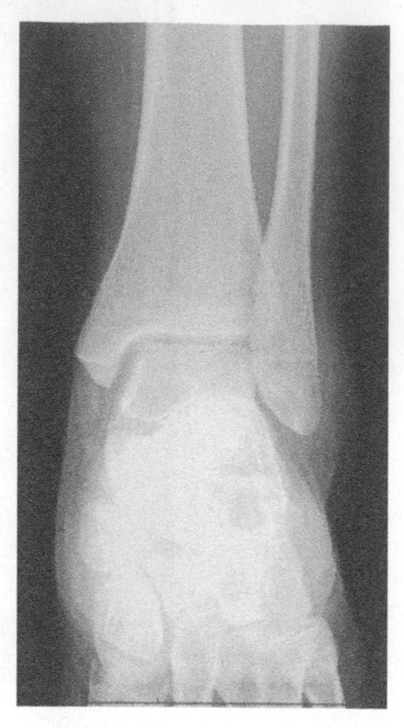

Radiograph 4 months prior, shows soft-tissue swelling at the lateral malleolus but no fracture.

Answers

1. A thickened anterior tibiofibular ligament with a "meniscoid" lesion is seen.
2. Tears of the anterior talofibular and anterior tibiofibular ligaments, and tears of the accessory anterior tibiofibular ligament (ligament of Bassett).
3. Inversion injury.
4. Posterolateral impingement is the least-common form of ankle impingement.
5. The initial examination should be a plain film ankle study. If anterolateral or anteromedial impingement is suspected, an MRI, or preferably an MR arthrogram, should be performed.

Pearls

- A normal anterior tibiofibular ligament is typically not seen.
- A "meniscoid" mass in the anterolateral gutter is the result of ligamentous injury and fibrosis.
- Osteophytes may be contributory, but in isolation does not result in anterolateral impingement.
- The accessory anterior tibiofibular ligament (or ligament of Bassett) may be injured and become thickened, contributing to anterolateral impingement.
- The anterior talofibular ligament is also frequently injured.
- Anterolateral impingement is the most common ankle impingement. The least common is posterolateral impingement.

Suggested Readings

Datir A, Connell D. Imaging of impingement lesions in the ankle. *Top Magn Reson Imaging.* 2010;21(1):15–23.

Robinson P, White LM. Soft-tissue and osseous impingement syndromes of the ankle: role of imaging in diagnosis and management. *Radiographics.* 2002;22(6):1457–1469.

Chronic dull pain in right groin

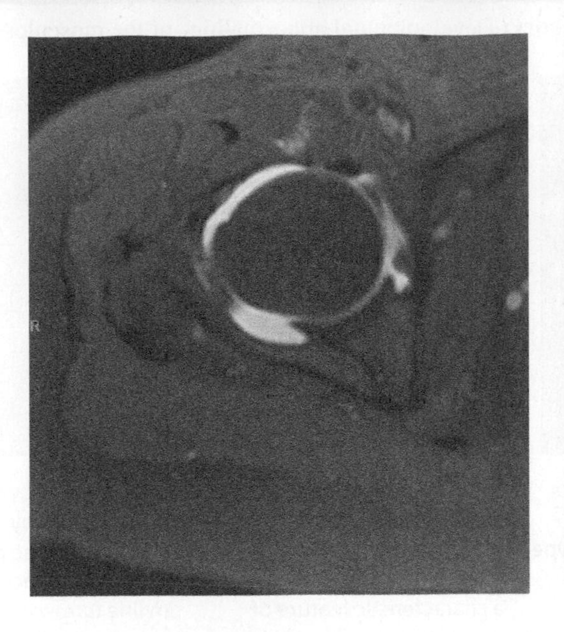

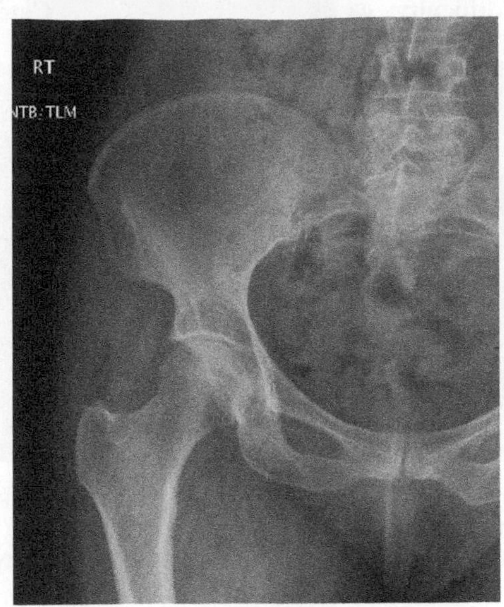

1. What is the most likely diagnosis?

2. What is the pattern of hyaline cartilage loss in this condition?

3. What is the pattern of labral damage with this condition?

4. What are the predisposing factors for this condition?

5. What is the name of the radiographic sign(s) associated with this abnormality?

Pincer-type femoroacetabular impingement (FAI) 2355

Case ranking/difficulty: 

Category: Developmental abnormalities of the musculoskeletal system

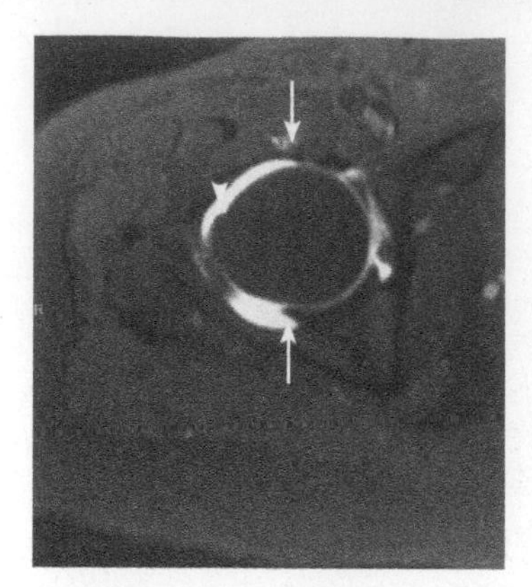

Axial T1 FS MRI arthrogram image demonstrates acetabular overcoverage, which is the hallmark of pincer-type FAI (*arrows*). Note the presence of the "linear indentation sign," which occurs as a result of mechanical injury and reactive change at the femoral neck (*arrowhead*).

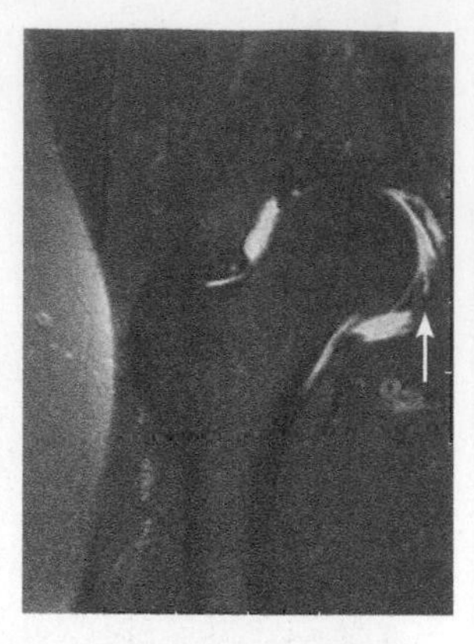

Contrecoup posteroinferior labral tearing (*arrow*) is a typical feature of pincer-type impingement.

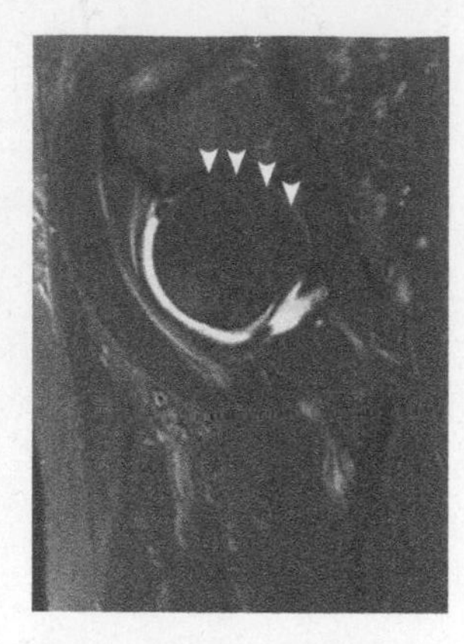

Diffuse acetabular hyaline chondrosis—appearing as high signal on T2 FS images (*arrowheads*)—is a characteristic feature of pincer-type impingement.

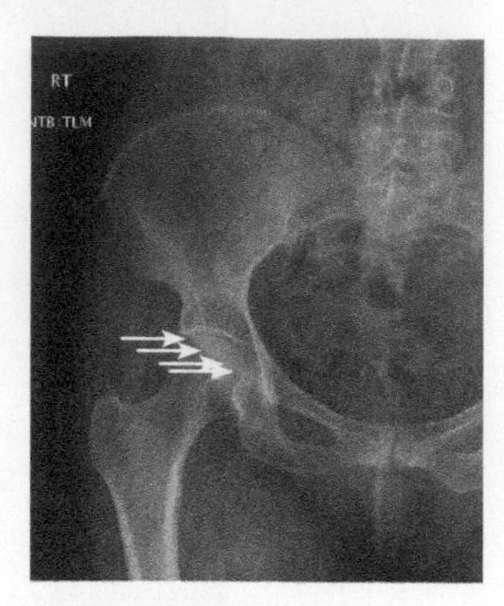

Acetabular retroversion is demonstrated by the crossover sign, which is the projection of the anterior acetabular rim line (*arrows*) lateral to the posterior rim line. A "figure-of-8" configuration results.

Answers

1. Acetabular retroversion is demonstrated on the plain radiograph with a "crossover" sign, and the MR arthrogram image demonstrates acetabular overcoverage, in conjunction with a characteristic tear of the anterosuperior labrum and contrecoup posteroinferior labrum. These are classical features of pincer-type impingement.
2. Diffuse chondrosis is a frequent finding with pincer-type femoroacetabular impingement (FAI). The cartilage loss is on the acetabular side. A more focal pattern of loss is seen on the anterosuperior acetabular cartilage at the chondrolabral junction where there is focal direct impact in cam-type FAI.
3. With pincer-type FAI, the abnormal femoral head motion as a consequence of the acetabular abnormalities leads to early degeneration of the posteroinferior labrum and tearing of the anterosuperior labrum. Cam-type impingement, however, results in more focal tearing of the anterosuperior and/or superolateral labrum.
4. Any factor that alters the morphology of the acetabulum and/or femoral head can potentially cause pincer FAI.

   Acetabular dysplasia, protrusio, coxa profunda, and acetabular nonunited fractures can lead to acetabular overcoverage or retroversion and hence to pincer-type FAI.

   Avascular necrosis including Perthes disease causes flattening of the femoral head, and thus indirectly leads to acetabular overcoverage.
5. An important radiographic abnormality in this condition is the "crossover" sign. It refers to the anterior acetabular rim line projecting lateral to the posterior rim line on a frontal view. The appearance of the anterior and posterior rim lines together produces a "figure of 8," which can easily be traced on the frontal view.

   Care must be taken to obtain a well-centered AP pelvis radiograph since isolated hip radiographs lead to spurious overdiagnosis of this sign.

Pearls

- Pincer-type FAI is one of the 2 main categories of FAI.
- Focal or generalized acetabular overcoverage or retroversion leads to excessive labral and hyaline cartilage wear.
- Contrecoup labral tearing typically occurs in the posteroinferior location and hyaline cartilage loss is diffuse, in contradistinction to the more focal anterosuperior cartilage loss seen with cam-type of FAI.
- Axial CT images are ideal for assessing acetabular version.
- Surgical correction may be considered in suitable, usually young candidates, with the aim of preventing premature osteoarthritis. This may involve resection of the impinging portion of acetabular rim, or more complex periacetabular osteotomy for correction of retroversion.

Suggested Reading

Tannast M, Siebenrock KA, Anderson SE. Femoroacetabular impingement: radiographic diagnosis—what the radiologist should know. *AJR Am J Roentgenol.* 2007;188(6):1540–1552.

Painful hip

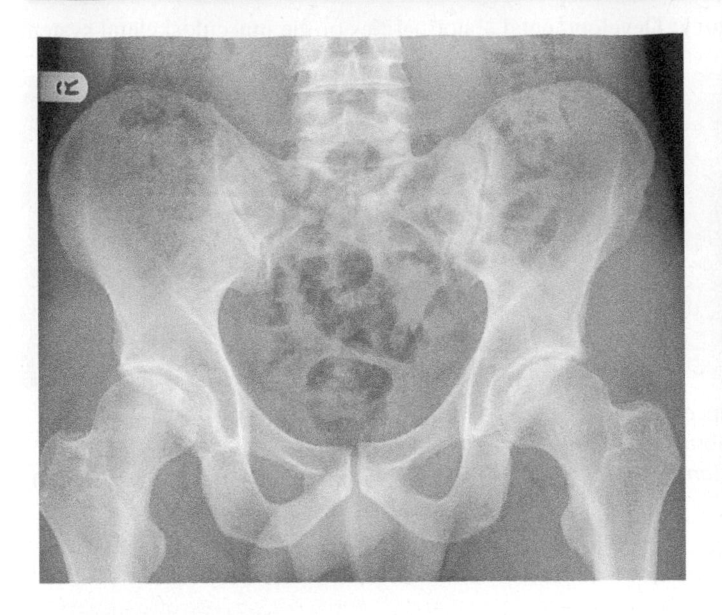

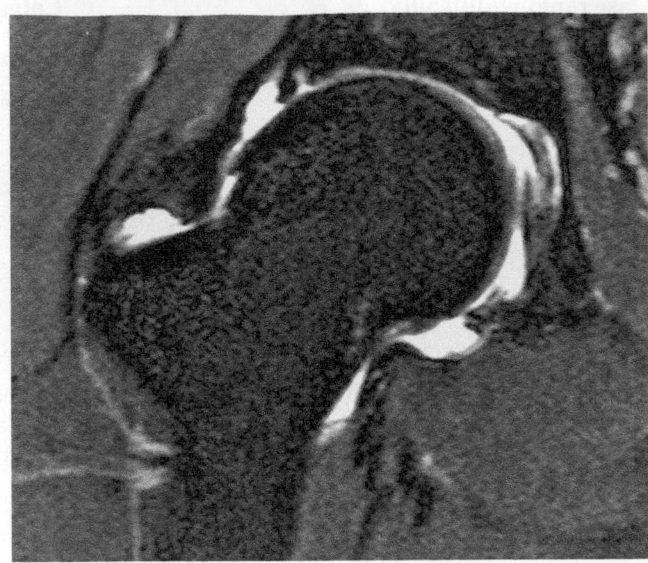

1. What are the plain film findings?
2. What are the MRI findings?
3. What are the different types of this condition?
4. What age group is affected in this condition?
5. What are the proposed etiologies?

Cam-type femoral acetabular impingement 1334

Case ranking/difficulty: 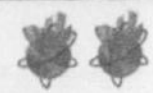 **Category:** Developmental abnormalities of the musculoskeletal system

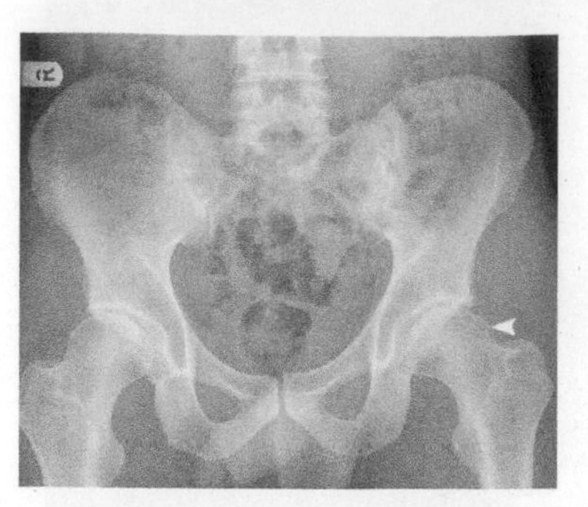

There are bilateral abnormal femoral shaft and neck angles with bony protuberances of the lateral aspect of the neck of femur (best seen on the left, *arrowhead*). There is an osteophyte on the superolateral aspect of the acetabulum.

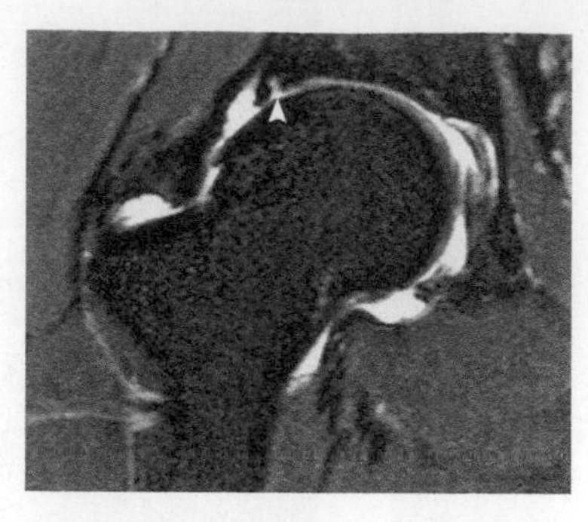

MRI arthrogram of hip: cam-type impingement with labral tear at the superolateral aspect (*arrowhead*).

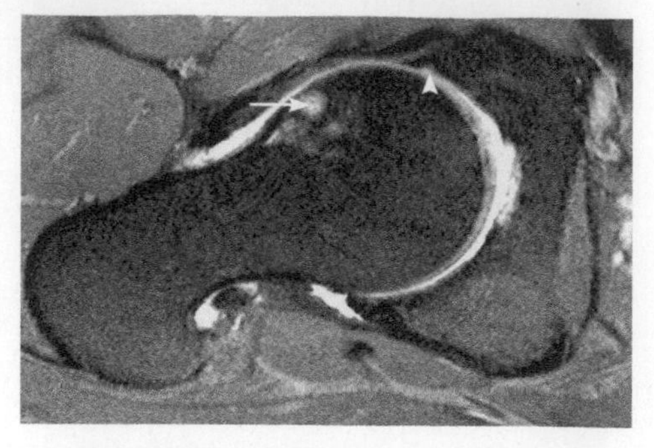

MRI arthrogram of the hip: axial image showing cam-type impingement and labral tear (*arrowhead*). Note herniation pits (*arrow*), which can be seen in femoroacetabular impingement.

Answers

1. Asymmetrical head and neck configuration is the key finding, with an associated osseous projection at the head and neck junction.

   Herniation pits are not specific features, but when present may suggest underlying femoroacetabular impingement (FAI).

2. There is an abnormal head and neck angle with anterior superior labral tear with labral detachment. The alpha angle is >55 degrees. There is no cartilage loss and secondary osteoarthritic changes in this case, but in the later stages these are expected findings.

3. Cam, pincer, and mixed are the main 3 types of FAI. The most common is actually a mixed cam and pincer type.

   Although there is no specific slipped femoral epiphysis subtype, one of the presumed etiologies of cam FAI is a subclinical form of a slipped upper femoral epiphysis.

4. Young males are more commonly affected in the cam form of FAI. Middle-aged females are most often affected in pincer FAI.

5. Some theories suggest it is developmental and represents subclinical slipped capital femoral epiphysis. Other theories suggest growth disturbances leading to eccentric closure or delayed closure of the physis between the femoral head and neck.

Pearls

- Cam FAI is a type of FAI syndrome. The other types of FAI include pincer type and mixed type. The mixed type is a combination of cam and pincer types.
- There is an abnormal morphology of the femoral head and neck junction leading to abnormal offset. This results in repetitive friction on the acetabular labrum, and ultimately anterosuperior labral tear and/or detachment with secondary osteoarthritic changes.
- The plain film shows an abnormal femoral head and neck angle with a bony spur at the junction. Degenerative changes may also be demonstrated.
- A lateral synovial herniation pit may or may not be seen.
- MRI and MR arthrography demonstrates an abnormal alpha angle (>55 degrees) at the femoral head and neck. There is also an abnormal morphology of the femoral head and neck, with labral tears and secondary degenerative changes.
- Treatment includes hip arthroscopy and labral tear repair if no arthritis. However if there are associated arthritic changes, hip replacement is performed.

Suggested Readings

Kassarjian A, Yoon LS, Belzile E, Connolly SA, Millis MB, Palmer WE. Triad of MR arthrographic findings in patients with cam-type femoroacetabular impingement. *Radiology.* 2005;236(2):588–592.

Pfirrmann CW, Mengiardi B, Dora C, Kalberer F, Zanetti M, Hodler J. Cam and pincer femoroacetabular impingement: characteristic MR arthrographic findings in 50 patients. *Radiology.* 2006;240(3):778–785.

Pain in the foot and ankle

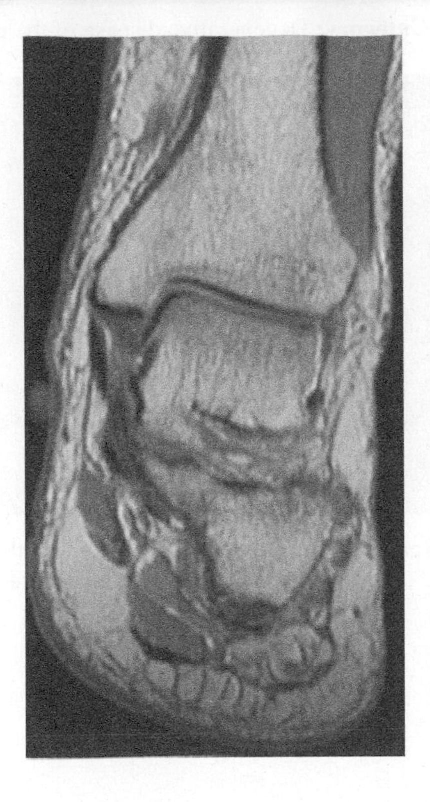

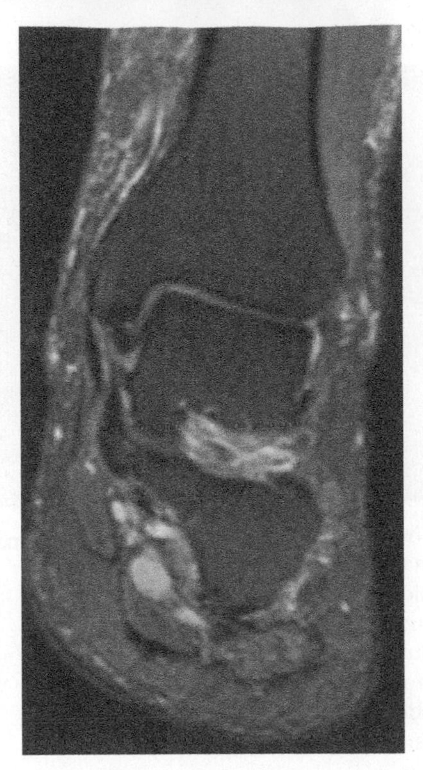

1. What are the MRI findings?

2. What is the etiology of the main finding?

3. What conditions are associated with this finding?

4. What are the sites of entrapment of the inferior calcaneal nerve?

5. What is the management?

Baxter neuropathy 1451

Case ranking/difficulty: 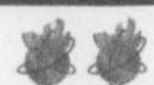

Category: Degenerative disease of the musculoskeletal system

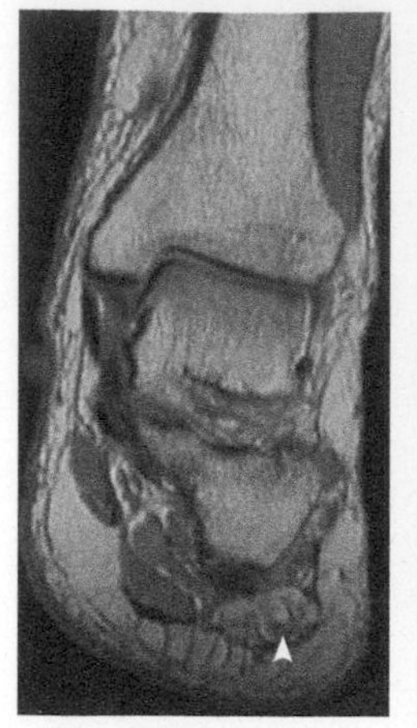

There is fatty atrophy of the abductor digiti minimi muscle (*arrowhead*).

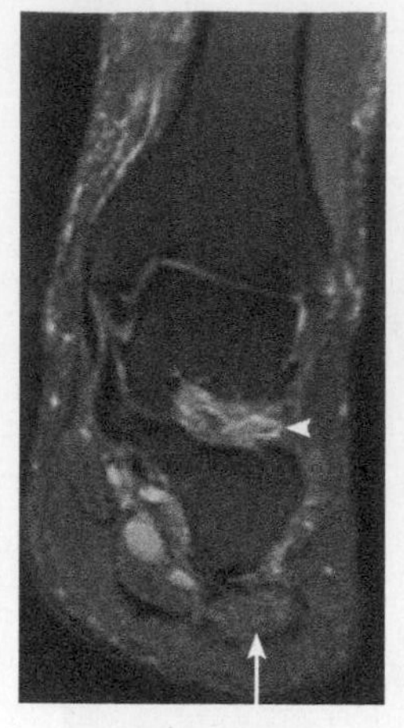

There is mild edema in the abductor digiti minimi muscle suggesting subacute atrophy (*arrow*). There is also incidental edema in the sinus tarsi (*arrowhead*).

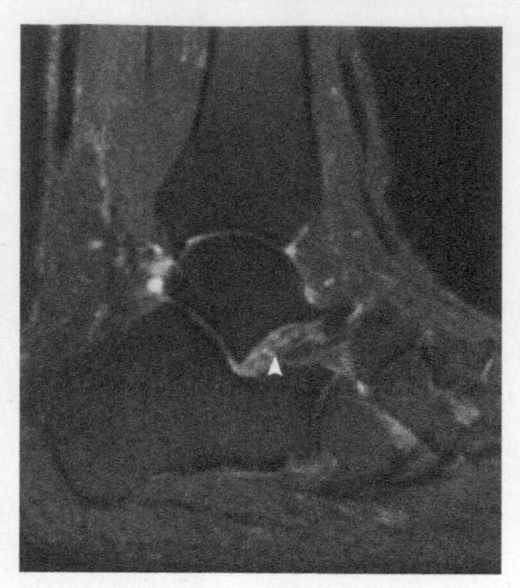

Sinus tarsi edema again noted.

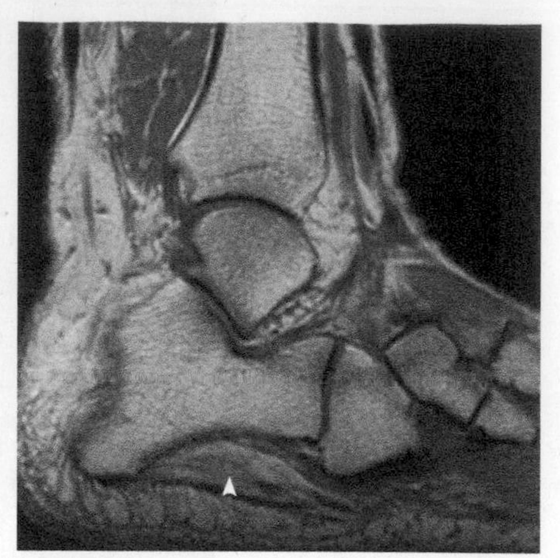

Fatty atrophy of the abductor digiti minimi muscle is again seen (*arrowhead*).

Answers

1. There is fatty atrophy of the abductor digiti minimi muscle. Incidental mild sinus tarsi edema is seen.
2. Entrapment of the inferior calcaneal nerve results in denervation atrophy of the abductor digiti minimi muscle, or Baxter neuropathy.
3. Calcaneal spurs, plantar fasciitis, ganglion cysts, and hypertrophy of the abductor hallucis and quadratus plantae muscles may all cause impingement on the inferior calcaneal nerve.
4. Common sites of entrapment of the inferior calcaneal nerve are the fascial edge of the abductor hallucis muscle, medial calcaneal tuberosity, and the medial edge of the quadratus plantae muscle.
5. Although the management is initially conservative with orthotics or steroid injection, the definitive management is with neurolysis (release of the nerve).

Pearls

- Baxter neuropathy is related to entrapment of the inferior calcaneal nerve.
- There are 3 sites of impingement: fascial edge of the abductor hallucis, medial edge of the quadratus plantae, and the medial calcaneal tuberosity. The latter is most common.
- Plantar fasciitis and calcaneal spurs predispose to impingement.
- MRI will show changes of denervation atrophy of the abductor digiti minimi muscle, with fatty replacement in chronic cases.
- A contributory mass lesion such as a neurofibroma or ganglion can also be seen on MRI.

Suggested Readings

Delfaut EM, Demondion X, Bieganski A, Thiron MC, Mestdagh H, Cotten A. Imaging of foot and ankle nerve entrapment syndromes: from well-demonstrated to unfamiliar sites. *Radiographics*. 2003;23(3):613–623.

Donovan A, Rosenberg ZS, Cavalcanti CF. MR imaging of entrapment neuropathies of the lower extremity. Part 2. The knee, leg, ankle, and foot. *Radiographics*. 2010;30(4):1001–1019.

Chronic right shoulder pain

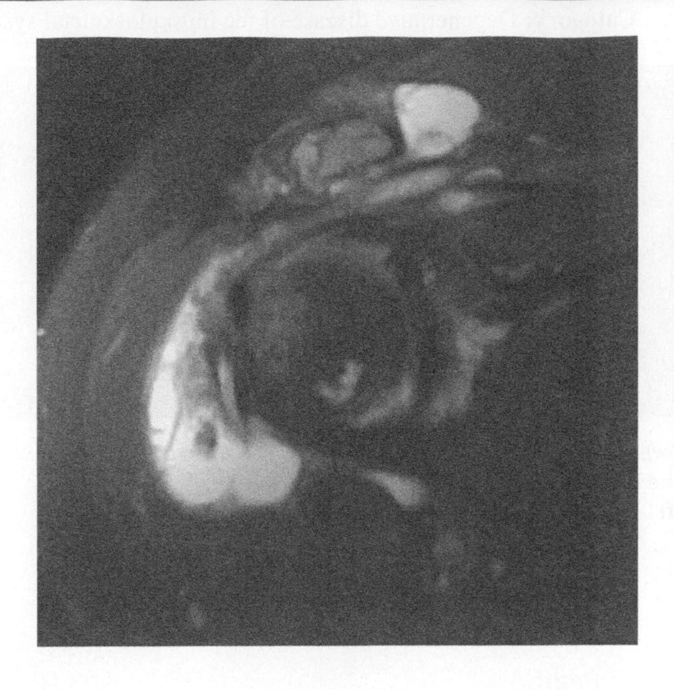

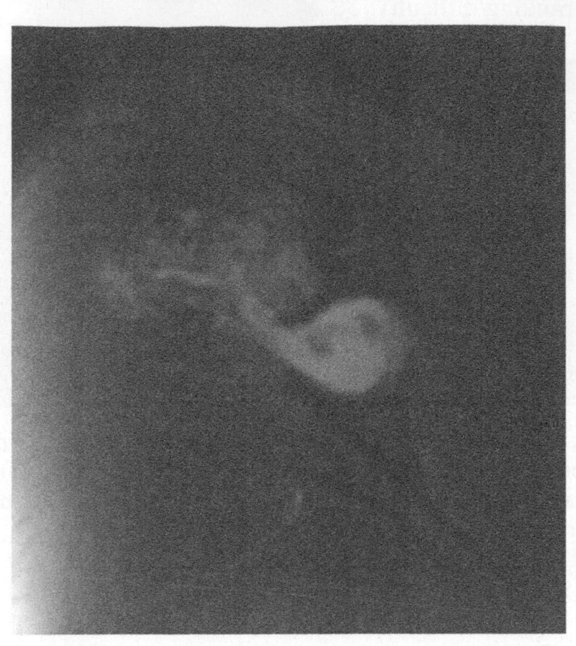

1. What are the MRI findings?

2. What is the cystic lesion located above the AC joint?

3. What is the proposed etiology?

4. What is the management for the cystic lesion?

5. What are the other abnormalities at the acromion and their etiology?

MRI geyser sign; os acromiale 1389

Case ranking/difficulty:  **Category:** Degenerative disease of the musculoskeletal system

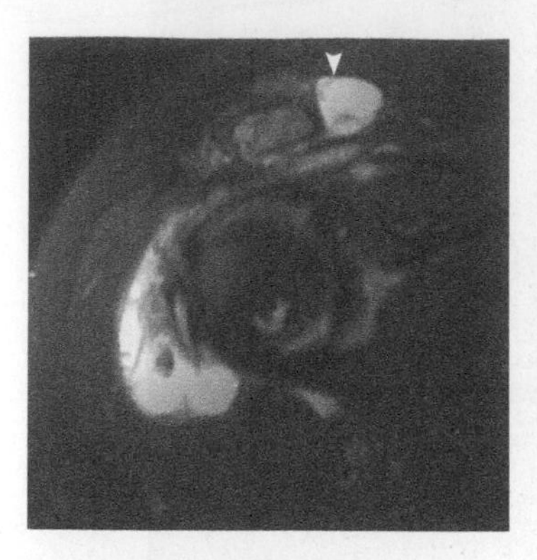

There is a full-thickness supraspinatus tear, with fluid in the subacromial–subdeltoid bursa dissecting into the AC joint and above it (*arrowhead*).

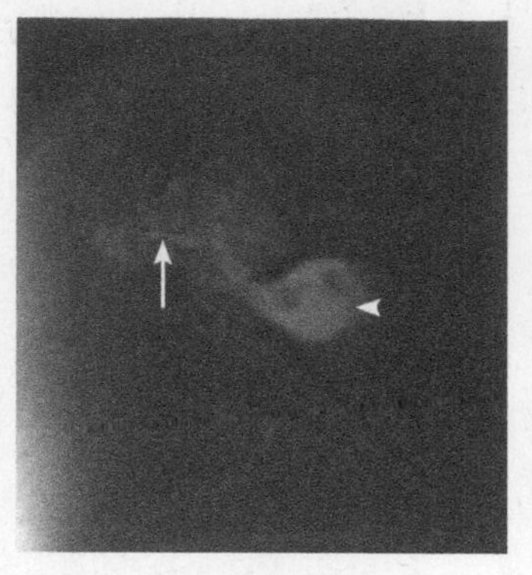

An os acromiale is seen (*arrow*), with fluid dissecting out of the AC joint into the superior soft tissues (*arrowhead*).

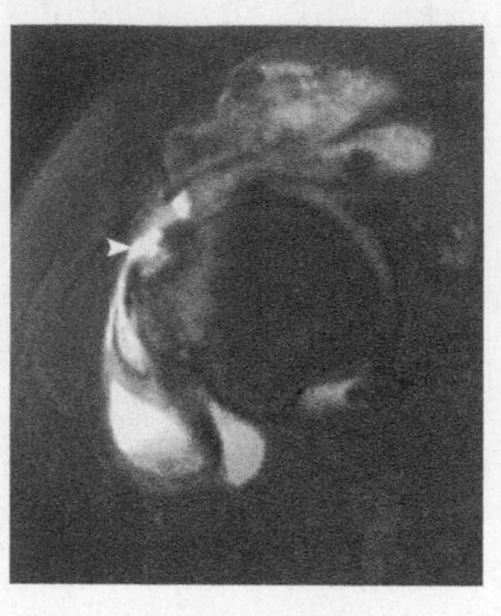

The supraspinatus tear (*arrowhead*) and bursal distension are well identified.

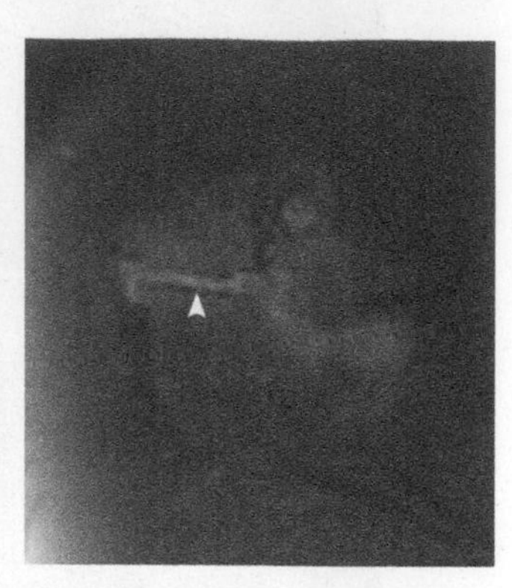

The os acromiale is seen.

Answers

1. Large rotator cuff tear involving the entire supraspinatus and the anterior infraspinatus with fluid in the subacromial–subdeltoid bursa, and a large cyst is seen superior to the AC joint communicating with the AC joint. There is an os acromiale and AC joint osteoarthritis.

2. The cystic lesion communicates with the AC joint and is a result of glenohumeral synovial joint fluid dissecting into the AC joint (geyser sign).

3. The cyst located above the AC joint is a result of a high-riding humeral head from a large rotator cuff tear, causing mechanical attrition of the AC joint capsule and allowing joint fluid to enter the AC joint. This geyser sign was initially described on conventional arthrography, where contrast entered the AC joint after glenohumeral injection. This is the MR equivalent.

4. Treatment is surgical repair of the rotator cuff. In some cases, excision arthroplasty of the AC joint with removal of the cyst base is indicated. Cyst aspiration should not be performed because of the risk of recurrence and sinus tract formation.

5. There is AC joint osteoarthritis. There is also an unfused acromial apophysis, known as an *os acromiale*. Typically the ossification centers of the acromion fuse at ages 22 to 25 years, and the persistent unfused apophysis (os acromiale) may lead to rotator cuff impingement.

Pearls

- The MRI geyser sign is a cystic fluid collection in or above the acromioclavicular joint.
- It results from a chronic rotator cuff tear, with the high-riding humeral head causing mechanical attrition on the AC joint capsule.
- The cyst may be unilocular or multilocular.
- Treatment is by rotator cuff repair or excision arthroplasty.
- Os acromiale occurs when the apophysis of the acromion does not fuse. It occurs in 8% of the population.
- Fusion of the apophyses occurs at ages 22 to 25 years.
- There are four main types of os acromiale: pre, mesa, meta, and basi. The most common are the mesa and meta types.
- Os acromiale may lead to subacromial impingement.

Suggested Readings

Ouellette H, Thomas BJ, Kassarjian A, et al. Re-examining the association of os acromiale with supraspinatus and infraspinatus tears. *Skeletal Radiol.* 2007;36(9):835–839.

Tshering Vogel DW, Steinbach LS, et al. Acromioclavicular joint cyst: nine cases of a pseudotumor of the shoulder. *Skeletal Radiol.* 2005;34(5):260–265.

Recurrent dislocation with discomfort

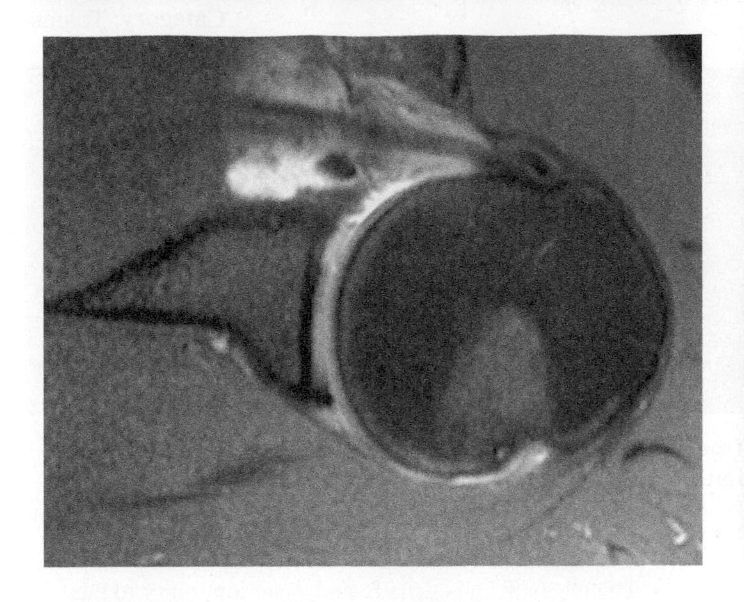

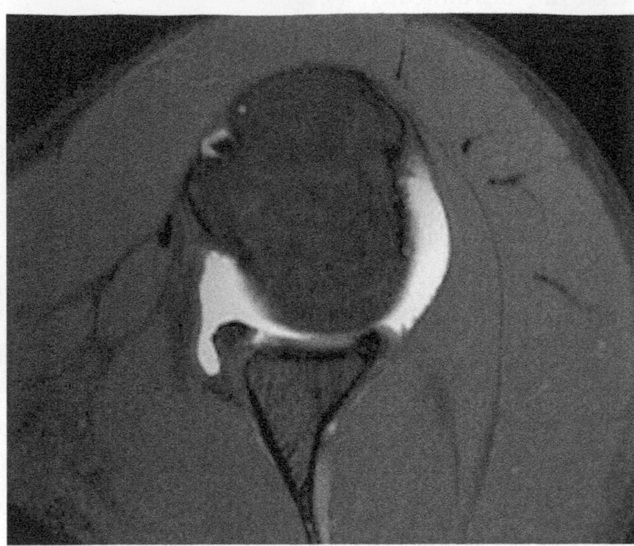

1. What are the MR arthrogram findings?
2. What is the differential diagnosis?
3. What is the most likely diagnosis?
4. What labral injuries are stable?
5. What lesions are a result of injuries of the inferior glenohumeral ligament?

Glenoid labral articular disruption (GLAD) lesion 1547

Case ranking/difficulty: 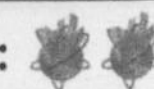 **Category:** Trauma

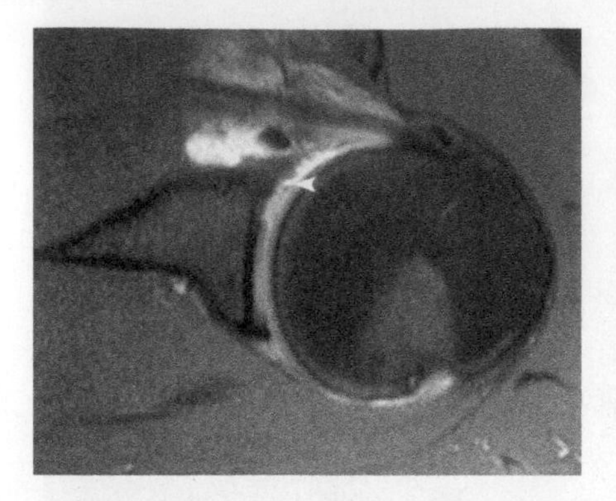

Anterior inferior glenoid labral tear with a focal cartilage defect.

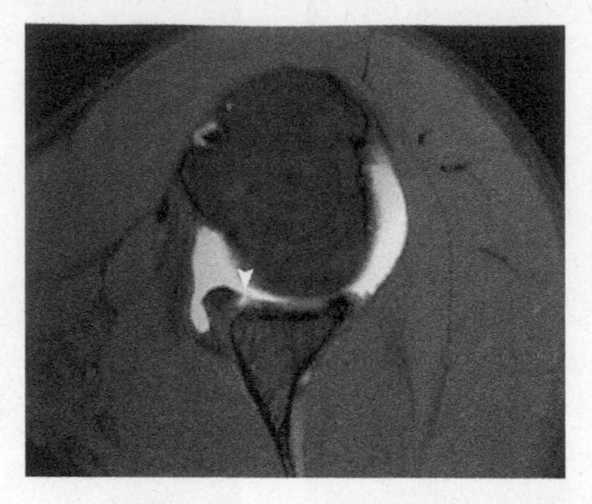

MRI arthrogram of the shoulder showing glenoid labral and articular cartilage defect.

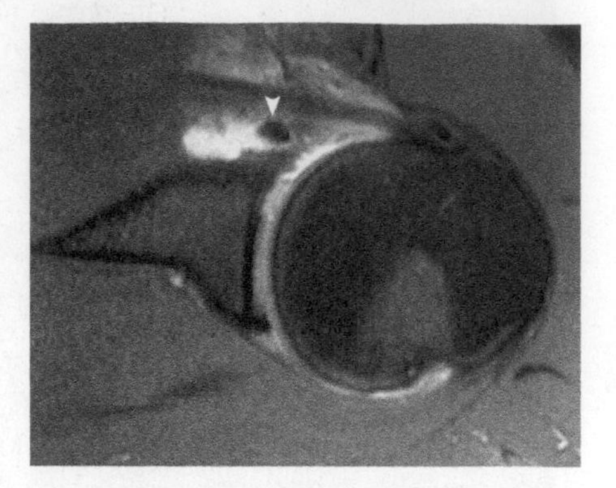

The middle glenohumeral ligament (*arrowhead*) should not be confused with a detached labral fragment.

Answers

1. There is a superficial anteroinferior glenoid labral tear, with a focal glenoid articular cartilage defect.
2. The differential diagnoses include ALPSA (anterior labroligamentous periosteal sleeve avulsion) lesion, SLAP (superior labral anterior to posterior) lesion, Perthes lesion, Bankart lesion, and GLAD lesion.
3. The combination of a focal hyaline cartilage defect with an anterior inferior labral tear is consistent with a GLAD lesion.
4. GLAD lesions are stable lesions. SLAP tears are also generally stable but not always.
5. The humeral avulsion of the glenohumeral ligament (HAGL) lesion is a tear of the humeral attachment of the anterior band of the inferior glenohumeral ligament. If there is associated bony avulsion, it is a BHAGL lesion. A PHAGL lesion is similar to a HAGL lesion but involves the posterior band of the inferior glenohumeral ligament. A GAGL lesion is similar to HAGL, but the tear is at the glenoid attachment of the anterior band of the inferior glenohumeral ligament, and not the humeral. Another similar lesion is an axillary pouch injury, involving the axillary fibers of the IGHL.

Pearls

- The glenolabral articular disruption (GLAD lesion) is an articular hyaline cartilage lesion of the anteroinferior aspect of the glenoid, with an associated tear of the anterior inferior glenoid labrum.
- The mechanism is usually an impaction injury to the glenohumeral joint, especially when the shoulder is abducted and externally rotated.
- No capsular or periosteal stripping is seen. There is no shoulder instability, as the anterior band of the inferior glenohumeral ligament remains intact.
- MR arthrogram demonstrates a cartilage defect ranging from softening and fibrillation to a detached loose fragment, which sometimes remains attached to the anterior labrum. MRI also rules out other important features such as periosteal or glenohumeral ligament injuries.
- The treatment usually is conservative, or with an arthroscopic surgical repair.

Suggested Readings

Amrami KK, Sperling JW, Bartholmai BJ, Sundaram M. Radiologic case study. Glenolabral articular disruption (GLAD) lesion. *Orthopedics.* 2002;25(1):29:95–96.

Waldt S, Burkart A, Imhoff AB, Bruegel M, Rummeny EJ, Woertler K. Anterior shoulder instability: accuracy of MR arthrography in the classification of anteroinferior labroligamentous injuries. *Radiology.* 2005;237(2): 578–583.

Recurrent anterior dislocations of shoulder

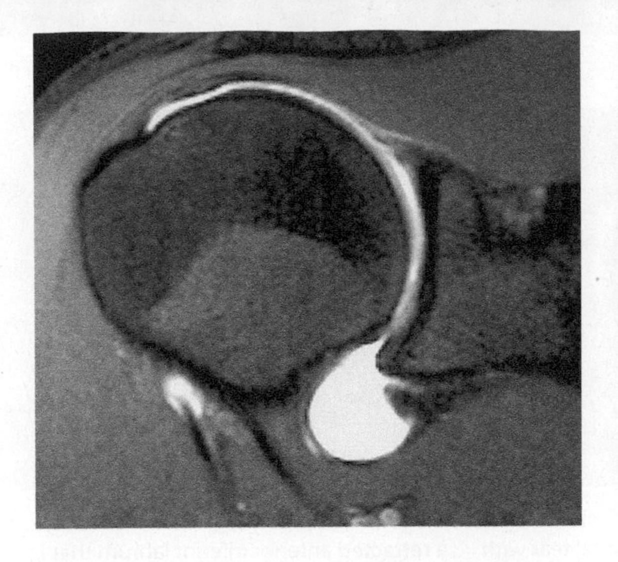

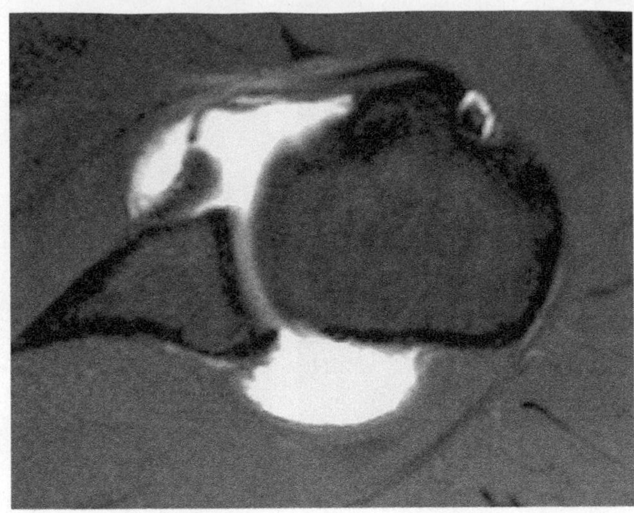

1. What are the MR arthrographic findings?

2. Which labral lesions are usually associated with instability of the shoulder joint?

3. What is the importance of an anterior labroligamentous periosteal sleeve avulsion (ALPSA) lesion?

4. What are the differential diagnoses?

5. What is the diagnosis?

Anterior labroligamentous periosteal sleeve avulsion (ALPSA lesion) 1398

Case ranking/difficulty: 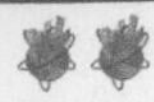

Category: Trauma

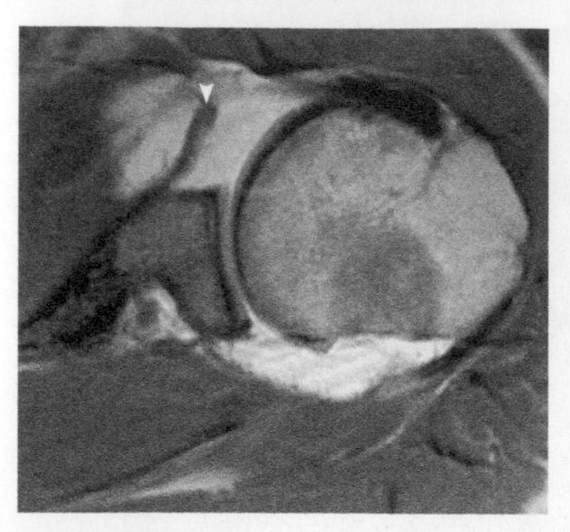

Another patient with an anterior labroligamentous tear of glenoid labrum, with intact periosteum (Perthes lesion).

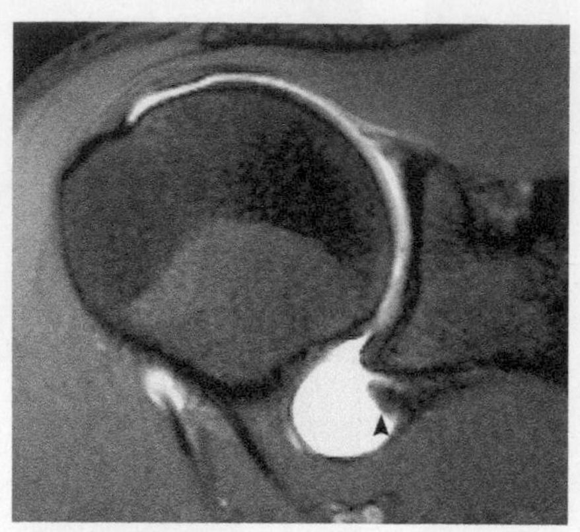

MR arthrogram showing an anterior and inferior detached glenoid labral tear with retraction.

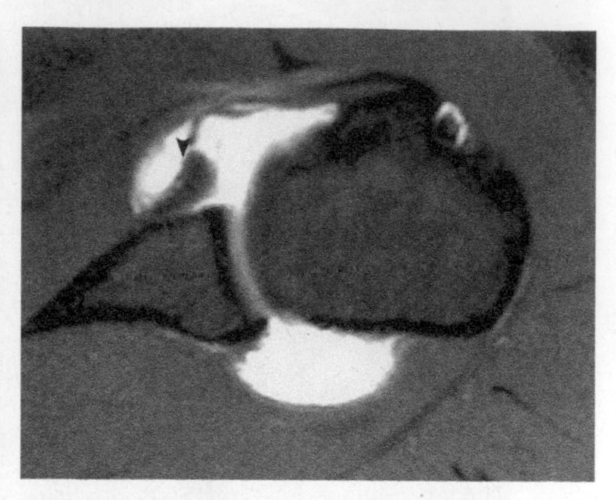

MR arthrographic image demonstrating a retracted anterior inferior labrum that is consistent with an ALPSA lesion.

Answers

1. MR arthrogram demonstrating an anterior inferior labral tear with retraction. No glenoid cartilage tear. The posterior labrum is intact.
2. Bankart and ALPSA lesions of the glenoid labrum are associated with instability of the shoulder. SLAP lesions, although associated with significant morbidity, are not all considered unstable. GLAD and Perthes lesions are stable labral injuries.
3. ALPSA lesions are unstable and result in recurrent instability of the shoulder. Because of resynovialization around the retracted labrum, the lesion may be difficult to diagnose arthroscopically, hence the importance of detecting it on MR arthrography.
4. The differentials include displaced Perthes, HAGL, GLAD, GLOM, ALPSA, and Bankart lesions.
5. The diagnosis is an ALPSA lesion.

Pearls

- Forty percent of primary shoulder dislocations result in recurrent dislocations.
- ALPSA is an important cause of recurrent dislocation of the shoulder.
- ALPSA lesions are unstable.
- It is important to distinguish it from other labroligamentous lesions such as a Perthes lesion or GLAD, as the management is different.

- MR arthrography is the investigative modality of choice for these lesions.
- In ALPSA lesions, the anterior glenoid labrum is displaced medially and retracted by the anterior band of the inferior glenohumeral ligament. Intra-articular contrast helps to identify this lesion. MRI at 3 Tesla has shown better diagnostic accuracy.
- Resynovialization around the retracted labrum makes the lesion sometimes difficult to appreciate arthroscopically, hence the importance of MR arthrography.
- These lesions are usually treated with arthroscopic repair.

Suggested Readings

Robinson G, Ho Y, Finlay K, Friedman L, Harish S. Normal anatomy and common labral lesions at MR arthrography of the shoulder. *Clin Radiol.* 2006;61(10):805–821.

Song HT, Huh YM, Kim S, et al. Anterior-inferior labral lesions of recurrent shoulder dislocation evaluated by MR arthrography in an adduction internal rotation (ADIR) position. *J Magn Reson Imaging.* 2006;23(1):29–35.

Waldt S, Burkart A, Imhoff AB, Bruegel M, Rummeny EJ, Woertler K. Anterior shoulder instability: accuracy of MR arthrography in the classification of anteroinferior labroligamentous injuries. *Radiology.* 2005;237(2):578–583.

Recurrent dislocations of shoulder after trauma, with pain

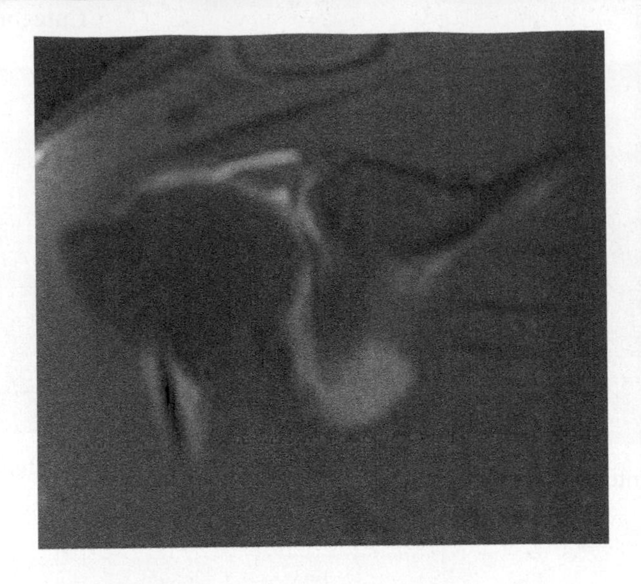

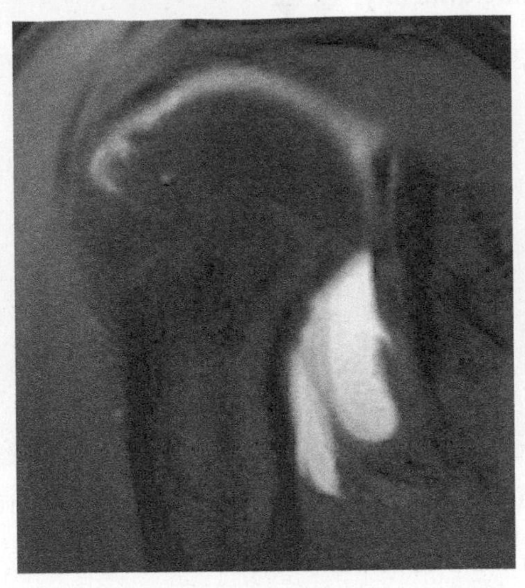

1. What are the MRI Findings?

2. Is there a bucket-handle labral (type III) tear?

3. What other MRI findings could help to distinguish a tear from a normal recess?

4. What is a type IV tear?

5. What is the most common type of this lesion?

Superior labral anterior to posterior (SLAP) type III tear 1333

Case ranking/difficulty: 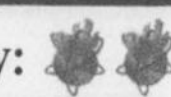

Category: Trauma

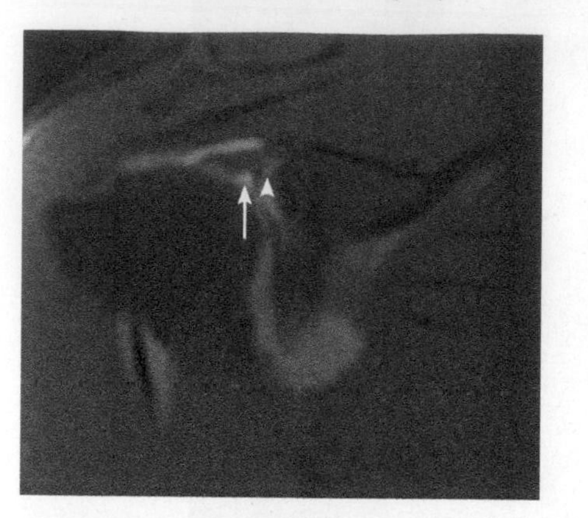

MR Arthrogram showing SLAP tear extending to the biceps anchor but not involving it. This demonstrates the described "double Oreo cookie" sign. *Arrowhead* points to the superior labral recess; *arrow* points to the labral tear.

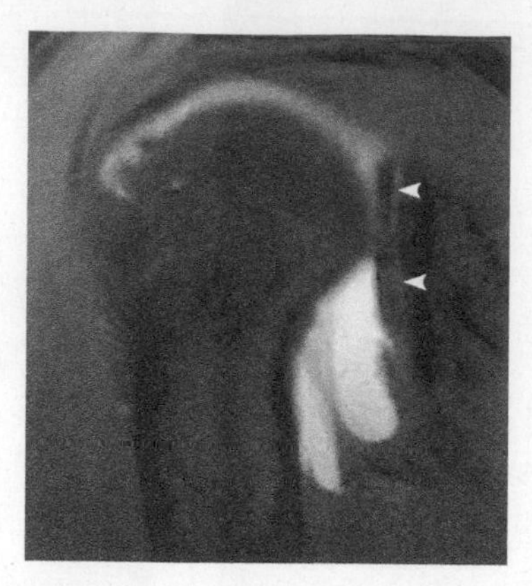

Extension into the posterior labrum.

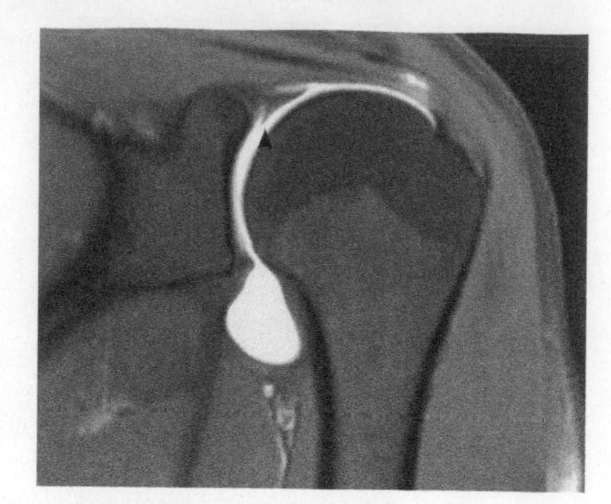

Another patient with a SLAP type II tear on MR arthrogram.

Answers

1. Superior labral tear from anterior to posterior, extending from 11 o'clock to 3 o'clock: a SLAP tear.
2. Yes. A bucket-handle tear is seen near the biceps anchor, and the glenoid labrum may be avulsed inferiorly between humeral head and articular margin. This is a SLAP type III tear.
3. Double line as in the "double Oreo cookie" sign, lateral position of the line, and extension along with involvement of the posterior one-third glenoid articular margin could help to distinguish a SLAP lesion from the normal superior labral recess.

   A "single Oreo cookie" sign can be seen in both a SLAP type II tear and a superior labral recess.
4. A type IV SLAP tear is a bucket-handle tear with extension into the biceps tendon.
5. Type II SLAP tears are the most common.

   In older patients there may be associated rotator cuff tears.

   Total of 10 types described (so far).

   Types 5 to 10 are also usually associated with type II SLAP tears.

Pearls

- SLAP lesions are labral tears at the biceps anchor extending from posterosuperior to anterosuperior, usually from the 11 o'clock position to 3 o'clock position.
- It is recognized as an important cause of shoulder disability but not always a cause of instability.
- There are at least 10 types described in the literature so far, but only 4 are commonly used.
  - Type I: Fraying and degeneration of the superior labrum.
  - Type II: Most common form, with detachment of the glenoid labrum. In older patients, there may be associated rotator cuff tears.
  - Type III: Bucket-handle tear with displaced labrum inferiorly between humeral head and articular margin.
  - Type IV: Tear extending into the long head of biceps.
- MR Arthrography is the investigative modality of choice.
- Two described signs in the literature on T2-weighted images or MR arthrogram are useful:
  1. Two high signal lines (double Oreo cookie sign) seen in a SLAP III tear.
  2. Irregular and laterally curved line, unlike the normal superior labral recess, which is curved medially and is smooth. This "single Oreo cookie" sign is seen in a normal superior labral recess, or a SLAP II tear.

Suggested Reading

Mohana-Borges AV, Chung CB, Resnick D. Superior labral anteroposterior tear: classification and diagnosis on MRI and MR arthrography. *AJR Am J Roentgenol.* 2003;181(6):1449–1462.

History of trauma

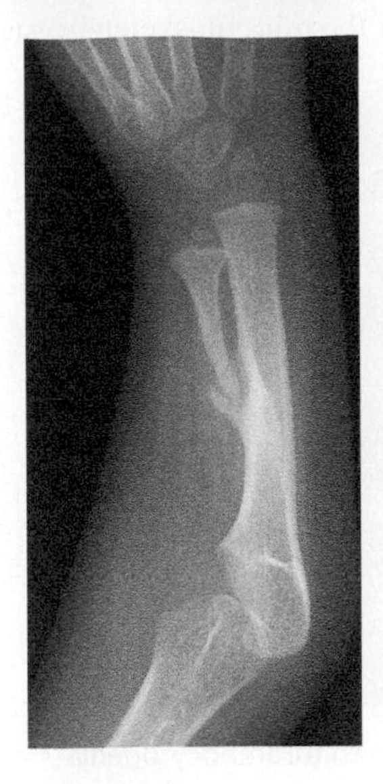

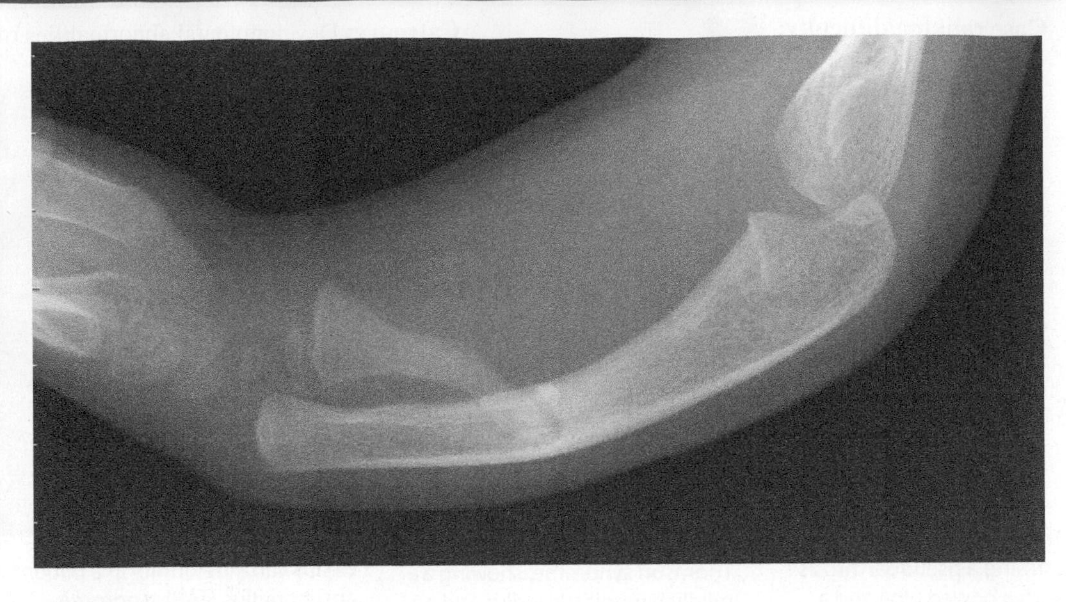

1. What are the radiographic findings?

2. What syndromes are associated with this finding?

3. What other clinical and radiological features are associated with this entity?

4. When performing a clinical workup of these patients, what is the most important condition that must be excluded?

5. What are the clinical features of thrombocytopenia-absent radius (TAR) syndrome?

Radial ray anomaly 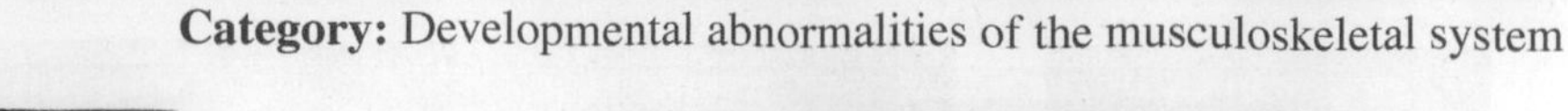

2344

Case ranking/difficulty: 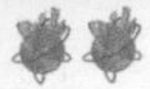 **Category:** Developmental abnormalities of the musculoskeletal system

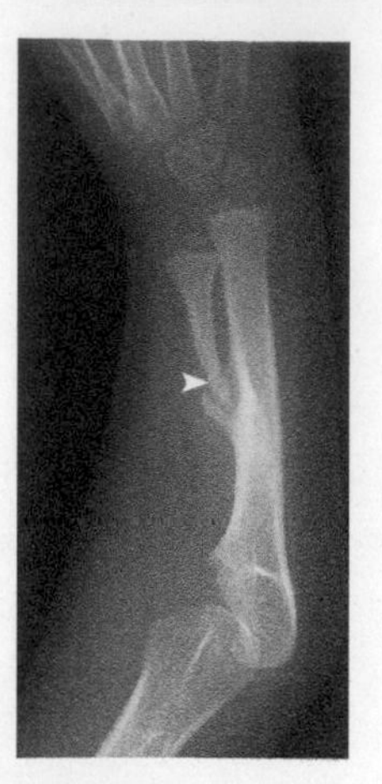

The radius is hypoplastic forming a pseudoarthrosis with a bowed ulna and a fracture of the hypoplastic radius (*arrowhead*).

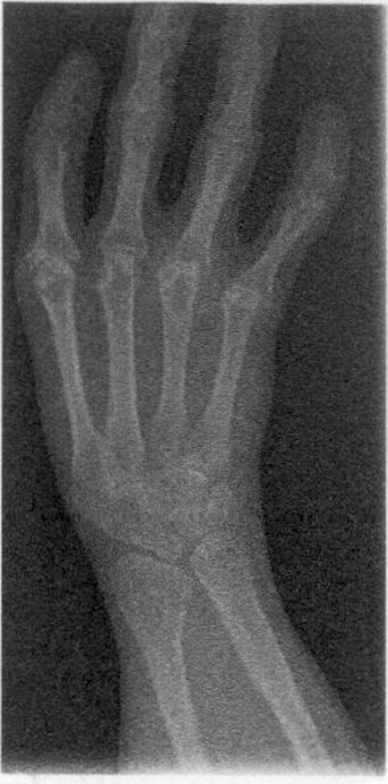

Patient with Rothmund-Thomson syndrome, showing a mildly hypoplastic radius and an absent thumb, trapezium, and scaphoid (preaxial deficiency).

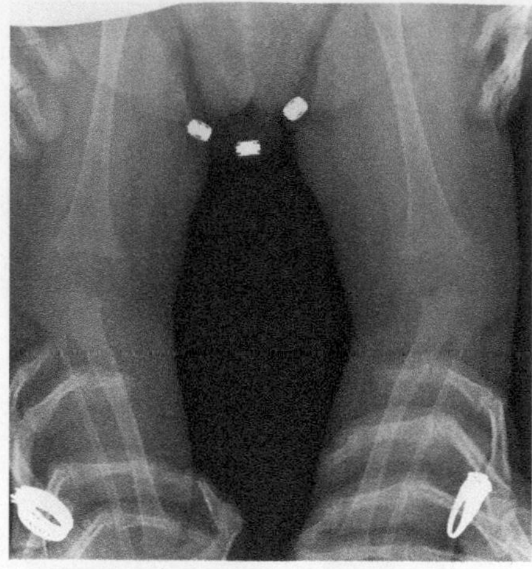

Genus varus deformity in a patient with thrombocytopenia-absent radius (TAR) syndrome.

Answers

1. The radius is hypoplastic with a nondisplaced fracture, and there is a bowed ulna. Although radial ray anomalies are associated with other preaxial deficiencies such as an absent thumb, they are not present in this case. The ulna is not dislocated, although the fibrous anlage predisposes individuals to elbow dislocation.

2. This patient had no syndromic features and was an isolated radial ray anomaly. Syndromes associated with preaxial deficiencies include VACTERL (vertebral, anal, cardiac, tracheal, esophageal, renal, limb), Holt Oram, Fanconi, thrombocytopenia-absent radius (TAR) and Rothmund-Thomson.

3. In preaxial deficiency, other preaxial structures may be absent. These include the thumb, scaphoid, and trapezium. An absent ulna is a postaxial deficiency.

4. Fanconi syndrome.

   Thrombocytopenia is seen in TAR syndrome, cardiac defects especially septal defects in Holt Oram, anal atresia in VACTERL, aplastic anemia in Fanconi syndrome, and osteosarcoma in Rothmund-Thomson syndrome. Because the aplastic anemia in Fanconi syndrome is invariably fatal without a bone marrow transplant, Fanconi syndrome must be excluded in all radial ray anomalies.

5. TAR syndrome is characterized by thrombocytopenia and an absent radius, typically bilateral. Other associated radiological and clinical features include absent menisci and cruciate ligaments, leading to unstable joints.

   The absence of the menisci also appears to affect the development of the osseous structures, leading to a convex proximal medial tibia and a saddle shaped distal medial femoral condyle. This may result in a genu varus deformity.

Pearls

- Radial ray anomalies may be isolated or syndromic.
- They are preaxial deficiencies, and can result in hypoplasia or absence of the radius, scaphoid, trapezium, and thumb.
- If unilateral, it is syndromic in 40%, and if bilateral, it is syndromic in 77% of cases.
- All patients with radial ray anomalies should be tested for Fanconi syndrome, as this is fatal without a bone marrow transplant.
- A hypoplastic or absent radius is the most common form.
- The radial nerve often ends at the elbow and is substituted for by the median nerve, and the radial artery is often absent.

Suggested Readings

Goldfarb CA, Wall L, Manske PR. Radial longitudinal deficiency: the incidence of associated medical and musculoskeletal conditions. *J Hand Surg Am.* 2006;31(7):1176–1182.

O'Rahilly R. Morphological patterns in limb deficiencies and duplications. *Am J Anat.* 1951;89(2):135–193.

History of injury to the leg

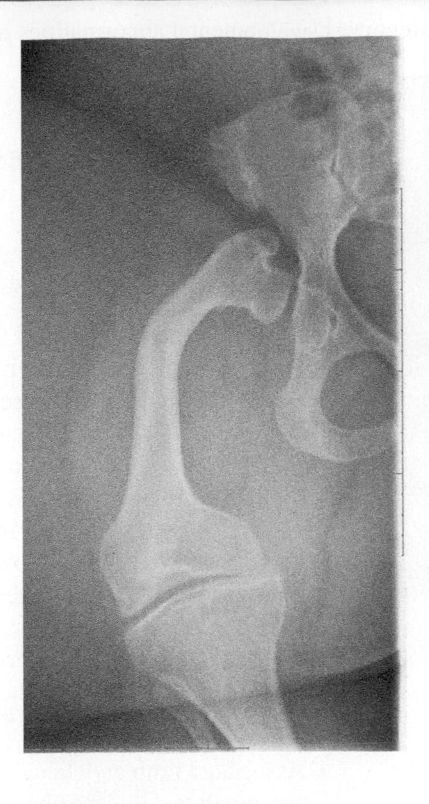

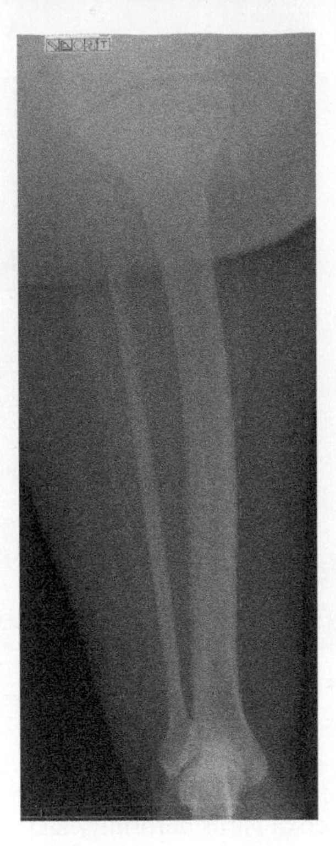

1. What are the pertinent radiographic features?

2. What is the most likely diagnosis?

3. In what percentage of patients is this condition bilateral?

4. What are some of the associations of this entity?

5. What is the best modality for investigating the severity of the disease?

Proximal focal femoral deficiency (PFFD) 2309

Case ranking/difficulty: 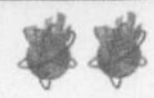

Category: Developmental abnormalities of the musculoskeletal system

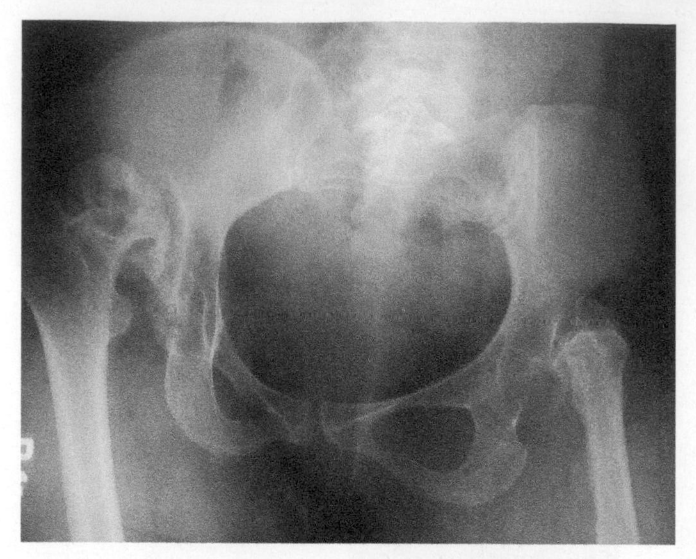

Another patient with bilateral PFFD, worse on the left side.

Answers

1. The femur is short with a coxa varus deformity and superior subluxation of the femur, with a dysplastic acetabulum. The fibula is also hypoplastic.
2. The radiographic features suggest proximal focal femoral deficiency (PFFD). Thalidomide given between the fourth and sixth weeks of gestation is a definite association with PFFD.
3. PFFD is bilateral in 15% of patients.
4. Cleft palate, club foot, fibula hemimelia, and other limb anomalies are frequently seen (up to 50%). Spinal anomalies, although rare, can occur.
5. MRI using conventional spin-echo and gradient-echo sequences is useful in establishing a fibrous or fibrocartilaginous connection between the proximal femur and shaft. It also aids in evaluating the acetabulum.

Pearls

- Proximal focal femoral deficiency (PFFD) is a condition characterized by a varying degree of femoral deficiency and shortening.
- The condition is classified from A to D, based on the radiographic characteristics:
    - Group A has a shortened femur ending at or slightly above the acetabulum, which is well developed. The femoral head is often absent but later ossifies.
    - Group B: The femoral head is present but ossification is delayed. There is no connection between the shaft and the proximal femur, with the proximal femur lying above the acetabulum
    - Group C: Markedly dysplastic acetabulum, with absence of the femoral head. The shaft is shorter than in B.
    - Group D: Most severe form with a severely shortened shaft, and a small irregular tuft of bone above the distal femoral epiphysis. The acetabulum is absent.
- Associated limb anomalies are very common, most commonly a deficient fibula.
- MRI is useful in establishing a fibrous or fibrocartilaginous connection between the head and shaft, as well as assessing the acetabulum.

Suggested Readings

Biko DM, Davidson R, Pena A, Jaramillo D. Proximal focal femoral deficiency: evaluation by MR imaging. *Pediatr Radiol.* 2012;42(1):50–56.

Hillmann JS, Mesgarzadeh M, Revesz G, Bonakdarpour A, Clancy M, Betz RR. Proximal femoral focal deficiency: radiologic analysis of 49 cases. *Radiology.* 1987;165(3):769–773.

1-month-old presenting with fever and irritability

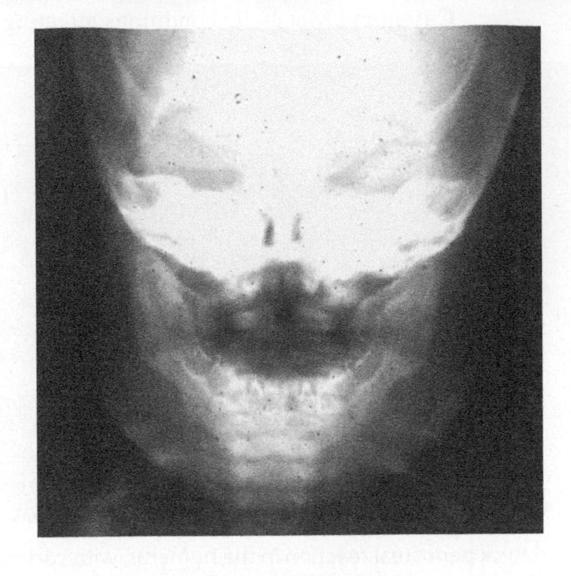

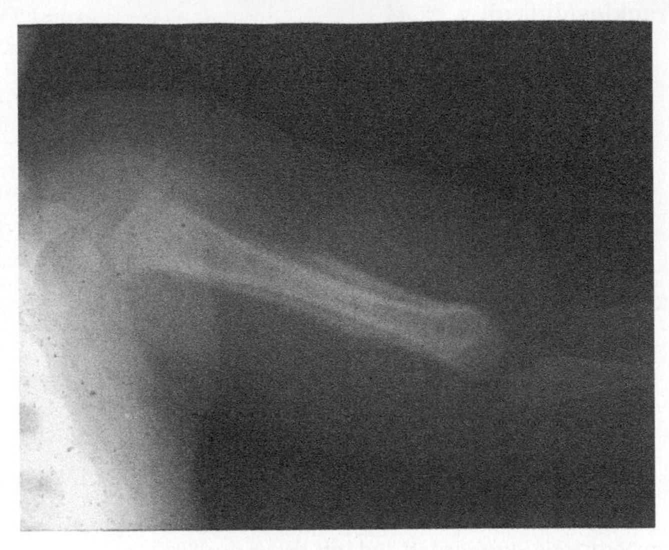

1. What are the radiograph findings?
2. What is the most likely diagnosis?
3. Most cases carry a poor prognosis.
   True or False?
4. Which bones are typically affected?
5. MRI is essential for the diagnosis of this entity.
   True or False?

Caffey disease (infantile cortical hyperostosis) 2311

Case ranking/difficulty: 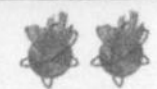

Category: Metabolic conditions affecting bone

Cortical hyperostosis (*arrowheads*) and soft-tissue swelling (*arrows*).

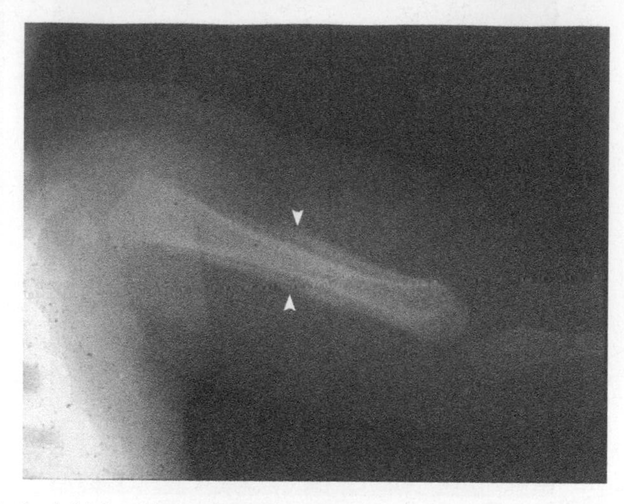

Marked thick periosteal reaction in the humerus, with cortical thickening. (Images courtesy of Dr. Akbar Bonakdarpour.)

Answers

1. There is soft-tissue swelling and cortical thickening in the mandible, with prolific periosteal reaction in the humerus. Although lytic bone changes may occur in Caffey disease, they are not demonstrated here.

2. Although prostaglandin E therapy and non-accidental injury may give similar findings, the age of the patient along with the clinical and radiological features suggest Caffey disease (infantile cortical hyperostosis).

3. False. The majority of cases of Caffey disease are self-limiting, although there is a rare prenatal form with a poor prognosis.

4. The flat bones are most often affected, including the mandible, skull, pelvis, and scapula. When tubular bones are affected, it is most often the ulna. Rarely, affected bones are the small bones of the hands and feet and the vertebral bodies.

5. False. Although MRI may detect the periosteal changes and soft tissue inflammation earlier than radiographs, the clinical picture along with radiographs are usually diagnostic.

Pearls

- Caffey disease has two forms: the rare prenatal form that has a poor prognosis and the more common infantile form that is usually self-limiting.
- Presentation is in the first five months of life, most commonly in the first two months.
- The classic presentation is fever, soft-tissue swelling, and hyperirritability.
- Radiographs show soft-tissue swelling, periosteal reaction, or cortical hyperostosis.
- Flat bones are most commonly affected, especially the mandible. Tubular bone involvement is most commonly in the ulna.
- Involvement of the radius and ulna may result in synostosis. Rib involvement may result in a pleural effusion.
- MRI may show the soft-tissue inflammation and periosteal reaction earlier than radiographs, but is usually not required.
- Nuclear medicine studies show intense uptake of radiopharmaceutical, with a "bearded child" appearance if the mandible is affected

Suggested Readings

Nemec SF, Rimoin DL, Lachman RS. Radiological aspects of prenatal-onset cortical hyperostosis [Caffey Dysplasia]. *Eur J Radiol.* 2012;81(4):e565–e572.

Oppermann HC. Original description of infantile cortical hyperostosis. *AJR Am J Roentgenol.* 1979;133(6):1208.

1-day-old female with a history of deformity

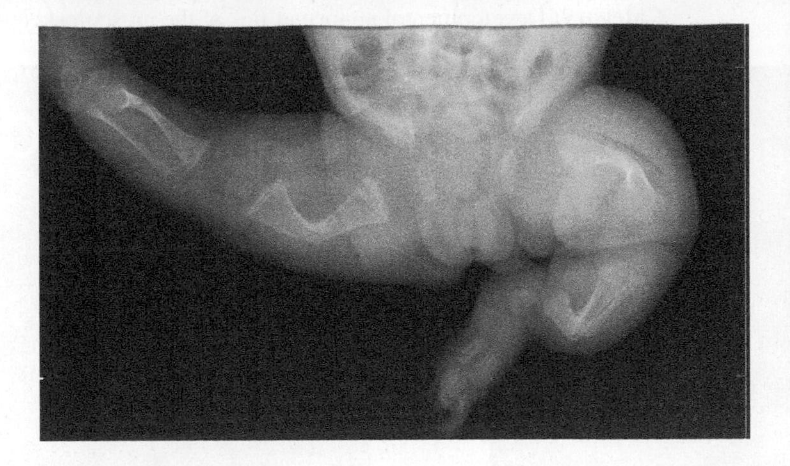

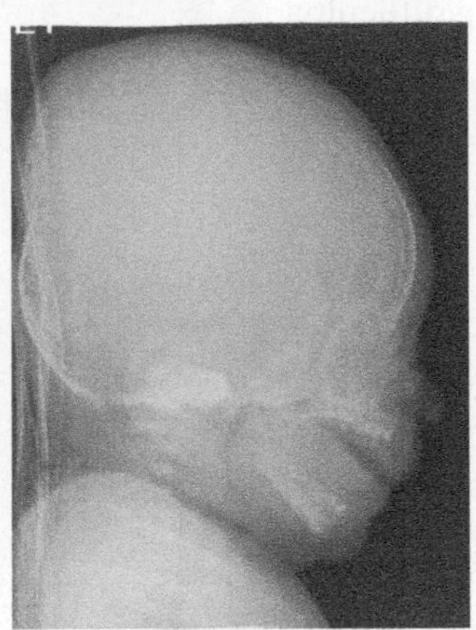

1. What features are demonstrated on the extremity radiograph?
2. What are the skull radiograph findings?
3. What is the most likely diagnosis?
4. What is the underlying abnormality in all types of this condition?
5. Which type of the disease is usually the most severe?

Osteogenesis imperfecta (type III) 1463

Case ranking/difficulty: 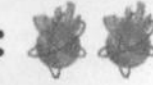

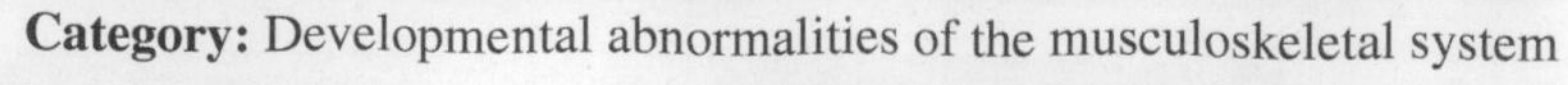

Category: Developmental abnormalities of the musculoskeletal system

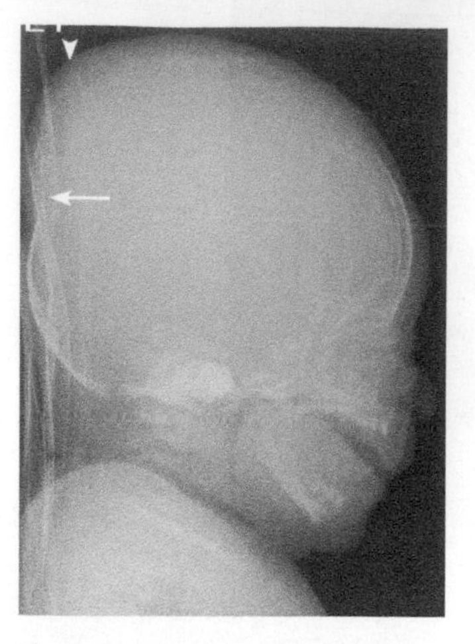

There is a depressed posterior skull fracture (*arrow*) and multiple wormian bones are seen (*arrowhead*).

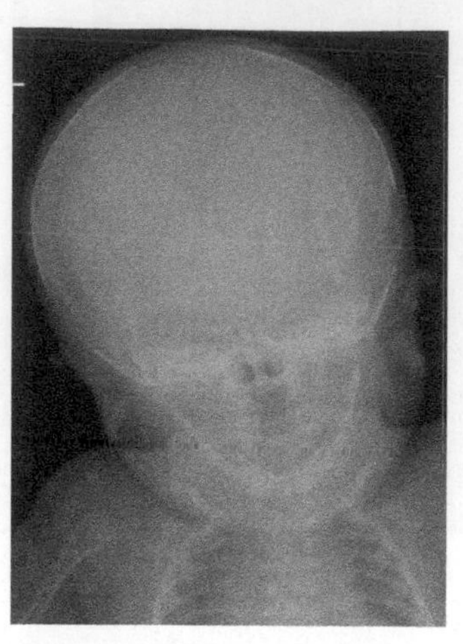

No upper rib fractures are identified.

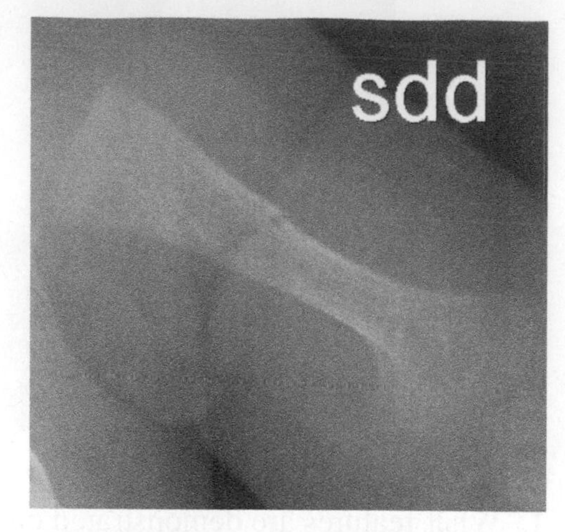

Ten months later there is an acute fracture of the mid left humerus.

Answers

1. The bones are osteopenic with multiple fractures and extensive deformity.
2. The bones are mildly osteopenic, with multiple wormian bones and a depressed posterior parietal skull fracture.
3. The constellation of findings and severity of disease in a newborn, but survival beyond the first year suggests osteogenesis imperfecta (OI) type III. Type I usually has much milder disease and usually presents later in life.
4. A defect in the quantity and/or quality of collagen is the underlying problem in OI, with a defect in the quality being more problematic. In the type II variant, both the quality and quantity of collagen is affected, accounting for the severity of disease.
5. Type II OI is the most severe type of osteogenesis imperfecta, with death in the first few weeks of life. Types V and VI are variants of type IV, and types VII and VIII are rare recessive forms.

Pearls

- OI is a disorder of either the quantity or quality of collagen, or both. Disorders of the collagen quality lead to more severe disease.
- The bones are osteopenic and are prone to fracture.
- Type I disease is mild, with propensity for fracture but no deformity. These patients have blue sclera and deafness.
- Type II is most severe and is incompatible with life.
- Type III is more severe than type I, with multiple fractures and deformity.
- Type IV is more severe than type I. This form is the type most often confused with non-accidental injury.
- Prenatal ultrasound may be diagnostic, with thin calvaria that are easily compressible or fractured. Increased acoustic through transmission occurs.

Suggested Readings

Ablin DS, Greenspan A, Reinhart M, Grix A. Differentiation of child abuse from osteogenesis imperfecta. *AJR Am J Roentgenol.* 1990;154(5):1035–1046.

Ablin DS. Osteogenesis imperfecta: a review. *Can Assoc Radiol J.* 1998;49(2):110–123.

Short stature

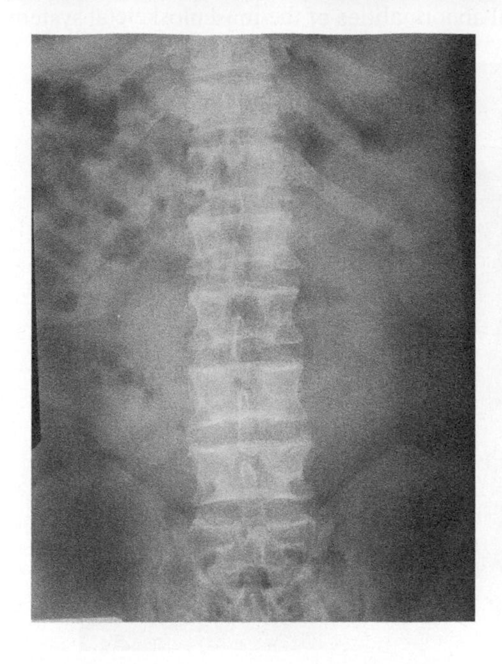

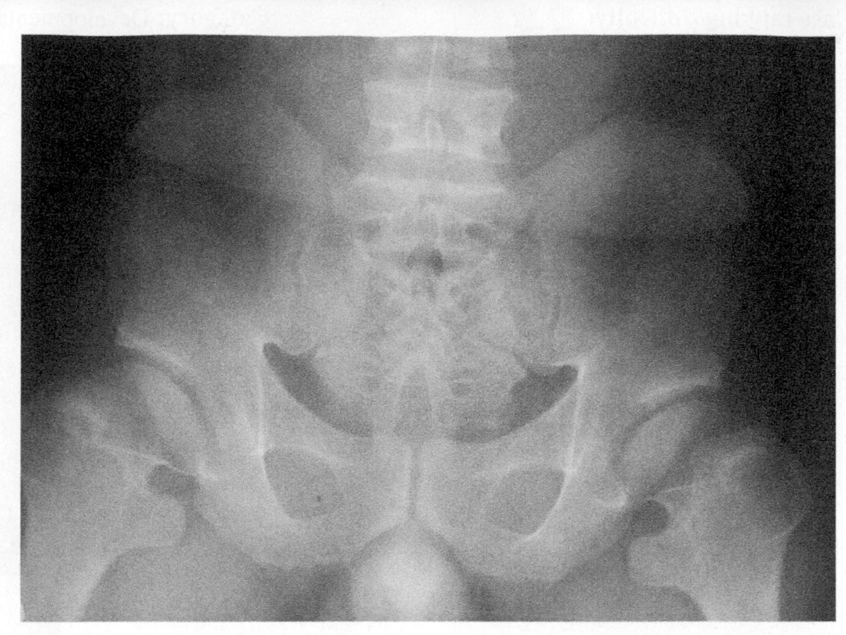

1. What are the radiograph findings?
2. What is the most likely diagnosis?
3. What form of dwarfism is demonstrated in this condition?
4. What is the inheritance pattern?
5. What are the main causes of mortality in these patients?

Achondroplasia 1460

Case ranking/difficulty: 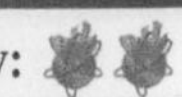

Category: Developmental abnormalities of the musculoskeletal system

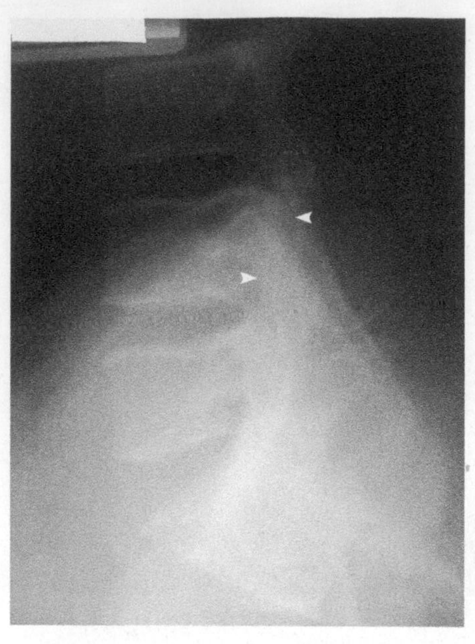

The pedicles are short and broad.

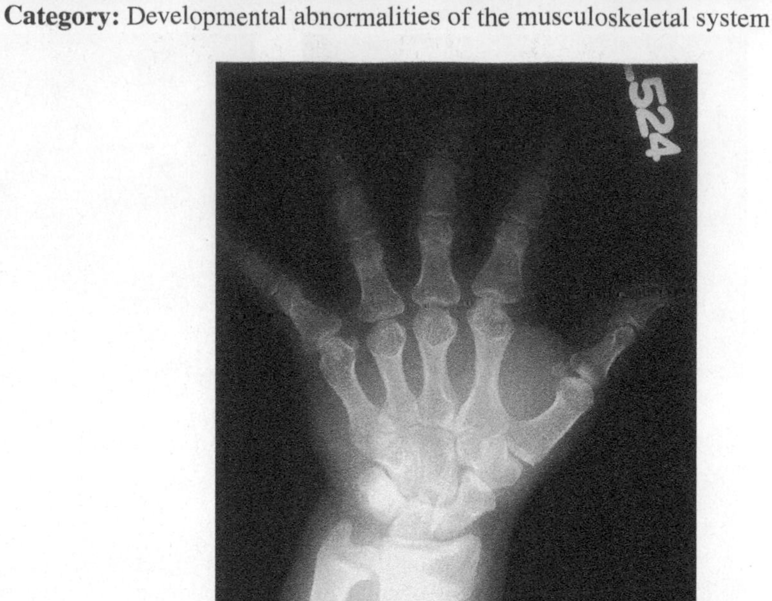

Short, broad metacarpals and phalanges with a trident hand.

Answers

1. Narrowed interpedicular distance, Champagne glass pelvis, horizontal sacrum and acetabulae with short, broad, femoral heads and necks.
2. The findings are consistent with achondroplasia.
3. Achondroplasia is a disproportionate rhizomelic (proximal) dwarfism.
4. Eighty-five percent of cases are a result of a spontaneous genetic mutation, and 15% are caused by an autosomal dominant inheritance.
5. In patients younger than age 4 years, brainstem compression is the leading cause of death. Between ages 5 and 24 years central nervous system and respiratory causes predominate, and between ages 25 and 54 years cardiovascular complications are the leading cause of death.

Pearls

- Achondroplasia is a proximal (rhizomelic) dwarfism.
- Endochondral ossification is affected, with normal periosteal and membranous bone growth.
- Affected bones are short with normal thickness.
- There is metaphyseal flaring with a ball in socket epiphysis.
- There are also trident hands, which are fingers of equal length that are widely opposed.
- The vertebrae are bullet-shaped with posterior scalloping and spinal stenosis. Brainstem compression may occur.
- A "champagne" glass pelvis is seen.
- The foramen magnum is narrowed, which can lead to brainstem compression.
- Mortality is increased, usually as a consequence of brainstem compression in young patients, and respiratory and cardiovascular complications appear in older patients.

Suggested Readings

Kao SC, Waziri MH, Smith WL, Sato Y, Yuh WT, Franken EA. MR imaging of the craniovertebral junction, cranium, and brain in children with achondroplasia. *AJR Am J Roentgenol.* 1989;153(3):565–569.

Song HR, Choonia AT, Hong SJ, et al. Rotational profile of the lower extremity in achondroplasia: computed tomographic examination of 25 patients. *Skeletal Radiol.* 2006;35(12):929–934.

Extra digits noted at birth

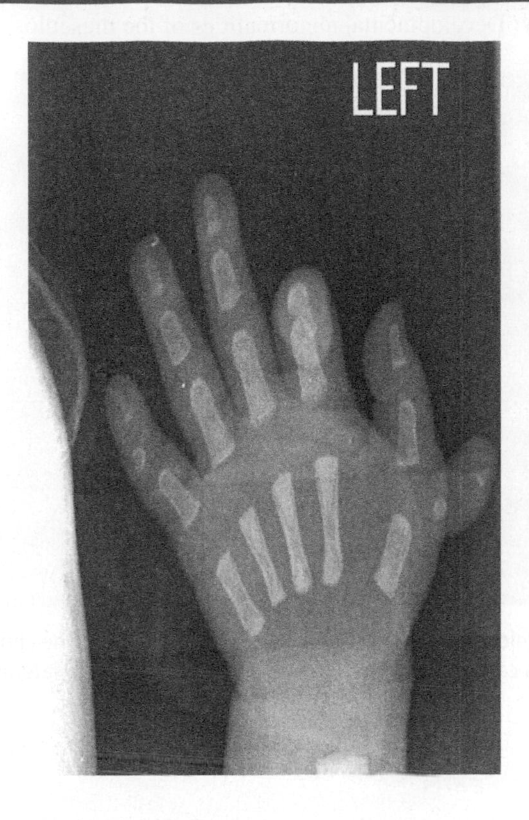

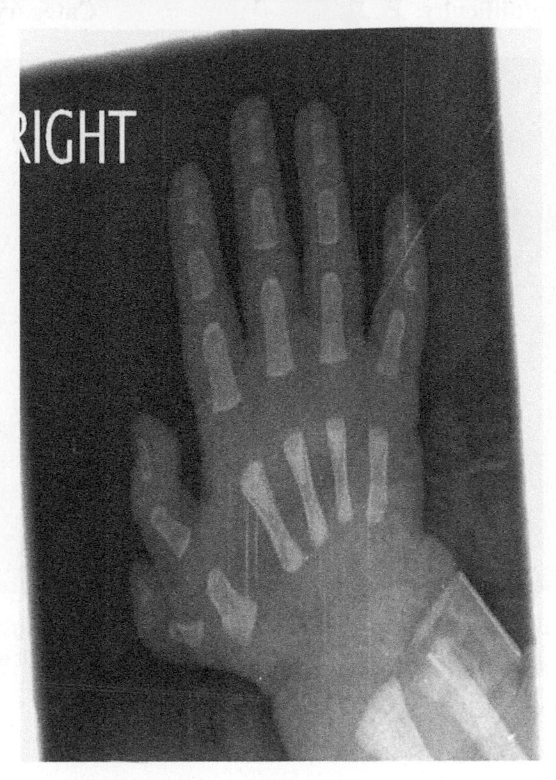

1. What are the radiograph findings?

2. What terminologies are used to describe the primary abnormality shown?

3. What is meant by preaxial, central, and postaxial forms of the condition?

4. Which form of this condition is most common?

5. What are the demographics of the condition?

Preaxial polydactyly 1461

Case ranking/difficulty: 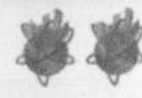

Category: Developmental abnormalities of the musculoskeletal system

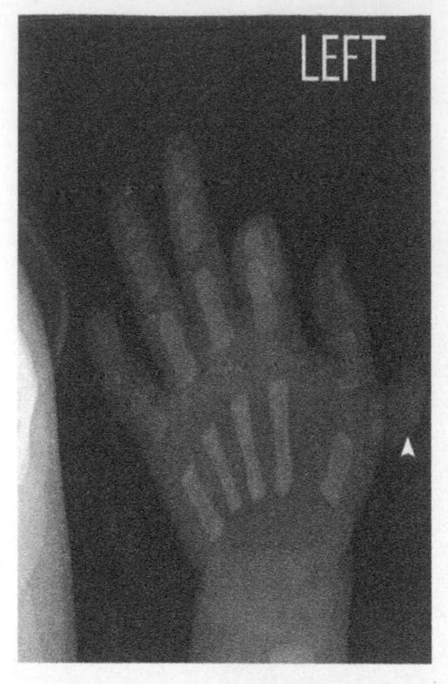

There is preaxial polydactyly and clinodactyly.

Incurving middle phalanx of the fifth digit is called clinodactyly.

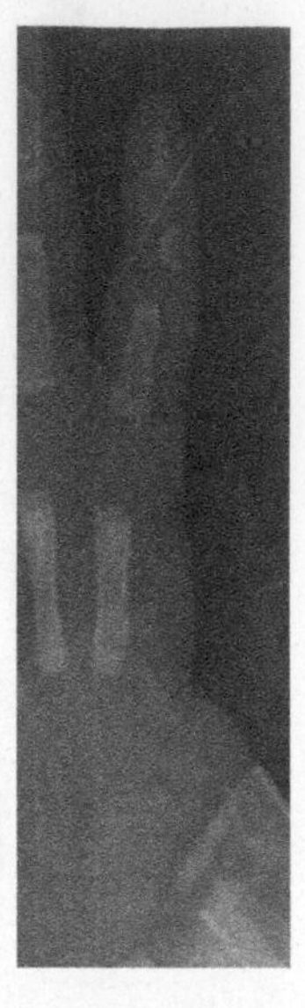

The clinodactyly is bilateral.

Answers

1. There are bilateral supernumerary digits at the thumbs. Incurved middle phalanges of the fifth digits are noted (clinodactyly).
2. The condition where there is a supernumerary digit is called *polydactyly*. There are 3 main types: preaxial, postaxial, and central.
3. Preaxial polydactyly means a supernumerary digit at the thumb or great toe, postaxial at the fifth digit, and central between the two.
4. Postaxial polydactyly with a single supernumerary digit (hexadactyly) is most common. Ectrodactyly is a deficiency of 1 or more central digits.
5. Postaxial polydactyly is 10 times more common in African-Americans as compared to whites and is usually incidental. It is usually syndromic in whites. Preaxial polydactyly is most common among whites and Asians.

Pearls

- An extra digit is called *polydactyly*.
- Polydactyly is preaxial if the supernumerary digit is adjacent to the thumb or great toe.
- Polydactyly is postaxial if the supernumerary digit is adjacent to the fifth digit.
- It is central polydactyly if located in between the first and fifth digits.
- Postaxial polydactyly is 10 times more common in African-Americans than in whites and is usually incidental.
- Postaxial polydactyly in whites tend to be syndromic.
- Clinodactyly refers to incurving of the fifth digit towards the fourth digit.

Suggested Readings

Bromley B, Benacerraf B. Abnormalities of the hands and feet in the fetus: sonographic findings. *AJR Am J Roentgenol.* 1995;165(5):1239–1243.

Klaassen Z, Choi M, Musselman R, Eapen D, Tubbs RS, Loukas M. A review of supernumerary and absent limbs and digits of the upper limb. *Surg Radiol Anat.* 2012;34(2):101–106.

Incidental finding

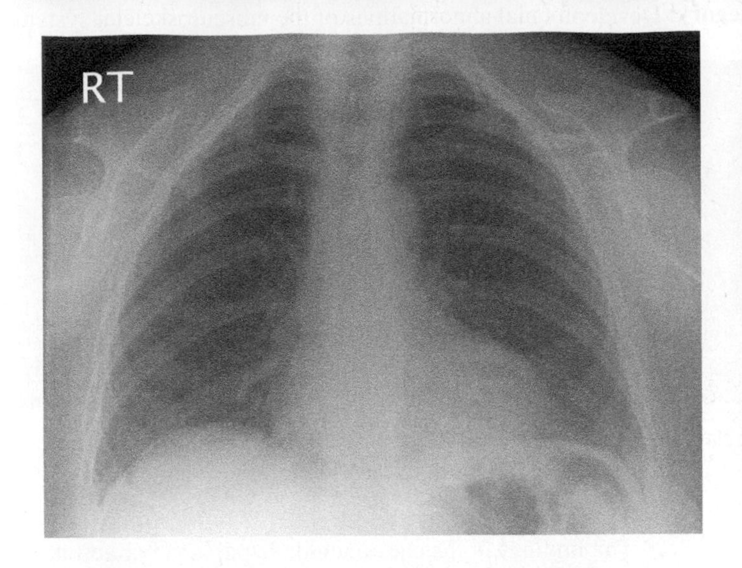

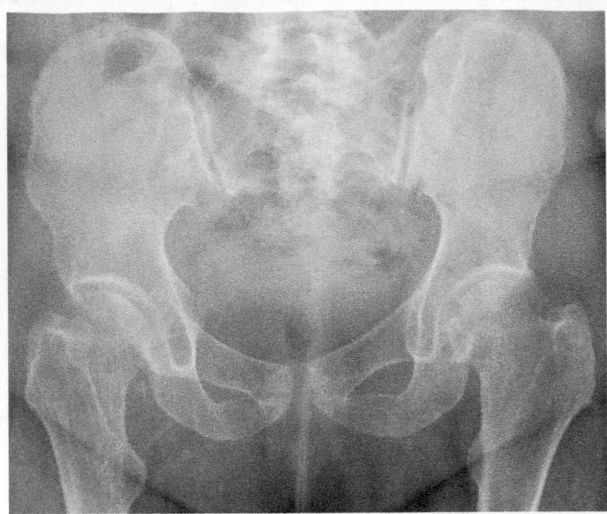

1. What are the expected chest X-ray findings in this condition?
2. What are the expected pelvic X-ray findings in this condition?
3. What are the skull manifestation of this condition?
4. What are the extremity findings in this condition?
5. What is the inheritance pattern?

Cleidocranial dysostosis 1436

Case ranking/difficulty: 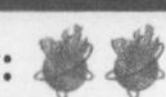

Category: Developmental abnormalities of the musculoskeletal system

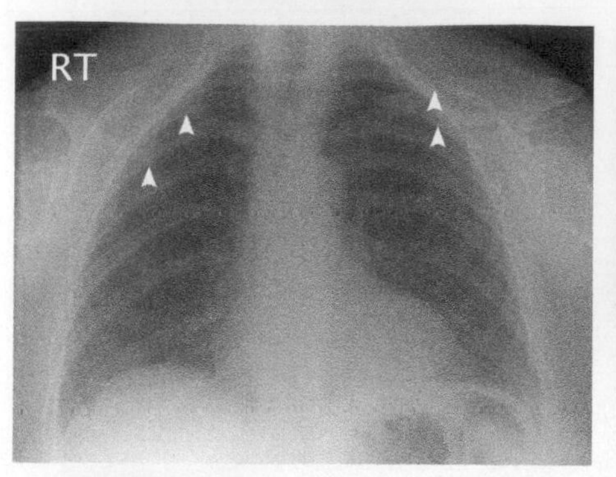

Hypoplastic clavicles.

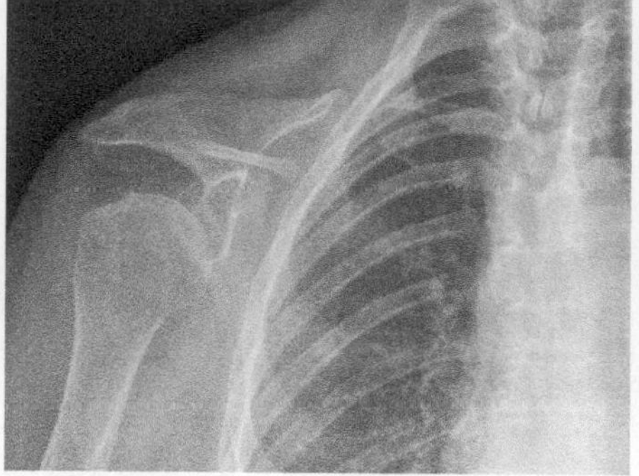

Hypoplastic right clavicle.

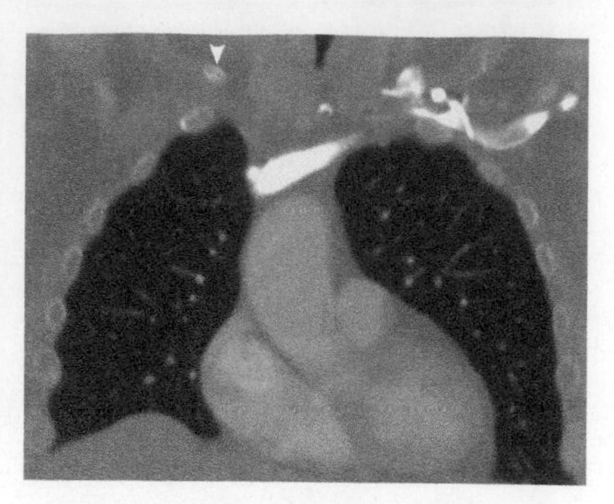

CT coronal image shows the hypoplastic right clavicle.

Answers

1. Hypoplastic or absent (10%) clavicles. The right side is most commonly affected.

   Other features include a narrowed and bell-shaped thorax, supernumerary ribs and an incompletely ossified sternum.

2. Hypoplastic iliac bones and sacrum and widened pubic symphysis are common features.
3. The main skull manifestations include wormian bones, enlarged head, and widened fontanelle with delayed closure of the cranial sutures. Other important features include delayed dentition and hypoplastic paranasal sinuses.
4. There is an elongated second metacarpal, pseudoepiphysis of the metacarpals, pointed terminal tufts, coned epiphysis, and coxa varus deformity.
5. Inheritance is autosomal dominant; Forty percent are sporadic mutations.

Pearls

- Rare, congenital hereditary dysplasia affecting membranous and enchondral bones such as the skull bones and clavicle.
- Male and females are equally affected.
- Autosomal dominant inheritance, but 40% are sporadic mutations.
- The skull findings are large fontanelles with delayed closure, wormian bones, supernumerary teeth, high-arched palate, persistent metopic sutures and non-union of the mandibular symphysis, hypoplastic paranasal sinuses, and delayed dentition.
- The findings in the chest include hypoplastic or absent clavicles (in 10%) leading to a bell-shaped appearance, and hypermobile shoulders.
- In the pelvis, delayed ossification of the symphysis pubis, hypoplastic ilium, and sacrum.
- Within the extremities, there is a coxa vara deformity caused by deformed or absent femoral necks, short or rarely absent radius, elongated second metacarpals, short hypoplastic distal phalanges, coned epiphysis, accessory epiphyses, and pointed terminal tufts.
- The treatment is mainly of dental problems requiring regular oral care. Genetic counseling and family planning are also required.

Suggested Readings

Golan I, Baumert U, Held P, Feuerbach S, Müssig D. Radiological findings and molecular genetic confirmation of cleidocranial dysplasia. *Clin Radiol.* 2002;57(6): 525–529.

Gonzalez GE, Caruso PA, Small JE, Jyung RW, Troulis MJ, Curtin HD. Craniofacial and temporal bone CT findings in cleidocranial dysplasia. *Pediatr Radiol.* 2008;38(8): 892–897.

Genu vara

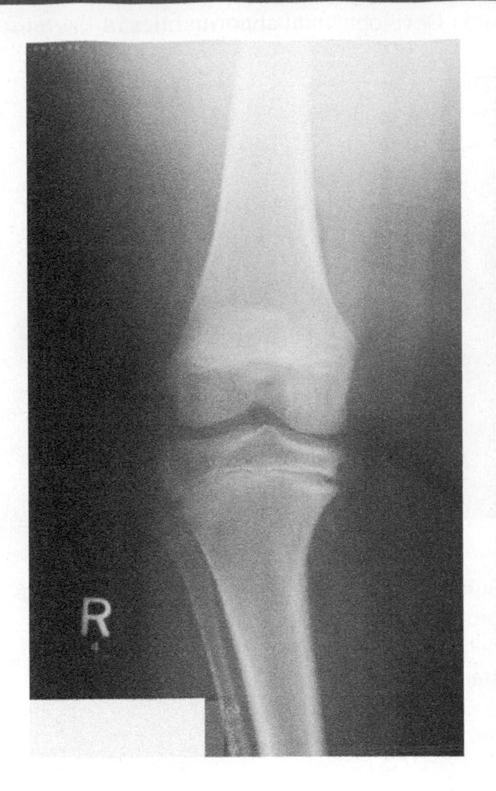

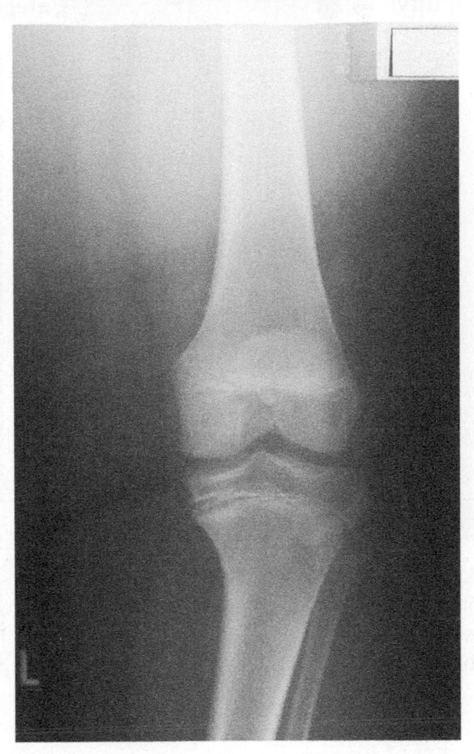

1. What radiological features characterize this entity?
2. What is the differential diagnosis for lower-extremity bowing?
3. What are the risk factors for this entity?
4. What is the proposed etiology?
5. The infantile form of this entity is rarely bilateral. True or False?

Blount disease

Case ranking/difficulty:

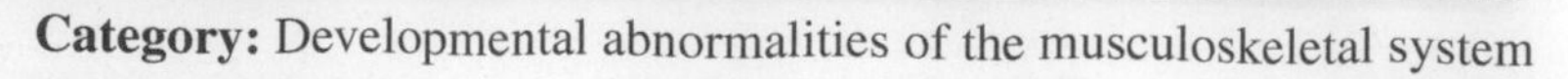

Category: Developmental abnormalities of the musculoskeletal system

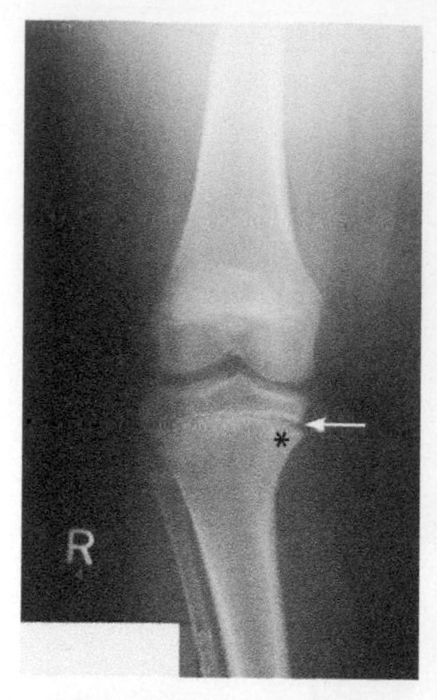

Varus angulation, medial downsloping of the proximal tibial metaphysis (*asterisk*), and medial widening of the physis (*arrow*) are demonstrated in the right knee.

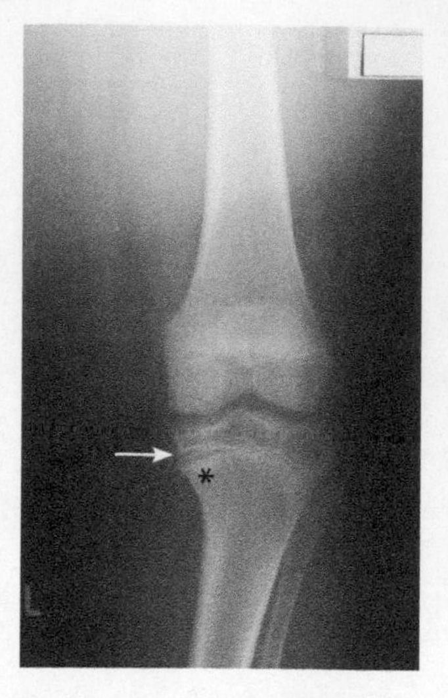

Radiograph of the left knee demonstrates similar findings.

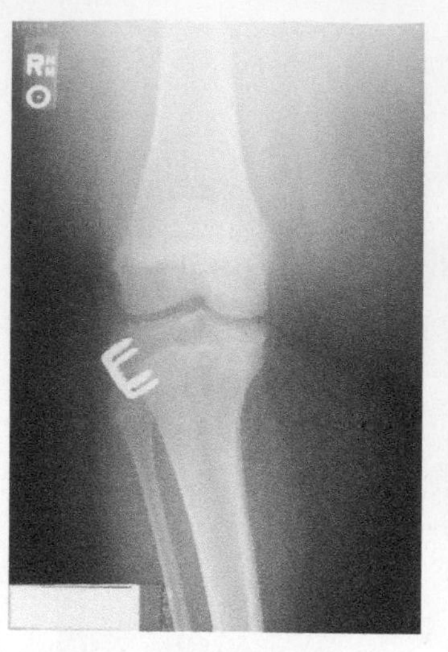

Surgical correction with proximal tibial lateral hemiepiphysiodesis using staples.

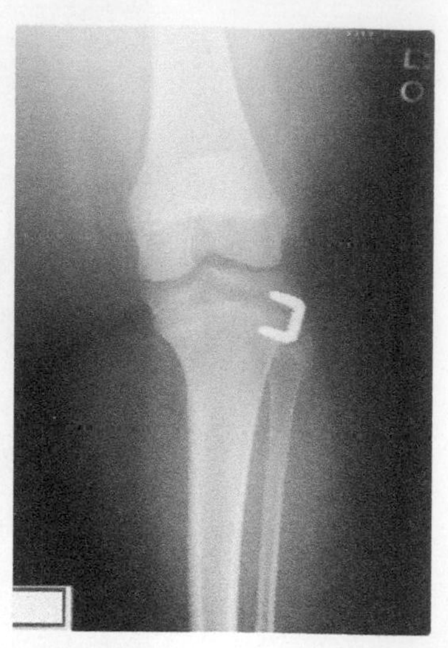

Similar surgical correction in the left knee.

Answers

1. Blount disease is characterized by genu varum, a result of growth suppression at the posteromedial proximal tibial physis.
2. Developmental bowing, Blount disease, congenital tibial bowing, rickets, and neurofibromatosis are all included in the differential for lower-extremity bowing.
3. Risk factors for Blount disease include early walking, obesity, and African American descent.
4. Blount disease is thought to be caused by abnormal stress on the proximal tibial physis, likely related to weight bearing.
5. False. The infantile form of Blount disease is bilateral in up to 60% of cases.

Pearls

- Blount disease, or tibia vara, is a common cause of varus angulation at the knees in pediatric patients.
- It is thought to be caused by abnormal stress on the proximal tibial physis, likely related to weight bearing.
- It is more common in obese children.
- The infantile form, which is more common, is bilateral in up to 60% of cases and typically affects obese children who start walking at an early age, particularly female African-American children.
- The adolescent form typically affects obese African American boys, and is usually unilateral.
- On frontal radiographs, Blount disease is characterized by tibia vara and posteromedial depression of the proximal tibial metaphysis.
- Lateral tibial subluxation and genu recurvatum may be evident in more advanced cases.

Suggested Readings

Cheema JI, Grissom LE, Harcke HT. Radiographic characteristics of lower-extremity bowing in children. *Radiographics.* 2003;23(4):871–880.

Sabharwal S. Blount disease. *J Bone Joint Surg Am.* 2009;91(7):1758–1776.

Unable to supinate or pronate arm, pain and deformity of right hand

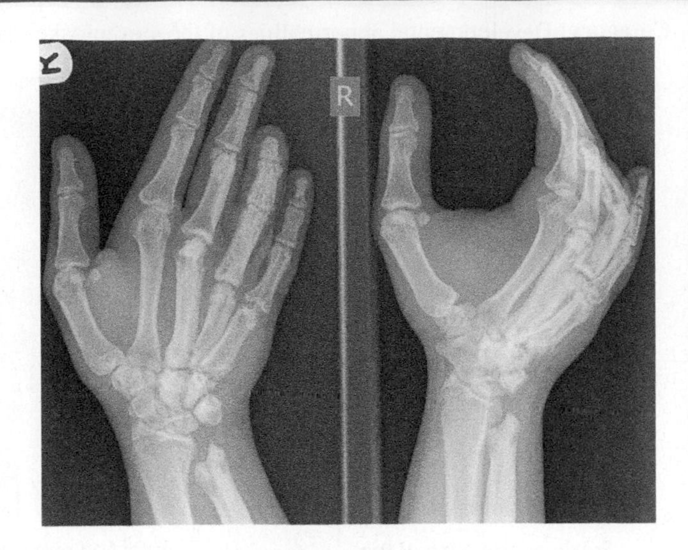

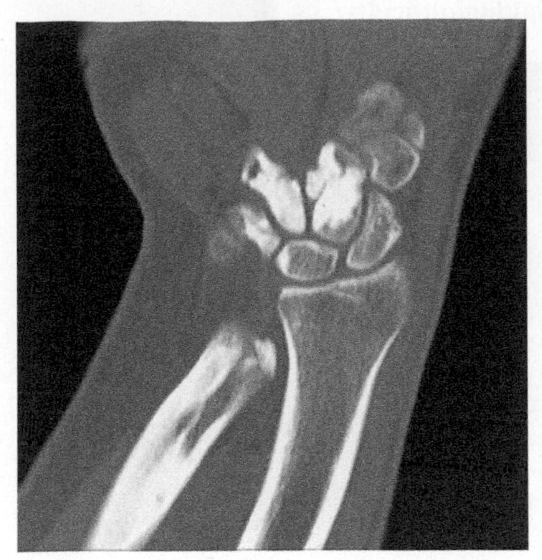

1. What are the radiograph findings?
2. What is the differential diagnosis?
3. What is the most likely diagnosis?
4. What particular anatomic pattern does this disease follow?
5. What are the associations of this entity?

Melorheostosis 1860

Case ranking/difficulty: 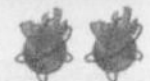 **Category:** Developmental abnormalities of the musculoskeletal system

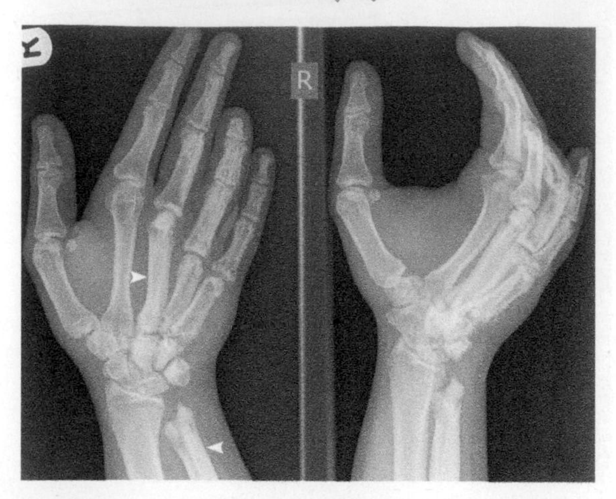

Hypoplastic ulna, fourth and fifth fingers with eccentric sclerosis, and cortical thickening in the fingers, carpus, and ulna giving a "dripping candle wax" appearance.

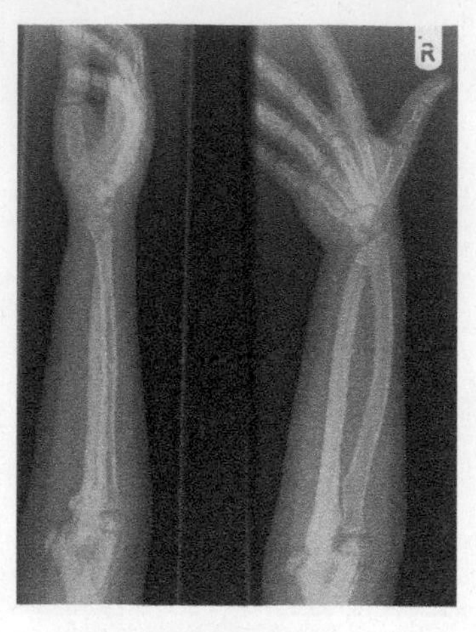

Proximal extension of the sclerosis crossing the elbow joint.

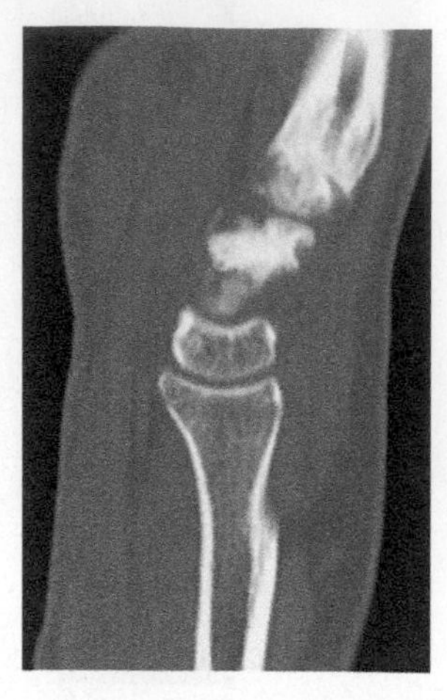

Carpal and metacarpal involvement.

Answers

1. There is a sclerosis of the ulnar aspect of the hand, wrist, and forearm with atrophy of the bones.
2. The differential diagnosis includes neurofibromatosis, fibrous dysplasia, tuberous sclerosis, melorheostosis, and Engelmann disease.
3. The sclerosis and cortical thickening in a sclerotome distribution, demonstrating a "dripping candle wax" appearance, is consistent with melorheostosis. Melorheostosis may cross a joint and result in a joint effusion.
4. The disease usually follows a sensory spinal nerve distribution. The most commonly affected bones are the diaphyses of long bones in the lower extremities but also in the upper extremities and the axial skeleton.
5. Melorheostosis is associated with vascular tumors and malformations of the blood vessels and lymphatics.

   Other sclerotic bone dysplasias such as osteopoikilosis, osteopathia striata, and mixed sclerosing bone dystrophy are associations.

Pearls

- Melorheostosis is a nonhereditary disease of unknown etiology. It is usually an incidental finding. Also known as Leri (first reported in 1922 by Leri and Joanny) disease.
- The condition is associated with mesenchymal dysplastic malformations such as AVM , hemangiomas, and glomus tumor. Young adults or children are commonly affected.
- There is soft tissue and skin thickening, which may be a predominant feature early in the disease.
- There is a typical sclerotic "dripping candle wax" appearance to the long bones, and this follows a spinal sensory nerve distribution. The changes may cross the joint and can cause a joint effusion.
- MR shows heterogeneous signal intensity as a result of a mixture of osseous, fibrous, adipose, and cartilaginous tissues within the lesion.
- The differential diagnosis include neurofibromatosis, fibrous dysplasia, tuberous sclerosis, and Engelmann disease.
- Usually the treatment is conservative, but in extreme cases surgery is required.

Suggested Readings

Abdullah S, Pang GM, Mohamed-Haflah NH, Sapuan J. Melorheostosis of the ulna. *J Chin Med Assoc.* 2011;74(10):469–472.

Ihde LL, Forrester DM, Gottsegen CJ, et al. Sclerosing bone dysplasias: review and differentiation from other causes of osteosclerosis. *Radiographics.* 2011;31(7):1865–1882.

Tekin L, Akarsu S, Durmuş O, Kiralp MZ. Melorheostosis in the hand and forearm. *Am J Phys Med Rehabil.* 2012;91(1):96.

History of deformity and wrist pain

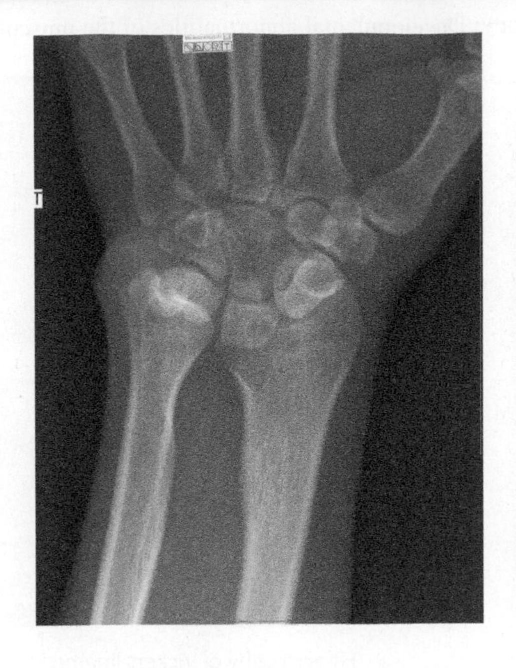

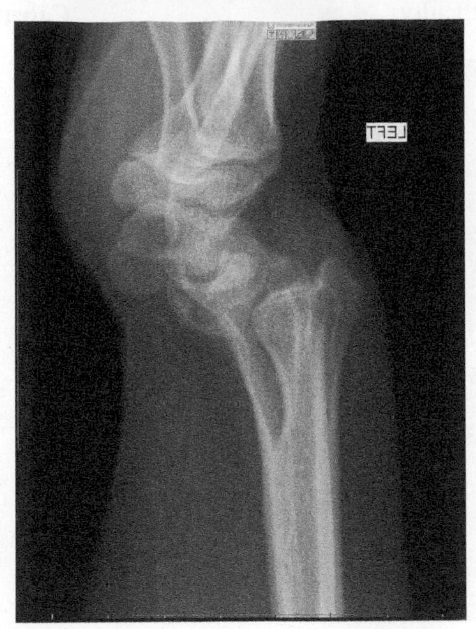

1. What are the radiograph findings?

2. What is the cause of soft-tissue swelling in the volar aspect of the wrist?

3. What are some of the associations of this deformity?

4. How often is this condition bilateral?

5. What are the accepted methods for treatment?

Madelung deformity 1339

Case ranking/difficulty: 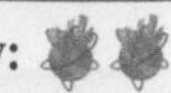

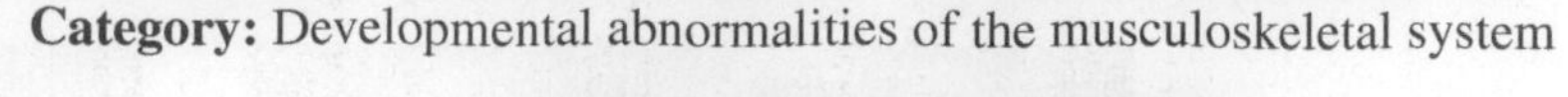

Category: Developmental abnormalities of the musculoskeletal system

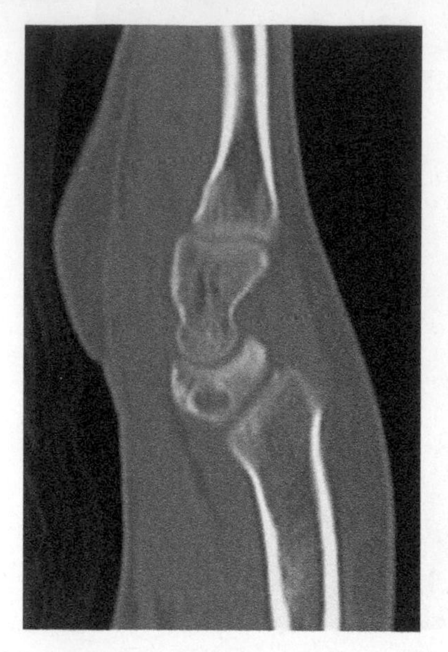

Volar inclination of the radial articular surface.

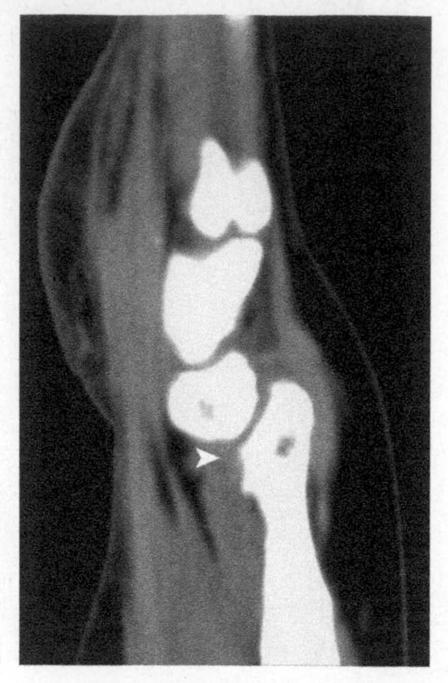

Hypertrophy of Vickers ligament is seen.

Answers

1. There is a "V"-shaped proximal carpal row, with mild relative lengthening and apparent dorsal dislocation of the distal ulna with an increase in the radial inclination, typical for a Madelung deformity.
2. Soft-tissue swelling is caused by hypertrophy of Vickers ligament, the anomalous volar radiolunate, and radiotriquetral ligaments.
3. Multiple hereditary exostoses, Ollier disease, achondroplasia, multiple epiphyseal dysplasia, and the mucopolysaccharidoses are all associations with Madelung deformity.
4. Madelung deformity is bilateral in 50% to 60% of patients.
5. Initially, management is conservative. With progressive or symptomatic disease, surgical techniques include distal ulnar resection, distal radius osteotomy, and the release of Vickers ligament.

Pearls

- Madelung deformity is a rare condition characterized by growth arrest of the medial and volar aspect of the distal radial epiphysis.
- It is bilateral in 50% to 60% of patients.
- This leads to an increased radial inclination, relative ulnar lengthening and apparent dorsal dislocation of the distal ulna. The migration of the proximal carpal row leads to a "V"-shaped configuration of the proximal carpus.
- Soft-tissue swelling in the volar ulnar aspect of the wrist is typically caused by hypertrophy of Vickers ligament (anomalous radiolunate and radiotriquetral ligaments).
- Primary Madelung' deformity is typically inherited as an autosomal dominant condition caused by a mutation on the X chromosome.
- Cases can be post-traumatic and can be seen in a variety of skeletal dysplasias, including multiple hereditary exostoses.

Suggested Readings

Berdon WE, Grossman H, Baker DH. Dyschondrostéose (Leri-Weill syndrome): congenital short forearms, Madelung-type wrist deformities, and moderate dwarfism. *Radiology.* 1965;85(4):677–681.

Landis MS, Etemad-Rezai R, Shetty K, Goldszmidt M. Case 143: Madelung disease. *Radiology.* 2009;250(3):951–954.

Ankle pain after twisting injury

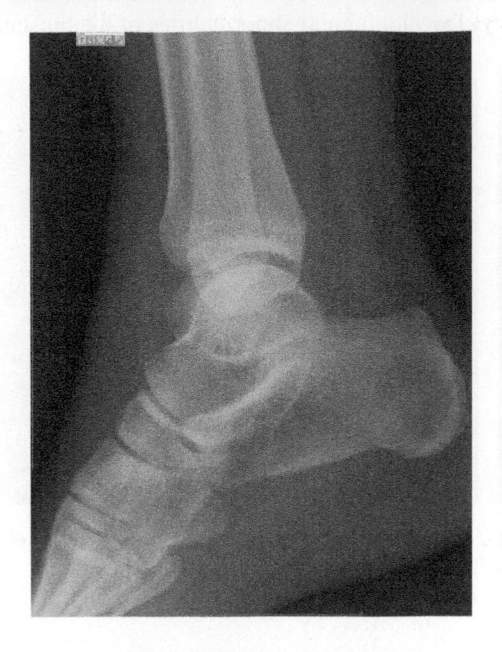

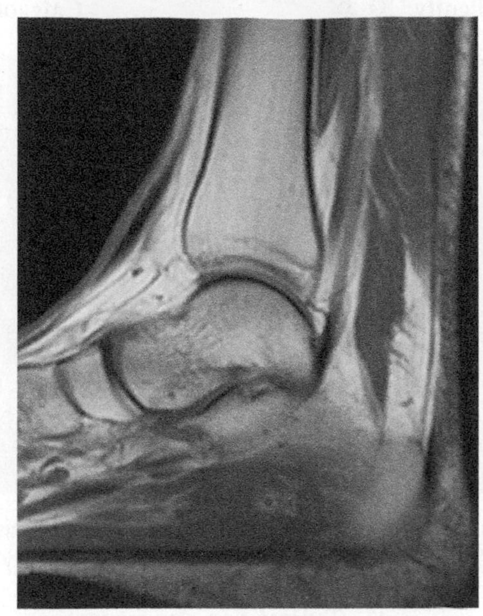

1. What are the plain film and MRI findings?
2. What is the differential diagnosis for this abnormality?
3. What is the most likely diagnosis?
4. How many types of this abnormality are reported in the literature?
5. What is the treatment?

Accessory soleus muscle 1430

Case ranking/difficulty: 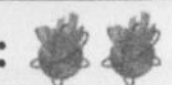 **Category:** Developmental abnormalities of the musculoskeletal system

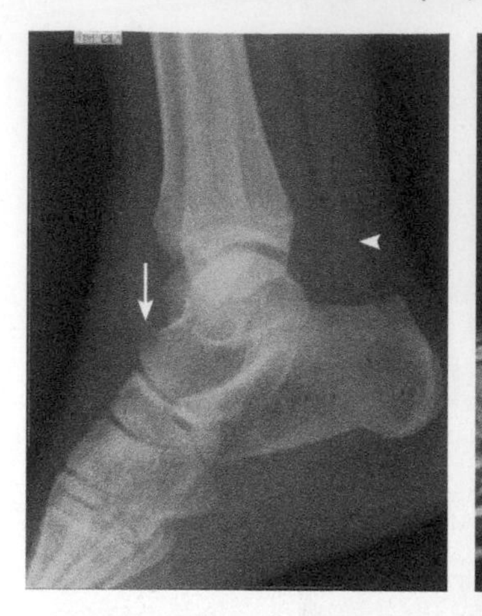

Soft-tissue density in the Kager fat pad (*arrowhead*). Talar neck avulsion fracture noted (*arrow*).

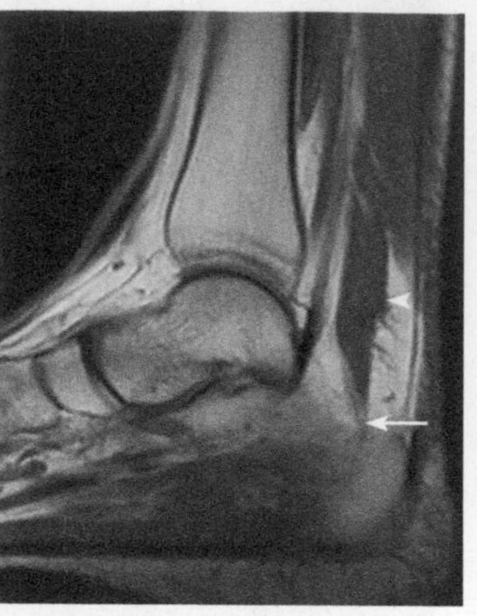

Sagittal T1-weighted image shows a "mass" of muscle signal intensity in the Kager fat pad (*arrowhead*). The insertion is on the superior medial calcaneus (*arrow*).

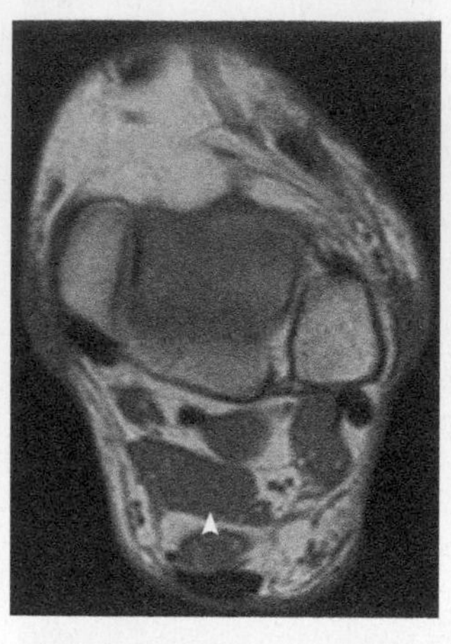

There is a soft-tissue "mass" of muscle signal intensity in the Kager fat pad.

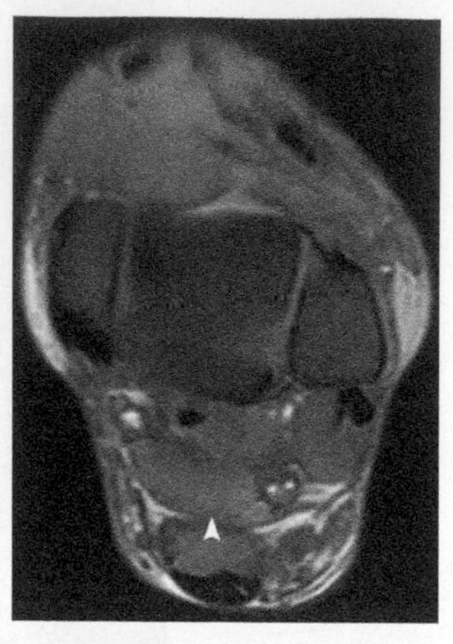

There is no edema in or around the "mass".

Answers

1. There is a soft-tissue abnormality anterior to the Achilles tendon in the Kager fat pad, which is confirmed on MRI to be of muscle signal intensity.
2. A muscle signal intensity lesion posterior to the tibia should suggest an accessory muscle. The tibiocalcaneus internus typically lies deep to the flexor retinaculum, while the accessory soleus lies external to it. The normal muscle signal characteristics make sarcoma unlikely.
3. Based on the signal characteristics and location, an accessory soleus is the most likely diagnosis.
4. Five types of accessory soleus, based on the insertion, are reported. One type is insertion into the Achilles tendon. The other insertions are onto the calcaneus either superiorly or medially. Both can have either a tendinous or muscular insertion.
5. No treatment is required for asymptomatic patients. If the patient develop a compartment syndrome, fasciotomy may be required. Excision or debulking is usually curative.

Pearls

- An accessory soleus is a normal variant that occurs in 0.7% to 5.5% of the population.
- Most patients are asymptomatic, but mass effect may cause a compartment type syndrome or nerve compression.
- The muscle may also be confused with a soft-tissue tumor, except the signal is that of skeletal muscle.
- Five types have been described on the basis of the insertion. These insertions include an insertion into the Achilles tendon or insertion on the superior or medial calcaneus with either a tendinous or fleshy muscular insertion for both.
- A soft-tissue mass of variable size will be seen in the Kager fat pad on plain films.
- The muscle demonstrates typical signal characteristics of muscle on MRI, deep to the Achilles and superficial to the flexor retinaculum more medially.
- Signal characteristics may vary because of trauma, ischemia, or atrophy.

Suggested Readings

Lorentzon R, Wirell S. Anatomic variations of the accessory soleus muscle. *Acta Radiol*. 1987;28(5):627–629.

Sookur PA, Naraghi AM, Bleakney RR, Jalan R, Chan O, White LM. Accessory muscles: anatomy, symptoms, and radiologic evaluation. *Radiographics*. 2008;28(2): 481–499.

Anterior knee pain

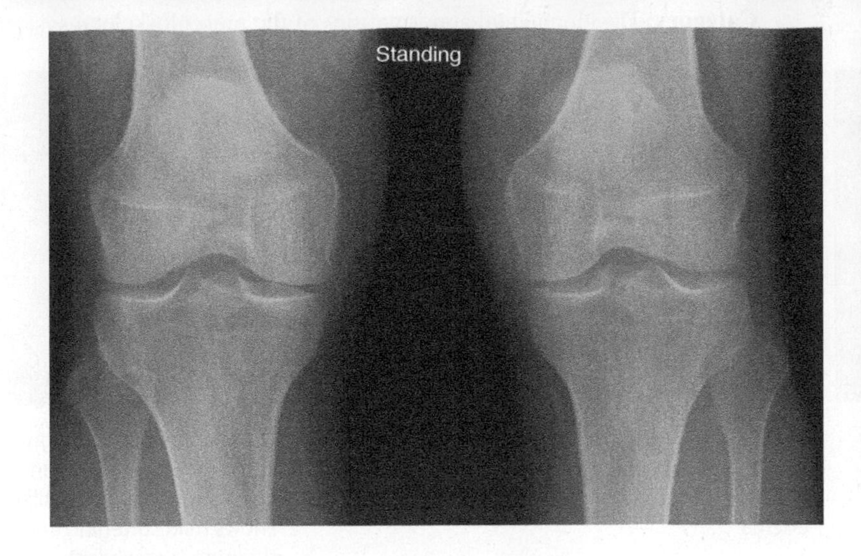

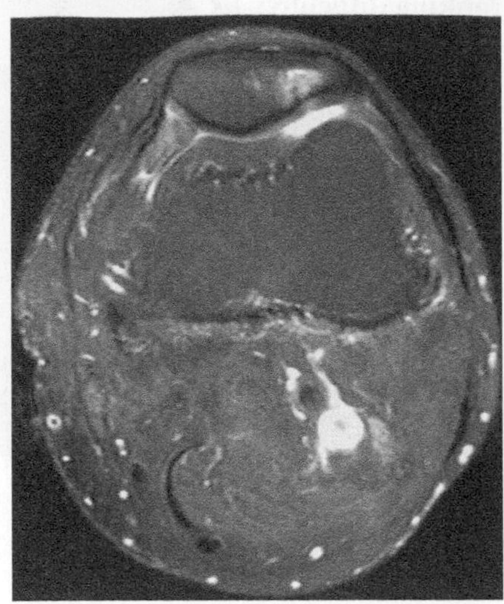

1. What are the radiograph and MRI findings?

2. What are the most likely differentials?

3. What is the proposed etiology of the lesion in the superolateral patella?

4. What are the typical radiological features of this lesion?

5. What is the management?

Dorsal defect of the patella 1349

Case ranking/difficulty: 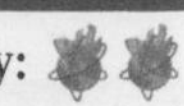

Category: Developmental abnormalities of the musculoskeletal system

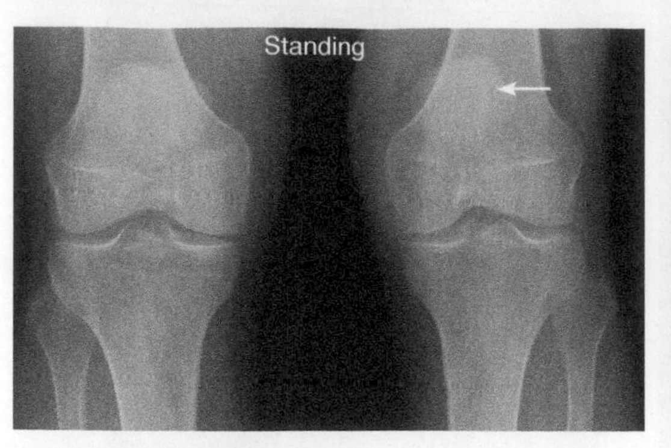

There is a well-defined lucency in the left superolateral patella with a sclerotic rim.

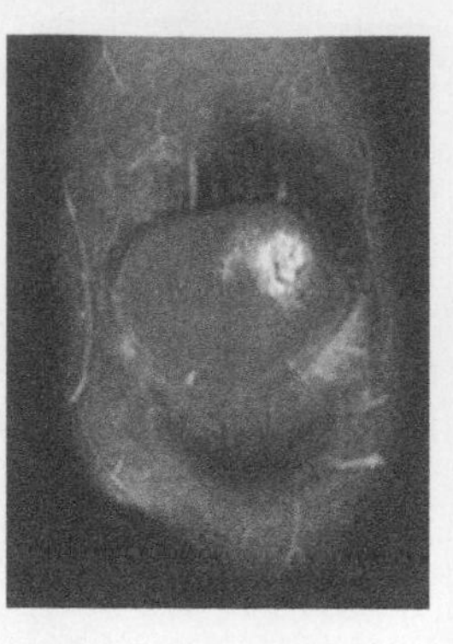

There is lobulated increased T2 signal with mild surrounding edema.

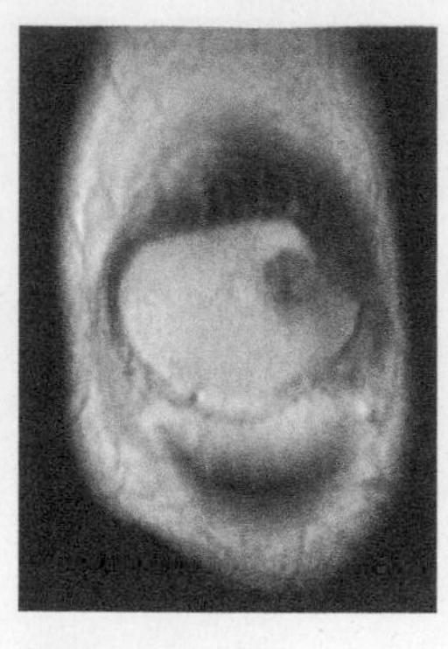

The lesion is T1 isointense to mildly hypointense.

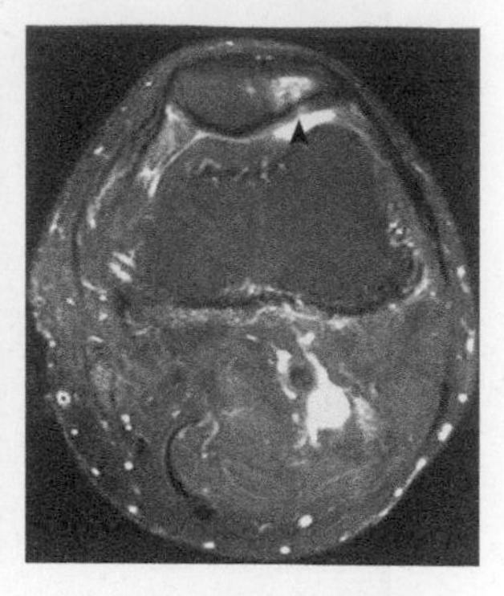

Lobular increased T2 signal with mild edema is again seen. The overlying cartilage shows mild softening and thinning (*arrowhead*).

Answers

1. The plain film shows a well-defined lucent lesion in the superolateral patella, with a sclerotic rim. MRI shows a T2 hyperintense lesion with minimal cartilage thinning over the lesion. There is associate moderate cartilage disease consistent with osteoarthritis in the medial patella facet.
2. The location and MRI findings strongly suggest a dorsal defect of the patella (DDP). Although intact cartilage is usually present over a DDP, it may be mildly thinned and a source of symptoms. The patient also has coincident osteoarthritic change, as evidenced by the more severe medial facet cartilage loss.

   Sinding-Larsen-Johansson syndrome and osteochondritis desiccans of the patella affects the lower pole, and chondromalacia usually affects the ridge between the medial and odd patella facets.
3. Dorsal defects of the patella are presumed to be developmental, although an ischemic etiology has also been proposed.
4. Dorsal defects of the patella are usually well-defined lucent lesions in the superolateral patella, with or without a sclerotic rim. MRI shows T1 hypointensity and T2 hyperintensity similar to the overlying cartilage. However, the T1 signal may be inhomogeneous as a result of fibrosis and necrosis. The overlying cartilage is usually intact, but may be mildly fissured or thinned.
5. Dorsal patella defects often undergo spontaneous resolution, and if symptomatic are treated conservatively. If conservative management fails, curettage of the lesion with debridement of the fibrillated cartilage may be performed.

Pearls

- DDP is likely a developmental phenomenon, but ischemia has also been proposed.
- Affects young patients, ages 10 to 20 years. Bilateral in 25% to 33%.
- Well-defined lesion in the superolateral patella with or without a sclerotic rim on plain films.
- On MRI, the lesion is T1 hypointense or inhomogeneous and T2 hyperintense, mirroring the overlying cartilage, which is generally intact, but which also may be thinned or fissured.
- The associated cartilage disease may be the source of anterior knee pain, not the DDP.
- Spontaneous resolution is typical

Suggested Readings

Hedayati B, Saifuddin A. Focal lesions of the patella. *Skeletal Radiol.* 2009;38(8):741–749.

Ho VB, Kransdorf MJ, Jelinek JS, Kim CK. Dorsal defect of the patella: MR features. *J Comput Assist Tomogr.* 1991;15(3):474–476.

Incidental finding on MRI scan for wrist pain

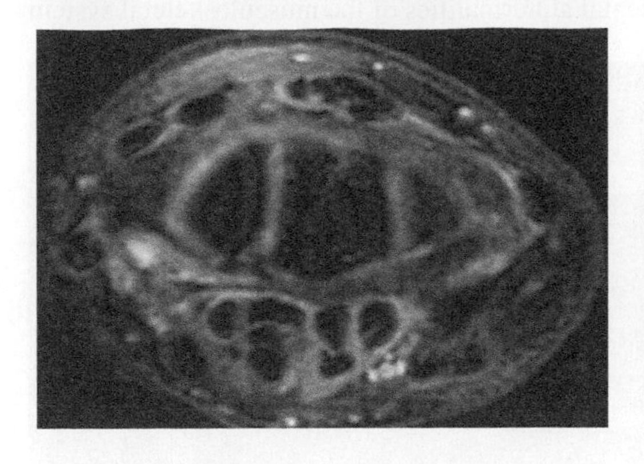

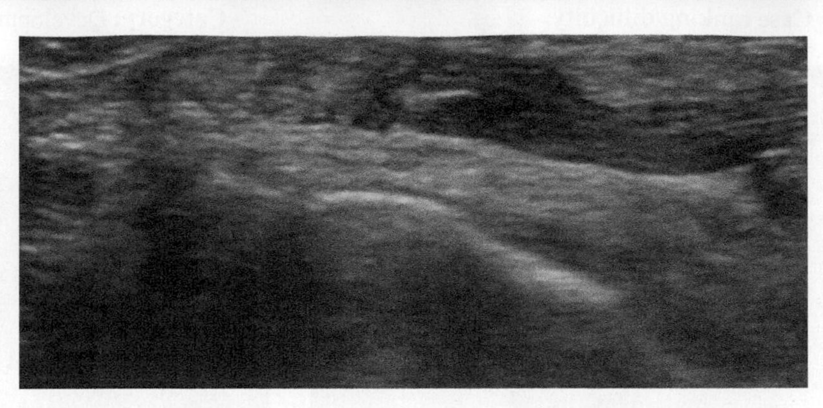

1. What is the abnormality?
2. What is the incidence of this anomaly?
3. What percentage of this anomaly is bilateral?
4. Which nerve is compressed in fourth extensor compartment syndrome?
5. What are the main differential diagnoses of this anomaly?

Extensor digitorum brevis manus (EDBM) 1449

Case ranking/difficulty: 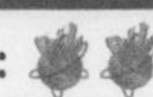 **Category:** Developmental abnormalities of the musculoskeletal system

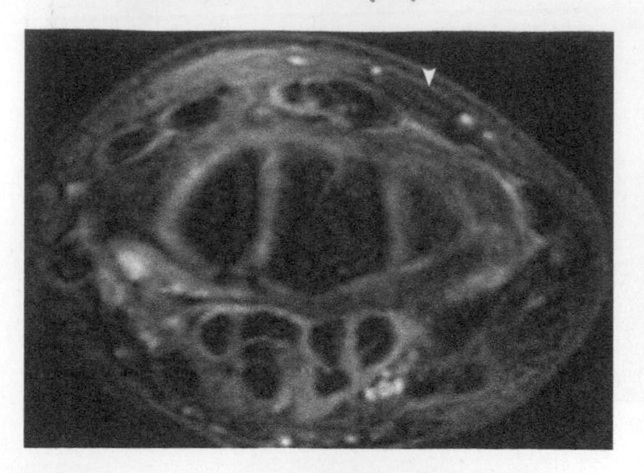

EDBM demonstrated on STIR images.

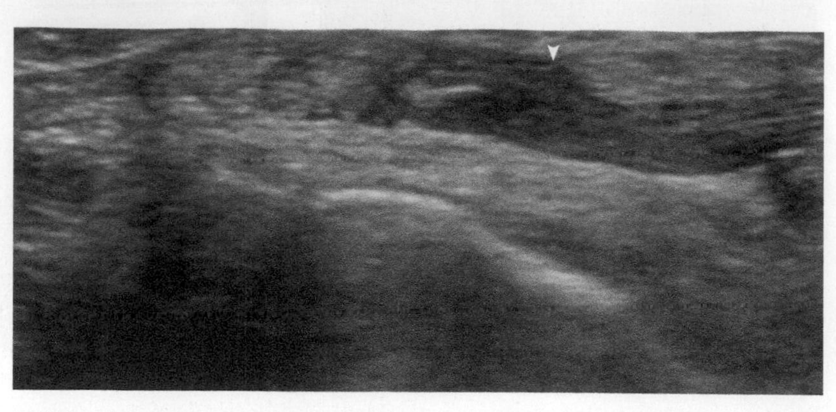

EDBM on longitudinal ultrasound images.

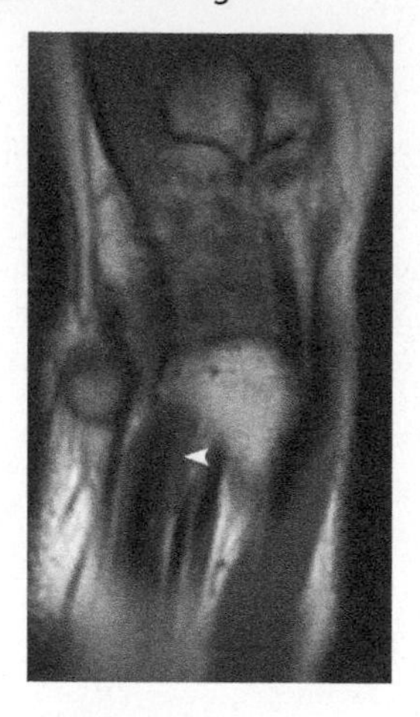

EDBM muscle.

Answers

1. Extensor wrist accessory muscle: the extensor digitorum brevis manus muscle (EDBM).
2. The incidence is 2% to 3% of the general population.
3. One-half to one-third of cases of EDBM are bilateral.
4. The posterior interosseous nerve is compressed in fourth compartment syndrome. One of the causes of this compartment syndrome is the EDBM anomalous muscle.
5. Ganglion cysts on the dorsum of the wrist and giant cell tumor are clinical differentials. Giant cell tumor (GCT) is difficult to differentiate on imaging, as it has similar low or intermediate signal on T1- and T2-weighted sequences to EDBM. However, on gradient-echo sequences, GCT typically shows susceptibility artifact.

   A soft-tissue sarcoma is also in the differential, although the muscle signal intensity and lack of edema in EDBM will differentiate it. Other anomalous muscles in this region include extensor pollicis indices accessorius and extensor indices et medii communis.

Pearls

- EDBM is a rare accessory muscle on the dorsum of the wrist.
- EDBM usually originates from the dorsum of the wrist capsule, dorsal wrist ligaments, and the scaphoid and lunate, and inserts into the ulnar aspect of the proximal phalanx of the index finger. It can also insert into the third, fourth, or fifth fingers.
- EDBM usually lies in the fourth compartment. The muscle can present as a mass or a ganglion clinically.
- It is slightly more common in males and is seen in 2% to 3% of the population. One-half to one-third of cases are reported to be bilateral.
- Ultrasound can be helpful. MRI is the gold standard and shows a low/isointense oval lesion on T1- and T2-weighted sequences, unless there is edema, for example, from trauma.
- If it is still difficult to confirm on standard imaging, then electromyography can be helpful.
- EDBM can cause fourth compartment syndrome by directly or indirectly compressing the posterior interosseous nerve.
- In such cases, decompression of the extensor retinaculum or excision of the EDBM is performed.

Suggested Readings

Anderson MW, Benedetti P, Walter J, Steinberg DR. MR appearance of the extensor digitorum manus brevis muscle: a pseudotumor of the hand. *AJR Am J Roentgenol.* 1995;164(6):1477–1479.

Ouellette H, Thomas BJ, Torriani M. Using dynamic sonography to diagnose extensor digitorum brevis manus. *AJR Am J Roentgenol.* 2003;181(5):1224–1226.

Irritable child

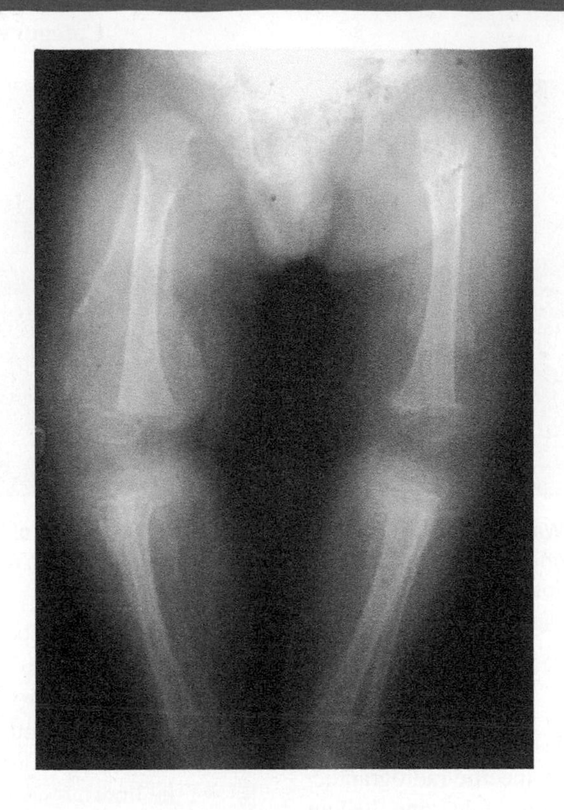

1. What are the radiographic features?

2. What is the differential diagnosis?

3. What are the expected MRI findings?

4. What is the diagnosis?

5. What are the risk factors for this condition?

Scurvy 1737

Case ranking/difficulty: 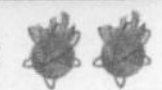

Category: Metabolic conditions affecting bone

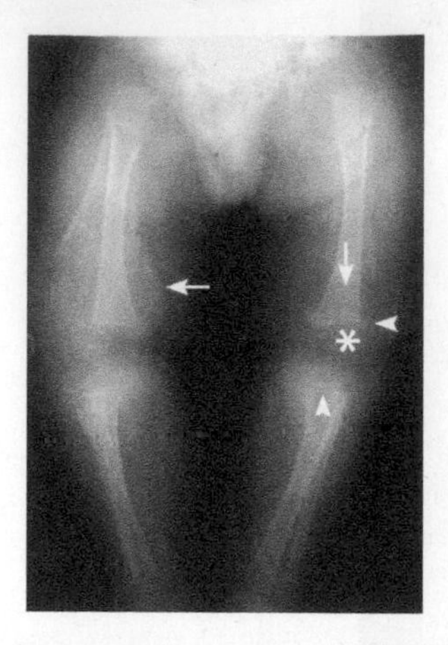

There is ground-glass osteopenic bone, Wimberger sign (*asterisk*), Frankel line (*arrowhead*), Trümmerfeld zone (*arrow*), and Pelkan spurs (*right arrowhead*). There is also periosteal detachment secondary to subperiosteal hemorrhage (*left arrow*).

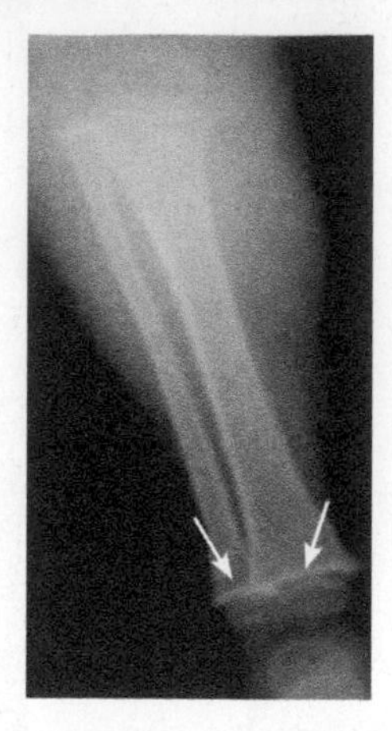

Prominent white lines of Frankel in the tibia and fibula (*arrows*). (Images courtesy of Dr. Akbar Bonakdarpour.)

Answers

1. There is a generalized "ground-glass" osteopenic appearance of the bones. There are specific radiographic features of a Wimberger sign, Trümmerfeld zone, Pelkan spur, Frankel line, and subperiosteal hematoma.
2. The differential diagnoses include scurvy, rickets, leukemia, infection, and neuroblastoma.
3. The MRI features are nonspecific and include heterogeneous T1- and T2-weighted marrow signal, metaphyseal signal changes, subperiosteal hematoma, and periostitis.
4. The clinical and radiographic appearance is consistent with a diagnosis of scurvy.
5. Unlike rickets, the risk factors include non-breastfed babies. It may also be present in alcoholics and smokers (smoking reducing vitamin C absorption and increases its catabolism). Patients with anorexia nervosa, thyrotoxicosis, and type 1 diabetes are also at a higher risk. Reduced dietary intake, inflammatory bowel disease, and malabsorption syndrome also increases the risk of vitamin C deficiency.

Pearls

- Scurvy is caused by vitamin C deficiency, and usually affects infants 6 to 9 months of age. Younger children are protected by maternal vitamin C.
- Vitamin C is important for collagen synthesis, hence its deficiency will lead to compromise of skin, vascular, bone, and joint integrity. The main clinical features are gum bleeding in an irritable child and pseudoparalysis of the limbs.
- Radiographically, there is a ground-glass osteopenic appearance of bones with decreased cortical thickness. In adults, sometimes osteoporosis is the only feature.
- The following are classic features of scurvy on X-ray.
  - Trümmerfeld zone, which is caused by subepiphyseal infarction, and manifests as a radiolucent zone on the metaphyseal side of the Frankel white line.
  - White line of Frankel, a dense metaphyseal line of provisional calcification.
  - Wimberger sign, a loss of epiphyseal density with a pencil-thin cortex.
  - Pelkan spurs caused by fractures at the lucent metaphysis, leading to a cupping appearance of the metaphysis.
  - Periosteal detachment caused by subperiosteal bleeding and hematoma.
- On MRI, there is a nonspecific heterogeneous bone marrow signal on T1- and T2-weighted images. There is also subperiosteal hematoma and periostitis.

Suggested Readings

Fain O. Musculoskeletal manifestations of scurvy. *Joint Bone Spine.* 2005;72(2):124–128.

Karthiga S, Dubey S, Garber S, Watts R. Scurvy: MRI appearances. *Rheumatology (Oxford).* 2008;47(7):1109.

Increasing pain in the shoulder

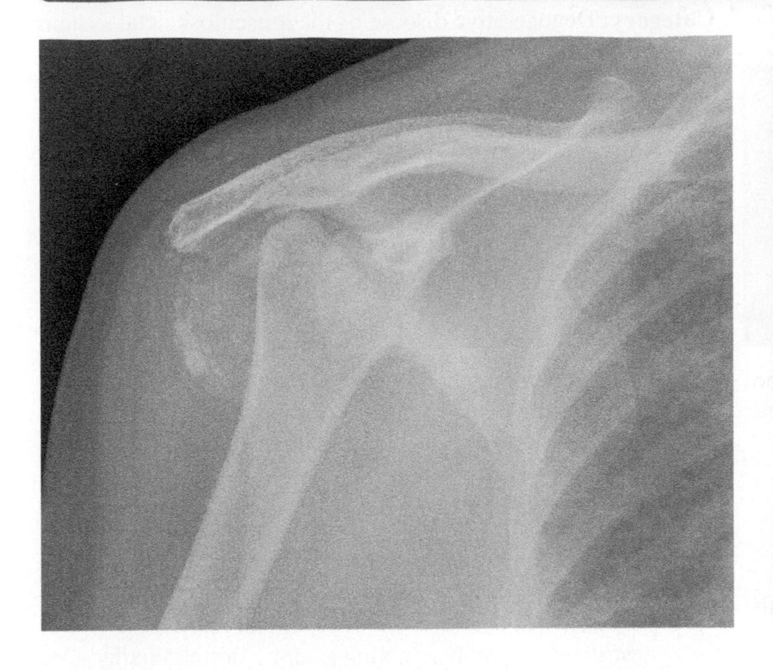

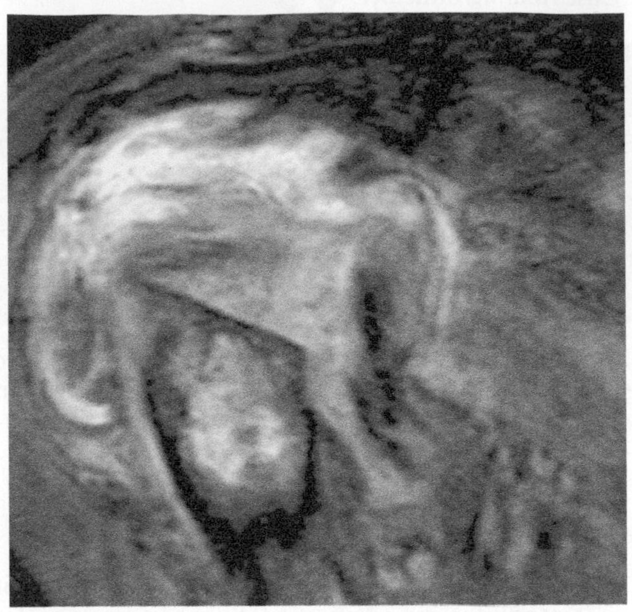

1. What are the pertinent radiograph findings?

2. What are the MRI findings?

3. What is the most likely diagnosis?

4. What is the likely etiology of this entity?

5. How is the diagnosis made?

Milwaukee shoulder 1548

Case ranking/difficulty: 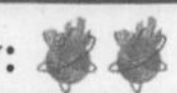

Category: Degenerative disease of the musculoskeletal system

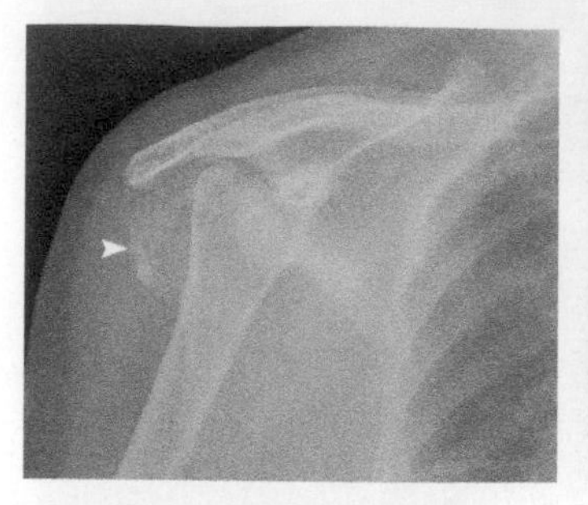

Destruction of the shoulder joint with calcifications (*arrowhead*) and joint effusion.

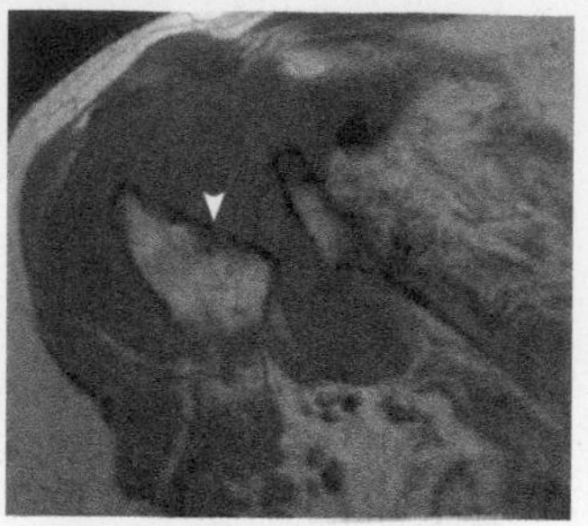

Rotator cuff tear, joint effusion and sharply demarcated bone destruction (*arrowhead*).

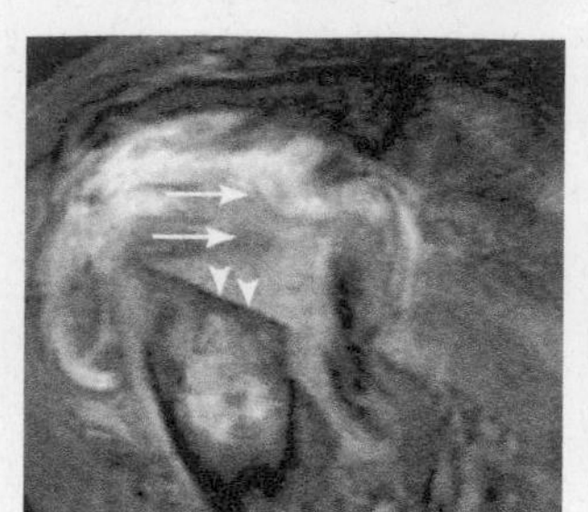

Destruction of the rotator cuff (*arrows*). Sharply demarcated subchondral bone destruction (*arrowheads*) with edema.

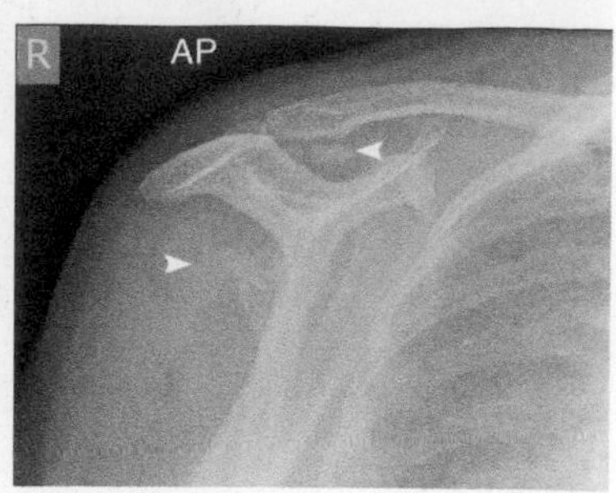

Y view of the shoulder confirming the calcifications in the rotator cuff and the shoulder joint.

Answers

1. There is a destruction of the proximal humeral head with joint effusion and calcification. A sharply demarcated destruction of the proximal humerus is seen.
2. There is a complete destruction of the rotator cuff with joint effusion, bone marrow edema, and calcification around and in the joint space.
3. The presence of periarticular calcifications with dramatic effusions and joint destruction is consistent with Milwaukee syndrome. Septic arthritis can have a similar appearance clinically and radiologically, and the sharply demarcated humeral destruction can also raise the possibility of atrophic neuroarthropathy. Avascular necrosis with collapse and fragmentation, or rapidly destructive osteoarthritis are also in the differential.
4. Milwaukee shoulder is believed to be a result of intra-articular deposition of calcium hydroxyapatite crystals. These crystals incite a dramatic inflammatory reaction, with the release of cytokines that causes bone and rotator cuff destruction. Trauma, CPPD (calcium pyrophosphate deposition disease), dialysis, and denervation have also been proposed as predisposing events.
5. The diagnosis is made with joint aspiration and is confirmed by alizarin red staining.

Pearls

- Milwaukee shoulder is a syndrome of shoulder destruction resulting from periarticular and intra-articular deposition of calcium hydroxyapatite crystals. The crystals present in the rotator cuff enter the joint space and incite a marked inflammatory response with the release of cytokines. This results in rapid bone destruction, often resembling a septic or neuropathic arthritis. The rotator cuff is also usually completely disrupted.
- This rapid destructive process usually affects elderly females. The clinical presentation is pain, stiffness, and swelling of the shoulder.
- Plain film radiography shows destructive changes, soft-tissue calcification, joint effusion, and superior migration of the humeral head as a result of a complete loss of the rotator cuff, with a sharp margin of the proximal humerus because of destruction of the subchondral bone. The sharp demarcating margin and rapid presentation can be confused with an atrophic neuropathic joint, or rapidly destructive osteoarthritis (RDO).
- MRI will confirm the complete rotator cuff tear as well demonstrate loose bodies and effusion. It also outlines marked marrow edema and cartilage loss on cartilage-sensitive sequences.
- The diagnosis can be confirmed with joint aspiration and staining with alizarin red staining.
- Treatment includes conservative measures, such as analgesics and steroids, and in extreme cases, partial or total arthroplasty.

Suggested Readings

McCarty DJ. Milwaukee shoulder syndrome. *Trans Am Clin Climatol Assoc.* 1991;102(102):271–283; discussion 283–284.

Nguyen VD. Rapid destructive arthritis of the shoulder. *Skeletal Radiol.* 1996;25(2):107–112.

Pain and stiffness of the second and third metacarpophalangeal joints

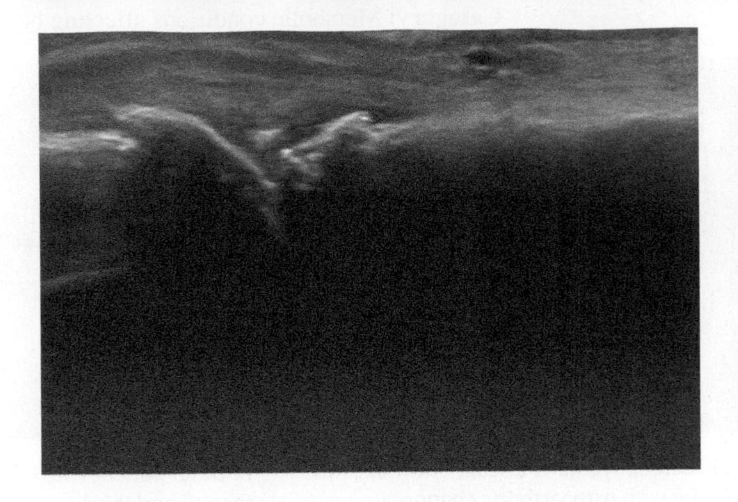

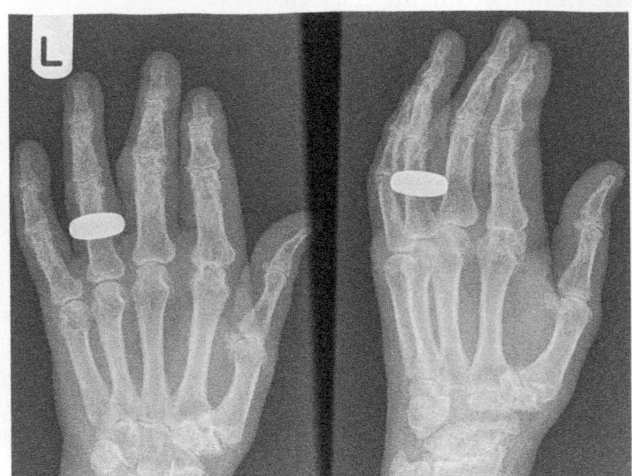

1. What are the radiographic findings?
2. What is the differential diagnosis?
3. What is the most likely diagnosis?
4. What other tests can be used to confirm this diagnosis?
5. What are the other complications of this condition?

Hemochromatosis-induced arthritis 1730

Case ranking/difficulty: 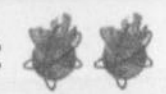

Category: Metabolic conditions affecting bone

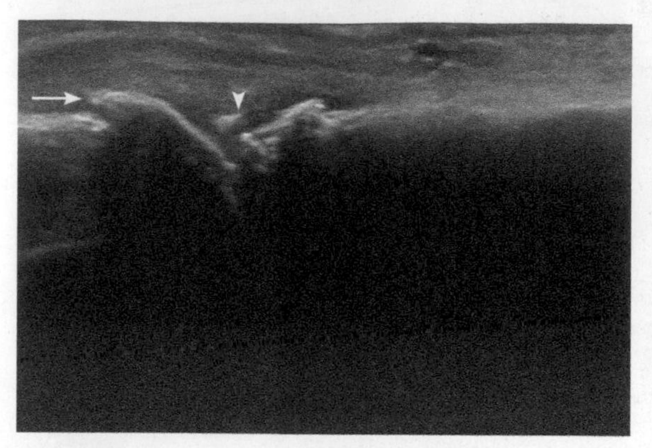

Degenerative changes with chondrocalcinosis (*arrowhead*) and a "hook" osteophyte (*arrow*).

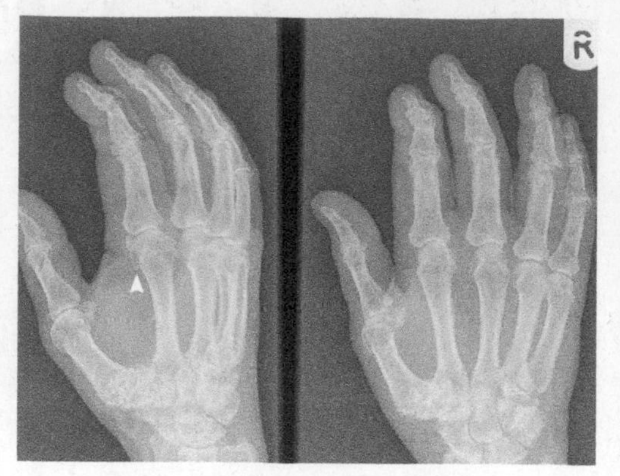

"Hook" osteophyte (*arrowhead*) at the second MCP joint with osteoarthritic changes.

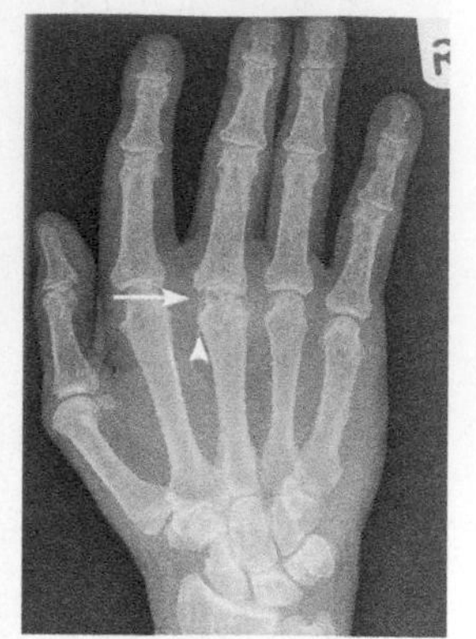

Another patient with second and third metacarpophalangeal joint osteoarthritic changes (*arrow*) and with "hook" osteophytes (*arrowhead*).

Answers

1. There are multiple subchondral cysts, subchondral sclerosis, and chondrocalcinosis with osteoarthritic change. There are "hook" osteophytes of the second and third MCP heads. No subluxation or erosions.
2. Osteoarthritis, gout, CPPD (calcium pyrophosphate dihydrate deficiency arthropathy), psoriasis, and hemochromatosis are included in the differential diagnosis.
3. The presence of second and third metacarpal joint osteoarthritis with "hook" osteophytes and chondrocalcinosis strongly suggests hemochromatosis. CPPD can also have a similar appearance, and distinction is often based on clinical features.
4. Serum ferritin level, liver MRI with T2* and inphase and outphase images. Ultrasound can show cirrhosis of the liver. Ultrasound guided biopsy also helps to obtain tissue for histological diagnosis.
5. Deposition of iron in the skin can result in a change in skin pigmentation. Deposition in the pancreas, myocardium, and liver can, respectively, cause diabetes (combined with a change in pigmentation, this is called "bronze" diabetes) congestive cardiac failure and cirrhosis of the liver. There is also a predisposition to hepatocellular carcinoma.

Pearls

- Hemochromatosis is a condition where there is an abnormal deposition of iron in nonreticuloendothelial cells.
- It could be either primary (autosomal recessive, short-arm chromosome 6 defect) or secondary as a result of multiple blood transfusions, increased intake of iron intake as in Bantu siderosis, or increased demands in thalassemic patients.
- Fifty percent have manifestations in skeletal system.
- Typically there are "hook-like" osteophytes on the radial aspect of the enlarged metacarpal heads of the second and third metacarpals. There are also associated degenerative changes within the second and third metacarpophalangeal joints
- Chondrocalcinosis is seen in the knee and wrist joints. Calcification of the triangular fibrocartilage (TFCC), Achilles tendon, and ligamentum flavum are also features of hemochromatosis.
- Treatment usually involves multiple phlebotomies and the use of chelating agents such as desferrioxamine. Five-year survival rate is 33% to 89%.

Suggested Readings

Dähnert W. *Radiology Review Manual*. Baltimore, MD: Lippincott Williams & Wilkins; (2007).

Mrabet D, Zouch I, Sahli H, et al. Rheumatic manifestations of genetic hemochromatosis [in French]. *Tunis Med.* 2011;89(12):891–895.

Schubert R, Mommsen C. Skeletal roentgen and scintigraphy findings in hemochromatosis [in German]. *Rofo.* 2012;184(2):143–145.

Generalized joint pain and soft tissue swelling

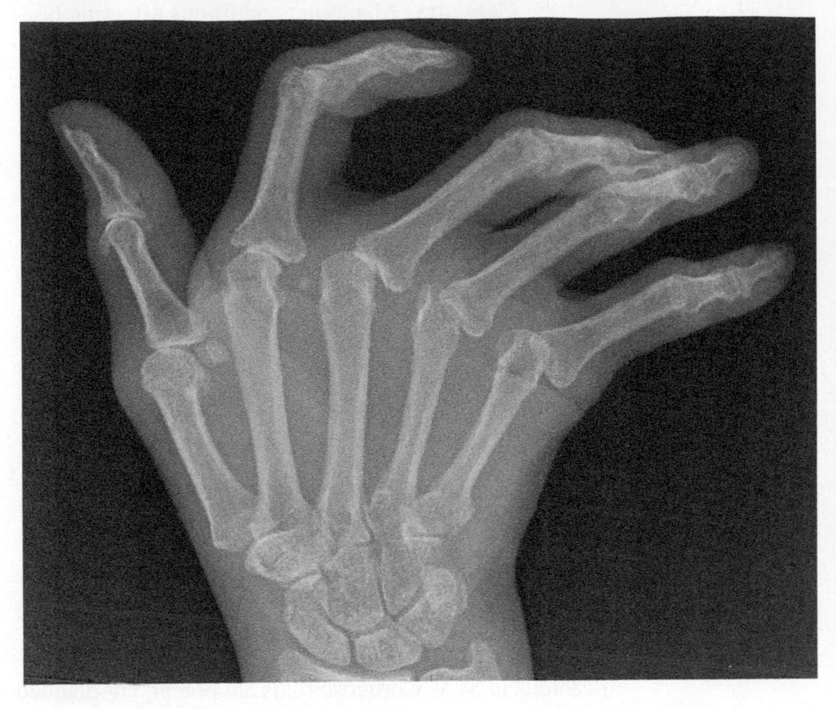

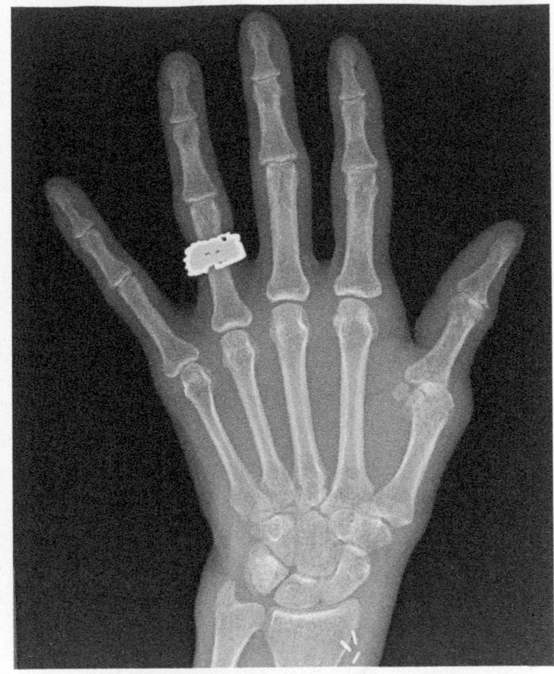

1. What are the clinical features of this entity?

2. What percentage of patients with this cutaneous disorder have musculoskeletal manifestations of the disease?

3. What is Jaccoud arthropathy?

4. What are the risk factors for this systemic disease?

5. What is the disease-suppressing drug of choice in this condition?

SLE arthritis 1718

Case ranking/difficulty: 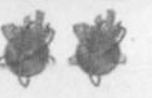

Category: Metabolic conditions affecting bone

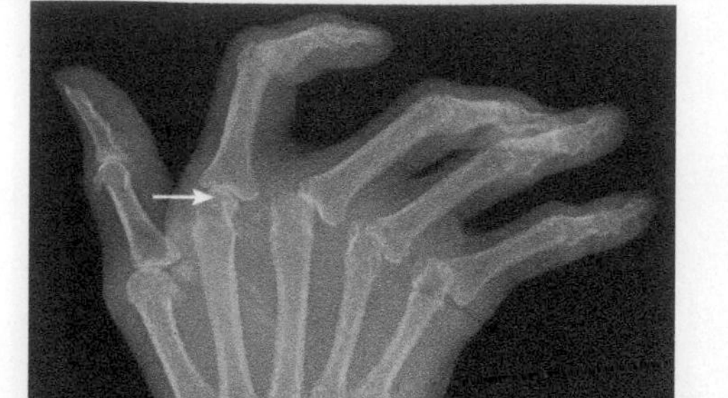

Deforming arthropathy at the MCP joints with ulnar deviation, a feature indistinguishable from rheumatoid arthritis. More commonly, SLE is a nondeforming arthropathy.

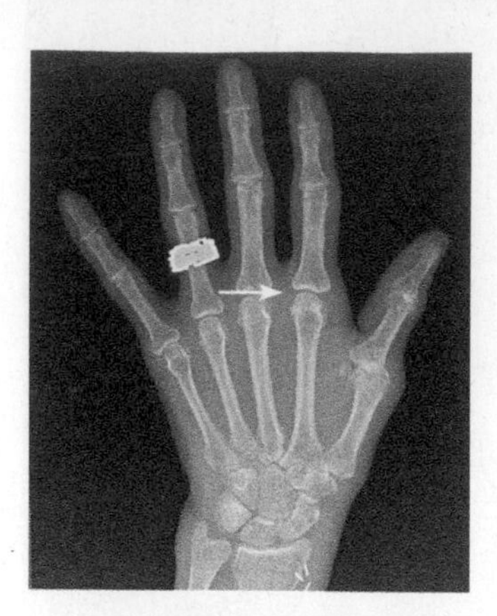

Soft-tissue swelling is noted at MCP joints.

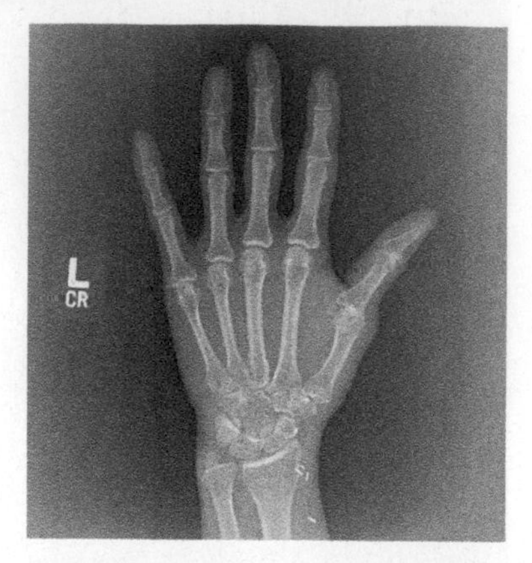

Normal hands are noted from this patient just 18 months previously, demonstrating the speed at which SLE arthritis can ensue.

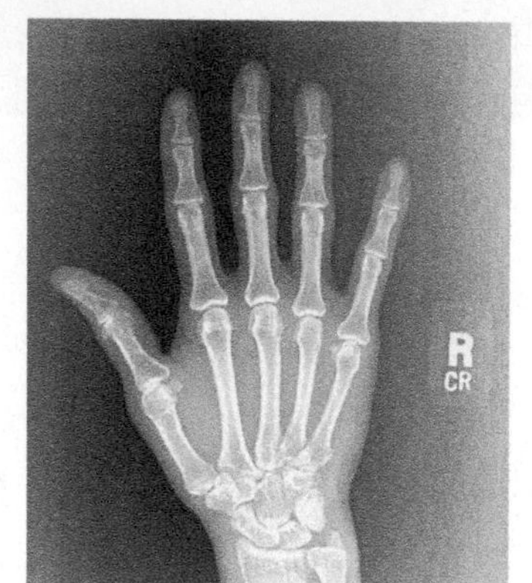

Normal hands previously.

Answers

1. Lupus arthritis is a symmetrical, usually non-deforming and non-erosive polyarthropathy. Occasionally it can be a deforming, non-erosive arthropathy. It is often clinically and radiologically indistinguishable from rheumatoid arthritis. Soft-tissue swelling, juxta-articular osteoporosis, and soft-tissue calcification are characteristic, although non-specific, features.
2. A large proportion of patients with SLE have musculoskeletal manifestations of the disease. These include a polyarthritis and osteonecrosis, although the latter may be in part related to corticosteroid usage.
3. Strictly speaking, Jaccoud arthropathy was initially described as a complication of recurrent rheumatic fever. It may be seen with erosive lupus arthritis but is more likely to be seen with rheumatoid and psoriatic arthritis.
4. SLE is more prevalent in females (90% of cases), those with a family history, Afro-Caribbean people and with high estrogen levels.
5. Hydroxychloroquine is an antimalarial, but particularly efficacious in SLE. Corticosteroids are potent, but plagued by a large side-effect profile, limiting their prolonged use.

Pearls

- SLE arthritis is clinically and radiologically difficult to separate from rheumatoid arthritis.
- Classical features are of a symmetrical, non-deforming, non-erosive arthropathy, in which soft-tissue swelling is a key finding.
- Some 10% of cases are erosive; these are indistinguishable from rheumatoid arthritis; 80% of all SLE sufferers will develop an arthritis.
- Complications of SLE include osteonecrosis, and this must be remembered when reading imaging studies in patients with this condition.
- Diagnosis of SLE is made by the presence of antinuclear antibodies (ANAs). Radiology is supportive, but not specific for this diagnosis.

Suggested Readings

Cronin ME. Musculoskeletal manifestations of systemic lupus erythematosus. *Rheum Dis Clin North Am.* 1988;14(1):99–116.

Salesi M, Karimifar M, Mottaghi P, Sayedbonakdar Z, Karimzadeh H. A case of SLE with bilateral osteonecrosis of femoral heads and bone infarct in distal of femur. *Rheumatol Int.* 2010;30(4):527–529.

van Vugt RM, Derksen RH, Kater L, Bijlsma JW. Deforming arthropathy or lupus and rhupus hands in systemic lupus erythematosus. *Ann Rheum Dis.* 1998;57(9):540–544.

History of chronic bilateral hand pain

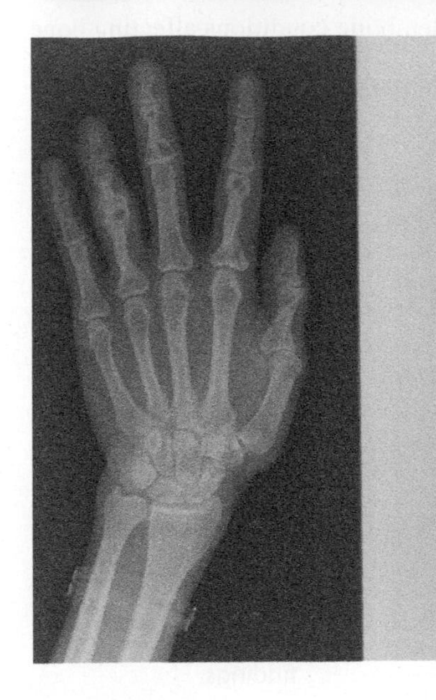
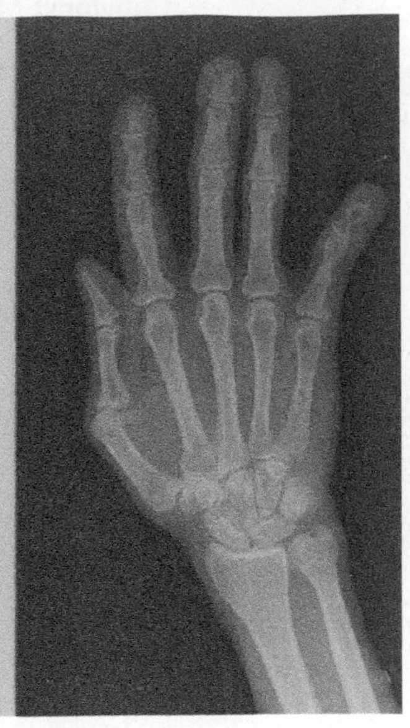
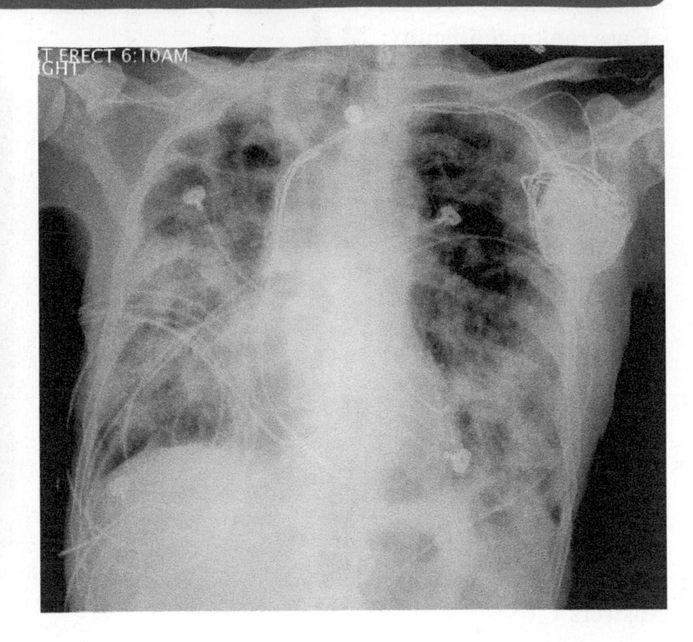

1. What are the demonstrated radiographic features?

2. What is the differential diagnosis?

3. What is the most likely diagnosis?

4. What features are included in Lofgren syndrome?

5. What are the MRI characteristics of intramuscular lesions in this entity?

Sarcoid 1534

Case ranking/difficulty: 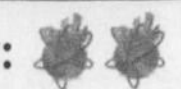

Category: Metabolic conditions affecting bone

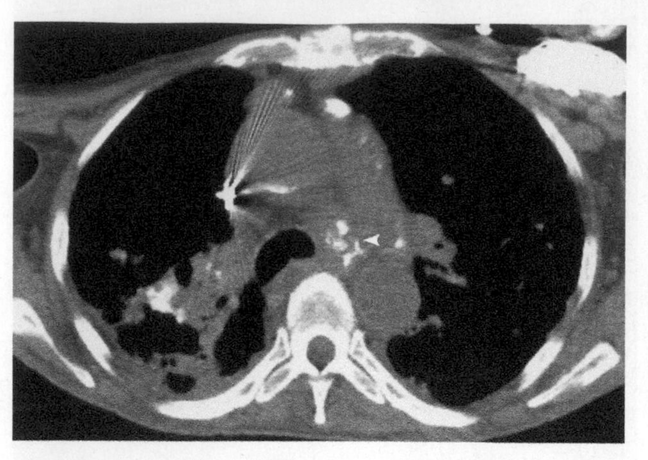

Calcified mediastinal adenopathy.

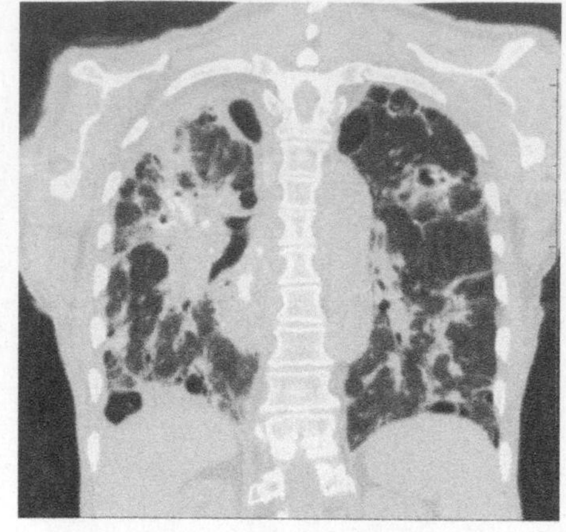

Extensive fibrotic lung disease.

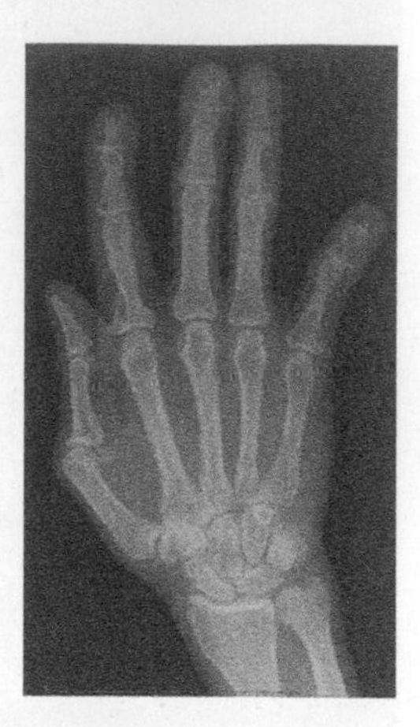

Radiograph of the right hand six years prior shows identical findings.

Answers

1. Lace-like trabecular pattern with intraosseous lucencies, acro-osteolysis, and bone sclerosis. The joint spaces are normal.
2. Sarcoid, hemangiomatosis, and multiple enchondromatosis are the likely differentials. Multiple lucencies with sclerotic rims would be very unusual for metastatic disease or infection. Fibrous dysplasia is possible, but this degree of bone destruction would be unlikely.
3. The most likely diagnosis is osseous sarcoid.
4. The combination of an acute arthritis, erythema nodosum, and lymphadenopathy in sarcoid is known as Lofgren syndrome.
5. Intramuscular sarcoid granulomas are centrally T1 and T2 hypointense, with peripheral T2 hyperintensity and contrast enhancement. This MR appearance has been called a "dark star."

Pearls

- Sarcoid results in the deposition of noncaseating granulomas in multiple organ systems.
- The lungs, skin, lymph nodes, and eyes are most affected, but the musculoskeletal system is also affected, usually in the presence of pulmonary or systemic disease.
- The distal bones of the hands and feet are most commonly affected.
- A lacelike trabecular pattern with multiple well-defined "cysts" are seen.
- Intracortical tunneling, bony remodeling and acro-osteolysis are features. Joint spaces are preserved.
- Bones may appear sclerotic in chronic cases.
- Patients may develop an acute or chronic arthritis.
- Acute arthritis, erythema nodosum, and lymphadenopathy together is known as Lofgren syndrome.
- Radiographic manifestations of chronic arthritis are uncommon, but mild osteopenia and erosions of the knees, ankles, and PIP joints may be seen.
- Myositis and muscles granulomas can occur. The "dark star" appearance of muscle granulomas is central T1 and T2 hypointensity, with peripheral T2 hyperintensity and contrast enhancement.

Suggested Readings

Jelinek JS, Mark AS, Barth WF. Sclerotic lesions of the cervical spine in sarcoidosis. *Skeletal Radiol.* 1998;27(12):702–704.

Pires-Gonçalves L, Watt I. Osseous sarcoidosis. *Acta Reumatol Port.* 2011;36(2):187–188.

Back pain and stiffness

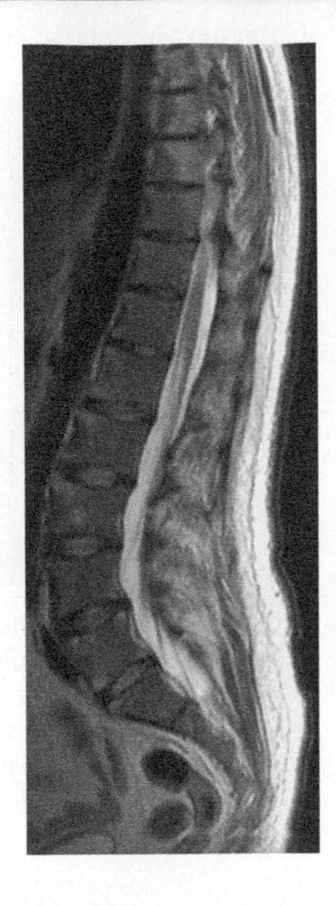

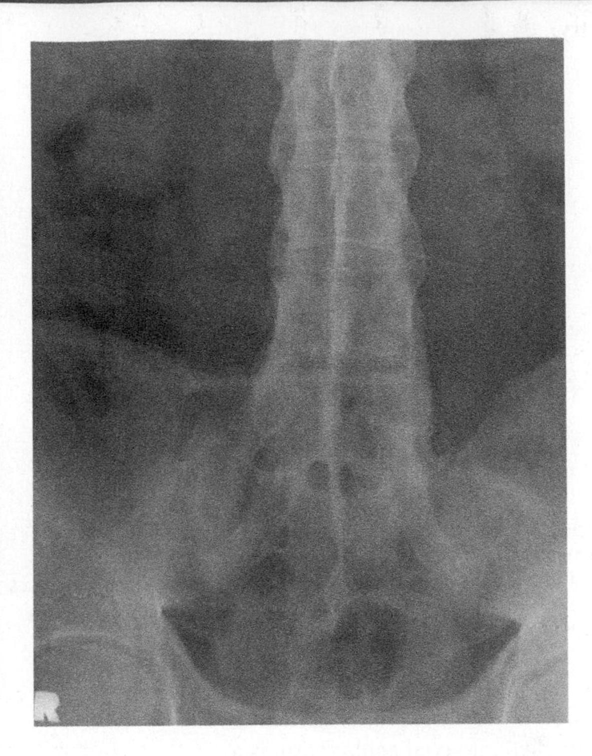

1. What are classical features of this condition?

2. Which diseases are associated with HLA-B27 positivity?

3. What are the possible treatments of this condition?

4. What are the local and systemic complications of this condition?

5. Which groups of patients have the highest levels of HLA-B27 concordance?

Ankylosing spondylitis 467

Case ranking/difficulty: 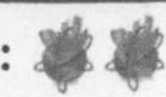

Category: Metabolic conditions affecting bone

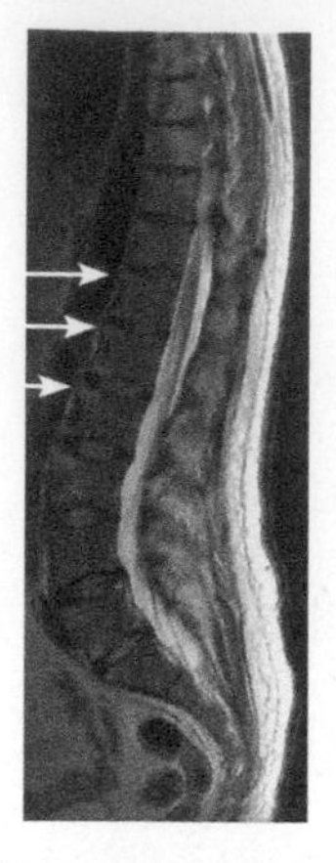

Sagittal T1 images demonstrate multiple Romanus lesions at anterior corners of vertebral bodies.

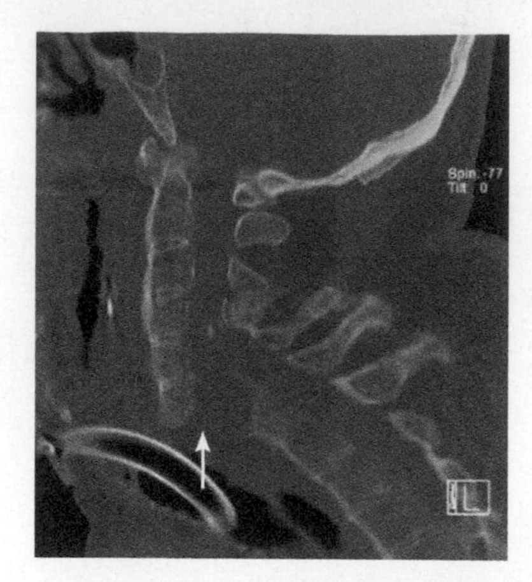

Chance fracture of C6/7 with trauma. The ankylosed spine is particularly vulnerable to fractures through the ossified intervertebral discs, as these are the points of mechanical weakness.

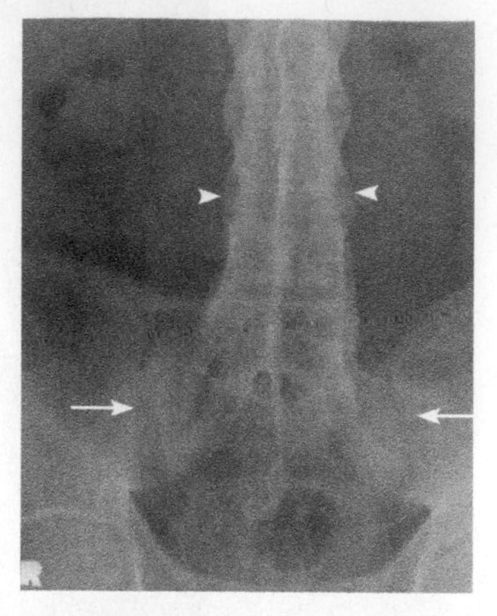

Classical features of ankylosing spondylitis with fused sacroiliac joints (*arrows*) and syndesmophyte formation (*arrowheads*) leading to a "bamboo spine." An ossified posterior longitudinal ligament is projected as a continuous central sclerotic line.

Answers

1. Entheseal inflammation is the basic pathology of ankylosing spondylitis. Atlantoaxial subluxation is a feature of rheumatoid arthritis. Sacroiliitis is usually bilateral; unilateral causes include infection. Peripheral joint ankylosis is not a feature.
2. Seronegative spondyloarthropathies include ankylosing spondylitis, psoriasis, inflammatory bowel disease, and Reactive disease.
3. Treatment for ankylosing spondylitis is generally directed at symptom control. Surgical correction of a kyphotic deformity is not generally performed. Novel approaches include anti-TNF therapy which is intended to treat active inflammation mediated by TNF-α cytokines.
4. Ankylosing spondylitis can predispose to spinal fracture and cord compression. Plantar fascitis is an association.

   Only 1% of cases are associated with an apical lung fibrosis, although this fact is beloved of radiology examiners!
5. More than 90% of whites with ankylosing spondylitis are HLA-B27 positive. The incidence of male-to-female is 3:1.

Pearls

- Bilateral symmetrical sacroiliitis is highly suggestive of ankylosing spondylitis.
- Because of the high relative incidence of the condition relative to other causes of sacroiliitis, unilateral or asymmetric sacroiliitis is still more likely to be caused by ankylosing spondylitis than a result of other disorders.
- Classical features include syndesmophytes, Romanus lesions, squaring of vertebral bodies, Andersson lesions, and bamboo spine.
- Syndesmophyte formation is caused by ossification of the outer fibers of the annulus fibrosus. It is best assessed on a frontal radiograph.
- Chance fractures can occur through ossified intervertebral discs with relatively little trauma, as these are the sites of mechanical weakness.
- Early spinal features include inflammation at costovertebral and costotransverse joints, which is best assessed on a fluid-sensitive MRI sequence.
- It is important to look for extraarticular features and associated features of HLA-B27 disorders, for example, apical lung fibrosis, enthesitis, inflammatory bowel disease, and psoriasis, in radiology examinations (and routine clinical practice).

Suggested Readings

Braun J, Baraliakos X. Imaging of axial spondyloarthritis including ankylosing spondylitis. *Ann Rheum Dis.* 2011;70 Suppl 1:i97–i103.

Ostergaard M, Poggenborg RP, Axelsen MB, Pedersen SJ. Magnetic resonance imaging in spondyloarthritis–how to quantify findings and measure response. *Best Pract Res Clin Rheumatol.* 2010;24(5):637–657.

History of trauma, now with severe neck pain

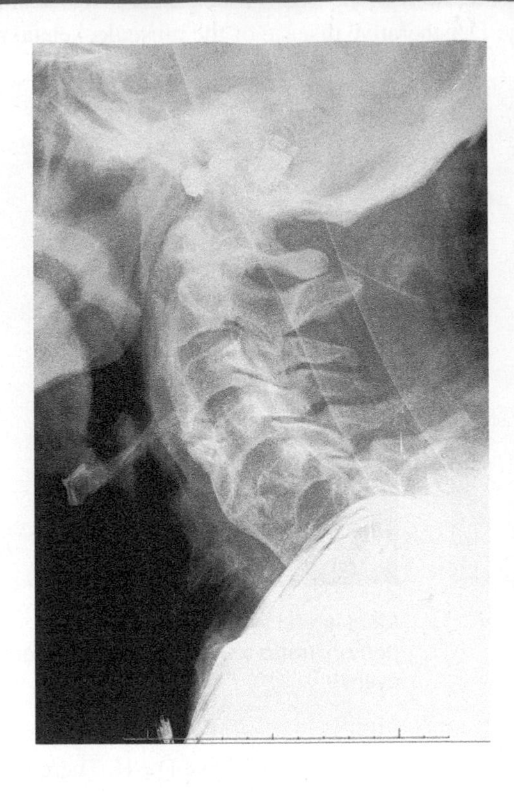

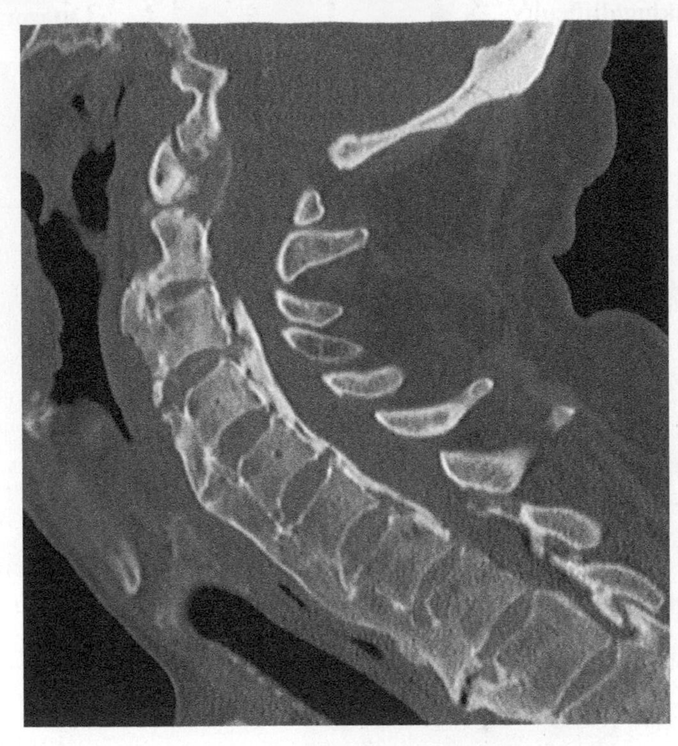

1. What are the radiographic findings?

2. What is the epidemiology of the findings in the spinal canal?

3. What is the natural history of the intraspinal finding?

4. What is the best imaging modality to use when investigating this finding?

5. What are the other associations of the intraspinal finding?

Ossification of the posterior longitudinal ligament (OPLL) 1342

Case ranking/difficulty: 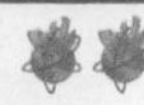 **Category:** Degenerative disease of the musculoskeletal system

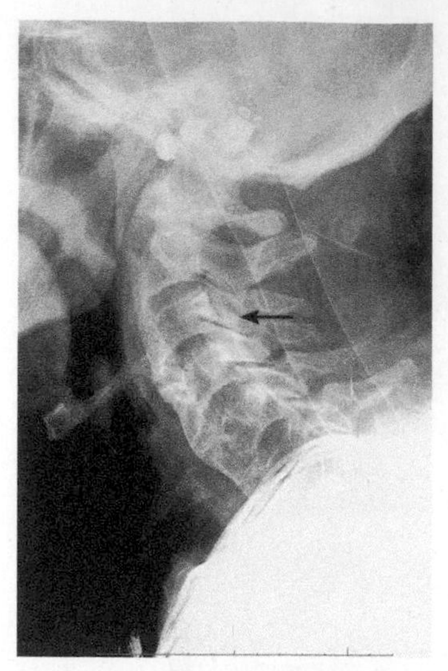

Extensive DISH changes with ossification of the posterior longitudinal ligament (*arrow*).

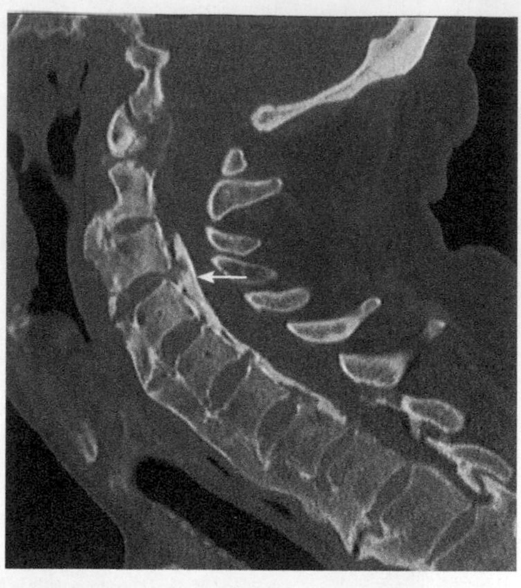

The ossification of the posterior longitudinal ligament (OPLL) is well demonstrated.

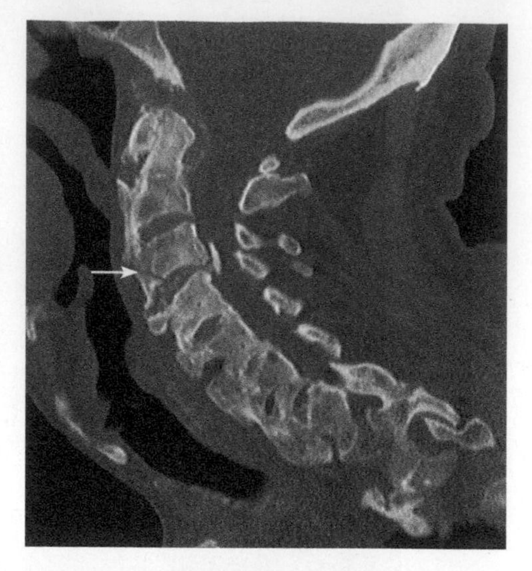

More lateral sagittal image better demonstrates a C3 fracture, the presenting event.

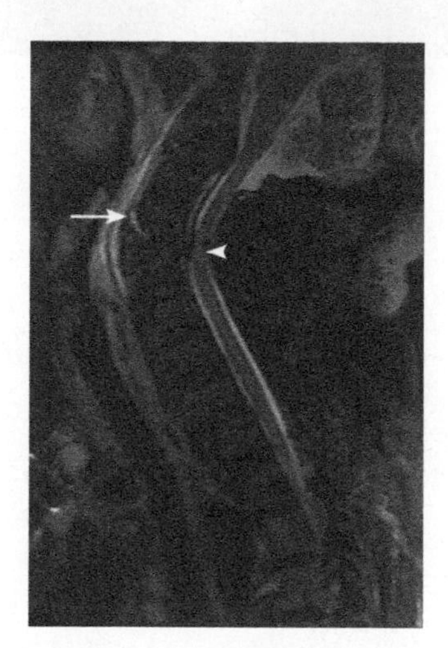

C3 body fracture (*arrow*), OPLL, and cord compression with mild cord edema (*arrowhead*) are well demonstrated.

Answers

1. There is ossification of the posterior longitudinal ligament (OPLL), and anterior paraspinal ossification consistent with DISH. The acute presenting feature was an acute traumatic fracture of the anterior inferior C3 vertebral body, not demonstrated in these radiographs.
2. OPLL is most common in older Japanese males.
3. OPLL is progressive and may result in spinal stenosis.
4. MRI is the best imaging modality, as it will indicate the extent of OPLL as well as show the degree of spinal stenosis. It will also show cord changes of edema and myelomalacia.
5. Of patients with OPLL, 50% have DISH. There is also an association of OPLL with the spondyloarthropathies.

Pearls

- OPLL occurs most commonly among Japanese.
- It may be classified as continuous or noncontinuous.
- The cervical spine at C3-C5 is most commonly affected.
- Plain film and CT show linear ossification posterior to the vertebral bodies and possibly discs, separated by a lucent line. CT will also show the degree of spinal stenosis.
- On MRI, OPLL shows T1 and T2 hypointensity with possible central T1 hyperintensity if marrow fat is present. MRI has the advantage of also showing cord changes.
- MRI will also show spinal stenosis or cord changes.

Suggested Readings

Munday TL, Johnson MH, Hayes CW, Thompson EO, Smoker WR. Musculoskeletal causes of spinal axis compromise: beyond the usual suspects. *Radiographics.* 1994;14(6):1225-1245.

Widder DJ. MR imaging of ossification of the posterior longitudinal ligament. *AJR Am J Roentgenol.* 1989;153(1):194-195.

3 to 4 months history of pain in the right hip

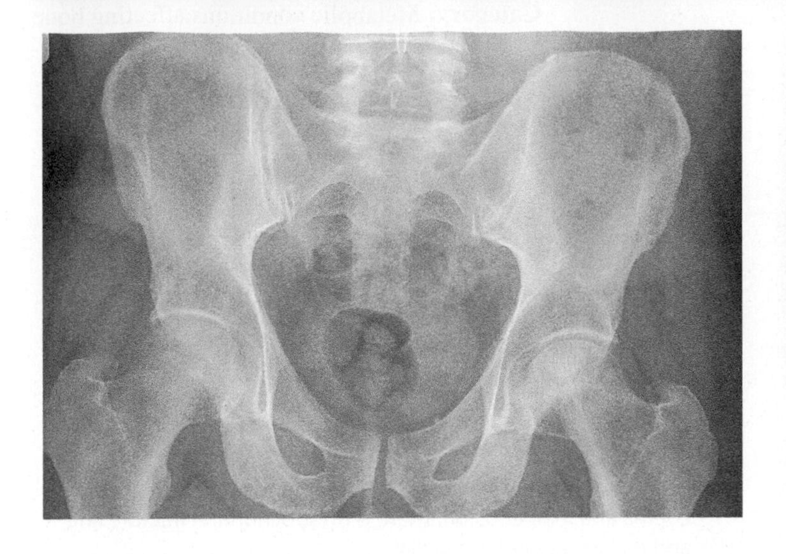

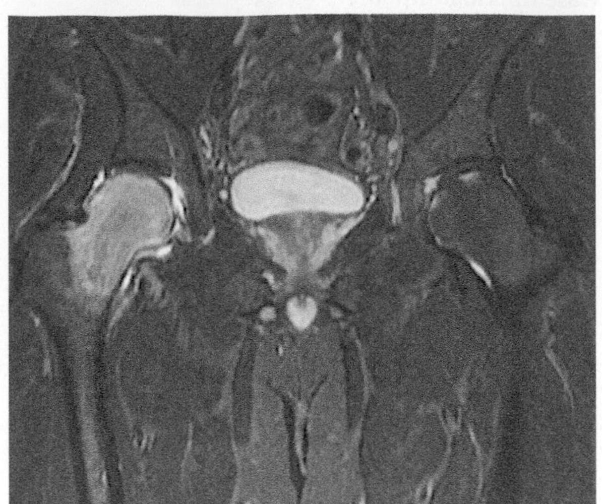

1. What are the radiograph findings?
2. What are the MRI features?
3. What is the differential diagnosis?
4. What are the risk factors for this condition?
5. What is the treatment for this condition?

Transient osteoporosis of hip 1435

Case ranking/difficulty: 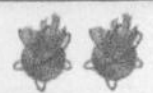

Category: Metabolic conditions affecting bone

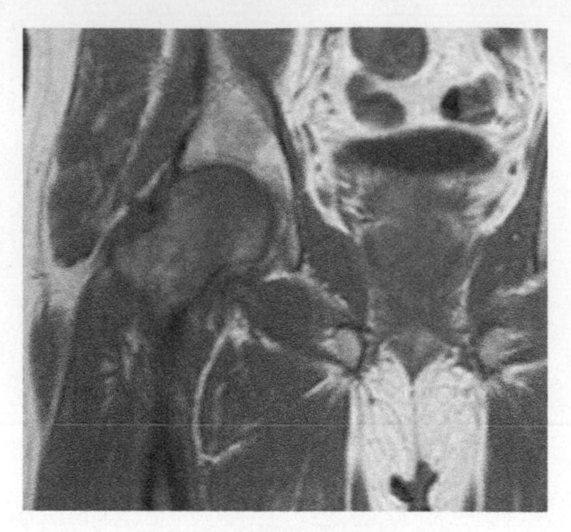

Low T1 signal intensity in the right hip.

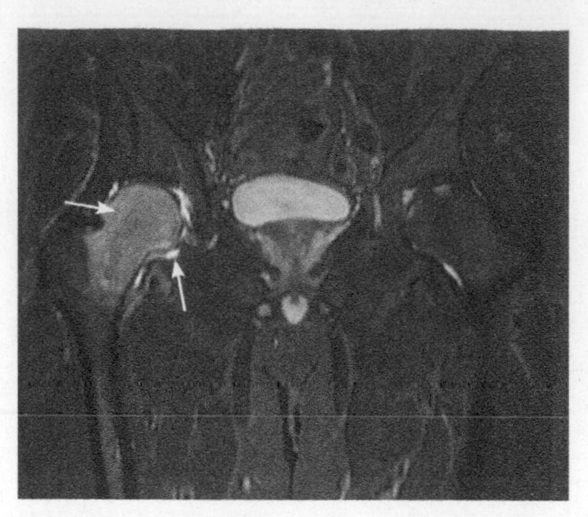

STIR coronal image of the right hip demonstrates high signal edema and joint effusion. There is no subchondral fracture line and the acetabulum is normal.

Answers

1. There is diffuse osteopenia and subcortical bone loss in the right hip, with preserved joint spaces and no collapse of the head.
2. MRI features include decreased marrow signal on T1-weighted images, with high T2 marrow signal suggesting bone marrow edema. Minimal joint effusion.
3. Avascular necrosis, stress fracture, and septic arthritis are the main differential diagnoses.
4. The risk factors include males 40 to 50 years old and women in the third trimester of pregnancy.
5. This condition is self-limiting and resolves after 6 to 12 months. Consequently, nonsurgical conservative treatment is usually recommended. Analgesics and protected weight bearing are the main treatment options.

Pearls

- Transient osteoporosis of the hip is a self-limiting disorder of unknown etiology. It occurs in the 40 to 55 years age group and is 3 times more common in males.
- It also affects women in the third trimester of pregnancy.
- The differential diagnosis includes avascular necrosis, stress fracture, and septic arthritis.
- Some patients develop similar findings in the opposite hip or other joints, and this is called *regional migratory osteoporosis*.
- X-rays are normal initially and become abnormal within 4 to 8 weeks, demonstrating femoral head and neck subchondral cortical loss and osteopenia with or without joint effusion. The joint space is always maintained.
- MRI shows bone marrow edema in the femoral head and neck region which will show low T1 and high T2 signal. In extreme cases, early subchondral fracture lines can be seen. These are usually thinner than 4 mm and less than 12.5 mm in length, unlike the subchondral fractures of avascular necrosis. However, at this stage, differentiation radiologically and clinically from avascular necrosis is difficult.
- Bone scan shows increased uptake in the femoral head and neck region.
- The treatment is supportive and includes analgesics and protected partial weight bearing. This condition is usually self-limiting and regresses clinically and radiologically within 6 to 12 months.

Suggested Readings

Miyanishi K, Kaminomachi S, Hara T, et al. A subchondral fracture in transient osteoporosis of the hip. *Skeletal Radiol.* 2007;36(7):677-680.

Toms AP, Marshall TJ, Becker E, Donell ST, Lobo-Mueller EM, Barker T. Regional migratory osteoporosis: a review illustrated by five cases. *Clin Radiol.* 2005;60(4):425-438.

Vande Berg BC, Lecouvet FE, Koutaissoff S, Simoni P, Malghem J. Bone marrow edema of the femoral head and transient osteoporosis of the hip. *Eur J Radiol.* 2008;67(1):68-77.

Pain and swelling in the right arm, with fever and severe constitutional symptoms

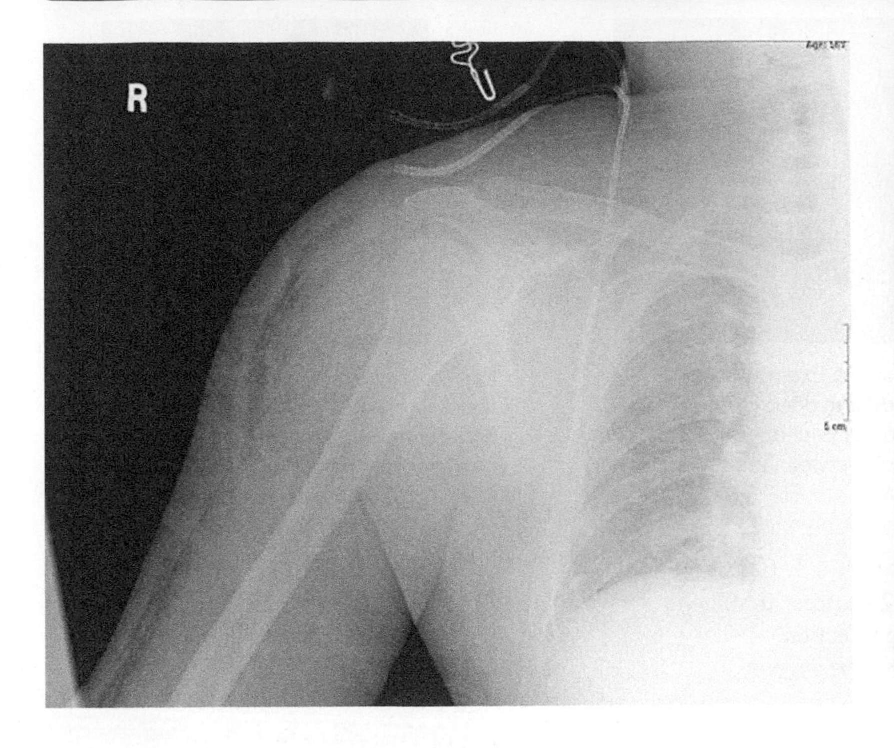

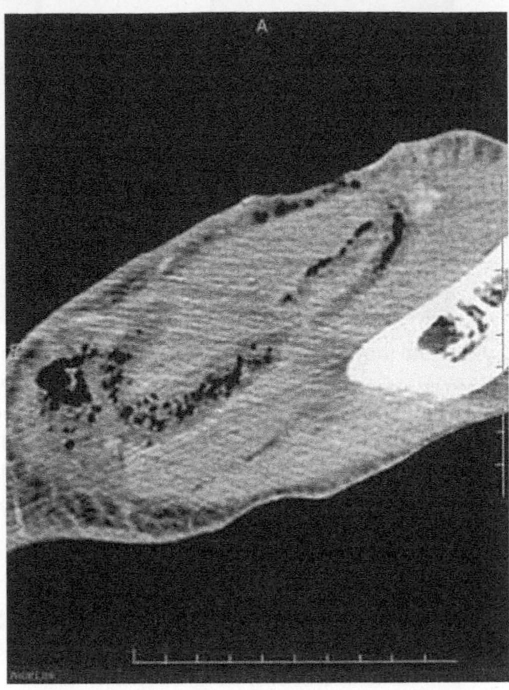

1. What is the most relevant finding demonstrated?

2. What is the most common causative agent?

3. What is the role of ultrasound in the diagnosis?

4. What entities are associated with a poor outcome?

5. What are the typical MRI characteristics?

Necrotizing fasciitis 2368

Case ranking/difficulty: 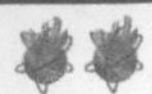

Category: Infections in the musculoskeletal system

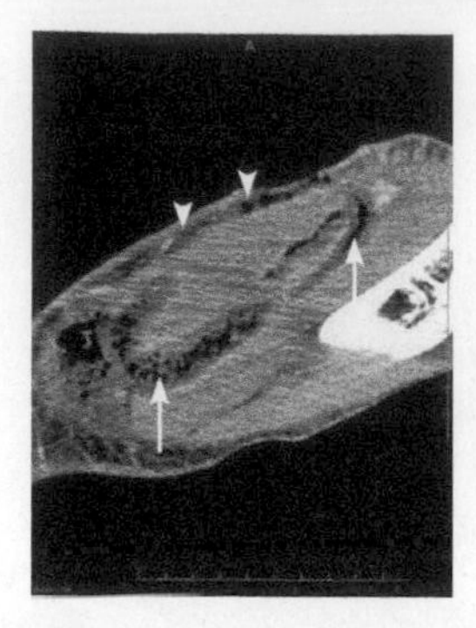

Superficial (*arrowheads*) and deep (*arrows*) fascial fluid with gas.

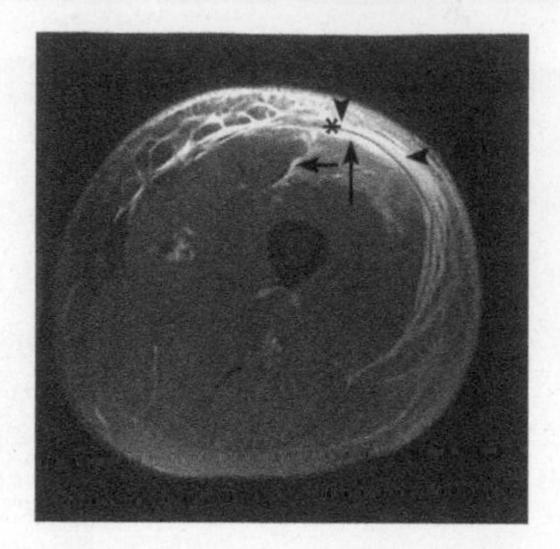

Another patient. Extensive superficial (*arrowheads*) and deep (*arrows*) fascial fluid in another patient. *Asterisk* marks the demarcation between the superficial and deep fascia.

Post-contrast enhancement in the fascial layers with a fluid collection (*arrowhead*), and areas of non-enhancement indicating the overestimation of disease on T2-weighted images, or non-viable tissue (*arrows*).

Answers

1. Gas in the soft tissues can only come from 2 sources: an open wound or ulcer, or from a gas-forming infection. The latter is typically caused by *Clostridium perfringens*, and indicates necrotizing fasciitis.

2. Although *C. perfringens* is the classic gas-forming organism, the most common infection is polymicrobial. The most common single causative agent is group A streptococcus, well known in the press as the "flesh-eating" organism.

3. Ultrasound has limited utility in adults, but is very useful in the pediatric population. Ultrasound features included turbid fluid collections in the superficial and deep fascia, with a thickened and distorted fascia. Although gas may cause dirty shadowing which can obscure fluid collections, the presence of gas in the fascia is conversely useful in making the diagnosis. Ultrasound is also useful in draining fluid collections.

4. Minor insults can predispose to necrotizing fasciitis, including minor wounds and surgery, insect bites, furuncles, and diverticulitis in otherwise seemingly healthy individuals.

   Immunocompromised states, such as diabetes and HIV, as well as old (and very young) age, peripheral vascular disease, alcoholism, and obesity, are associated with poor outcomes. Overall mortality ranges from 30% to 70%, usually from multiorgan failure.

5. Because of its superior contrast resolution and multiplanar imaging capabilities, MRI is the imaging modality of choice. However, treatment should not be delayed to await imaging.

   MRI features included extensive fluid in the superficial and deep fascia, gas, and non-enhancement of non-viable tissue. Although cellulitis can demonstrate fluid in the superficial fascia, it is more extensive in necrotizing fasciitis, and gas is not present in cellulitis.

Pearls

- Necrotizing fasciitis is a rapidly progressive inflammatory infection of the fascia, with secondary necrosis of the subcutaneous tissues.
- The superficial fascia is the connective tissue in the subcutaneous fat, and the deep fascia is the tissue surrounding and between the musculature.
- Immunocompromised patients are at greatest risk, but the infection can occur in otherwise healthy individuals.
- Three subtypes have been recognized: polymicrobial with a *Vibrio* subtype, group A streptococcus, and *Clostridium* infection.
- Gas in the soft tissues is the hallmark radiologically, but is only seen in a minority of patients. Fluid in the deep fascial layers, and extensive subcutaneous fluid pockets are seen on CT and MRI T2-weighted images.
- T2-weighted images overestimate the severity of disease as a consequence of reactive edema, and post-contrast T1-weighted images underestimate the disease because of non-enhancement of dead tissue.
- Gas is best appreciated on gradient echo images.
- Treatment is with urgent fasciotomy, and should not be delayed to await imaging.

Suggested Readings

Fayad LM, Carrino JA, Fishman EK. Musculoskeletal infection: role of CT in the emergency department. *Radiographics*. 2007;27(6):1723-1736.

Fugitt JB, Puckett ML, Quigley MM, Kerr SM. Necrotizing fasciitis. *Radiographics*. 2004;24(5):1472-1476.

Back pain radiating down leg in a young man with fever

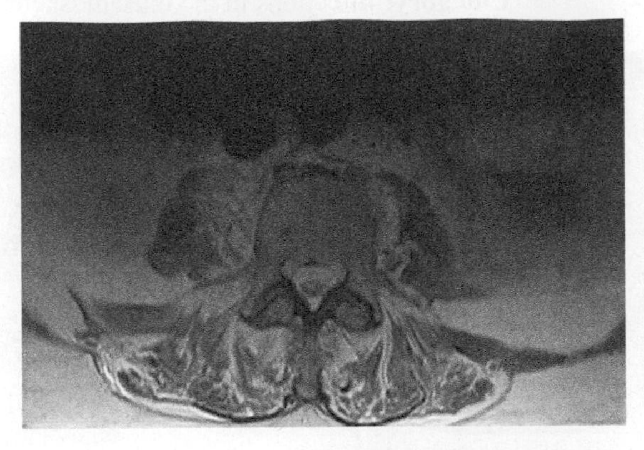

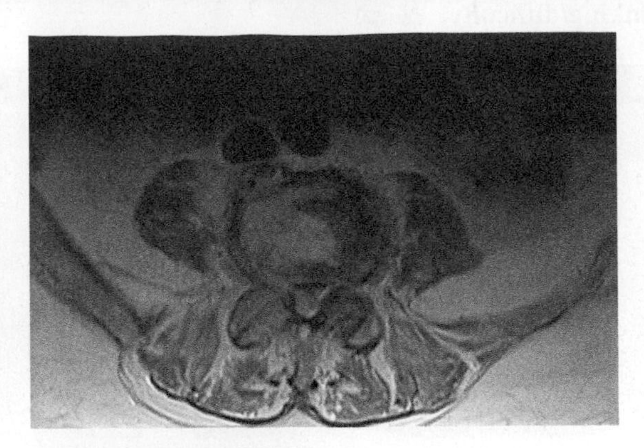

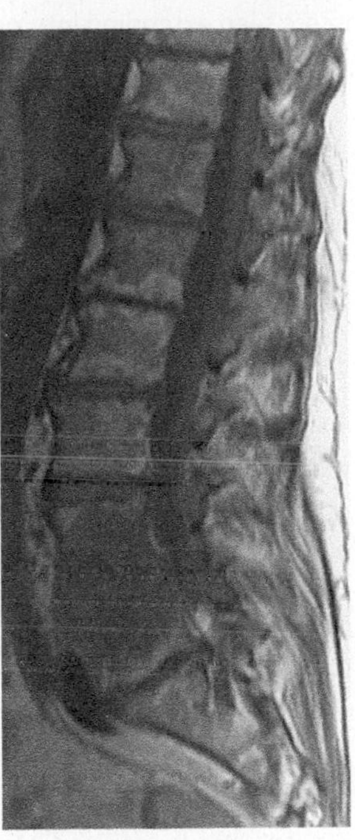

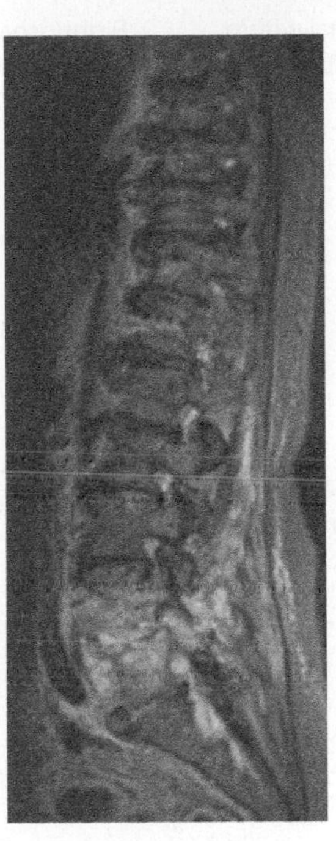

1. What are the imaging features of the right paravertebral abnormality?
2. What are the possible etiologies for this condition?
3. What other entities should be considered in the differential diagnosis?
4. What are the common infectious agents relevant to this entity?
5. What is the treatment of choice?

Psoas abscess—tuberculosis 1716

Case ranking/difficulty: 

Category: Infections in the musculoskeletal system

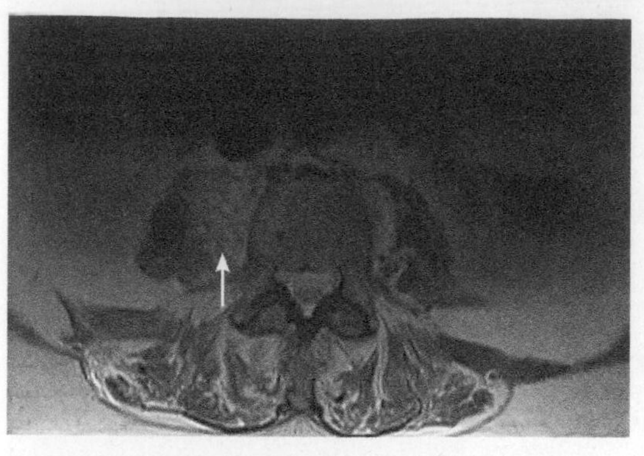

Asymmetric enlargement and high signal within right psoas muscle consistent with an abscess.

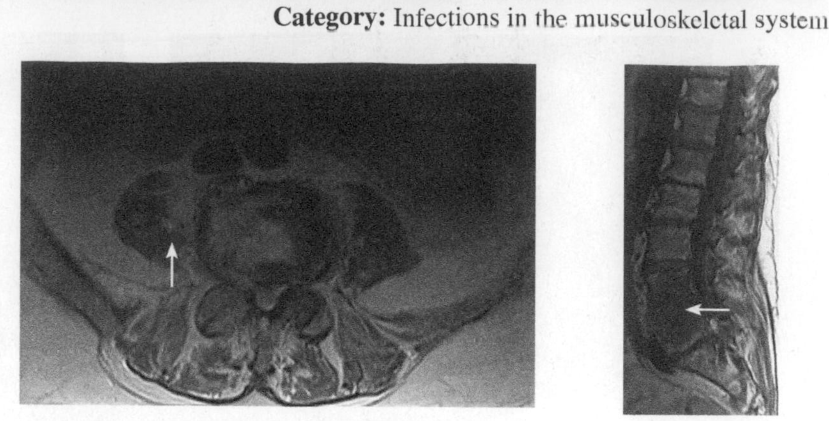

Right psoas abscess seen extending into pelvis along fascial planes.

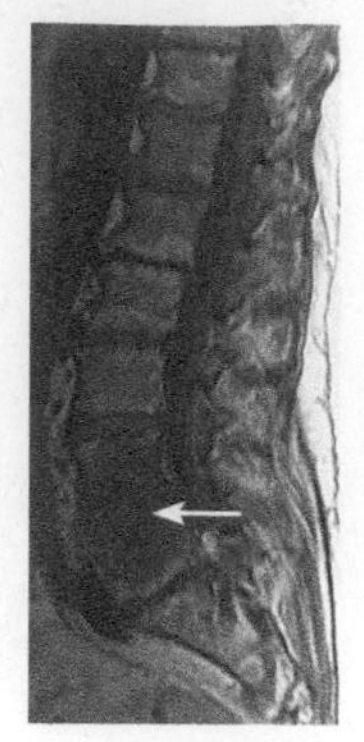

Spondylodiscitis at L4/5 is the source of the psoas abscess in this patient.

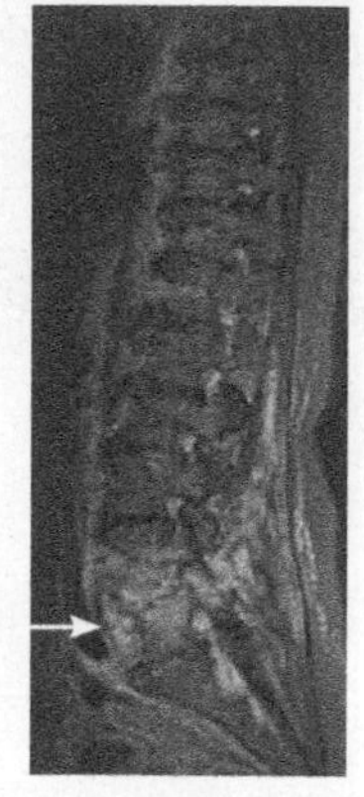

Abnormally high signal within L4/5 consistent with discitis. There is high signal in the adjacent L4 and L5 vertebral bodies. Infection from the spine extends and tracks down the right psoas muscle.

Answers

1. The investigative modality of choice for diagnosing and determining the extent of a psoas abscess is MRI. Ultrasound may reveal the pathology, although its utility is dependent on operator skill and patient body habitus. A plain radiograph may show loss of the psoas shadow, although this is not a sensitive test for detecting psoas pathology.
2. Any infective pathology within the retroperitoneum or paravertebral region can cause secondary extension into the psoas sheath with abscess formation. Local pathology in the pelvis or groin may also be implicated.
3. A psoas abscess can mimic a retroperitoneal mass or collection or a groin mass.
4. Pathogens that cause osteomyelitis or urinary tract or gastrointestinal infections may be implicated in psoas abscesses.
5. Percutaneous drainage guided by CT imaging is the treatment of choice for a psoas abscess. Early cases may be treated with IV antibiotics, although a sample should be obtained for microbiological culture and cytology.

Pearls

- Psoas abscess should be considered in the differential diagnosis of a tender groin mass.
- The retroperitoneal location of the psoas muscles explains why abdominal (retroperitoneal) and spinal pathology may present with a psoas (groin) abscess.
- The etiology may be related to retroperitoneal infection (pyelonephritis, diverticulitis, pancreatitis, retrocecal appendicitis) or spondylodiscitis. An increasingly prevalent cause is local groin pathology, for example, infected hematoma post-coronary intervention and infection in IV drug users.
- An extremely common worldwide cause of psoas abscess—though perhaps less so in developed countries—is a tuberculous "cold abscess" which is usually the result of tracking infection from a spondylodiscitis.
- Diagnosis is best made on MRI, although ultrasound is an acceptable alternative to guide a percutaneous sample.
- CT with contrast is an acceptable alternative to MRI if there are contraindications, for example, cardiac pacemaker.

Suggested Readings

Goni V, Thapa BR, Vyas S, Gopinathan NR, Rajan Manoharan S, Krishnan V. Bilateral psoas abscess: atypical presentation of spinal tuberculosis. *Arch Iran Med.* 2012;15(4):253-256.

Tamaki H, Kishimoto M, Okada M. Clinical Images: iliopsoas bursa rupture mimicking psoas muscle abscess. *Arthritis Rheum.* 2010;62(6):1769.

Tonolini M, Campari A, Bianco R. Common and unusual diseases involving the iliopsoas muscle compartment: spectrum of cross-sectional imaging findings. *Abdom Imaging.* 2012;37(1):118-139.

Knee pain and swelling for several weeks

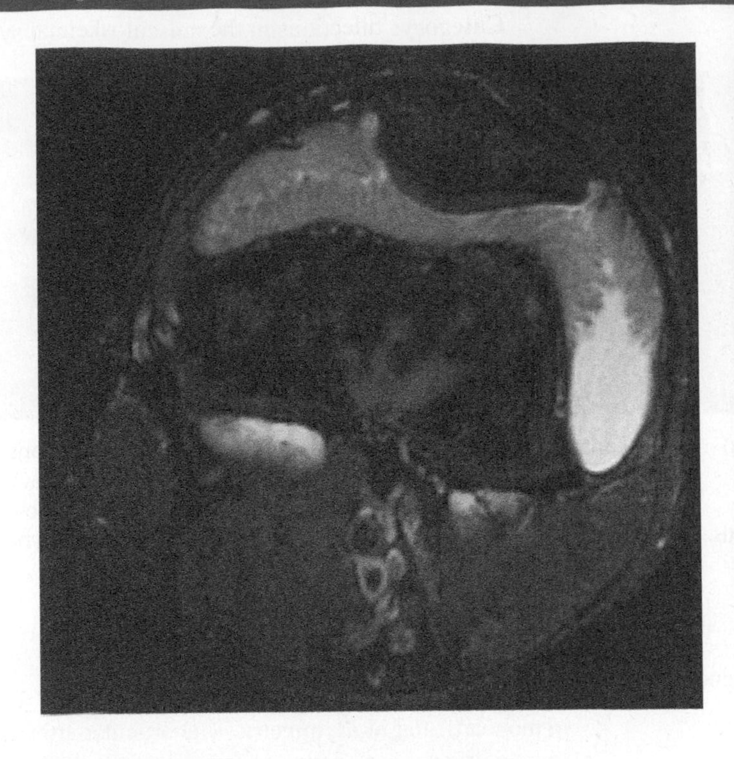

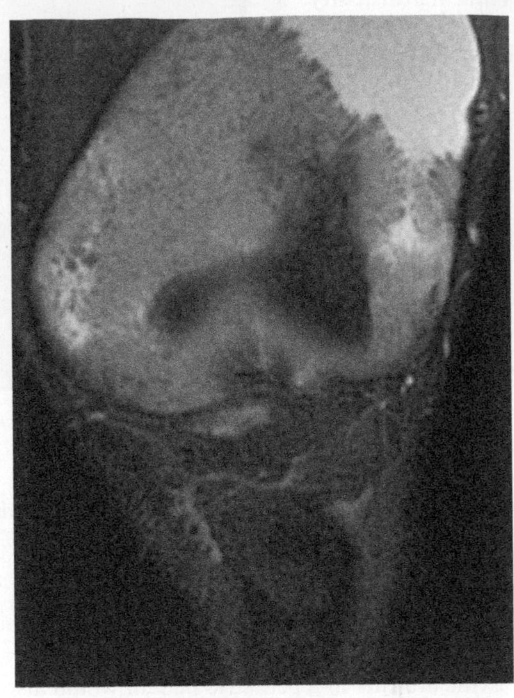

1. What is in the differential diagnosis in this 17-year-old patient?

2. What is the causative agent in the entity depicted?

3. What organ systems are typically affected in this disease?

4. What joints are commonly involved in pediatric patients with this disease?

5. In which geographic regions of the United States is this entity most common?

Lyme arthritis 1340

Case ranking/difficulty: 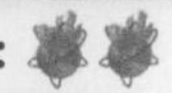

Category: Infections in the musculoskeletal system

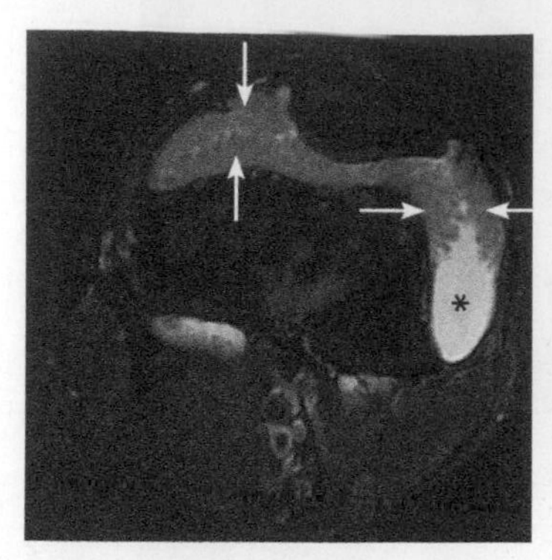

MRI demonstrates a large effusion (*asterisk*) and marked synovial thickening (*arrows*) consistent with synovitis.

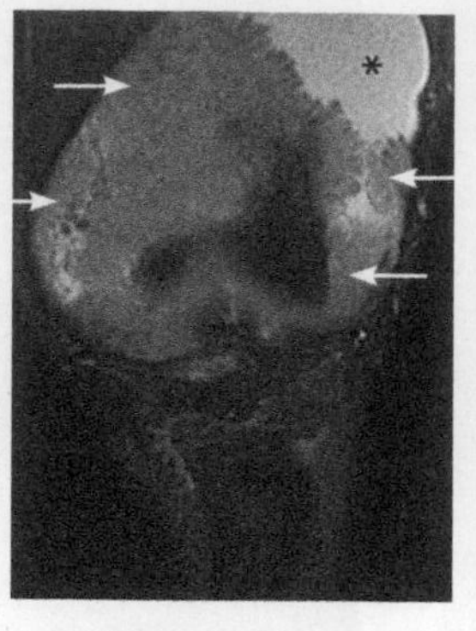

Large effusion (*asterisk*) and marked synovial thickening (*arrows*) consistent with synovitis.

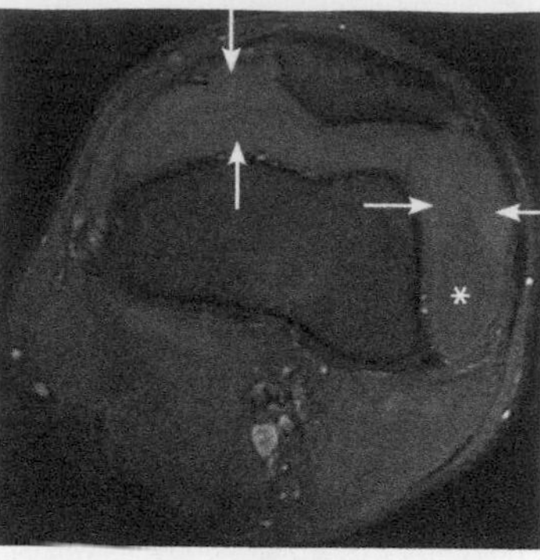

Pre-contrast image shows a large effusion (*asterisk*) and synovial thickening (*arrows*) consistent with synovitis.

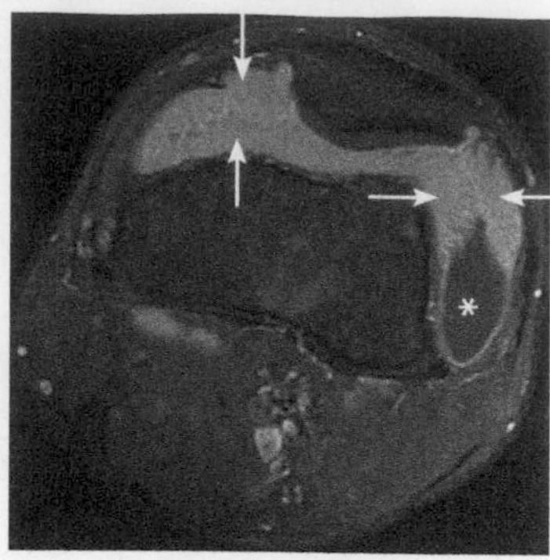

Post-contrast Image demonstrates an effusion (*asterisk*) and avidly enhancing, thickened synovium (*arrows*) consistent with synovitis.

Answers

1. This patient has Lyme disease. The differential diagnosis for Lyme arthritis in a pediatric patient would also include septic arthritis, juvenile rheumatoid arthritis, and psoriatic arthritis.
2. Lyme disease is caused by the spirochete *Borrelia burgdorferi* and transmitted by the bite of the Ixodes (deer) tick.
3. Patients with Lyme disease have a characteristic skin lesion, erythema migrans. If untreated, Lyme disease results in neurologic, cardiac, or musculoskeletal manifestations. Hepatobiliary involvement is not a common manifestation of Lyme disease.
4. In pediatric patients, Lyme arthritis involves the knee in 86% of cases, the hip in 11%, the elbow in 3%, and the ankle in 1%.
5. Most cases of Lyme disease in the United States occur in the Northeastern and North Central regions, in the months of May through August.

Pearls

- Lyme disease is a multisystem illness caused by the spirochete *Borrelia burgdorferi* and transmitted by the bite of the Ixodes (deer) tick.
- Lyme disease is the most common vector-borne disease in the United States.
- Up to 90% of patients develop a characteristic skin lesion, erythema migrans, at the site of the tick bite.
- Most patients experience constitutional symptoms.
- In the musculoskeletal system, Lyme disease may result in monoarticular or asymmetric oligoarticular arthritis.
- In pediatric patients, Lyme arthritis involves the knee in 86% of cases, the hip in 11%, the elbow in 3%, and the ankle in 1%.
- Lyme arthritis may resolve spontaneously or persist, resulting in chronic arthritis of 1 or 2 large joints, such as the knees.
- Clinically, Lyme arthritis in children may resemble septic arthritis and juvenile rheumatoid arthritis.
- MRI and ultrasound in patients with Lyme arthritis may demonstrate effusions, synovitis, cartilage damage, or popliteal cysts.

Suggested Readings

Davidson RS. Orthopaedic complications of Lyme disease in children. *Biomed Pharmacother.* 1989;43(6):405-408.

Thompson A, Mannix R, Bachur R. Acute pediatric monoarticular arthritis: distinguishing lyme arthritis from other etiologies. *Pediatrics.* 2009;123(3):959-965.

Pain and swelling of distal tibia

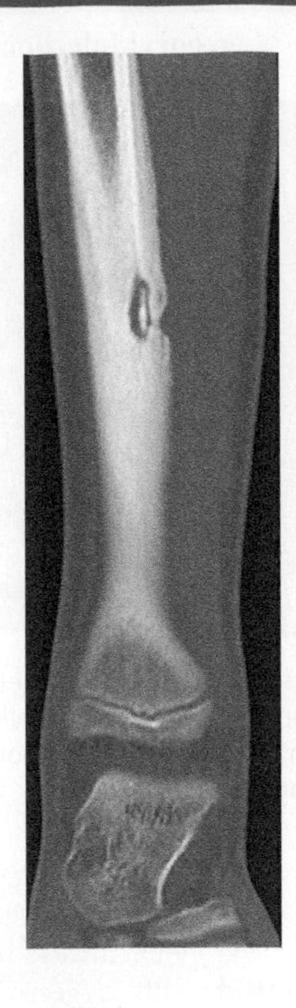

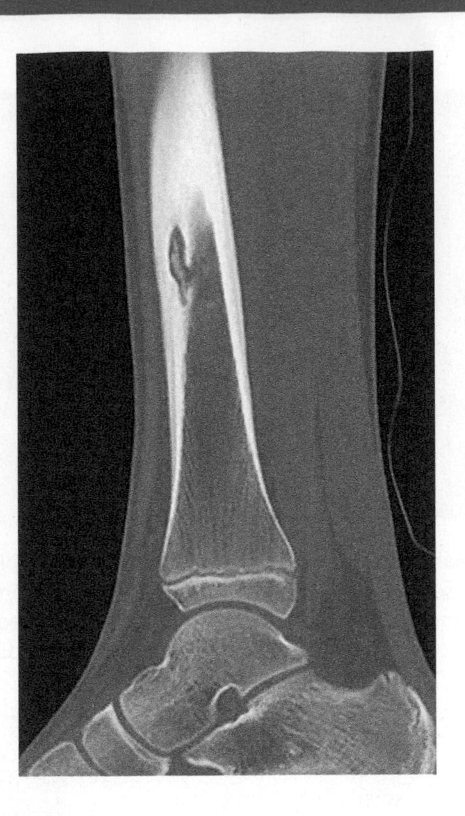

1. What is the differential diagnosis?

2. What is the term used to describe the sclerotic lesion on the lateral aspect of the tibial cortex?

3. What is the treatment of this entity?

4. What is the likely etiological agent?

5. What is the eponymous name given to this condition?

Brodie abscess 229

Case ranking/difficulty: 

Category: Infections in the musculoskeletal system

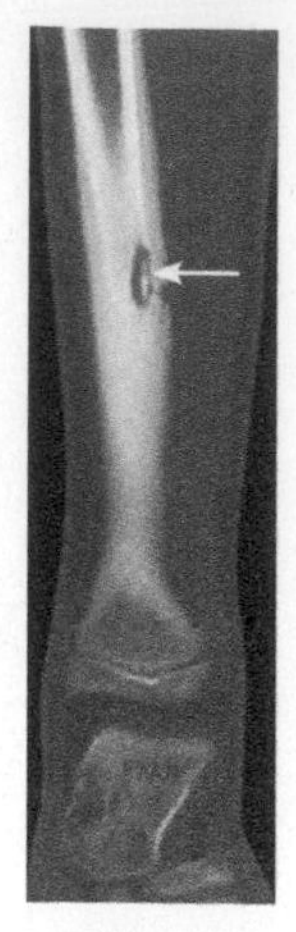

Sequestrum and surrounding involucrum is seen with a sinus tract leading into it.

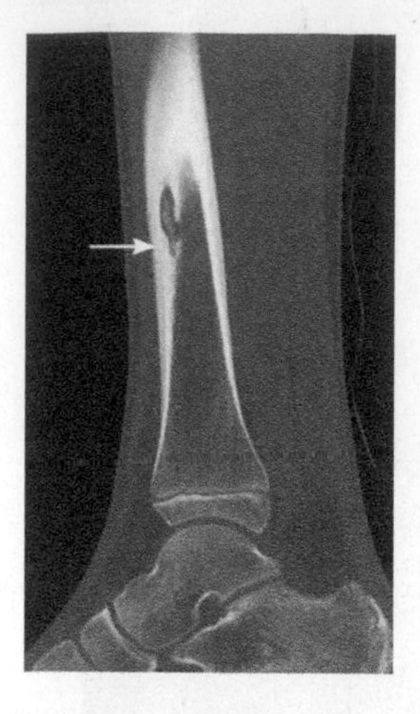

Marked cortical sclerosis is seen surrounding the Brodie abscess.

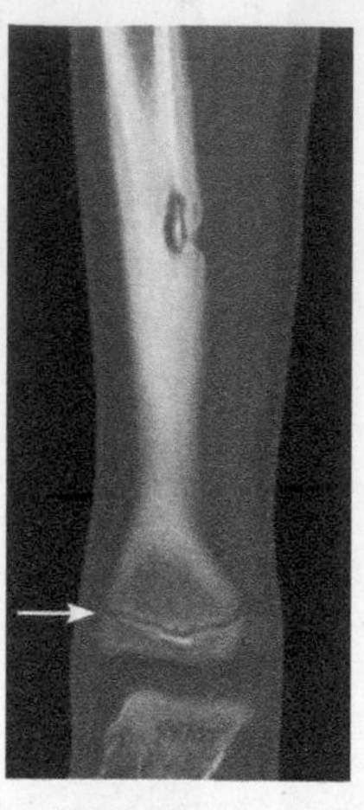

The unfused epiphyses indicate the common incidence of osteomyelitis in the pediatric population.

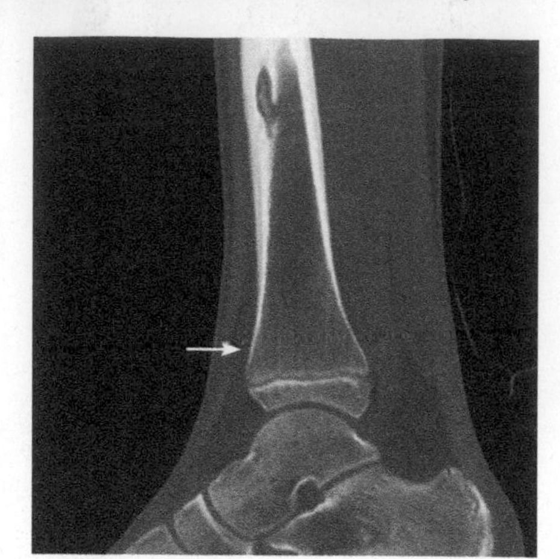

The metaphysis is not involved which is usually the most common site of infection in the pediatric patient.

Answers

1. The main differential for a sclerotic cortically based lesion with profound reactive sclerosis is between a Brodie abscess and an osteoid osteoma. The latter is significantly smaller (less than 1 cm) with a small nidus. Clinical history is suggestive. A metaphyseal location may favor osteomyelitis.
2. A sequestrum is an area of devitalized bone secondary to chronic osteomyelitis. Involucrum is the formation of periosteal new bone in chronic osteomyelitis, as pus strips off the periosteum and expands the bone.
3. With the presence of a sequestrum, surgical excision of devitalized bone, removal of sinus tracts, curettage, and packing with bone graft may be required. Antibiotics alone are unlikely to be successful at this stage.
4. The most likely organism to cause osteomyelitis is *Staphylococcus aureus*.
5. A sequestrum within a sinus cavity is a Brodie abscess and a characteristic feature of chronic osteomyelitis.

Pearls

- A well-defined lucent lesion in the tibia with surrounding reactive sclerosis is suspicious for a Brodie abscess.
- The differential includes osteoid osteoma and a stress fracture. Appropriate history, examination, and a distal tibial location favors a Brodie abscess over the other entities.
- As the vast majority of cases are in children, this diagnosis should always be entertained in the pediatric population with suggestive imaging features and clinical history.
- A Brodie abscess may be diagnosed by plain films, ultrasound, CT, or MRI. However, CT and MRI are the investigative modalities of choice, as the sinus tract can be well visualized. MRI is particularly useful in assessing the extent of marrow abnormality and soft-tissue involvement.
- A sequestrum may be found on CT and is highly suggestive of chronic infection. An involucrum is rarely found in developed countries unless osteomyelitis is left untreated.
- Treatment is incision and drainage. Antibiotics may be used; however, successful treatment is rare because of difficulty in penetrating the abscess cavity.

Suggested Readings

Abbas A, Idriz S, Thakker M, Sheikh FT, Rubin C. Brodie's abscess. *Emerg Med J.* 2012;29(1):27.

Datir A, Lidder S, Pollock R, Tirabosco R, Saifuddin A. High-grade chondrosarcoma mimicking Brodie's abscess. *Clin Radiol.* 2009;64(9):944-947.

Olasinde AA, Oluwadiya KS, Adegbehingbe OO. Treatment of Brodie's abscess: excellent results from curettage, bone grafting and antibiotics. *Singapore Med J.* 2011;52(6):436-439.

Discharging foot ulcer in a diabetic patient

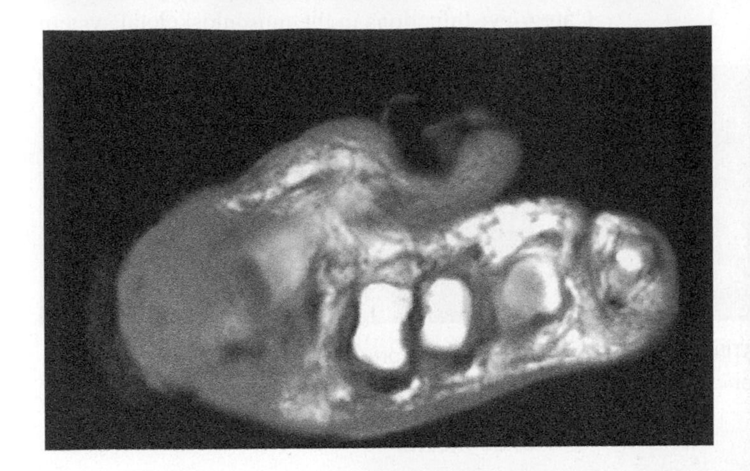

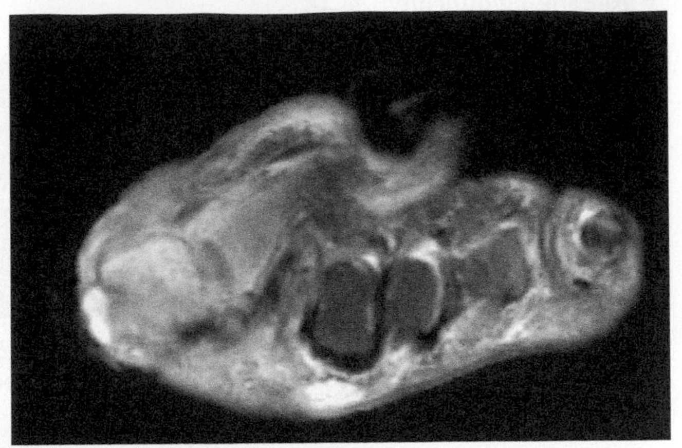

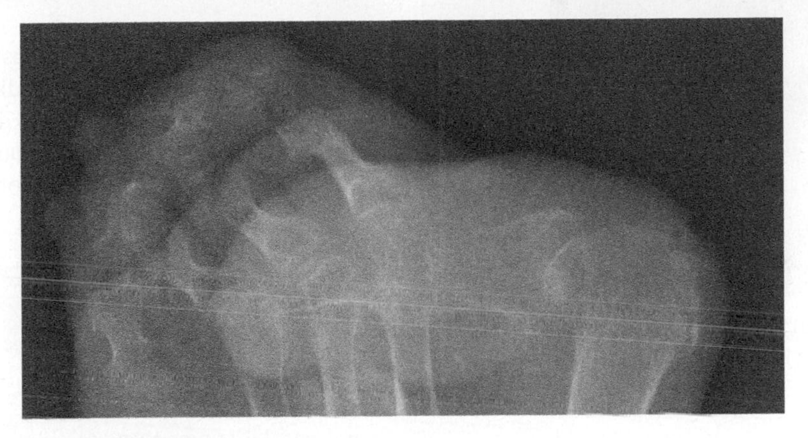

1. What is the differential diagnosis?

2. What is the imaging modality of choice in this entity?

3. What are useful associated findings when diagnosing this entity?

4. What are the common etiological agents in a diabetic patient?

5. After what period would X-rays be useful in diagnosing this entity?

Diabetic osteomyelitis of foot 1701

Case ranking/difficulty: 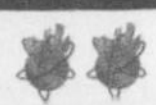

Category: Infections in the musculoskeletal system

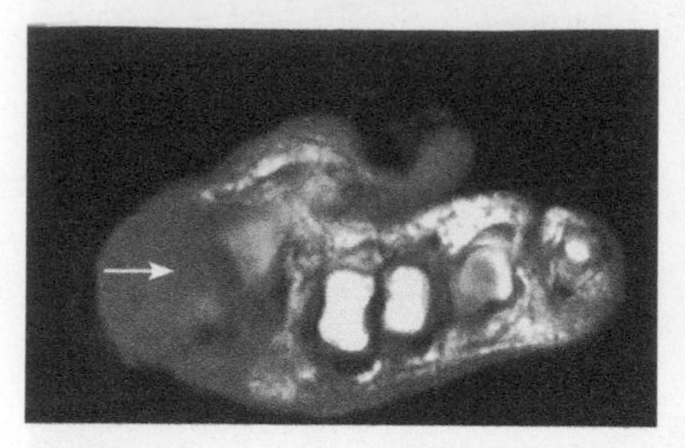

Loss of normal high T1 marrow signal and cortical destruction consistent with osteomyelitis.

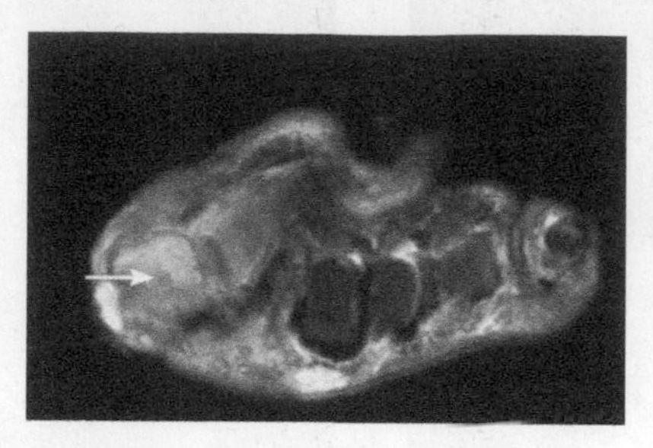

Corresponding high STIR signal is seen within the affected bone.

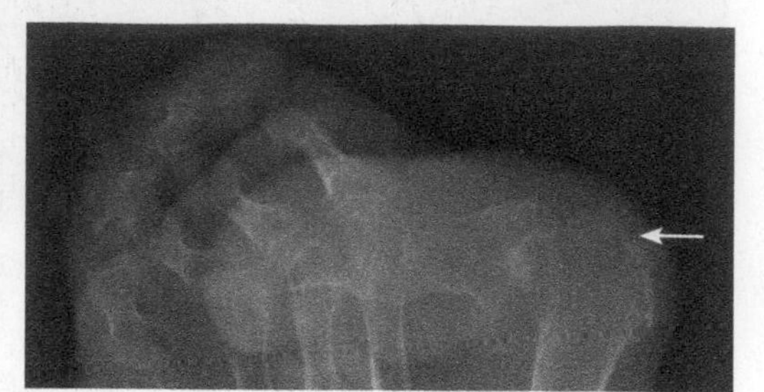

X-ray shows soft tissue gas and ulceration adjacent to the first metatarsal head, a feature that may suggest the presence of underlying osteomyelitis.

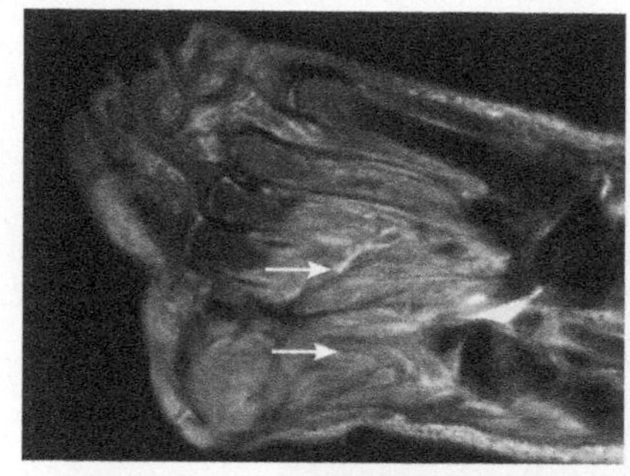

Subcutaneous edema is seen throughout the plantar surface of the foot—a common finding in the diabetic foot—although this is not specific for infection.

Answers

1. Osteomyelitis and neuropathic arthritis can have similar appearances in diabetic patients. The distribution may help, as osteomyelitis is found more commonly in the calcaneum and distal bones, whereas neuropathic arthritis most commonly involves the tarsometatarsal and metatarsophalangeal joints.

   There is likely to be extension of infection from a plantar ulcer in osteomyelitis. In addition there is invariably cortical destruction and loss of marrow signal on T1 images.

2. MRI is the imaging investigation of choice for diagnosing osteomyelitis.
3. A sinus tract and collection may be helpful in differentiating osteomyelitis from other entities, for example, neuropathic arthropathy and cellulitis.
4. *Staphylococcus aureus* is an important cause of acute osteomyelitis in diabetic and nondiabetic individuals. However, diabetics are also susceptible to other pathogens in chronic osteomyelitis, including *Bacteroides fragilis*, *Escherichia coli*, Group A and Group B streptococci, and *Proteus mirabilis*. *Pseudomonas aeruginosa* is a colonizer, but not actually a pathogen.
5. Soft-tissue swelling and periosteal reaction are features of osteomyelitis on a plain radiograph, but may not become apparent for 10 to 14 days. MRI and bone scans are sensitive very early (24 hours or less), although they may not be entirely specific for the diagnosis.

Pearls

- Diabetic osteomyelitis must be distinguished from cellulitis, osteitis, and Charcot neuropathy, although the entities often coexist.
- Useful distinguishing features are a loss of the normal T1 marrow signal, erosion of cortex, periosteal reaction, sinus tract extending from a skin ulcer, and location (distal to TMT joint or calcaneum).
- The presence of tenosynovitis should be commented on as it may be infective.
- MRI is the investigation of choice. T1-weighted sequences are most useful for evaluating marrow.
- Plain films are not sensitive for diagnosing early osteomyelitis, although care must be taken with MRI interpretation as the changes observed with osteomyelitis are nonspecific.
- Diagnostic confidence can increase by the presence of an adjacent soft-tissue ulcer, cortical destruction, and soft-tissue abscess or collection.

Suggested Readings

Donovan A, Schweitzer ME. Use of MR imaging in diagnosing diabetes-related pedal osteomyelitis. *Radiographics*. 2010;30(3):723-736.

Loredo R, Rahal A, Garcia G, Metter D. Imaging of the diabetic foot diagnostic dilemmas. *Foot Ankle Spec*. 2010;3(5):249-264.

Persistent deep pain in gluteal region

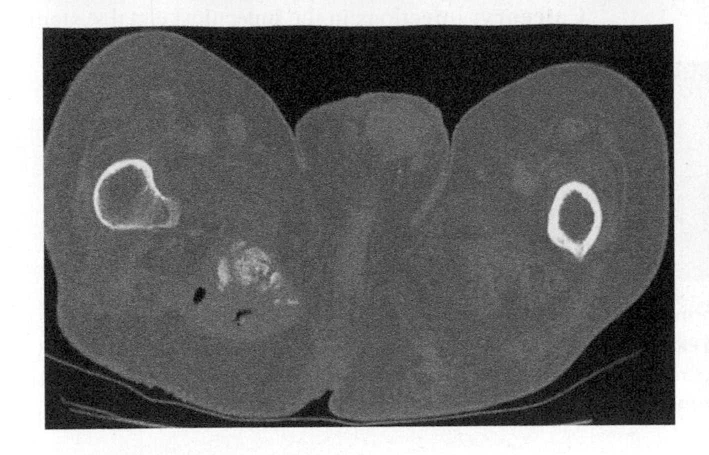

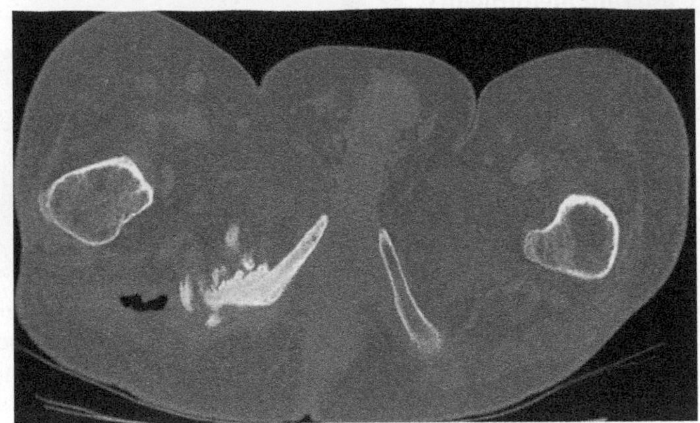

1. What is the most common etiological agent seen in this condition?

2. What are the imaging features of this condition?

3. What are the advantages of MRI over CT in the imaging of this condition?

4. What are the possible treatments for this condition?

5. What is the differential diagnosis of a soft-tissue mass with areas of irregular ossification within and around it?

Chronic osteomyelitis of ischium 1722

Case ranking/difficulty: 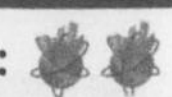 **Category:** Infections in the musculoskeletal system

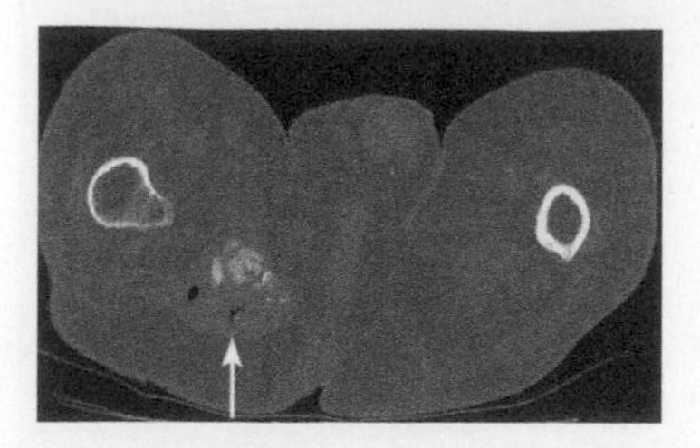

Gas-containing gluteal abscess seen on CT. Note adjacent irregular ossification within abscess consistent with heterotopic ossification.

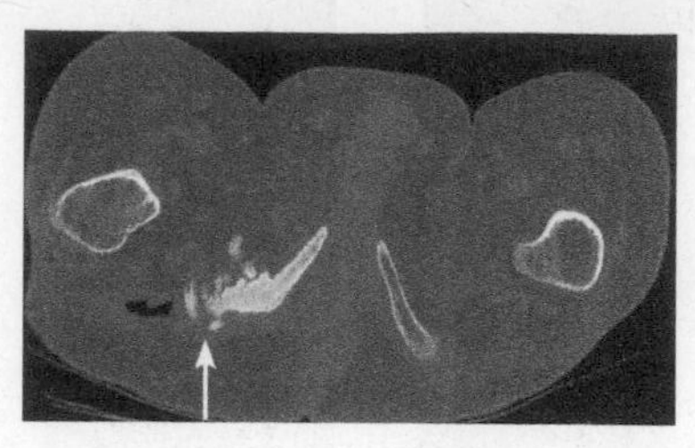

More cranial image demonstrates irregular cortical overgrowth and expansion of ischiopubic ramus compared to normal left side, consistent with chronic osteomyelitis.

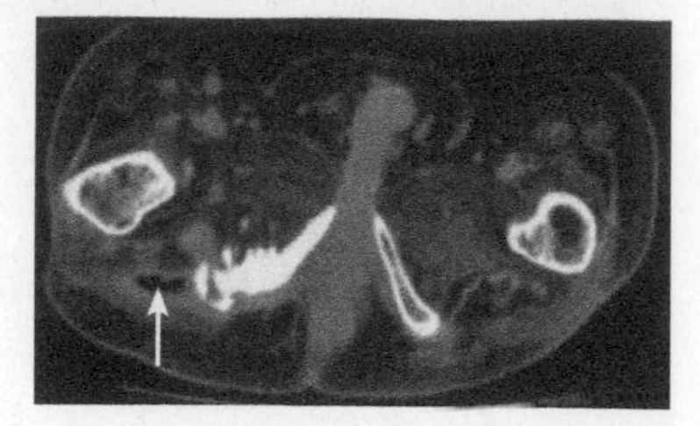

Soft-tissue windows demonstrate the large gas-containing soft-tissue abnormality lying adjacent to the abnormal ischium.

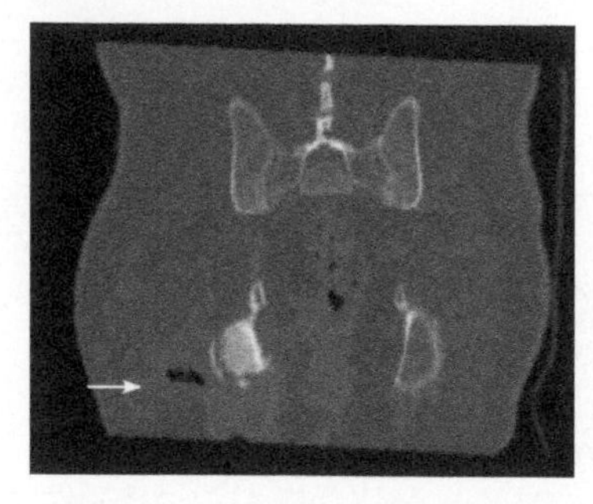

Coronal image shows the large extent of the gluteal abscess.

Answers

1. The same species that are implicated in acute osteomyelitis may result in chronic osteomyelitis if inadequately treated. Hence *Staphylococcus aureus* remains the most likely diagnosis in both acute and chronic forms of the condition.

2. Chronic osteomyelitis is clearly demonstrated on plain films. Acute osteomyelitis, if imaged very early, may not have radiographic changes. This is not the case for chronic cases where there has been significant cortical overgrowth and periosteal new bone formation. Typical features are sequestra (areas of dead bone because of loss of the overlying periosteal blood supply), involucrum (reactive new bone formation), and sinus tracts.

3. MRI is more sensitive than CT or plain film in detecting osteomyelitis, although it is inferior at detecting the presence and size of sequestra. MRI has the advantage of better contrast resolution and allowing the full extent of marrow abnormality to be assessed. CT does have faster scanning times and easier availability, but no ionizing radiation is an important benefit of MRI.

4. Although treatment should include systemic antibiotics, consideration should be made of underlying causes, for example, associated soft-tissue infection. Debridement is important to facilitate healing, including any sequestra.

5. Heterotopic ossification (formerly known as myositis ossificans), can often be misdiagnosed as malignancy. An area of trauma/inflammation containing areas of ossification should raise the possibility of this diagnosis. Other considerations for a soft-tissue mass with areas of ossification include a calcified hematoma, soft tissue sarcoma or chronic osteomyelitis.

Pearls

- Chronic osteomyelitis is characterized by periosteal new bone formation and cortical thickening.
- Associated causes should be sought, for example, adjacent soft-tissue abscess, immunodeficiency.
- Imaging should be performed to look for the complications, for example, sequestrum, soft-tissue abscesses, and sinus tracts.
- CT is superior to MRI for evaluating sequestra, but overall, MRI remains the investigative modality of choice because of better contrast resolution, no ionizing radiation, and better sensitivity for osteomyelitis.
- Periosteal new bone formation in chronic osteomyelitis should be distinguished from heterotopic ossification, although the two conditions may co-exist.

Suggested Readings

Forsberg JA, Potter BK, Cierny G, Webb L. Diagnosis and management of chronic infection. *J Am Acad Orthop Surg.* 2011;19 Suppl 1:S8-S19.

Hankin D, Bowling FL, Metcalfe SA, Whitehouse RA, Boulton AJ. Critically evaluating the role of diagnostic imaging in osteomyelitis. *Foot Ankle Spec.* 2011;4(2):100-105.

Kim SB, Jung WK, Song DI, Lee SH. Vesicocutaneous fistula presenting groin abscess and chronic osteomyelitis in pubic bone. *Clin Orthop Surg.* 2009;1(3):176-179.

Painful and swollen finger for several weeks, getting worse

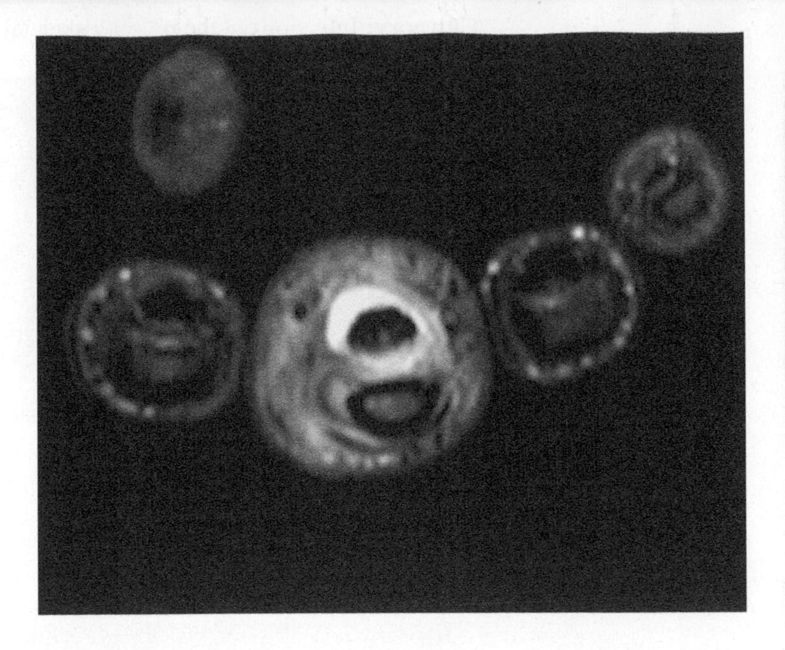

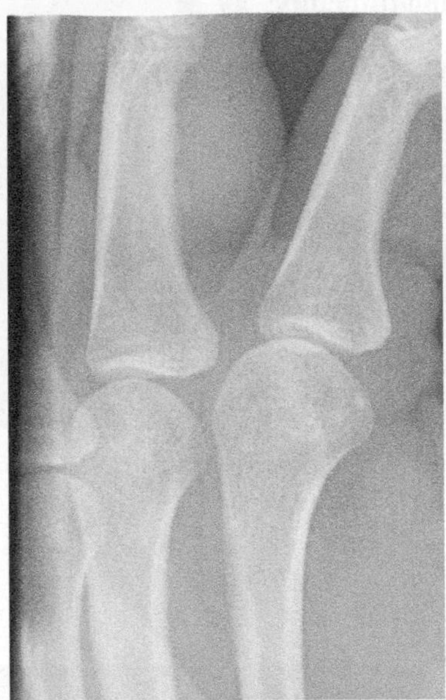

1. What are the plain radiograph findings?

2. What are the MRI findings?

3. What is the differential diagnosis?

4. What modalities are useful to detect subclinical inflammatory arthritis?

5. Psoriatic and rheumatoid arthritis can be differentiated on MRI. True or False?

Infectious flexor tenosynovitis 1332

Case ranking/difficulty: 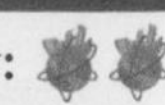

Category: Infections in the musculoskeletal system

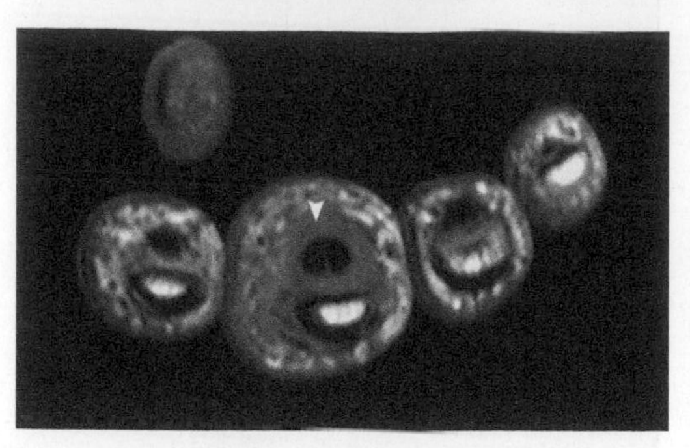

There is a low T1 signal intensity fluid around the flexor digitorum longus tendon.

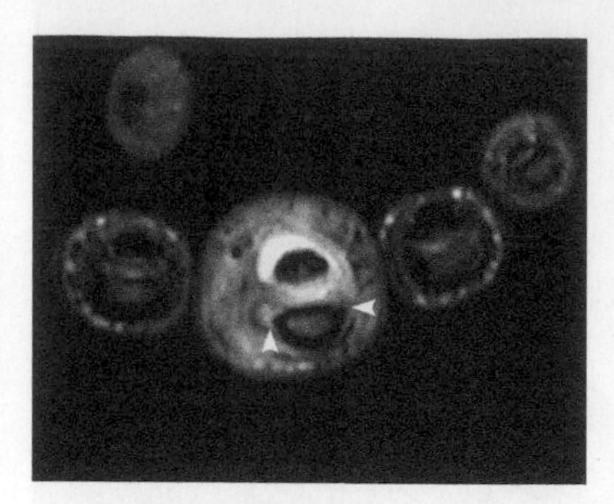

Fluid around the flexor tendon (FDP) of the middle finger. Associated edema and periosteal reaction (*arrowhead*) and subperiosteal collection (*left arrowhead*), of the proximal phalanx.

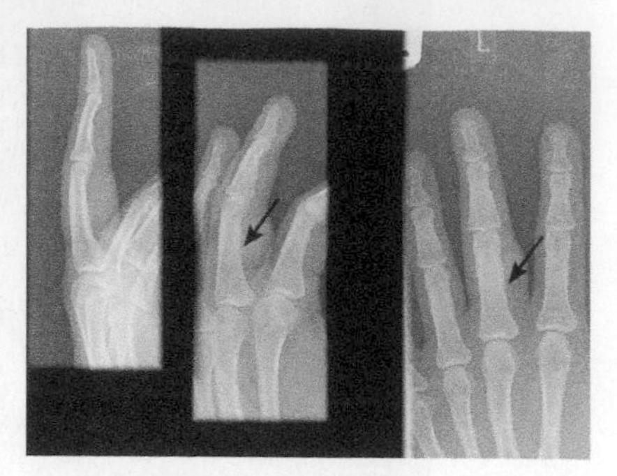

Arrow shows the periosteal reaction in the adjacent bone.

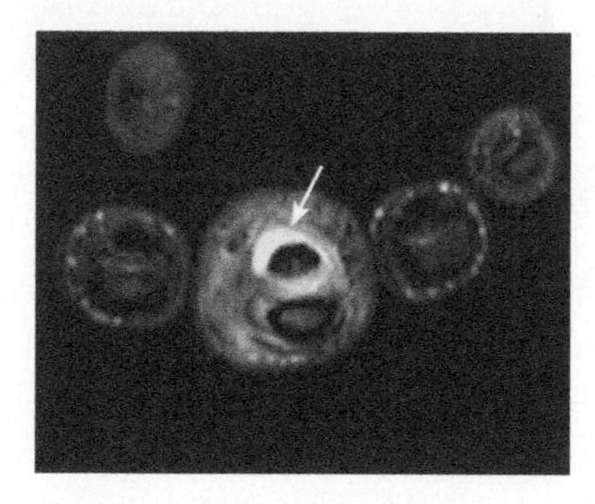

Axial image shows the fluid within the flexor tendon sheath.

Answers

1. Periosteal reaction and soft-tissue swelling is demonstrated.
2. Low T1 and high T2 signal intensity fluid collection within the flexor tendon sheath. There is mild associated bone marrow edema, and periosteal reaction with a subperiosteal fluid collection.
3. The causes for flexor tenosynovitis are either infective or inflammatory. This case was infective tenosynovitis.
4. Ultrasound can detect early subclinical synovitis. It is well recognized that MRI can demonstrate early rheumatoid arthritis changes, by showing tenosynovitic changes in the early stage of disease.
5. True. MRI can help to differentiate between rheumatoid and psoriatic arthritis, with the ability to look for specific changes. The presence of enthesitis or extensive diaphyseal bone marrow edema and pronounced soft tissue edema spreading to the subcutaneous tissues, favors psoriatic arthritis.

   The flexor tendons are also more commonly involved in psoriatic rather than rheumatoid arthritis.

Pearls

- Flexor tenosynovitis is an inflammatory condition of the flexor tendon sheath.
- It can be either secondary to infection, or autoimmune diseases such as rheumatoid arthritis.
- Plain film may show periosteal reaction in the adjacent bone in infectious tenosynovitis.
- MRI shows low T1 signal in the tendon sheath and high signal fluid on T2-weighted images with edema and sometimes collections of purulent material. In infectious causes, the synovial proliferation may be thick and irregular. The tendon may be enlarged with tendinosis, and uncommonly may become infarcted and tear.
- Conservative treatment includes IV or oral antibiotics. However, most surgeons consider this an emergency, and exploration and washout in conjunction with IV or oral antibiotics is performed to prevent rapid spread of infection to the palmar spaces, and tendon necrosis.
- A felon is considered as a fingertip closed space infectious collection, and requires urgent drainage. It is not a tendon sheath infection.

Suggested Readings

Eshed I, Feist E, Althoff CE, et al. Tenosynovitis of the flexor tendons of the hand detected by MRI: an early indicator of rheumatoid arthritis. *Rheumatology (Oxford).* 2009;48(8):887-891.

Tehranzadeh J, Ashikyan O, Anavim A, Tramma S. Enhanced MR imaging of tenosynovitis of hand and wrist in inflammatory arthritis. *Skeletal Radiol.* 2006;35(11): 814-822.

Back pain with fever and bladder and bowel incontinence

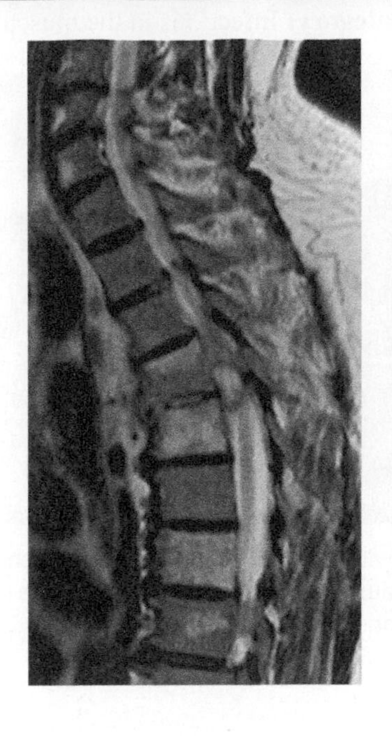

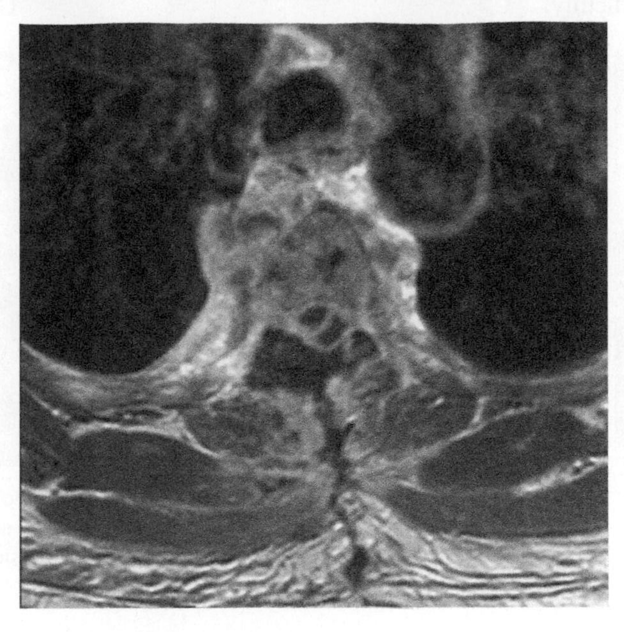

1. What are the MRI findings?

2. What are the differential diagnoses?

3. What is the diagnosis?

4. What are the pathways for spread of this disease?

5. Is periosteal reaction typically present in this condition?

Tuberculous epidural abscess with cord compression 988

Case ranking/difficulty: 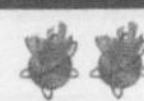

Category: Infections in the musculoskeletal system

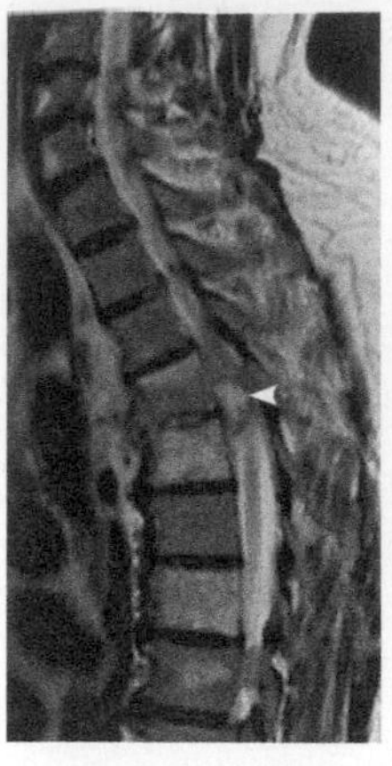

There is an epidural abscess (*arrowhead*) with osteomyelitis/discitis at the T3 and T4 levels of thoracic spine.

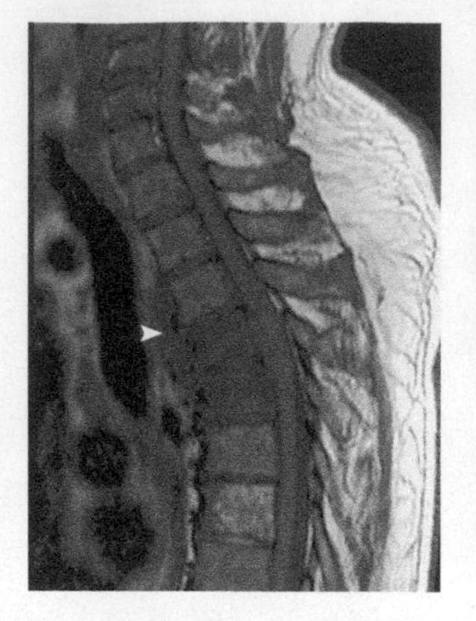

Paraspinal collection at T3/T4 with osteomyelitis.

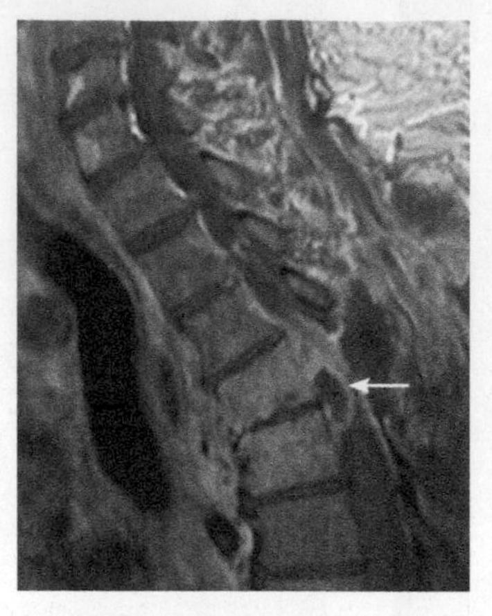

Post-contrast image showing the epidural collection causing thoracic cord compression.

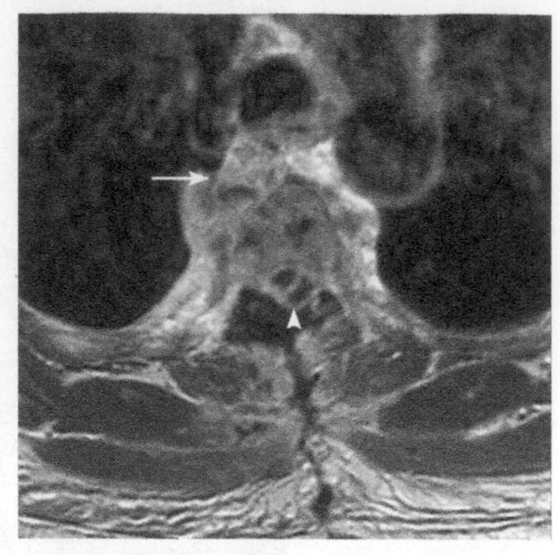

Post-contrast image showing epidural (*arrowhead*) as well as paraspinal (*arrow*) collection.

Answers

1. There is a paraspinal and epidural abscess, discitis, and cord compression.
2. There is cord compression that could be a result of metastatic infiltration, osteoporotic collapse, or discitis secondary to the TB or pyogenic infection. Lesions such as lymphoma, myeloma, brucellosis, and sarcoidosis should also be considered, but would be considered less likely.
3. The diagnosis is TB osteomyelitis with paravertebral abscess. Multilevel contiguous involvement and preserved discs until the end stage supports the diagnosis. Post-contrast image shows the epidural collection, with cord compression.
4. Contiguous subchondral endplate, subligamentous spread behind the anterior and posterior longitudinal ligaments, and spread along the venous plexus of Batson is typical for TB.
5. Periosteal reaction and bone sclerosis are typically absent until late in the disease process, and are inconstant features.

Pearls

- Tuberculosis of the spine is the most common skeletal manifestation of *Mycobacterium tuberculosis* infection, comprising 50% of skeletal TB cases.
- It commonly affects young children in developing countries, where paraspinal abscess and neurological symptoms are the common presentation. In the Western world it affects the older population, where a neurological presentation is not a common feature.
- Risk factors includes malnutrition, poor immunity, HIV, and previous TB exposure.
- The most common site is in the thoracolumbar spine.
- Radiographs may show a gibbus deformity.
- Periosteal reaction and bone sclerosis are typically absent or minimal, and is a late feature.
- The infection spreads along the periosteum and under the anterior longitudinal ligament. Subchondral bone involvement leads to weakening and to central disc prolapse.
- Spinal TB often presents as a paraspinal and/or prevertebral abscess. In rare cases, it can lead to an epidural collection and cord or cauda equina compression.

Suggested Readings

Jinkins JR, Gupta R, Chang KH, Rodriguez-Carbajal J. MR imaging of central nervous system tuberculosis. *Radiol Clin North Am*. 1995;33(4):771-786.

Shikhare SN, Singh DR, Shimpi TR, Peh WC. Tuberculous osteomyelitis and spondylodiscitis. *Semin Musculoskelet Radiol*. 2011;15(5):446-458.

Slow-growing mass in the neck

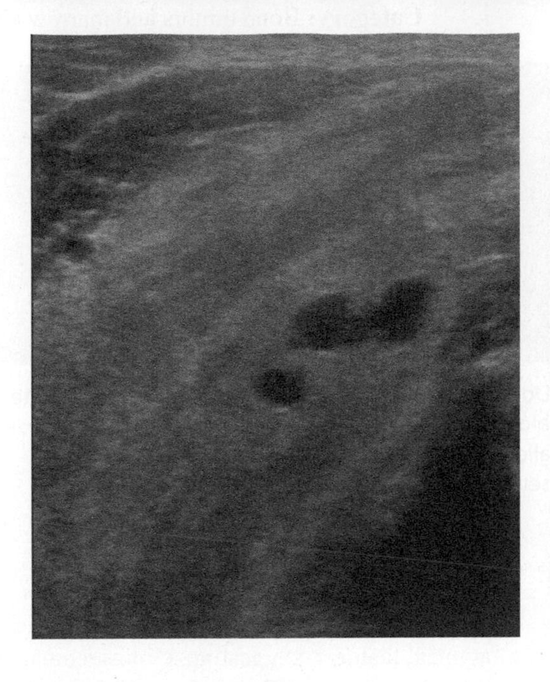

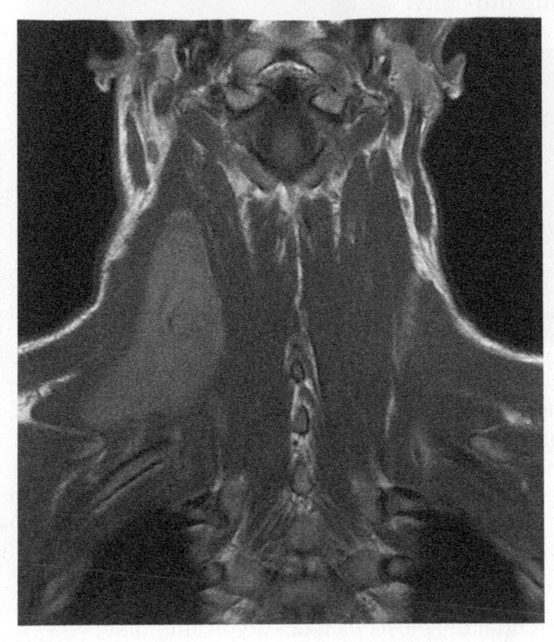

1. What is the differential diagnosis?
2. From where does this lesion arise?
3. What are the most common locations for this lesion?
4. What is the vascularity of this lesion on ultrasound and MRI?
5. What is the enhancement pattern after intravenous contrast?

Hibernoma 1596

Case ranking/difficulty: 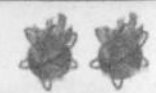 **Category:** Bone tumors and marrow abnormalities

Large intramuscular T2 hyperintense lesion in the right side of neck, showing linear septations (*left arrowhead*) and increased vascularity (*right arrowhead*).

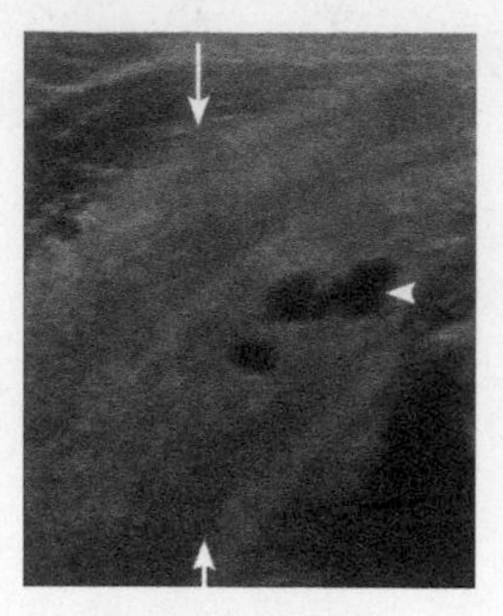

Ultrasound shows hyperechogenic lesion (*arrows*) with septations and vessels (*arrowhead*).

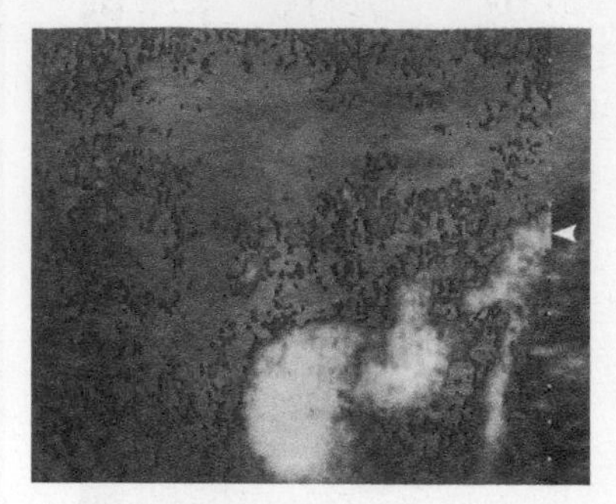

Doppler image shows increased blood flow within the lesion, even allowing for the suboptimal gain settings.

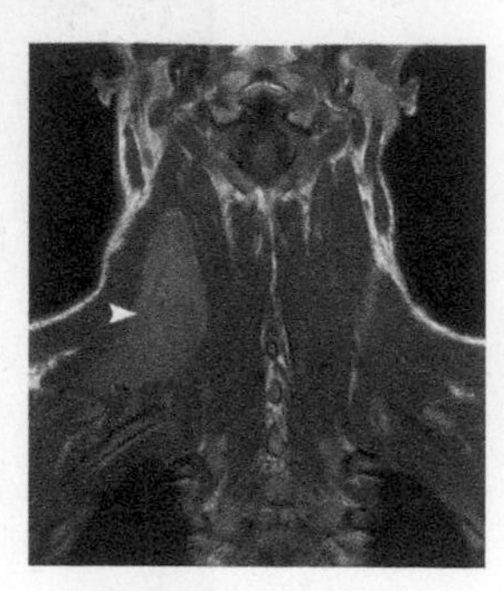

T1 hyperintense mass in the right side of neck.

Answers

1. The differential diagnosis includes atypical lipoma, low-grade liposarcoma, and hibernoma.
2. Hibernomas arise from the vestiges of fetal brown fat.
3. They are typically located in the thigh, back, neck, shoulders, and arms.
4. Hibernomas show increased Doppler signal with hypervascularity and arteriovenous shunting.
5. Increased vascularity within the lesion generally (but not always) results in contrast enhancement. This makes it difficult to differentiate from liposarcoma, hence excision biopsy is usually required.

Pearls

- A hibernoma is a rare benign soft-tissue tumor arising from fetal brown fat.
- It usually affects patients 20 to 50 years old and is commonly seen around the thigh, shoulder, back, neck, and arm.
- It is a slow-growing and vascular fatty tumor.
- Ultrasound shows a hyperechogenic lesion with atypical features, suggesting a liposarcoma. On MRI, it has high T1 and T2 signal, which is not completely saturated on fat-saturated images. There is increased vascularity with serpentine low T1 and T2 signal intensity vessels within the lesion.
- Histology makes the final diagnosis.
- Surgical excision is the treatment of choice. Hibernomas are not known to recur or metastasize.

Suggested Readings

Anderson SE, Schwab C, Stauffer E, Banic A, Steinbach LS. Hibernoma: imaging characteristics of a rare benign soft tissue tumor. *Skeletal Radiol.* 2001;30:590-595.

Bai S, Mies C, Stephenson J, Zhang PJ. Intraosseous hibernoma: a potential mimic of metastatic carcinoma. *Ann Diagn Pathol.* 2012 Aug 10 [Epub ahead of print].

Furlong MA, Fanburg-Smith JC, Miettinen M. The morphologic spectrum of hibernoma: a clinicopathologic study of 170 cases. *Am J Surg Pathol.* 2001;25(6):809-814.

Painful mass in the foot

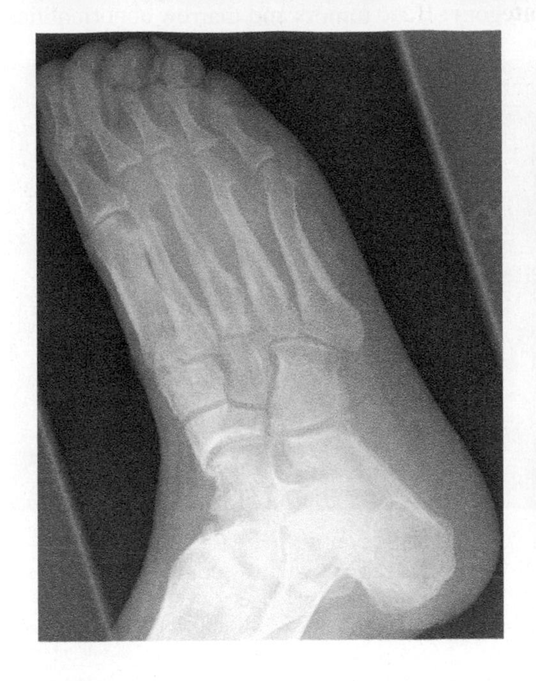

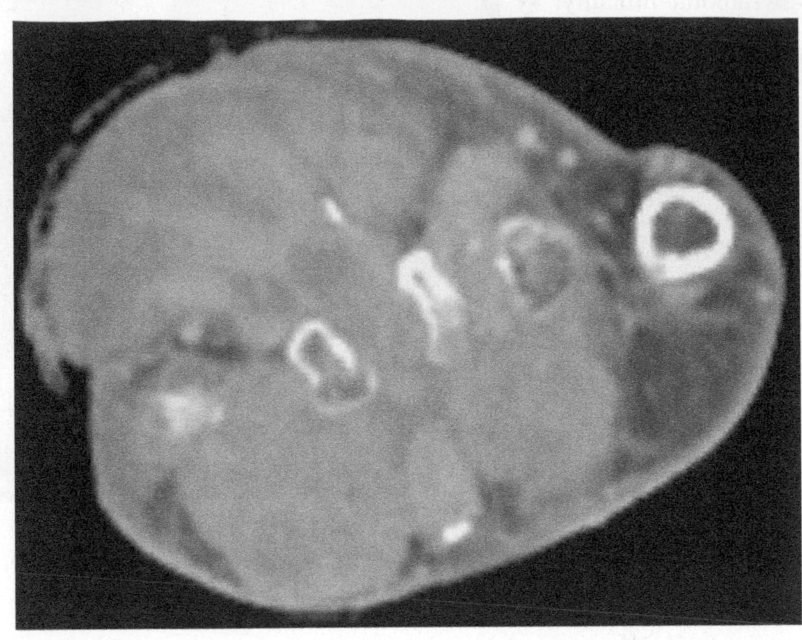

1. What are the radiograph and CT findings?

2. What may you expect to see on MRI?

3. What is included in the differential diagnosis in this case?

4. What is the most likely diagnosis?

5. What percentage of these tumors show calcification?

Synovial sarcoma 1562

Case ranking/difficulty: 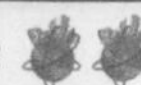

Category: Bone tumors and marrow abnormalities

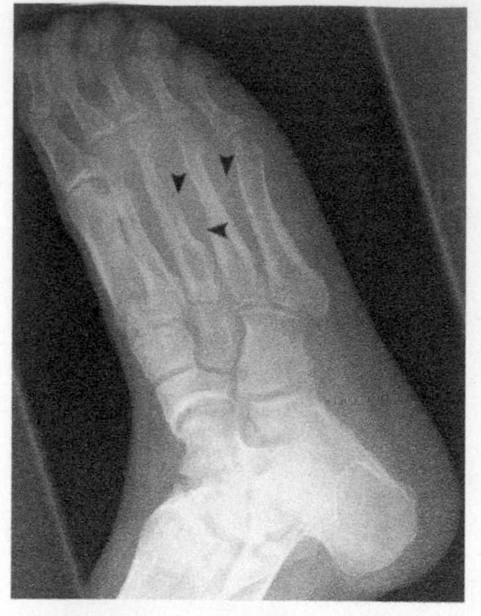

Soft-tissue mass with calcification (*arrowhead*), and remodeling of several metatarsals but no bone destruction.

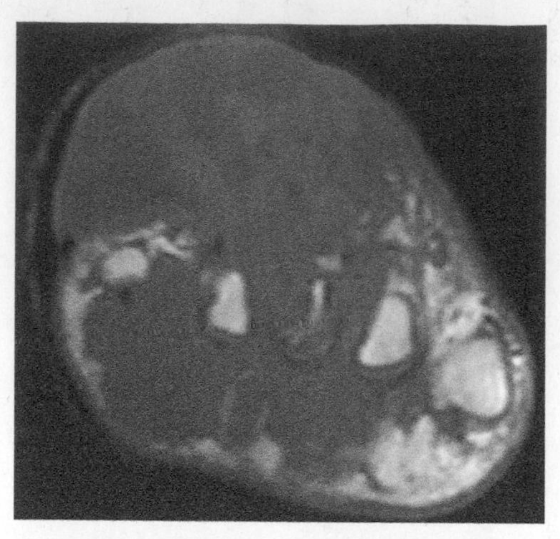

Heterogenous soft-tissue mass invaginating between the metatarsals.

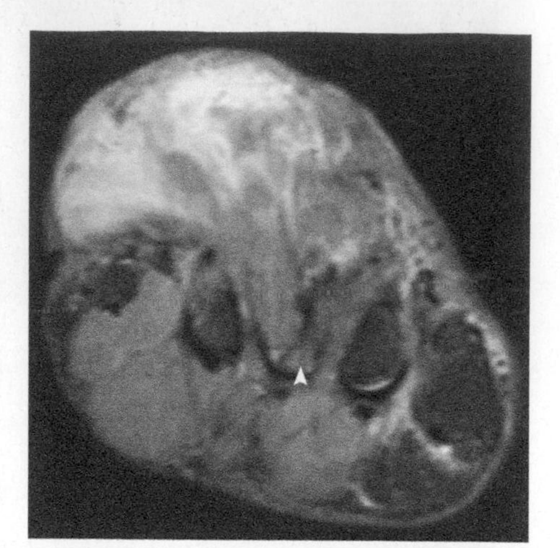

Heterogenously increased signal. Mild reactive bone marrow edema in the third metatarsal (*arrowhead*).

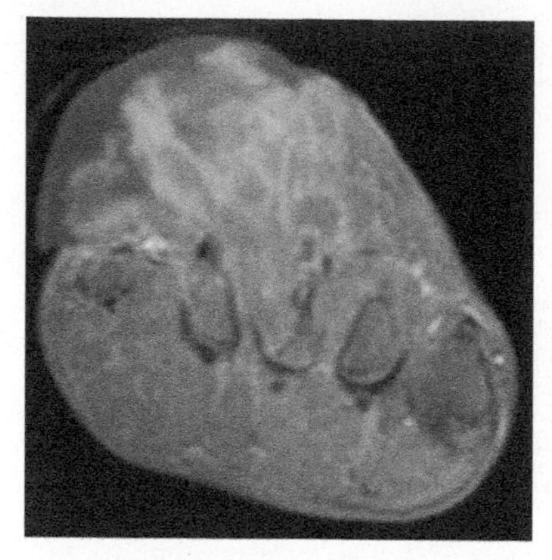

Marked heterogenous enhancement.

Answers

1. There is a large soft-tissue mass with internal calcification and remodelling but no destruction of bone.
2. MRI signal characteristics are highly variable, and may show a "triple signal" pattern as a result of fibrosis and necrosis and variable enhancement.
3. The differential includes malignant fibrous histiocytoma (MFH) and synovial sarcoma. Soft-tissue metastasis, deep fibromatosis, and clear cell sarcomas would not be expected to calcify.
4. Based on the age of the patient, location in the feet and calcifications, the most likely diagnosis is synovial sarcoma.
5. Thirty percent to 50% of synovial sarcomas show calcification.

Pearls

- Synovial sarcomas are the most common malignant soft-tissue tumors in the feet.
- The age peak is at 30 years, but tumors typically occur from ages 10 to 50 years.
- The lesions appear well defined, but infiltrate adjacent soft tissues.
- Calcification is seen in 30% to 50% of cases.
- Pressure effects on bone is common, but frank destructive changes are not.
- Up to one-third of cases will show the "triple-signal" pattern with T2 hypointensity caused by fibrosis, areas of isointensity to muscle, and areas of T2 hyperintensity caused by necrosis. Enhancement with contrast is typical, although heterogeneity is common.
- Periosteal reaction is seen in 20% of patients.

Suggested Readings

Jones BC, Sundaram M, Kransdorf MJ. Synovial sarcoma: MR imaging findings in 34 patients. *AJR Am J Roentgenol.* 1993;161(4):827-830.

Murphey MD, Gibson MS, Jennings BT, Crespo-Rodríguez AM, Fanburg-Smith J, Gajewski DA. From the archives of the AFIP: imaging of synovial sarcoma with radiologic-pathologic correlation. *Radiographics.* 2006;26(5):1543-1565.

Slow-growing mass in the hand

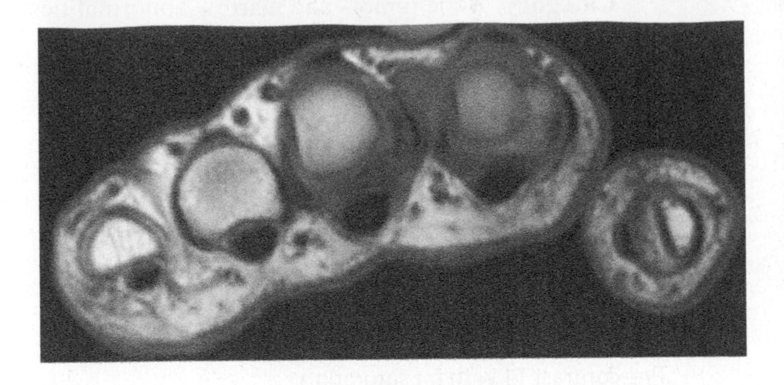

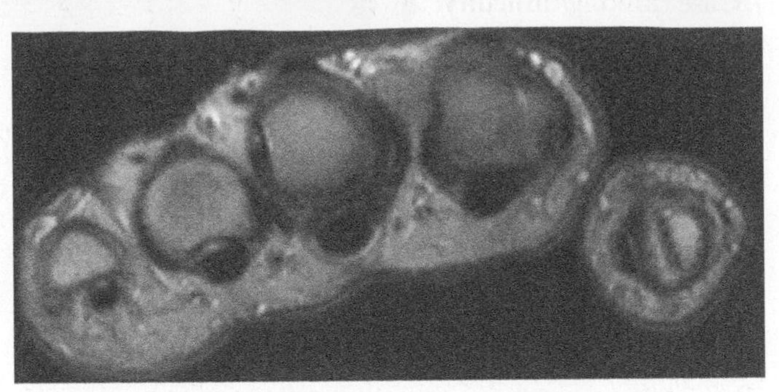

1. What are the MRI findings?

2. What is the most likely diagnosis?

3. What is the most common location of this lesion?

4. What additional test would be most useful in confirming the diagnosis?

5. What are the typical ultrasound characteristics of the lesion?

Giant cell tumor of the tendon sheath 1556

Case ranking/difficulty: 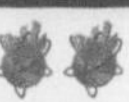

Category: Bone tumors and marrow abnormalities

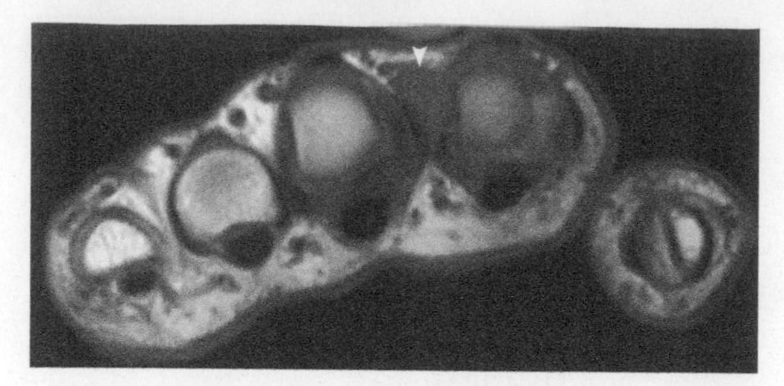

T1 isointense to mildly hypointense soft-tissue lesion located between the second and third metacarpal heads.

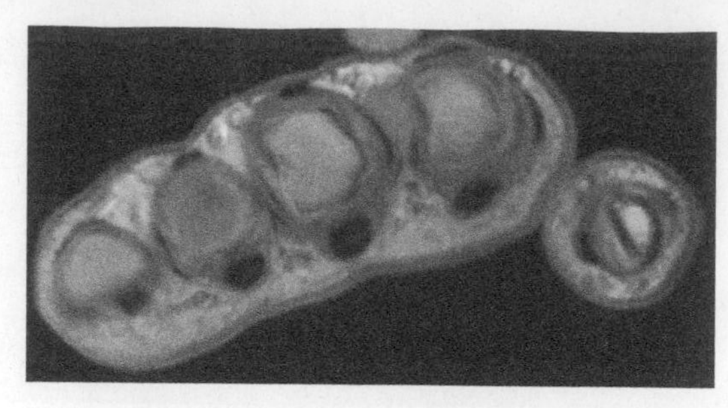

Pre-contrast T1 with fat saturation.

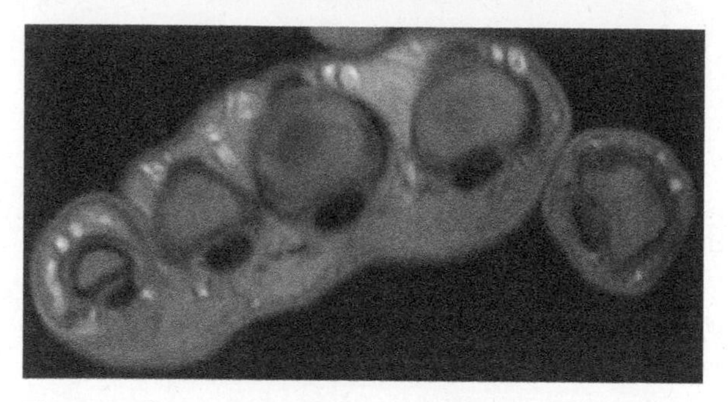

There is enhancement after contrast.

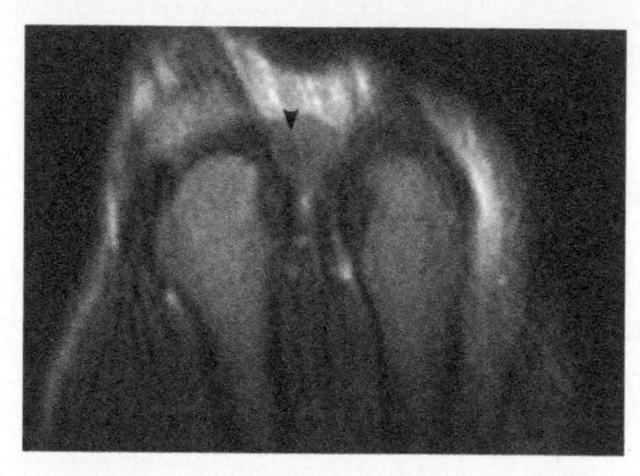

The lesion is mildly T2 hyperintense relative to muscle with foci of low signal, suggesting hemosiderin (*arrowhead*).

Answers

1. There is a soft-tissue mass that shows T1 hypo-/isointensity, mildly heterogenous T2 hyperintensity, and well-defined margins.
2. Giant cell tumor (GCT) of the tendon sheath.
3. The hands are the most common location for a GCT.
4. A gradient-echo sequence will show blooming, which is suggestive of intralesional hemosiderin.
5. A giant cell tumor of the tendon sheath is typically hypoechoic on ultrasound, with no posterior acoustic enhancement. Internal Doppler signal is typical.

Pearls

- GCTs of the tendon are the second most common soft-tissue lesion of the hands and feet after ganglion cysts.
- Lesions are much more common in the hands rather than feet.
- Weightbearing and degenerative joint disease may at least be contributory.
- Local forms are more common than the rare diffuse form. The diffuse form parallels the distribution of joint PVNS, that is, large joints such as knees or ankles, and is considered its soft-tissue counterpart.
- Plain film changes are uncommon and include pressure remodelling of bone and intraosseous cysts.
- Ultrasound typically shows a hypoechoic soft-tissue mass with internal vascularity and no posterior acoustic enhancement.
- MRI typically shows a soft-tissue lesion attached to a tendon that is T1 and T2 hypointense, and enhances with intravenous contrast. The amount of T2 hypointensity depends on the amount of hemosiderin present and is variable.
- The lesions bloom on gradient echo sequences because of hemosiderin. Fat-laden macrophages may cause signal heterogeneity, with tiny foci of increased T1 signal.
- Recurrence is common in up to 45% of patients, but with careful wide resection can be reduced to 10% to 20%.

Suggested Readings

Llauger J, Palmer J, Monill JM, Franquet T, Bagué S, Rosón N. MR imaging of benign soft-tissue masses of the foot and ankle. *Radiographics*. 1998;18(6):1481-1498.

Middleton WD, Patel V, Teefey SA, Boyer MI. Giant cell tumors of the tendon sheath: analysis of sonographic findings. *AJR Am J Roentgenol*. 2004;183(2):337-339.

History of foot mass that has slightly increased in size, possible history of trauma

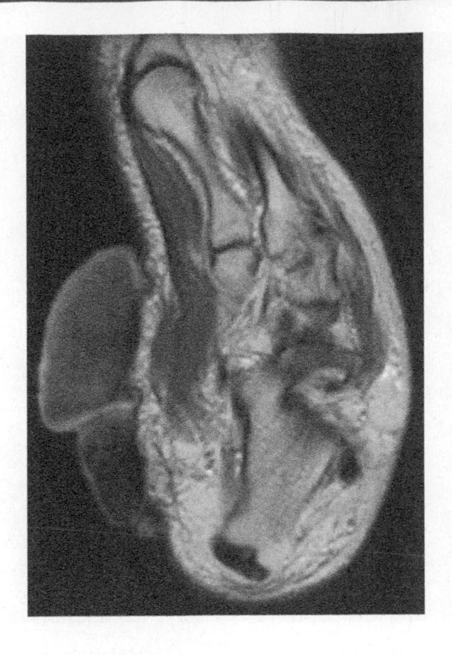

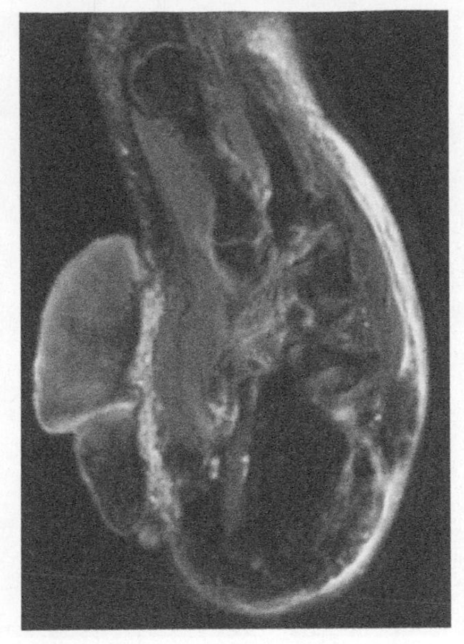

1. What are the MRI findings?
2. What can be expected to be seen on contrast-enhanced MRI?
3. What would you expect PET-CT to show in this lesion?
4. What is included in the differential diagnosis?
5. What is the most likely diagnosis?

Keloids 1550

Case ranking/difficulty: 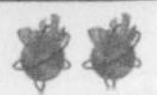

Category: Trauma

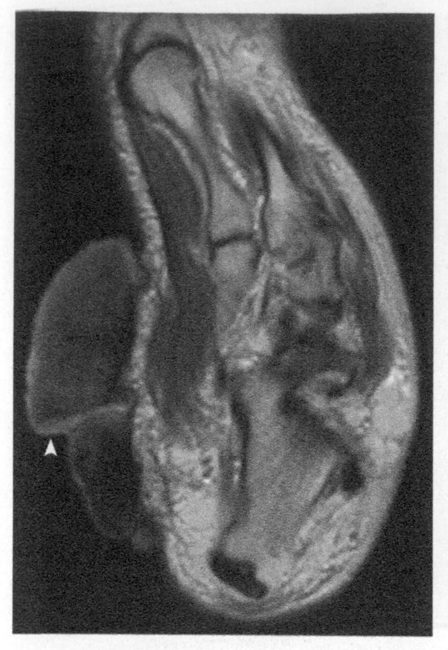

Multilobulated, predominantly T1 hypointense lesion in the skin of the medial foot.

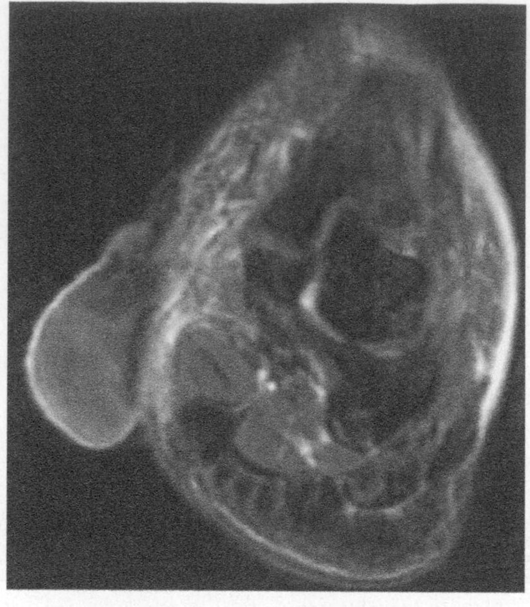

Lobulated, heterogenous, predominantly T2 hypointense lesion arising from the skin.

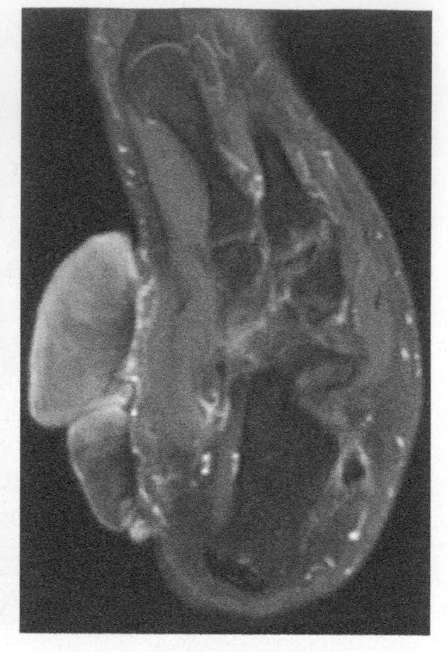

Heterogenous enhancement is seen.

Answers

1. There is an exophytic mass with T1 hypointensity, T2 hyperintensity, and heterogeneity with mild dermal edema.
2. Keloids typically enhance with gadolinium, although mild heterogeneity is typical. In large lesions, areas of necrosis may occur.
3. PET-CT is generally not indicated, as the diagnosis is made clinically. Increased uptake is typical, showing the glucose metabolism of the lesion.
4. The differential includes hypertrophic scar, keloids, lobomycosis, dermatofibrosarcoma protuberans, and foreign-body granuloma.
5. Based on the history and imaging, keloid is the most likely diagnosis.

Pearls

- Keloids are a dense growth of fibrous tissue that extends beyond the area of injury.
- Hypertrophic scars do not extend beyond the area of injury.
- Keloids are 15 times more common in blacks and Hispanics, and in more pigmented races overall.
- Patients with earlobe keloids are not considered "keloid formers" from a surgical perspective.
- On MRI, the lesions are isointense to low signal on T1-weighted images, and variable but generally decreased signal on T2-weighted images. This example is mildly T2 hyperintense, possibly reflecting recent treatment and a relative paucity of collagen. Lesions typically enhance with contrast.
- Keloids are echogenic on ultrasound.
- They show variable but increased ^{18}F-FDG uptake on PET-CT.

Suggested Readings

Atiyeh BS, Costagliola M, Hayek SN. Keloid or hypertrophic scar: the controversy: review of the literature. *Ann Plast Surg.* 2005;54(6):676-680.

Cugno S, Rizis D, Cordoba C. Beyond the borders of keloid formation: a case report. *Can J Plast Surg.* 2011;19(1):e10-e11.

Ankle pain

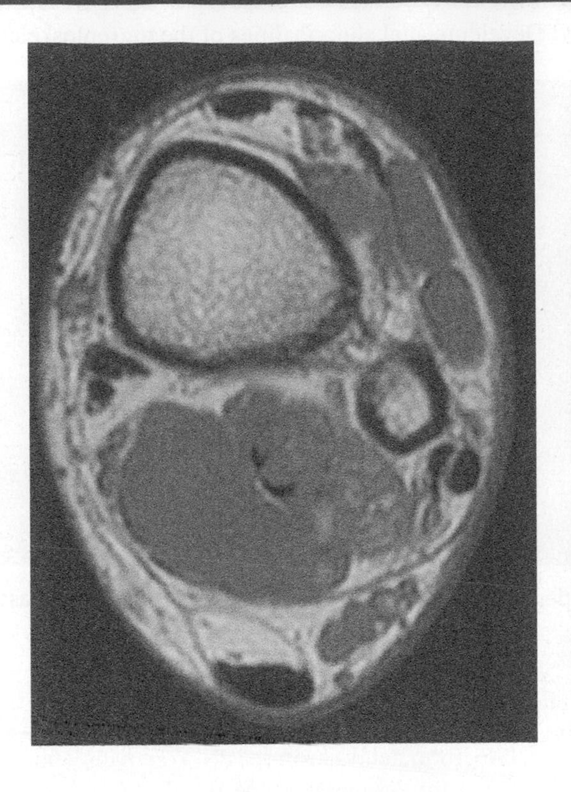

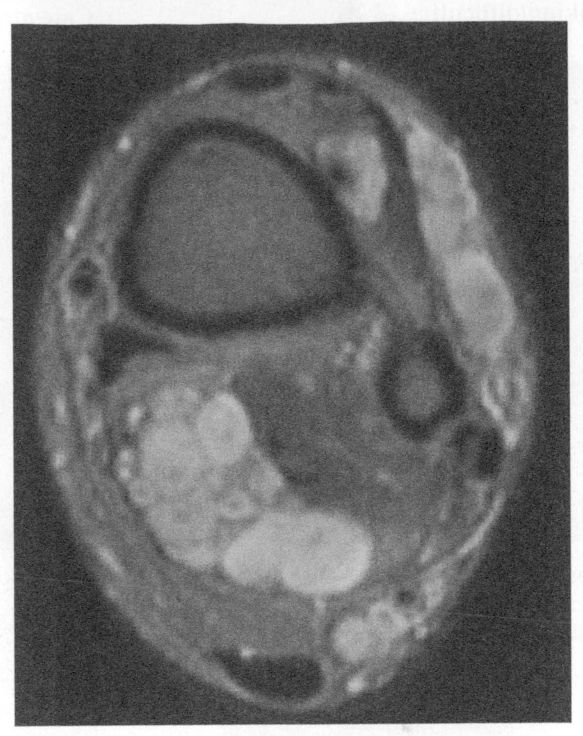

1. What features does MRI demonstrate?

2. What is included in the differential diagnosis?

3. What is the most likely diagnosis?

4. What is the target sign?

5. A plexiform neurofibroma is pathognomonic for what condition?

Plexiform neurofibroma 1549

Case ranking/difficulty: 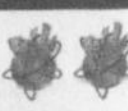

Category: Developmental abnormalities of the musculoskeletal system

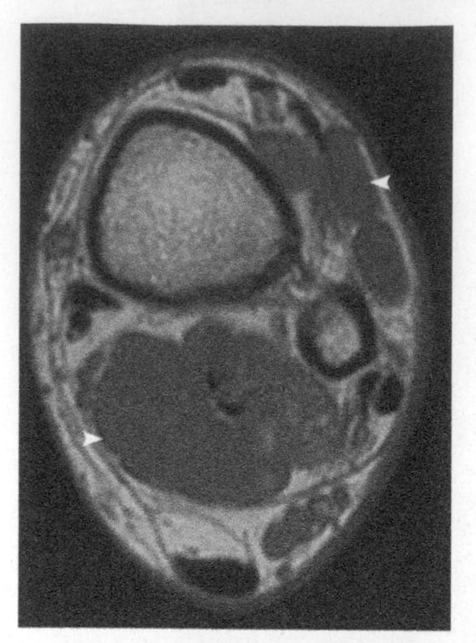

Large masses that are T1 isointense to mildly hypointense in the posteromedial and anterolateral ankle.

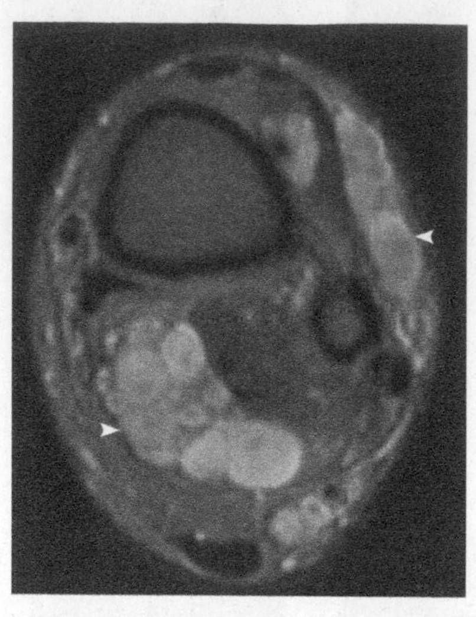

Multiple target signs are demonstrated.

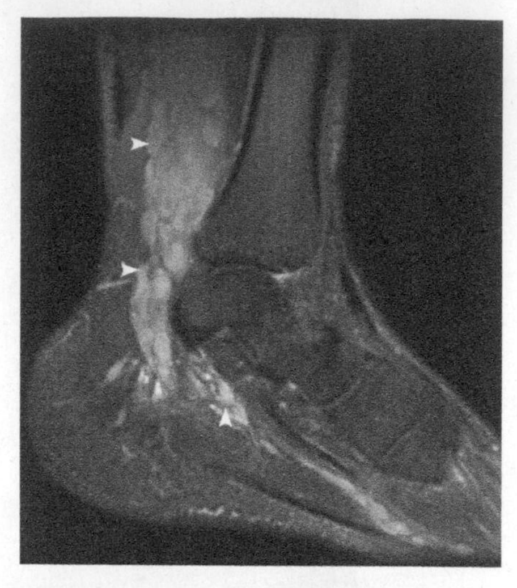

The extensive nature of the masses are demonstrated.

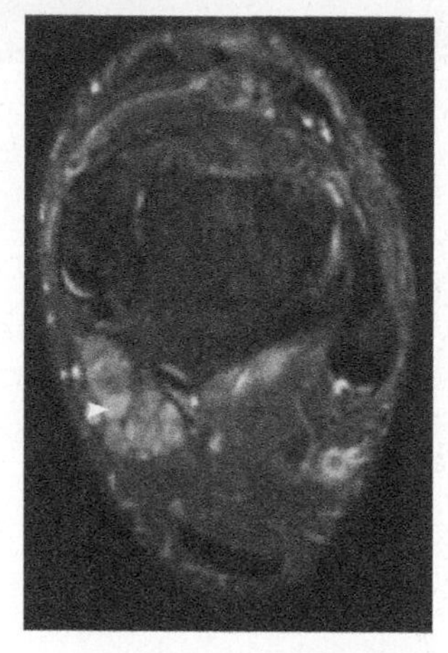

The lesion extends into the tarsal tunnel.

Answers

1. Multiple soft-tissue masses that demonstrate target signs are demonstrated.
2. Based on the morphology and multiplicity of lesions, the differential diagnosis includes hemangioma, lymphangioma, and plexiform neurofibroma.
3. Given the morphology of the lesions and the presence of numerous "target" signs, the most likely diagnosis is plexiform neurofibroma.
4. Central T1 hypointensity caused by collagen and peripheral T2 hyperintensity is characteristic of the "target" sign seen in nerve sheath tumors.
5. A plexiform neurofibroma is pathognomonic for neurofibromatosis type 1.

Pearls

- Plexiform neurofibromas (PNs) are pathognomonic for neurofibromatosis type 1.
- The most common nerve affected is the fifth cranial nerve.
- Superficial and deep variants of PN have been described.
- The deep variants are larger, better defined, and demonstrate the classic "target" appearance.
- The superficial variant most commonly does not have a target appearance. Contrast enhancement is variable.
- The diagnosis of neurofibromatosis is made if 2 of the following criteria are met:
  - Six or more café-au-lait spots
  - Two or more neurofibromas or 1 plexiform neurofibroma
  - Multiple freckles in the inguinal or axillary region
  - Characteristic osseous lesion such as pseudoarthrosis or sphenoid dysplasia
  - Optic glioma
  - Two or more iris hamartomas
  - A first-degree relative with neurofibromatosis (NF)
- Treatment is with surgical debulking if indicated.

Suggested Readings

Lim R, Jaramillo D, Poussaint TY, Chang Y, Korf B. Superficial neurofibroma: a lesion with unique MRI characteristics in patients with neurofibromatosis type 1. *AJR Am J Roentgenol.* 2005;184(3):962-968.

Woertler K. Tumors and tumor-like lesions of peripheral nerves. *Semin Musculoskelet Radiol.* 2010;14(5):547-558.

History of mass in the posterior knee

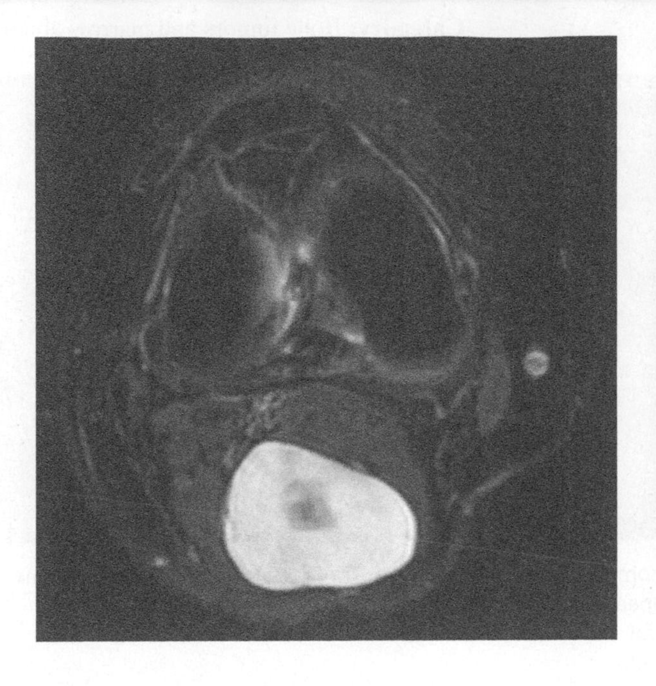

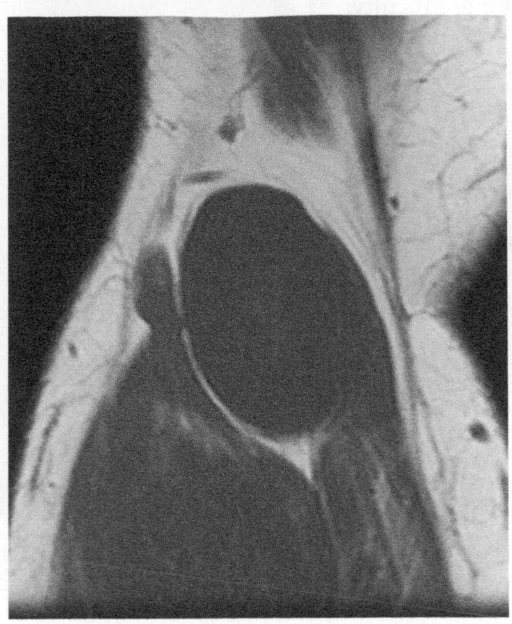

1. What are the pertinent MRI findings?

2. What is the differential diagnosis?

3. What is the most likely diagnosis?

4. What is the target sign?

5. What MRI features are more suggestive of schwannoma rather than neurofibroma?

Neurofibroma 1442

Case ranking/difficulty: 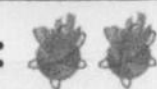

Category: Bone tumors and marrow abnormalities

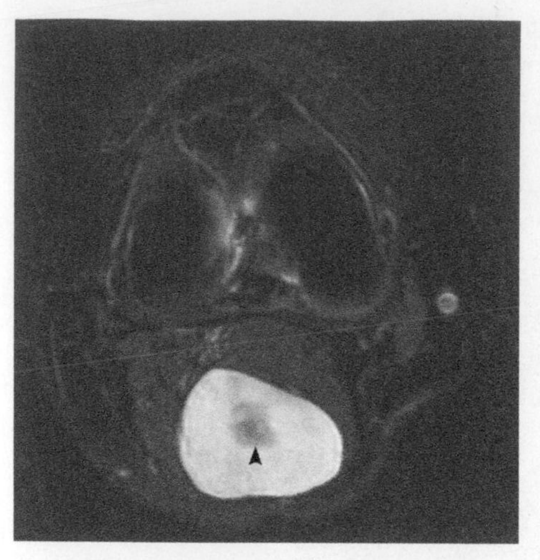

There is a well-defined soft-tissue mass with peripheral hyperintensity, and central hypointensity (*arrowhead*). This is known as the "target" sign.

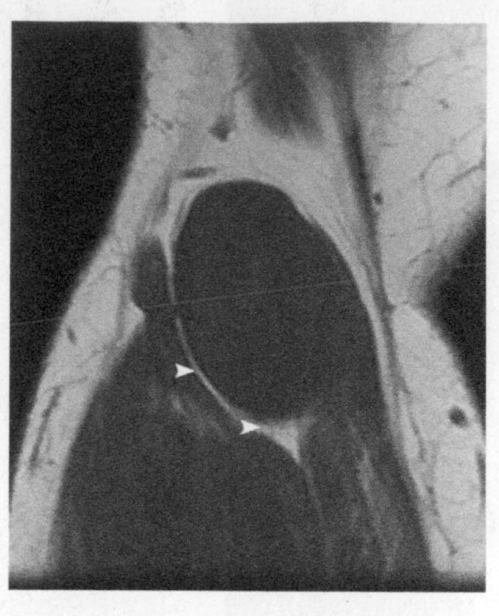

The lesion is homogenously low signal, and appears to "split" the hyperintense fat, the so-called split-fat sign (*arrowhead*).

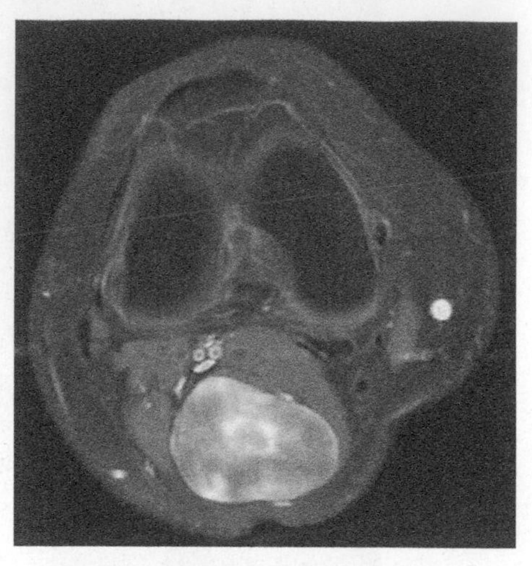

There is heterogenous enhancement.

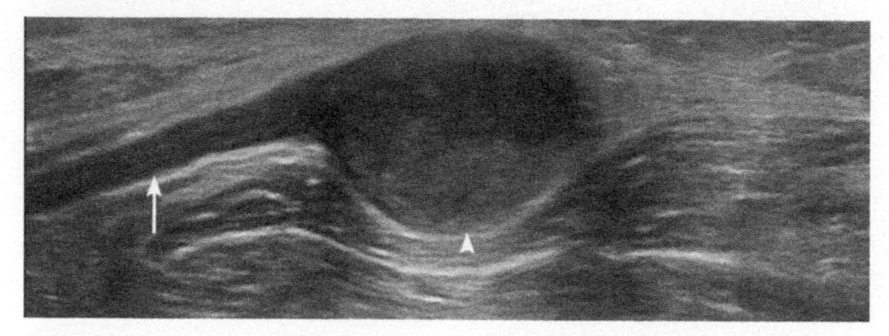

Neurofibroma on high-resolution ultrasound (another patient). *Arrowhead* points to the neurofibroma; *arrow* points to the normal nerve.

Answers

1. There is a T1 hypointense soft-tissue mass, with central T2 hypointensity and peripheral T2 hyperintensity. A "split-fat" sign is demonstrated.
2. The findings suggest a peripheral nerve sheath tumor. A sarcoma and lymphoma are unlikely, but still included in the differential.
3. The presence of "target" and "split-fat" signs suggests a peripheral neurofibroma.
4. The target sign is T2 central hypointensity caused by collagen, and peripheral T2 hyperintensity. It is seen in neurofibromas.
5. A fascicular appearance, a peripheral T2 hyperintense rim, and homogenous enhancement are more suggestive of a schwannoma.

Pearls

- Neurofibromatosis type 1 (NF1) accounts for 90% of cases of neurofibromatosis.
- Peripheral nerve sheath tumors in NF1 include neurofibromas, schwannomas, and plexiform neurofibromas.
- MR features of neurofibromas include the target and split-fat signs.
- A target sign is seen on T2-weighted images, with a central collagenous area that is T1 hypointense and peripherally T2 hyperintense.
- Central enhancement is seen after contrast.
- Homogenous enhancement, a peripheral T2 hyperintense rim and a fascicular appearance favor a schwannoma over neurofibroma.
- Plexiform neurofibromas have a tortuous worm-like configuration that may appear infiltrative. They are T1 hypointense, T2 hyperintense, and enhance after contrast.

Suggested Readings

Jee WH, Oh SN, McCauley T, et al. Extraaxial neurofibromas versus neurilemomas: discrimination with MRI. *AJR Am J Roentgenol.* 2004;183(3):629-633.

Murphey MD, Smith WS, Smith SE, Kransdorf MJ, Temple HT. From the archives of the AFIP. Imaging of musculoskeletal neurogenic tumors: radiologic-pathologic correlation. *Radiographics.* 1999;19(5):1253-1280.

Chronic foot pain

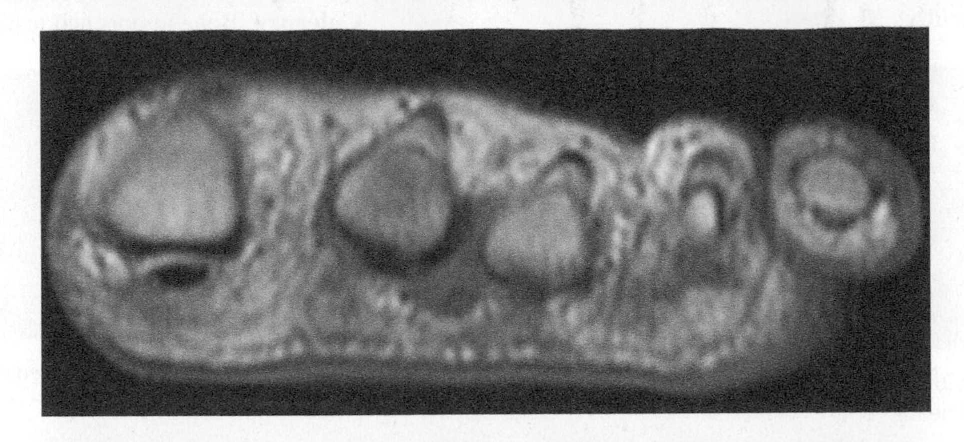

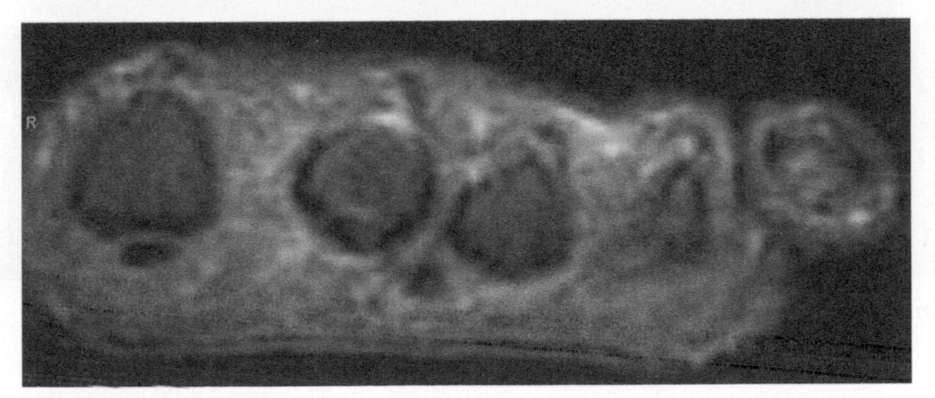

1. What are the MRI findings?
2. What is the differential diagnosis?
3. What is the most likely diagnosis?
4. What is the pathology of the lesion?
5. What are the ultrasound characteristics of this entity?

Morton neuroma 1419

Case ranking/difficulty: 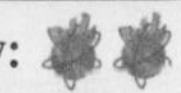

Category: Bone tumors and marrow abnormalities

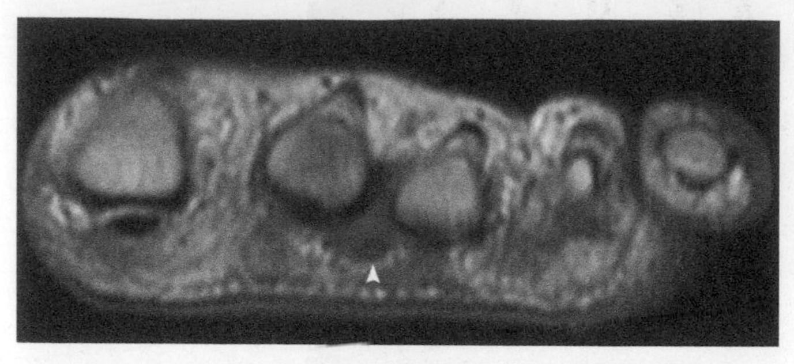

Focal low signal lesion located in the second interspace at the level of the metatarsal heads.

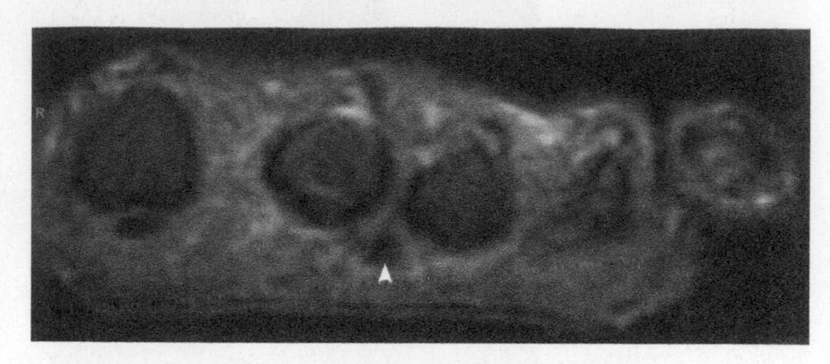

The lesion remains low signal on T2-weighted images.

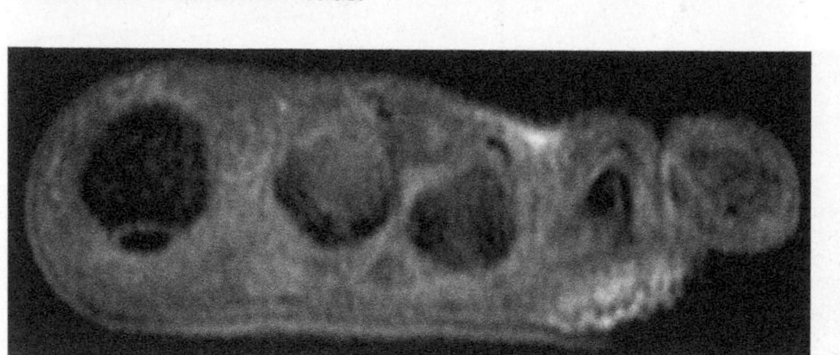

Fat-saturated T1 pre-contrast image shows the low signal lesion.

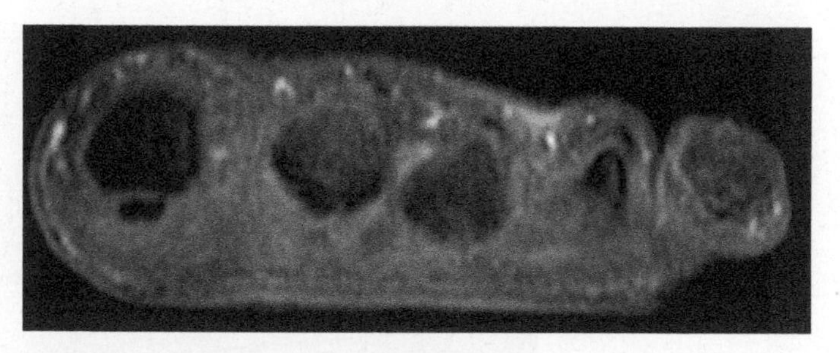

There is no enhancement after contrast.

Answers

1. Well-defined lesion in the plantar aspect of the second interspace, with T1 and T2 hypointensity. Typically there is contrast enhancement but there is variability, with this lesion showing no significant enhancement.
2. Morton neuroma, intermetatarsal bursitis, rheumatoid nodule, foreign-body granuloma, and giant cell tumor of the tendon sheath.
3. Based on the location and imaging characteristics, the most likely diagnosis is a Morton neuroma.
4. A Morton neuroma is the result of perineural fibrosis.
5. Typically hypoechoic, but uncommonly anechoic or mixed echogenic with increased Doppler signal. Lesions are contiguous with the fibrillary digital nerve.

Pearls

- Morton neuromas likely result from chronic repetitive injury, and are most commonly seen in women who wear high heels.
- Histology shows perineural fibrosis and the lesions are not true nerve sheath tumors.
- Lesions are most commonly located in the third intermetatarsal space, followed by the second space.
- Morton neuromas are most commonly hypoechoic on ultrasound and are continuous with the digital nerve. Lesions can be anechoic.
- MRI shows lesions that are low signal on both T1- and T2-weighted images, and typically enhance with contrast.
- The short axis plane is the best way of imaging these lesions on MRI.

Suggested Readings

Bencardino J, Rosenberg ZS, Beltran J, Liu X, Marty-Delfaut E. Morton's neuroma: is it always symptomatic? *AJR Am J Roentgenol.* 2000;175(3):649-653.

Walker EA, Fenton ME, Salesky JS, Murphey MD. Magnetic resonance imaging of benign soft tissue neoplasms in adults. *Radiol Clin North Am.* 2011;49(6):1197-1217, vi.

Knee joint swelling and pain

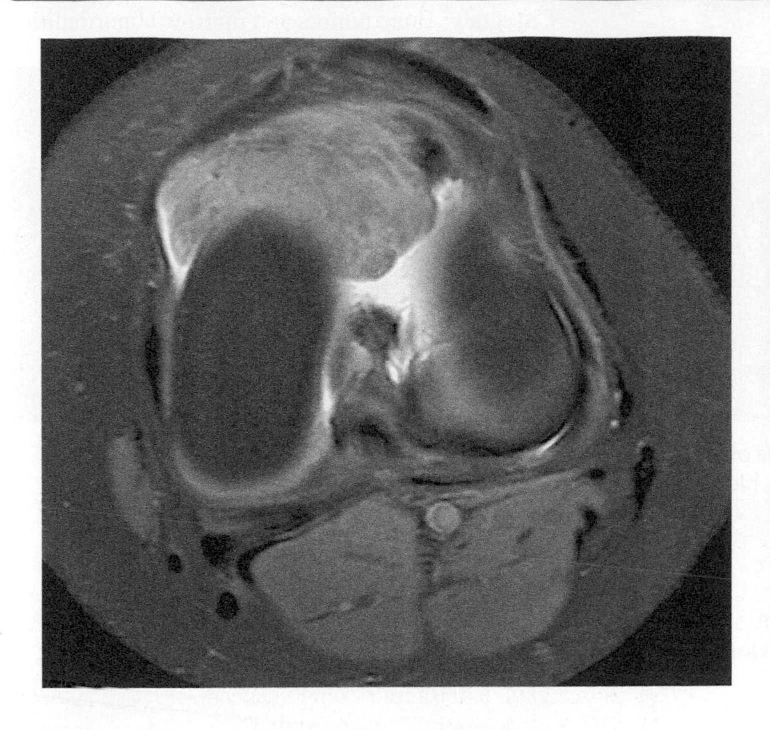

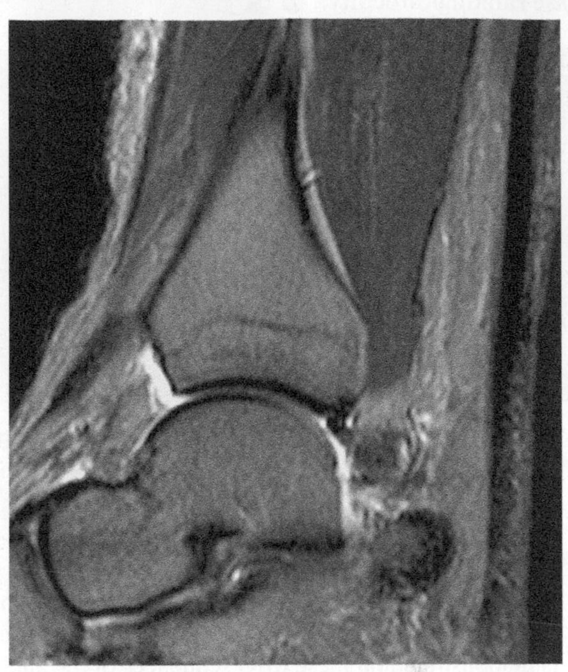

1. What are the MRI findings in both the ankle and knee joints?

2. What is the differential diagnoses?

3. What are the expected plain film findings?

4. What are the expected CT findings?

5. What are the treatment options?

Pigmented villonodular synovitis (PVNS) 1402

Case ranking/difficulty: 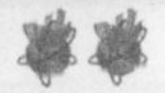

Category: Bone tumors and marrow abnormalities

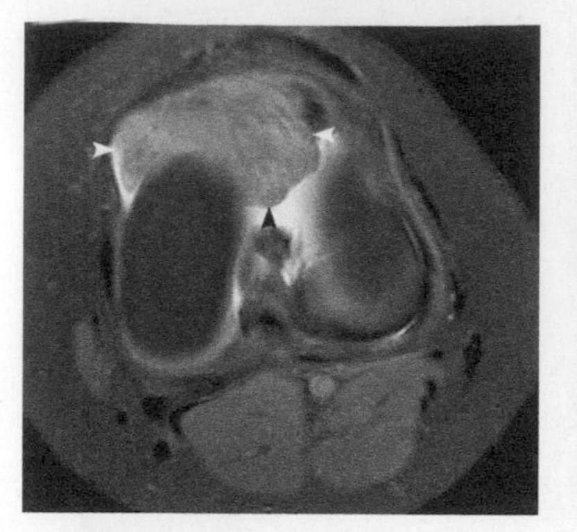

Low signal intensity synovial hypertrophy.

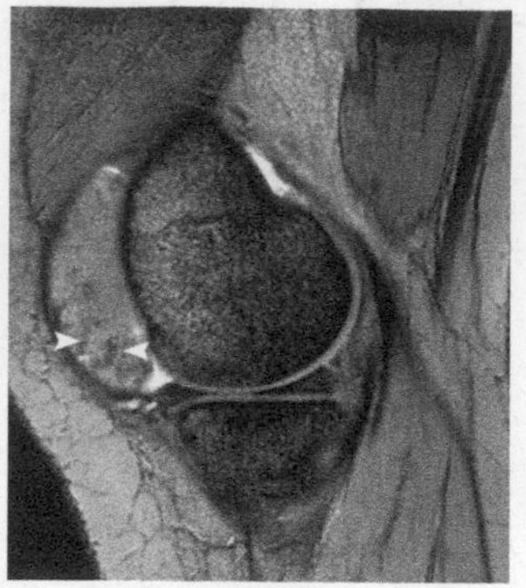

Gradient-echo image of the knee demonstrating blooming artifact.

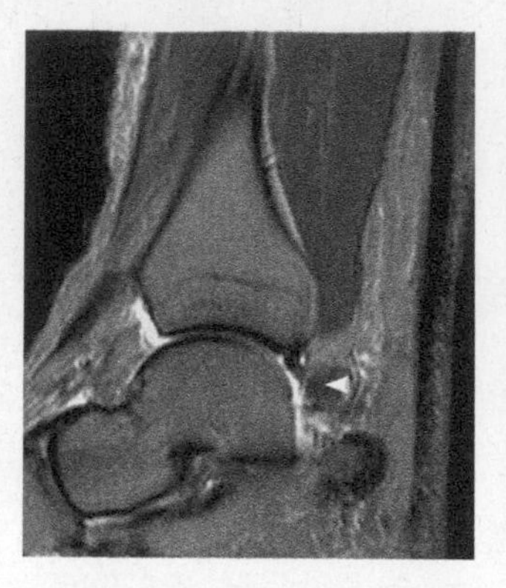

A different patient with similar changes of low signal intensity synovial proliferation and PVNS.

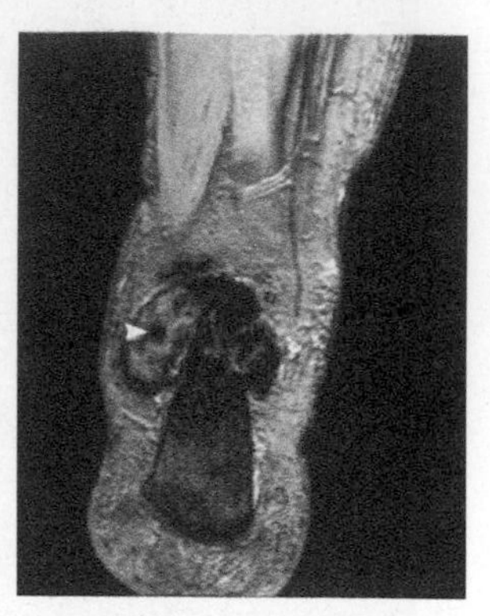

Blooming susceptibility artifact.

Answers

1. Low T1 and T2 signal intensity synovial proliferation, blooming effect on T2*GRE sequence and joint effusion is demonstrated on these MRI sequences of the ankle and knee joints. Marginal erosions are a feature of this condition, but not demonstrated in this case.
2. The differential diagnoses include synovial osteochondromatosis, synovial sarcoma, osteoarthritis, hemophilia, and PVNS. The overall findings are consistent with PVNS.
3. Although there are not many diagnostic findings on plain radiographs, joint effusion and marginal erosions or cysts can be appreciated.

   However, negative findings are important to exclude other conditions such as synovial osteochondromatosis.
4. Soft-tissue density mass is seen in 29% of cases, which is of higher attenuation than surrounding muscles as a result of hemosiderin deposition.

   There can be a knee effusion and marginal erosions. No calcifications or osteoporosis are usually seen.
5. The treatment options include complete synovectomy, arthrodesis, arthroplasty, intra-articular yttrium-90 and adjuvant external beam radiotherapy.

   There is a 20% chance of recurrence after complete synovectomy.

Pearls

- PVNS is a rare, benign, hyperplastic disorder of the synovium, leading to synovial villous or nodular proliferation with hemosiderin deposition.
- PVNS can be focal or diffuse. It may also be intra-articular, or extra-articular in a bursa or tendon sheath, as in a giant cell tumor of tendon sheath.
- PVNS most commonly affects the knee joint.
- Clinically presents with pain, effusion, monoarthritis, and possibly a palpable mass.
- X ray: Usually nonspecific with a joint effusion that can appear somewhat dense as a result of hemosiderin. There is no calcification or osteoporosis, and no joint space narrowing until late-stage disease. There are marginal erosions and cystic change in some cases.
- CT: Joint effusion and soft-tissue mass of synovial hypertrophy that is denser than muscle as a result of hemosiderin. Possible erosions and cysts.
- MRI: T1 and T2 low to intermediate signal synovial proliferation. Gradient echo (T2*) will demonstrate a blooming susceptibility artifact with low signal intensity. There is variable post-contrast enhancement.

Suggested Readings

Heyd R, Micke O, Berger B, et al. Radiation therapy for treatment of pigmented villonodular synovitis: results of a national patterns of care study. *Int J Radiat Oncol Biol Phys.* 2010;78(1):199-204.

Masih S, Antebi A. Imaging of pigmented villonodular synovitis. *Semin Musculoskelet Radiol.* 2003;7(3):205-216.

Murphey MD, Rhee JH, Lewis RB, Fanburg-Smith JC, Flemming DJ, Walker EA. Pigmented villonodular synovitis: radiologic-pathologic correlation. *Radiographics.* 2009;28(5):1493-1518.

History of a slow-growing mass in the foot and pain

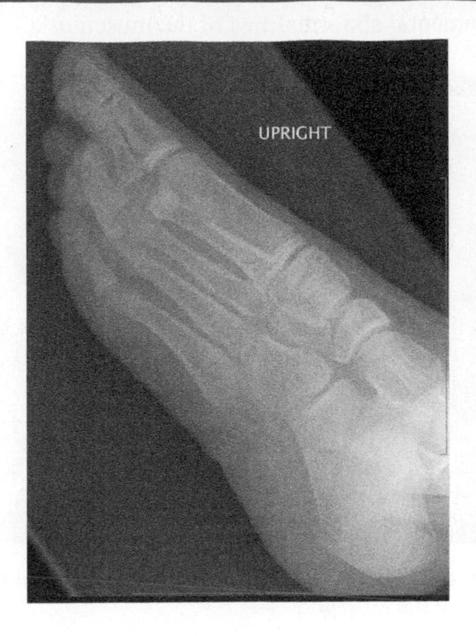

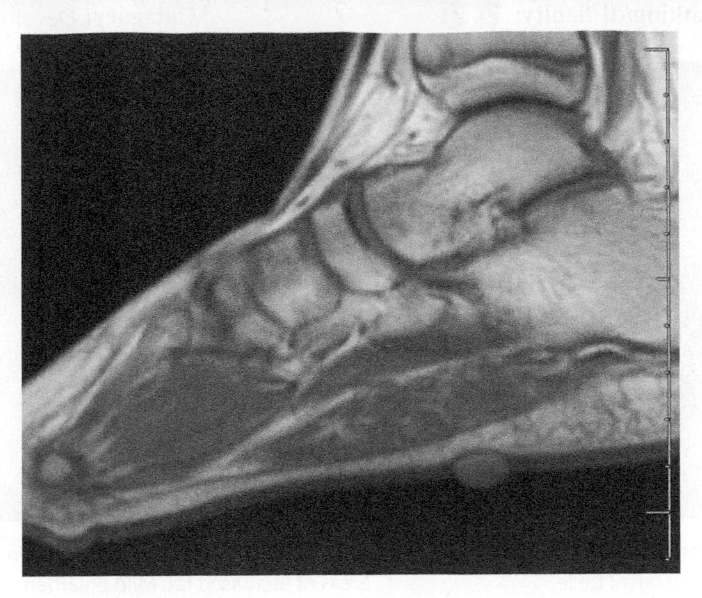

1. What are the radiograph findings?
2. What does the T1-weighted MR image show?
3. What is the most likely diagnosis?
4. What changes may be seen in Maffucci syndrome?
5. What are the features of Kasabach-Merritt syndrome?

Intramuscular hemangioma 1458

Case ranking/difficulty: 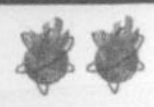

Category: Developmental abnormalities of the musculoskeletal system

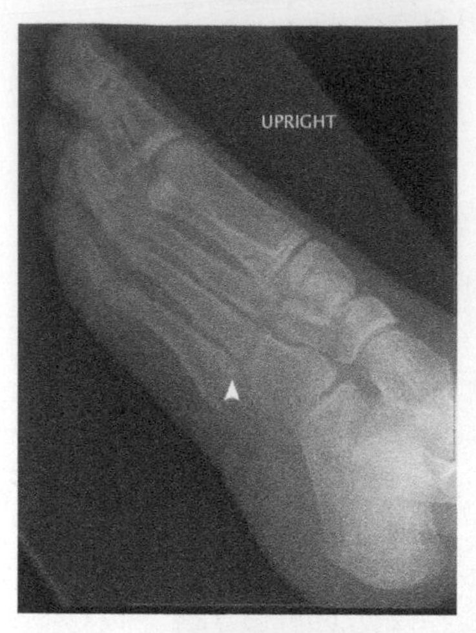

Single phlebolith is noted over the fifth metatarsal base.

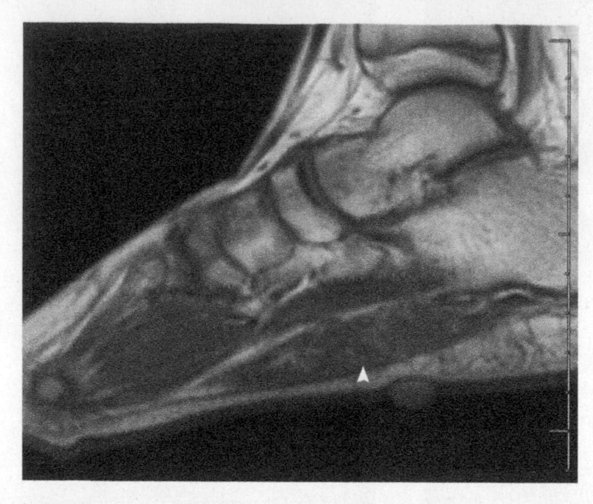

Heterogeneity of the flexor digitorum brevis muscle with areas of increased fat. Mild enlargement of the muscle.

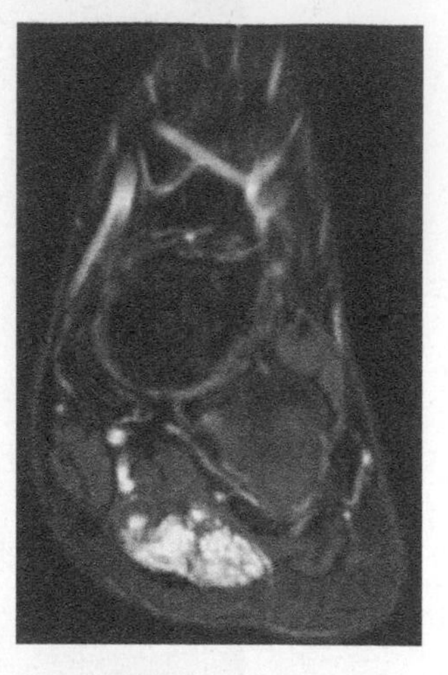

Lobular increased T2 signal.

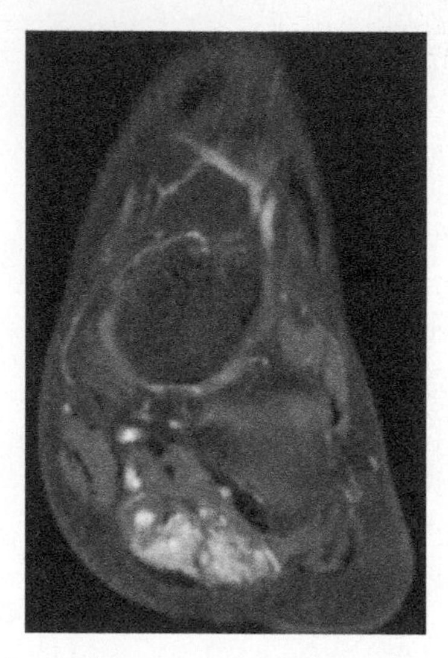

Marked serpiginous contrast enhancement is seen.

Pearls

- Hemangiomas in the musculoskeletal system are vascular malformations.
- Lesions may be capillary, cavernous, venous, arteriovenous, or mixed.
- Phleboliths are seen in 20% to 67% of cases but are nonspecific.
- Ultrasound shows a hyperechoic mass with variable vascularity.
- MRI shows a mass with areas of T1 hyperintensity as a result of entrapped fat or fatty hypertrophy. T2-weighted images will show increased T2 signal.
- Foci of low T1 and T2 signal are a result of fibrosis, hemosiderin, and calcified phleboliths.
- There is usually marked serpiginous enhancement after contrast.

Answers

1. Typical radiographic features include a soft-tissue mass, cortical thickening, periosteal reaction, and remodelling of adjacent bone. The only finding in this case is an isolated phlebolith.
2. Mass in the flexor digitorum brevis muscle with areas of fat, but no bony changes.
3. Intramuscular hemangioma.
4. Multiple soft-tissue hemangiomas and osseous enchondromas are seen in Maffucci syndrome. There is an increased risk for osseous sarcomatous transformation.
5. Thrombocytopenia, hemolytic anemia, hemangiomas, rapid growth, and a consumptive coagulopathy.

Suggested Readings

Ly JQ, Sanders TG, Mulloy JP, et al. Osseous change adjacent to soft-tissue hemangiomas of the extremities: correlation with lesion size and proximity to bone. *AJR Am J Roentgenol.* 2003;180(6):1695-1700.

Yuh WT, Kathol MH, Sein MA, Ehara S, Chiu L. Hemangiomas of skeletal muscle: MR findings in five patients. *AJR Am J Roentgenol.* 1987;149(4):765-768.

Pain in the shoulder with a sensation of fullness

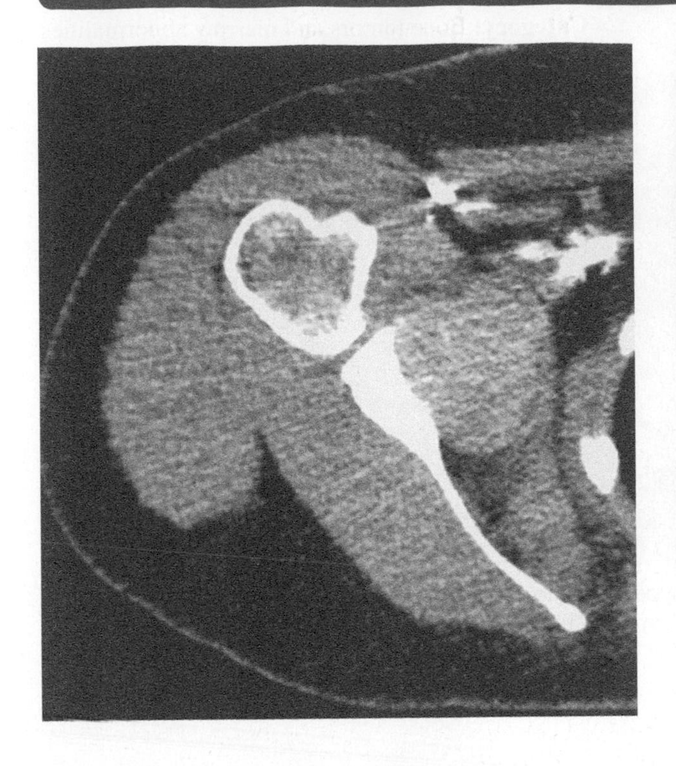

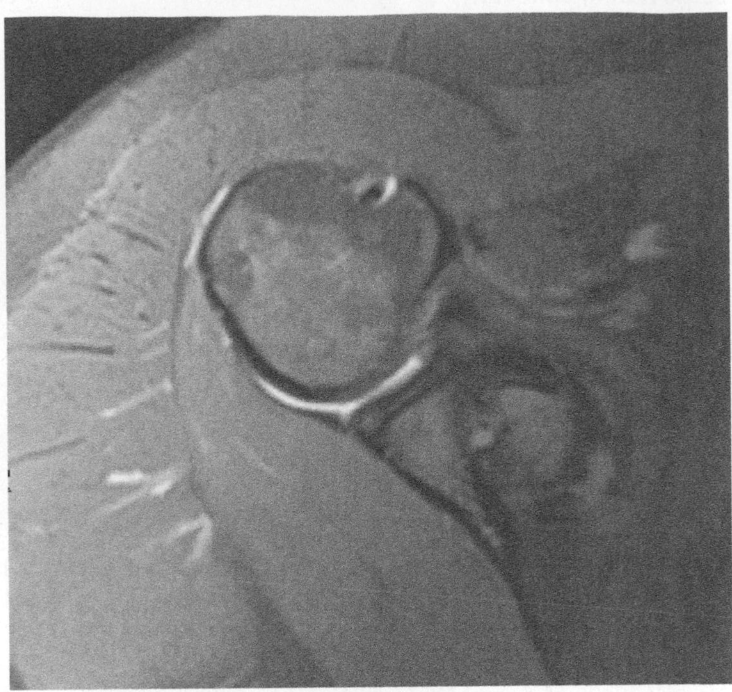

1. What are the CT findings?

2. What are the low signal intensity bands on the fat-saturated FSE T2-weighted images?

3. What entities are included in the general differential diagnosis?

4. What is the most likely diagnosis?

5. Patients with which syndrome have a much higher risk for developing these lesions?

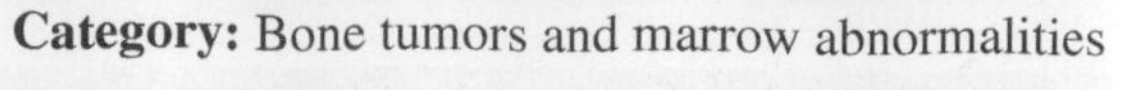

Fibromatosis: deep extra-abdominal 1454

Case ranking/difficulty: 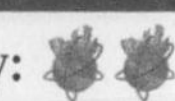

Category: Bone tumors and marrow abnormalities

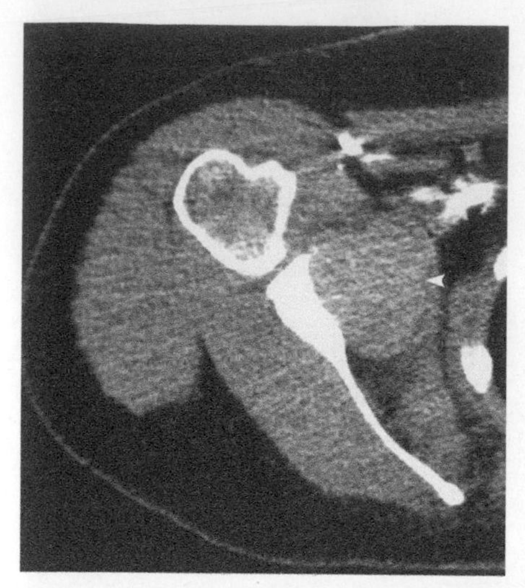

Mildly hyperdense soft-tissue mass deep to the subscapularis muscle with bony remodeling.

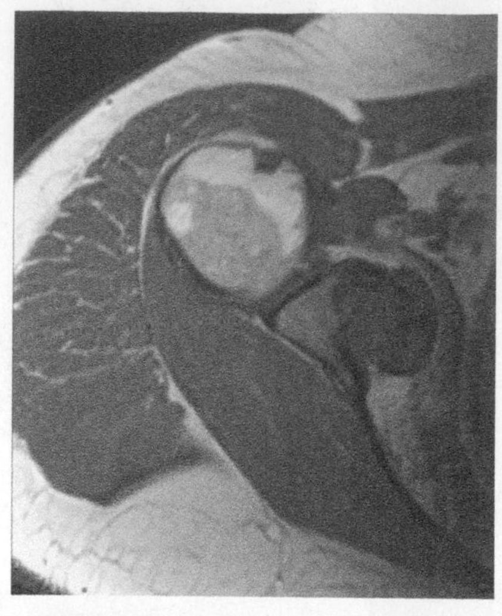

The mass is isointense to hypointense to muscle on T1 images, and remodels the scapular cortex.

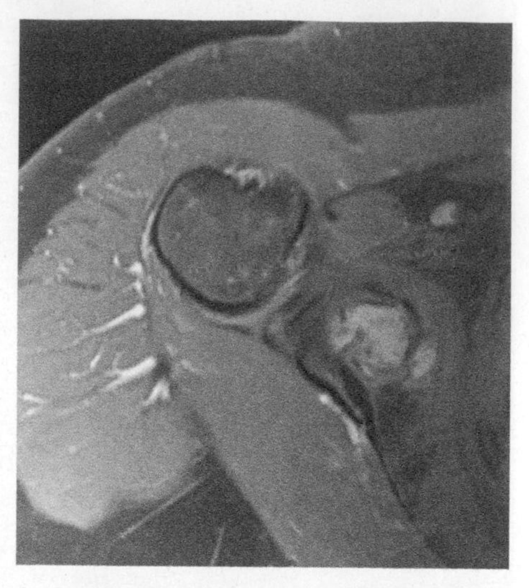

Post-contrast images show marked heterogenous enhancement.

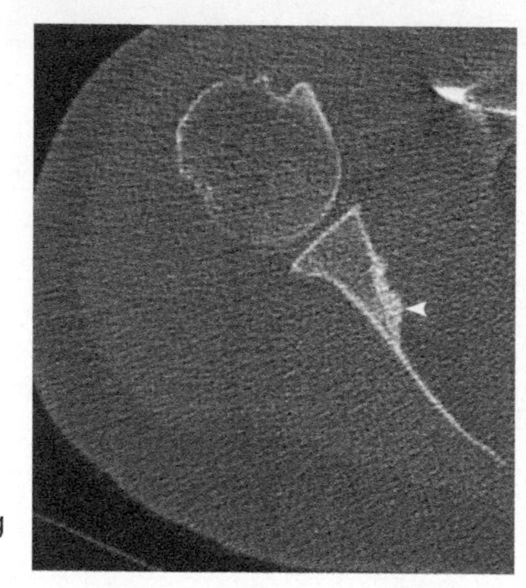

Bone windows show mild scapula cortical thickening and remodeling.

Answers

1. There is a subscapular soft-tissue mass that is mildly hyperdense relative to muscle, that displaces muscle but does not invade it. There is reactive cortical thickening.
2. The dark bands likely reflect collagen.
3. Desmoid tumor, malignant fibrous histiocytoma (MFH), giant cell tumor of tendon sheath, lymphoma, and elastofibroma dorsi are included in the differential.
4. Based on the patient's age, location of lesion, and imaging characteristics, the most likely diagnosis is a desmoid tumor. Elastofibroma dorsi would be more inferior, deep to the scapula muscles such as the serratus anterior and latissimus dorsi.
5. Patients with Gardner syndrome have multiple colonic polyps, osteomas and soft-tissue tumors. Up to 13% of these individuals will develop desmoid tumors.

Pearls

- The fibromatoses are benign tumors arising from musculoaponeurotic structures.
- They are locally aggressive and infiltrative, but have no metastatic potential.
- The deep fibromatoses are classified as intra-abdominal, abdominal, or extra-abdominal depending on the relationship to the abdominal wall.
- The superficial fibromatoses include plantar and palmar fibromas.
- CT shows a soft-tissue lesion that is isodense to hyperdense, with contrast enhancement. More collagenous components account for the hyperdensity.
- MRI shows low to isointensity on T1-weighted images.
- T2 signal is heterogenous, with areas of T2 hypointensity reflecting fibrous bands. T2 hyperintensity is a result of myxoid components.
- Most lesions show moderate to marked enhancement after intravenous contrast.
- Treatment is with wide surgical excision, with or without adjunctive radiation.

Suggested Readings

Murphey MD, Ruble CM, Tyszko SM, Zbojniewicz AM, Potter BK, Miettinen M. From the archives of the AFIP: musculoskeletal fibromatoses: radiologic-pathologic correlation. *Radiographics.* 2009;29(7):2143-2173.

Robbin MR, Murphey MD, Temple HT, Kransdorf MJ, Choi JJ. Imaging of musculoskeletal fibromatosis. *Radiographics.* 2009;21(3):585-600.

Non-painful mass on the palmar aspect of the wrist

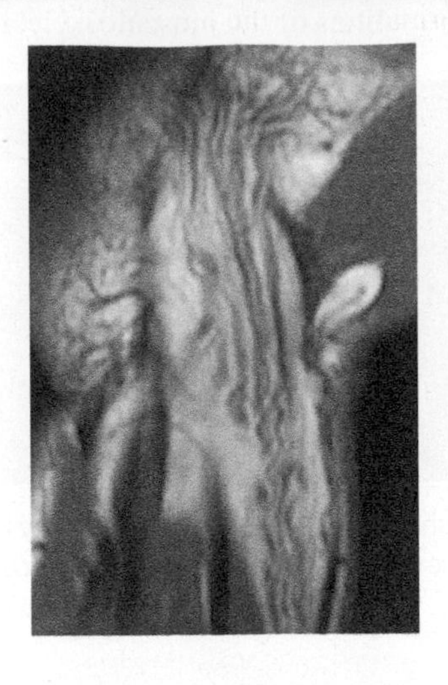

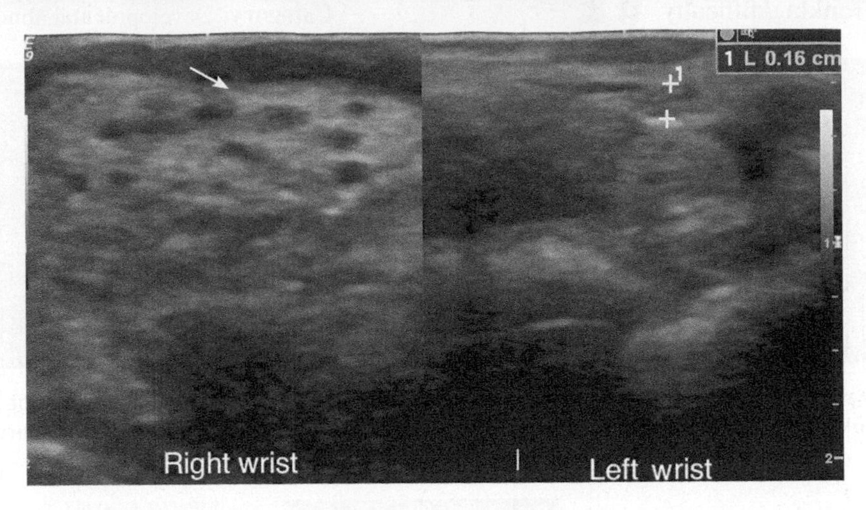

1. What are the MRI and ultrasound findings?
2. What are the differential diagnoses?
3. Which nerve is commonly affected in this condition?
4. What are the associations with this entity?
5. The lesion is associated with carpal tunnel syndrome. True or False?

Fibrolipoma of the median nerve 1446

Case ranking/difficulty: 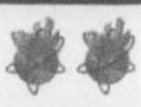

Category: Developmental abnormalities of the musculoskeletal system

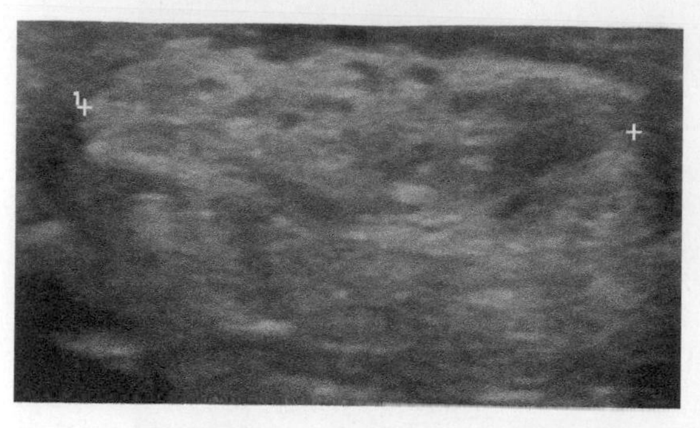

Abnormal fatty infiltration of the right median nerve with marked increased echogenicity.

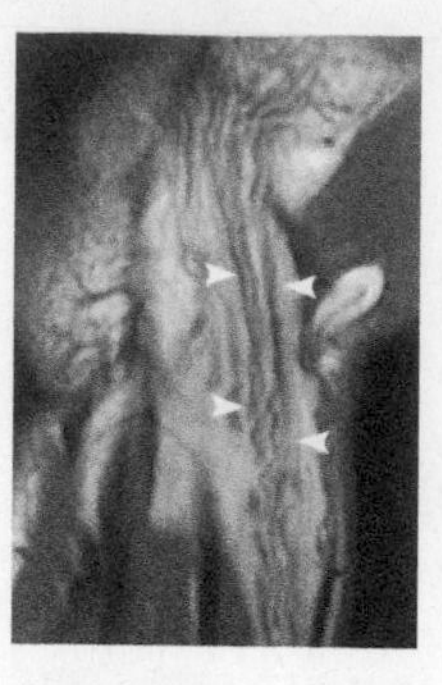

High T1 signal intensity fatty infiltration of the median nerve.

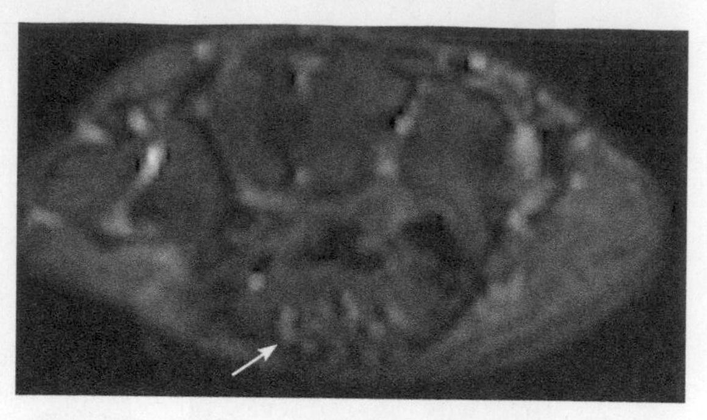

Axial image showing fat saturation of the fatty infiltrated median nerve with a "coaxial cable" appearance.

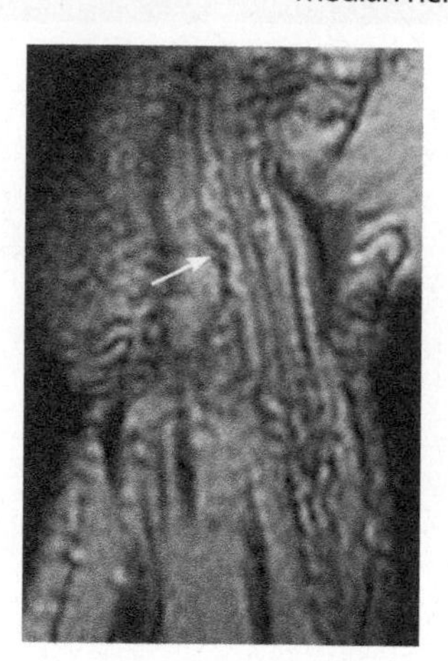

Coronal STIR image showing fat saturation and a "spaghetti string" appearance.

Answers

1. MRI showing high T1 and T2 signal intensity infiltration of the median nerve, which is saturated on fat-saturated images. No contrast enhancement. The median nerve is thickened. The above gives a cord-like appearance in the coronal plane, and coaxial cable-like appearance in axial images.

   Ultrasound image demonstrates a thickened right median nerve with hyperechogenic tissues. Note the normal left median nerve.

2. The differential diagnosis in this region includes nerve sheath tumor of the median nerve, vascular malformation, ganglion cyst, intraneural lipoma, and fibrolipoma of median nerve.

3. The median nerve is involved in 80% of cases. Other affected nerves include ulnar, radial, axillary, dorsal nerve of the foot, and the cranial nerves.

4. Macrodystrophia lipomatosa is seen in approximately 27% to 60% of cases of fibrolipoma.

5. Fibrolipoma of the median nerve often presents with symptoms of a carpal tunnel syndrome.

Pearls

- Lipofibromatous hamartoma or fibrolipoma of the median nerve is a rare benign lesion of the median nerve.
- It is thought to be congenital, although some researchers believe it could be a post-traumatic or post-inflammatory reaction.
- Eighty percent of cases affect the median nerve, but other nerves, such as ulnar, brachial, dorsum of foot, and cranial nerves, can be affected.
- It is usually seen in newborns or infants, but a late presentation could be seen, presenting as a carpal tunnel syndrome. Males and females are equally affected.
- Ultrasound can be diagnostic with a hyperechogenic mass infiltrating the median nerve and its thenar branches, giving the classic coaxial cable appearance.
- On MRI, the lesion is high signal intensity on both T1- and T2-weighted images, which is suppressed on fat-saturated images. There is no contrast enhancement.
- There is also enlargement of the nerve fascicles which is low signal intensity on T1- and T2-weighted images. This arrangement gives a "coaxial cable" appearance on axial images, and cord-like "spaghetti string" appearance on coronal images.
- Treatment is controversial, but carpal tunnel decompression helps symptomatically in 60% of cases. Debulking of lesion carries a risk of damage to the vascular supply to the nerve and risk of neurological deficit.

Suggested Readings

Amadio PC, Reiman HM, Dobyns JH. Lipofibromatous hamartoma of nerve. *J Hand Surg Am.* 1988;13(1):67–75.

Toms AP, Anastakis D, Bleakney RR, Marshall TJ. Lipofibromatous hamartoma of the upper extremity: a review of the radiologic findings for 15 patients. *AJR Am J Roentgenol.* 2006;186(3):805-811.

Elbow mass

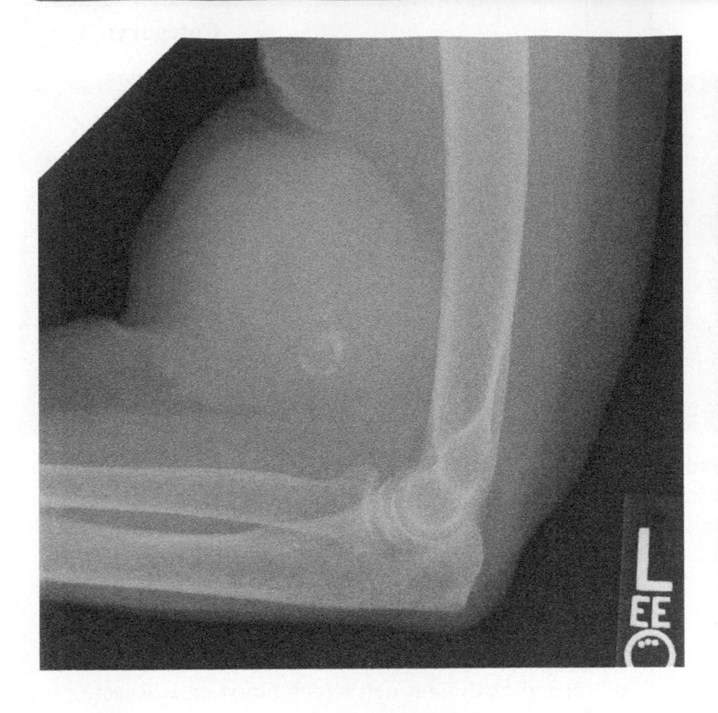

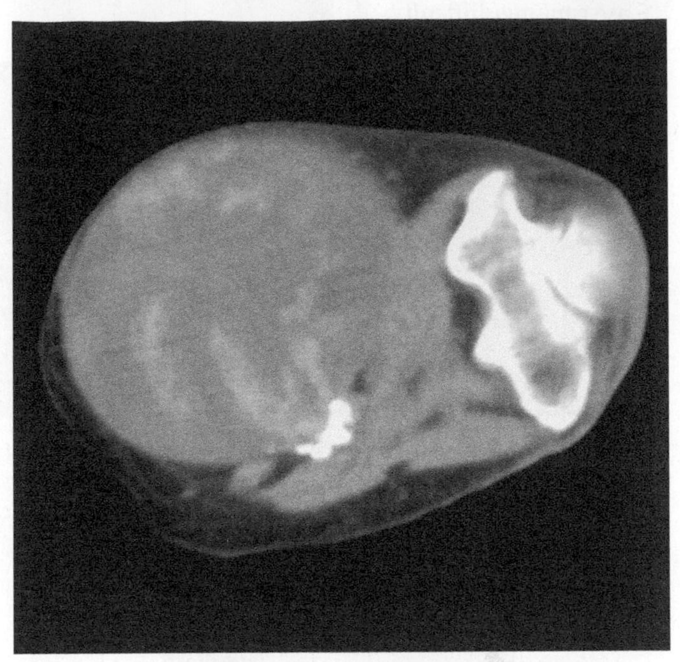

1. What is the most likely diagnosis?

2. What are treatment options for this entity?

3. What is the most common etiology for this entity?

4. Where is the most common location for this entity?

5. What are complications of this entity?

Pseudoaneurysm 1466

Case ranking/difficulty:

Category: Trauma

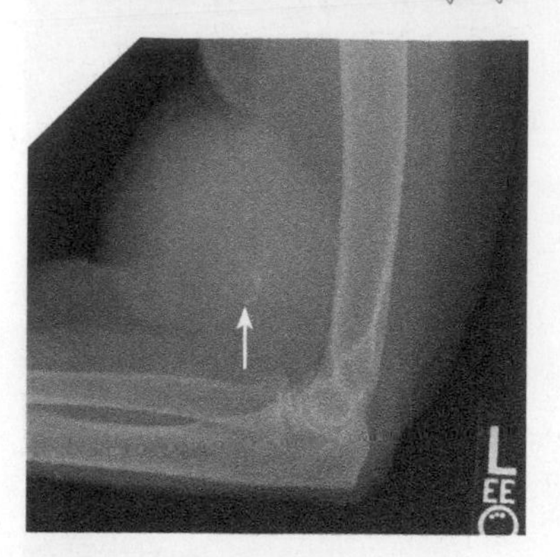

There is a soft-tissue mass in the anterior soft tissues. Calcification is seen within the mass (*arrow*).

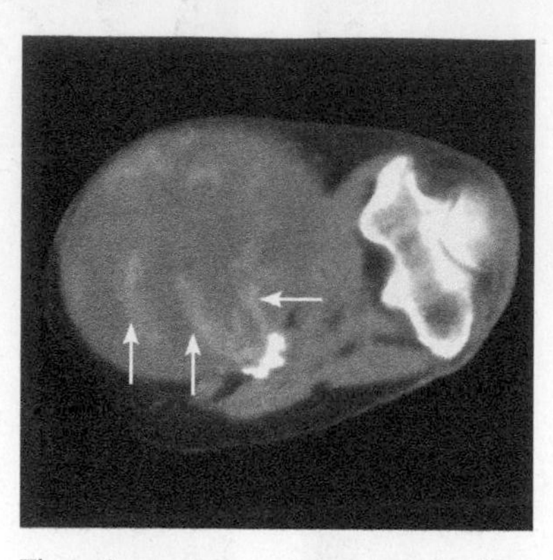

There is contrast enhancement of the mass (*arrows*). Large portions do not enhance because of thrombosis.

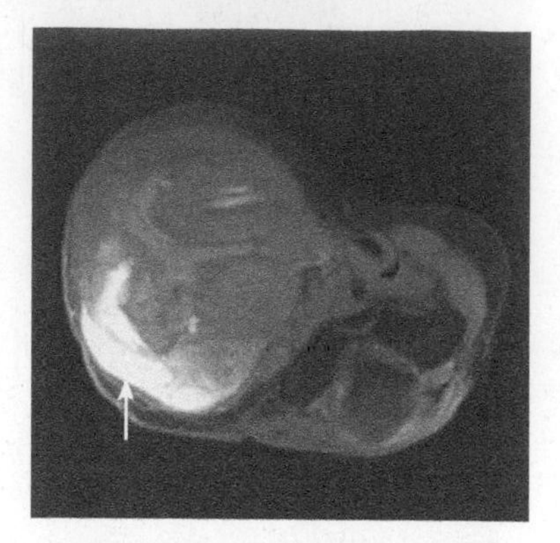

Inhomogeneous fat saturation is present at the medial, posterior aspect of the mass (*arrow*).

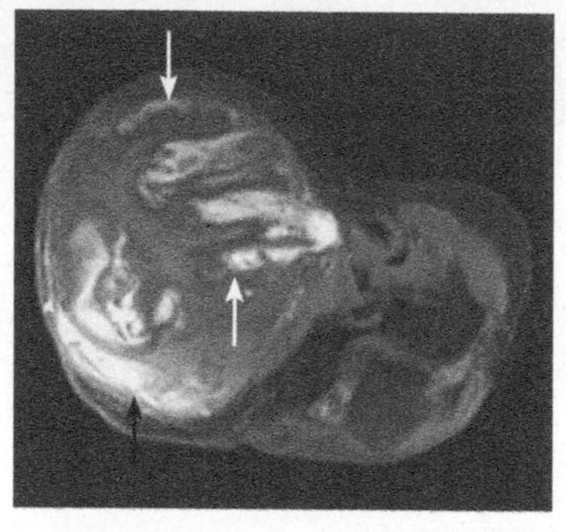

Contrast enhancement of the mass (*white arrows*), consistent with a pseudoaneurysm. Large portions of the mass do not enhance because of thrombosis. Inhomogeneous fat saturation persists (*black arrow*).

Answers

1. The calcified mass with contrast enhancement suggests a pseudoaneurysm. A soft tissue sarcoma is a less likely possibility. The history would help to differentiate the two entities.
2. Treatment options for pseudoaneurysms include thrombin injection, covered stent placement, surgical ligation and/or bypass, and ultrasound probe compression.
3. Most pseudoaneurysms are caused by iatrogenic trauma such as arterial catheterization, surgery, or percutaneous procedures, including biopsy and drainage.
4. The femoral artery is the most common location for pseudoaneurysm formation.
5. Complications of pseudoaneurysms include mass effect on adjacent structures such as nerves and veins and uncontrolled hemorrhage.

Pearls

- A pseudoaneurysm represents a defect in the arterial intima and media through which blood can dissect; it is contained within a sac formed by the adventitia and surrounding tissues.
- Pseudoaneurysms are usually iatrogenic, caused by procedures such as arterial catheterization, surgery, or percutaneous biopsy or drainage.
- The femoral artery is the most common site of pseudoaneurysm formation, as it is the most common site for catheterization.
- Ultrasound, CT, MRI, and angiography can be used to diagnose pseudoaneurysms.
- On ultrasound, CT, and MRI, a pseudoaneurysm typically appears as an eccentric saccular structure adjacent to an artery.
- Swirling blood flow within the pseudoaneurysm may create the characteristic bidirectional "ying-yang" sign on ultrasound.
- Variable CT/MRI contrast enhancement or flow within the pseudoaneurysm may be seen, depending on the presence and amount of thrombus.
- Complications include mass effect on adjacent structures such as nerves and veins, and rupture with uncontrolled hemorrhage.

Suggested Readings

Katzenschlager R, Ugurluoglu A, Ahmadi A, et al. Incidence of pseudoaneurysm after diagnostic and therapeutic angiography. *Radiology.* 1995;195(2):463-466.

Saad NE, Saad WE, Davies MG, Waldman DL, Fultz PJ, Rubens DJ. Pseudoaneurysms and the role of minimally invasive techniques in their management. *Radiographics.* 2005;25 Suppl 1:S173-S189.

History of a slowly enlarging jaw mass with pain

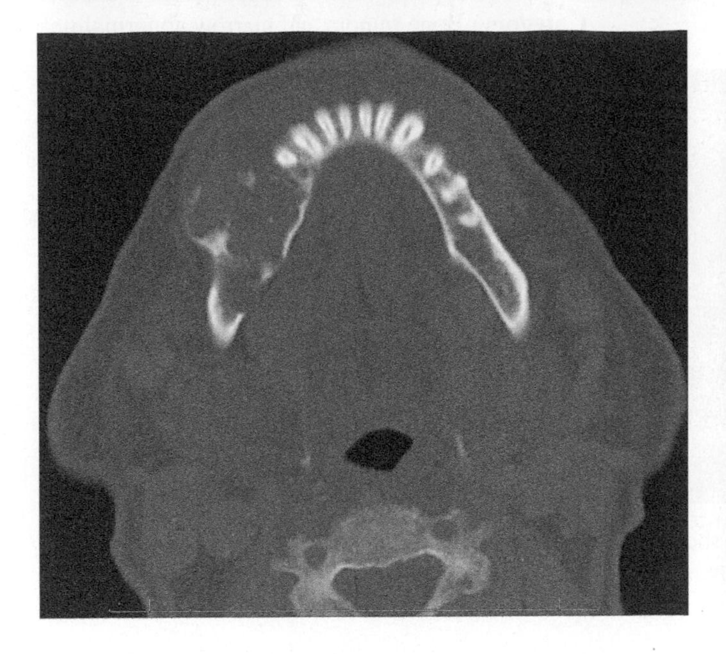

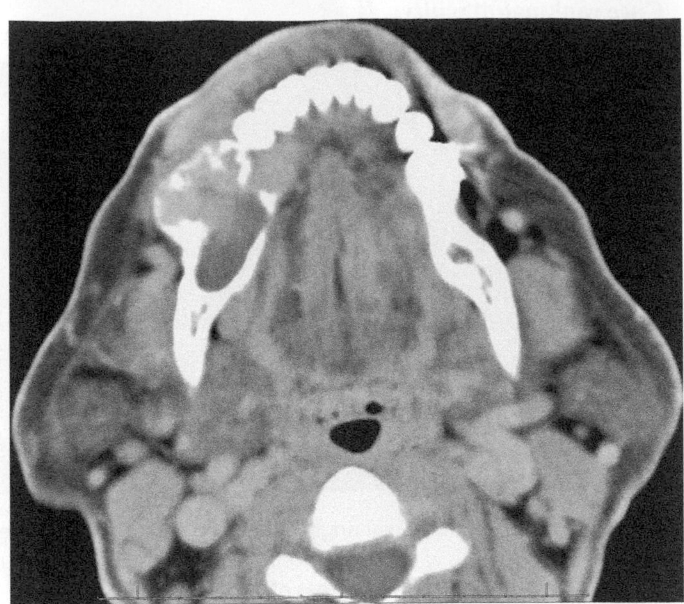

1. What are the CT findings?

2. What is included in the differential diagnosis?

3. What is the most likely diagnosis?

4. Is histology or cross-sectional imaging more useful in assessing local tumor invasion?

5. What is the malignant potential of this lesion?

Ameloblastoma 1551

Case ranking/difficulty: 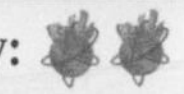

Category: Bone tumors and marrow abnormalities

Markedly expansile mandibular angle lesion, with no matrix or teeth within the lesion. Cortical thinning is marked, with areas of cortical breakthrough (*arrowheads*).

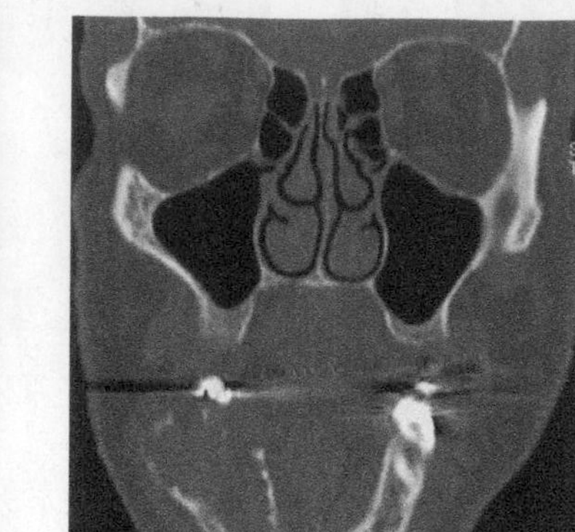

Coronal image shows the markedly expansile nature.

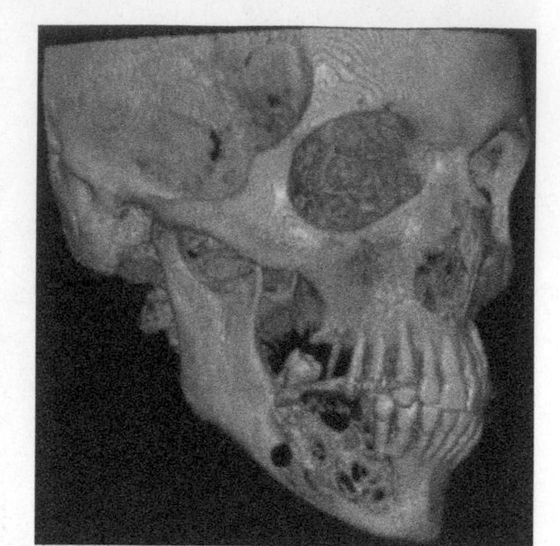

3D volume-rendered CT shows the "soap bubble" appearance.

Answers

1. There is a lucent expansile lesion in the mandibular angle with no matrix, but with cortical thinning and breakthrough and soft tissue infiltration. The lesion does not contain a tooth.
2. Differential includes odontogenic keratocyst, dentigerous cyst, ameloblastoma, metastasis, and plasmacytoma.
3. Based on the imaging characteristics including absence of a tooth in the lesion, the most likely diagnosis is an ameloblastoma.
4. CT and MRI underestimate soft-tissue infiltration by 2 to 8 mm. PET-CT is useful in assessing local infiltration, but the best assessment is on histology.
5. Metastases are rare, and foci typically show a benign cytological appearance.

Pearls

- Ameloblastomas are a benign tumor of odontogenic origin.
- They are associated with unerupted teeth, but a tooth is not typically seen in the lesion, unlike a dentigerous cyst.
- Lesions may be intraosseous or extraosseous.
- The angle of the mandible is the most common site.
- Bony expansion and cortical thinning with breakthrough is common.
- The degree of soft-tissue invasion is usually underestimated on imaging.
- Mixed solid and cystic variants are more aggressive.
- Lesions are benign but locally aggressive.
- Recurrence is common, and metastasis after excision has been reported although rare.
- When metastasis does occur, it is to the lungs.

Suggested Readings

Cankurtaran CZ, Branstetter BF, Chiosea SI, Barnes EL. Best cases from the AFIP: ameloblastoma and dentigerous cyst associated with impacted mandibular third molar tooth. *Radiographics.* 2010;30(5):1415-1420.

Scholl RJ, Kellett HM, Neumann DP, Lurie AG. Cysts and cystic lesions of the mandible: clinical and radiologic-histopathologic review. *Radiographics.* 2001;19(5):1107-1124.

Pain in the ankle

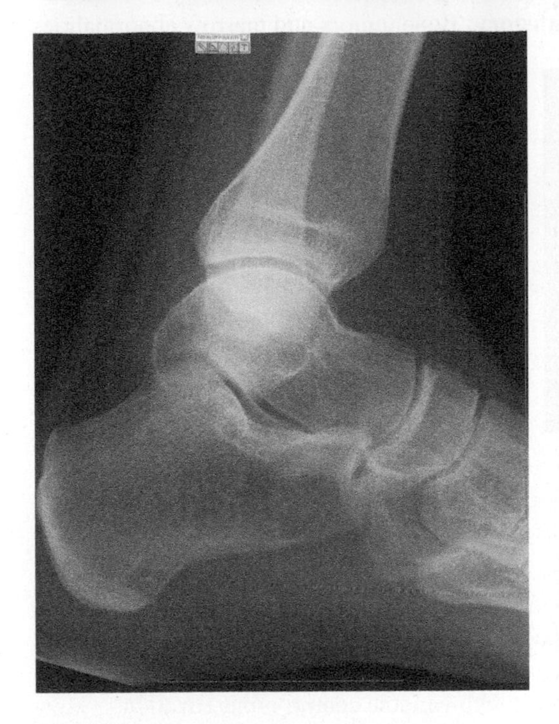

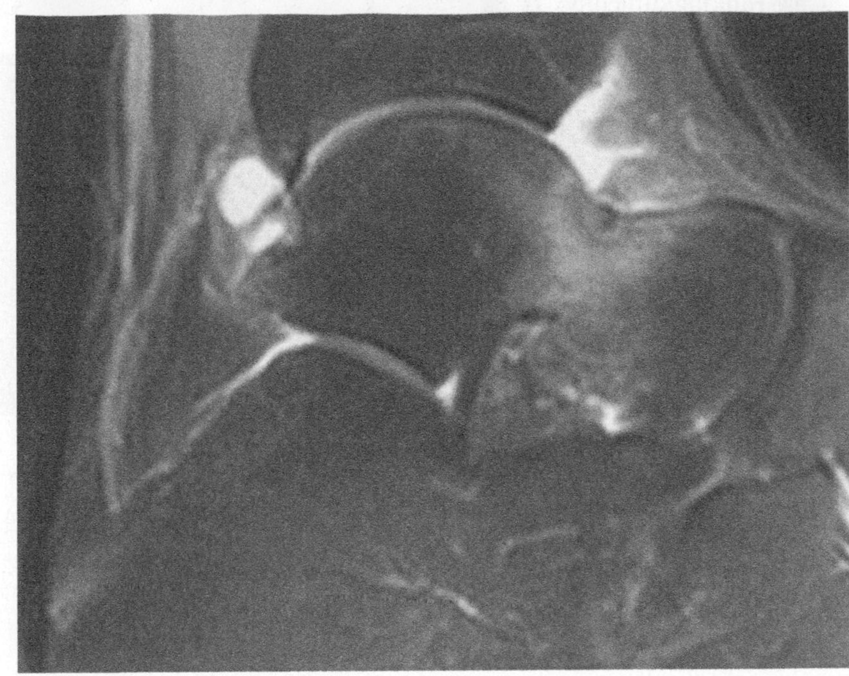

1. What are the radiograph and MRI findings?

2. What is the most likely diagnosis?

3. What are the different locations for this lesion?

4. What is the best imaging modality to identify the cancellous form of this lesion?

5. What is the common age group affected in this condition?

Osteoid osteoma 1391

Case ranking/difficulty:

Category: Bone tumors and marrow abnormalities

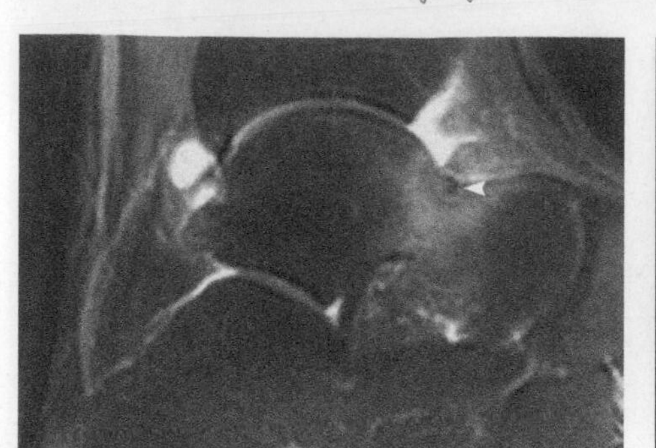

There is marked bone marrow edema in the neck of the talus, an ankle effusion, and a cortically based lesion with a central calcified nidus.

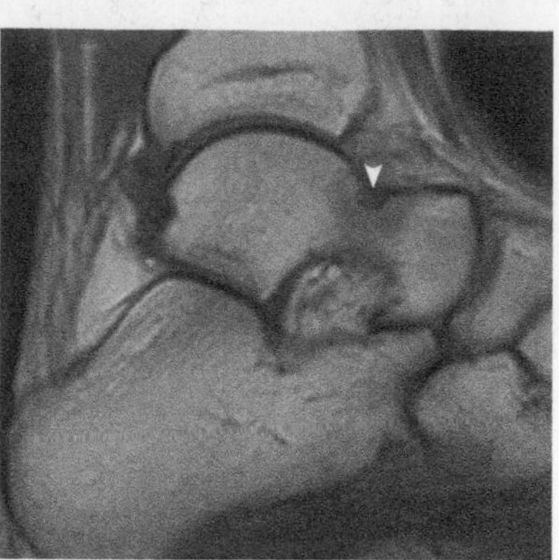

Central nidus is seen.

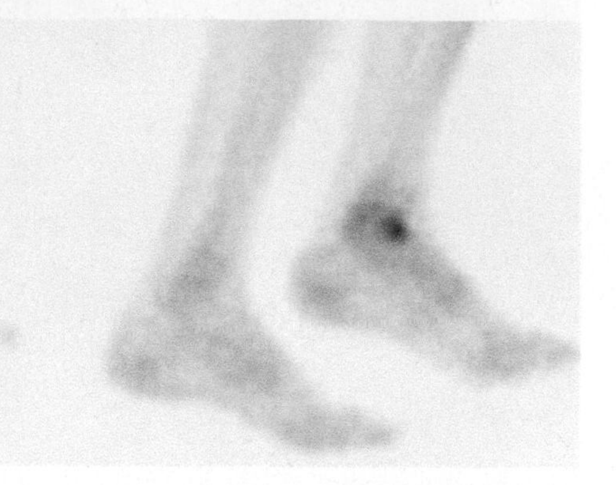

Radionuclide bone scan shows marked uptake of radiopharmaceutical in the talus neck.

Answers

1. Radiograph is normal. MRI shows a cortically based rounded lesion in the talar neck with intense surrounding bone marrow edema, and an ankle effusion. Central low intensity focus is consistent with a calcified nidus.
2. A rounded lesion in the cortex is consistent with an osteoid osteoma. There are no aggressive features to suggest osteosarcoma, and the lesion is not large enough to call an osteoblastoma.
3. Classic locations for an osteoid osteoma are intracortical, cancellous or subperiosteal.
4. CT best demonstrates an intracortical osteoid osteoma, but an MRI is the best modality to diagnose a cancellous lesion.
5. The most common age group for an osteoid osteoma is 10 to 30 years, with a peak in the early 20s.

Pearls

- Osteoid osteomas are benign tumors of woven bone and osteoid.
- Young adults are affected, with a 2:1 male-to-female ratio.
- They are located most commonly in the cortex, but also in cancellous bone and in a subperiosteal location.
- The typical lesion is less than 2 cm with a central lucent nidus, with variable central mineralization and surrounding sclerosis.
- CT best demonstrates a cortical lesion, whereas MRI best shows cancellous lesions.
- CT also may demonstrate the "vascular groove" sign, which is believed to be dilated feeding vessels around the tumor. This sign is fairly sensitive, but highly specific.
- Subperiosteal lesions can be difficult to identify on plain films because of the absence of reactive bone changes, but MRI will show the surrounding soft-tissue changes or synovial changes.
- Ultrasound has also been shown to be capable of detecting intra-articular lesions.

Suggested Readings

Liu PT, Kujak JL, Roberts CC, de Chadarevian JP. The vascular groove sign: a new CT finding associated with osteoid osteomas. *AJR Am J Roentgenol.* 2011;196(1):168-173.

Shukla S, Clarke AW, Saifuddin A. Imaging features of foot osteoid osteoma. *Skeletal Radiol.* 2010;39(7):683-689.

Incidental finding

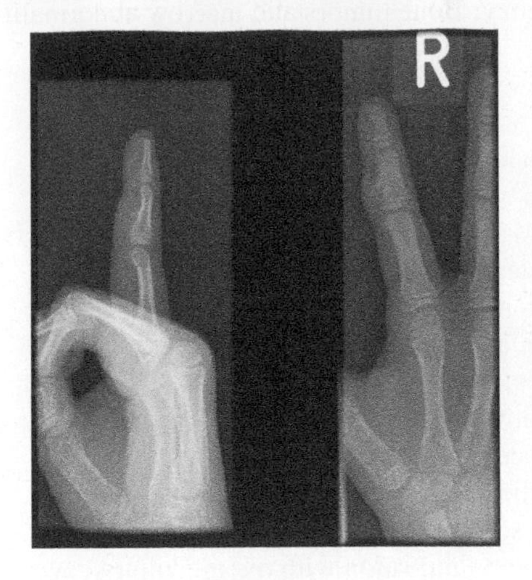

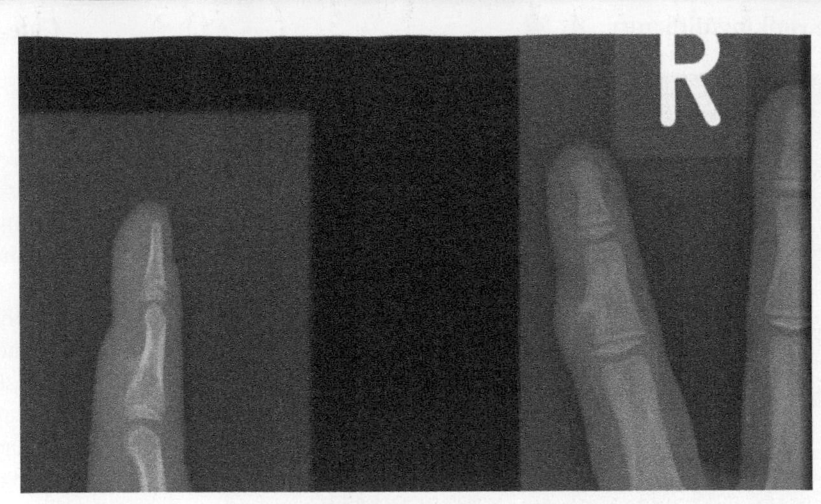

1. What are the radiograph findings?

2. What is the differential diagnosis?

3. What is the likely diagnosis?

4. What are the pertinent features of this condition?

5. This lesion has a high rate of recurrence after excision. True or False?

Bizarre parosteal osteochondromatous proliferation: Nora lesion 1536

Case ranking/difficulty: 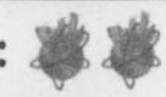

Category: Bone tumors and marrow abnormalities

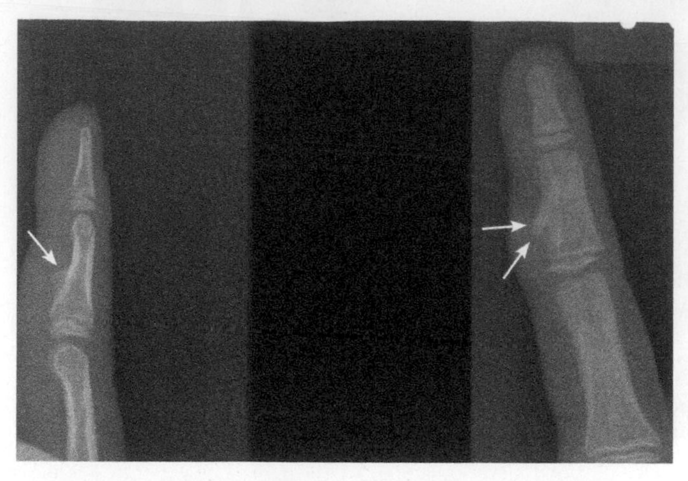

No marrow continuity and no orientation toward the physis. No aggressive features are seen.

Answers

1. There is a proliferative osseous lesion on the radial and volar aspect of the middle phalanx of the ring finger. It has no specific orientation away from the physis, and no medullary communication. In addition, the lesion is diaphyseal unlike a typical metaphyseal osteochondroma.
2. The differential diagnoses includes parosteal osteosarcoma, myositis ossificans, periostitis ossificans, osteochondroma, and Nora lesion.
3. Nora or bizarre parosteal osteochondromatous proliferation (BPOP) lesion is the diagnosis.
4. These well-defined lesions have non-aggressive features such as a narrow zone of transition, no medullary cavity connection, no orientation away from the physis, and no periosteal reaction. They do not have a cartilage cap. It affects males and females equally, and is most common in the phalanges although the long bones, skull, and mandible may also be affected.
5. BPOP has a 29% to 55% rate of recurrence, and therefore wide surgical excision of the lesion with the overlying pseudocapsule and periosteum is recommended.

Pearls

- Bizarre parosteal osteochondromatous proliferation lesion is also called a Nora lesion, and was first described in 1983.
- It affects males and females equally, and commonly affects the small bones, such as the middle and proximal phalanges, but can also affect the mandible or long bones. The etiology is unknown.
- Plain film shows a well-defined pedunculated or broad-based bony mass on the surface of a bone, extending outwards from the cortex to the surrounding soft tissues.
- There is no communication with the medullary cavity, and no orientation away from the adjacent physis as in an osteochondroma.
- CT scan confirms the plain film findings, and helps to differentiate it from other lesions.
- MRI shows a low T1 and a high T2 signal intensity well-defined lesion with a narrow zone of transition, unlike the mature signal characteristics of a benign osteochondroma, which does not show T2 hyperintensity. It has no cartilage cap.

Suggested Readings

Gursel E, Jarrahnejad P, Arneja JS, Malamet M, Akinfolarin J, Chang Y-J. Nora's lesion: Case report and literature review of a bizarre parosteal osteochondromatous proliferation of a small finger. *Can J Plast Surg.* 2008;16(4):232-235.

Nora FE, Dahlin DC, Beabout JW. Bizarre parosteal osteochondromatous proliferations of the hands and feet. *Am J Surg Pathol.* 1983;7(3):245-250.

Patient presented to the emergency room with a pathologic fracture; second film was obtained 15 months later

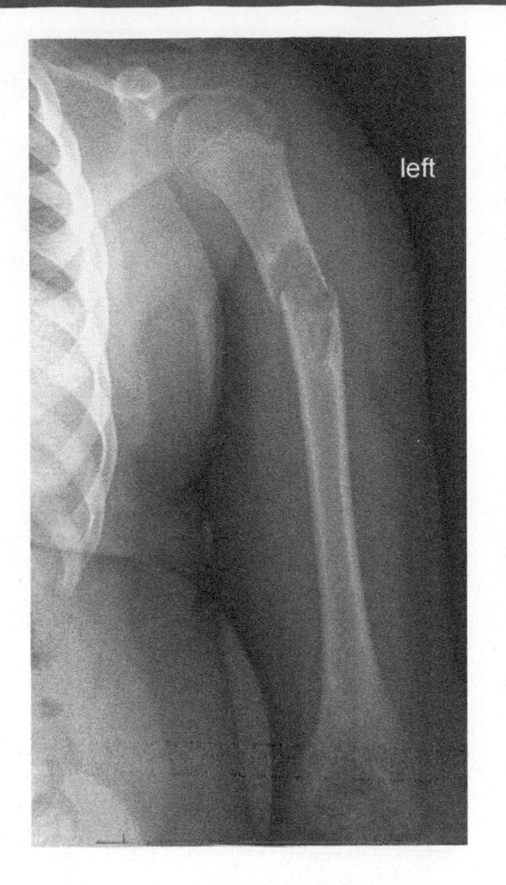

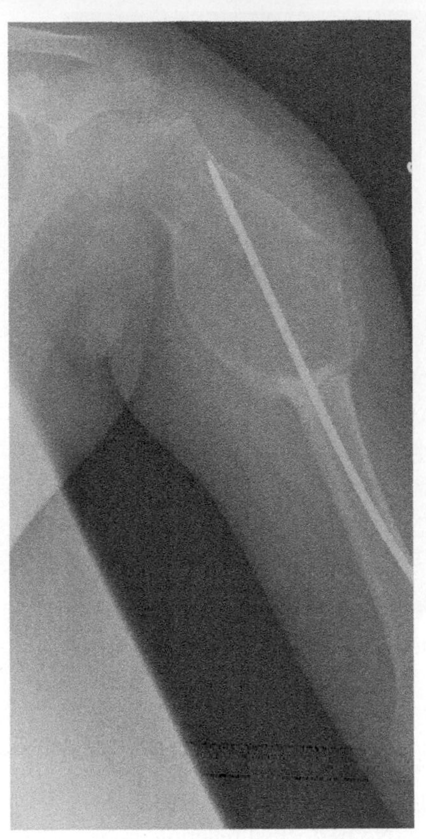

1. What does the first radiograph show?

2. What does the second radiograph, obtained 15 months later, show?

3. What is the most likely diagnosis?

4. What could you expect to see in an MRI of the lesion shown in the second radiograph?

5. What percentage of lesions shown in the second radiograph has an underlying lesion?

Aneurysmal bone cyst 1438

Case ranking/difficulty: 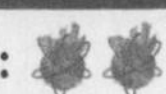

Category: Bone tumors and marrow abnormalities

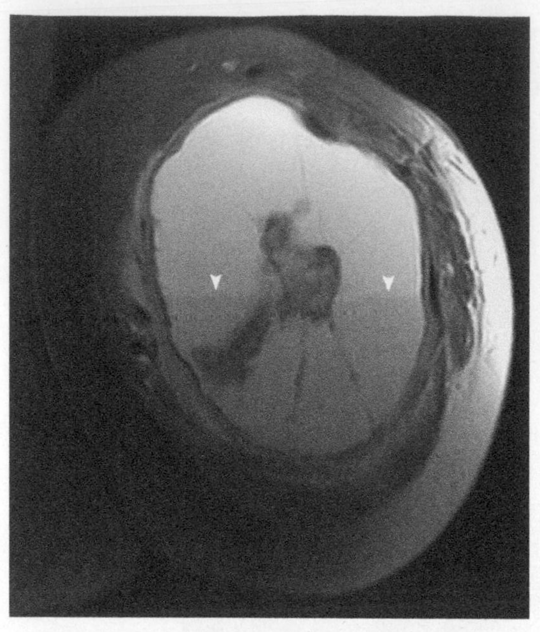

There are internal septae and multiple fluid–fluid levels, with no solid component.

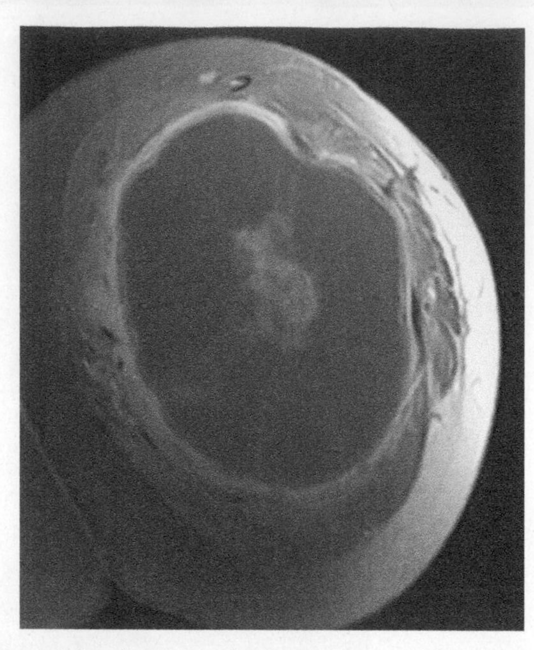

There is peripheral and septal enhancement, but no enhancing solid component.

Answers

1. Lytic nonexpansile metaphyseal lesion, with a pathologic fracture. No periosteal reaction, bone expansion, or matrix is demonstrated.
2. The lesion is now markedly expansile, with no internal matrix, cortical breach, or periosteal reaction. A rod from fracture fixation is seen.
3. This is most likely an aneurysmal bone cyst, secondary to the underlying unicameral bone cyst and/or the prior fracture.
4. Fluid–fluid levels, bone expansion, intraosseous hemorrhage, and no solid component are typical. A hypointense rim may be seen.
5. An underlying lesion is identified in 33% of aneurysmal bone cysts.

Pearls

- Aneurysmal bone cysts (ABCs) are lytic expansile lesions eccentrically located in the metaphysis or metadiaphysis.
- ABCs are thought to result from vascular occlusion and intraosseous hemorrhage.
- An underlying lesion is seen in 33% of cases, most commonly a giant cell tumor.
- The cortex can be markedly expanded and thinned resembling an aggressive lesion.
- The lesion may have a "soap bubble" appearance.
- Most commonly there is no periosteal reaction, unless there is a pathologic fracture.
- MRI can show fluid–fluid levels consisting of blood products of variable age. This is, however, nonspecific.

Suggested Readings

Beltran J, Simon DC, Levy M, Herman L, Weis L, Mueller CF. Aneurysmal bone cysts: MR imaging at 1. T. *Radiology.* 1986;158(3):689-690.

Hudson TM. Fluid levels in aneurysmal bone cysts: a CT feature. *AJR Am J Roentgenol.* 1984;142(5):1001-1004.

Pain in the knee

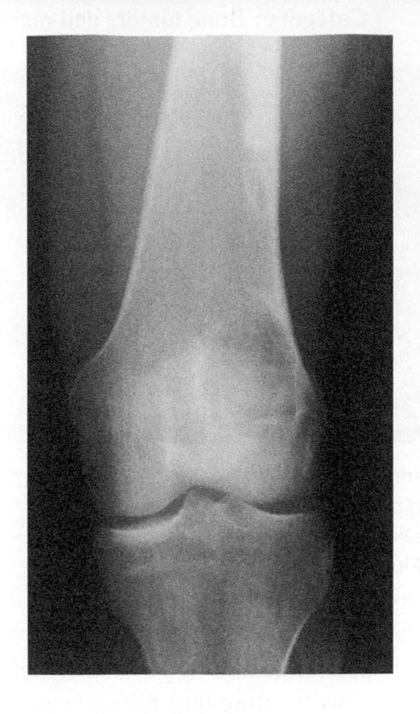

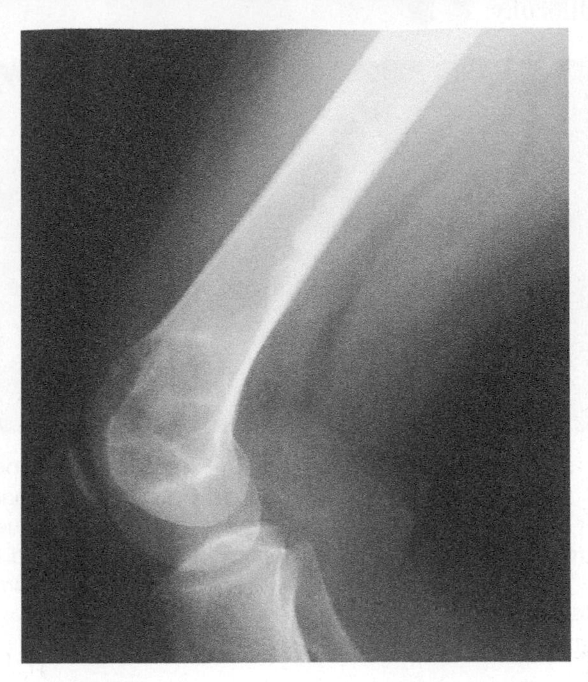

1. What are the radiograph findings?
2. What is the differential diagnosis?
3. Based on the imaging, what is the most likely diagnosis?
4. This entity may occur secondary to what condition?
5. What are the MRI signal characteristics of the lesion?

Giant cell tumor 1413

Case ranking/difficulty: 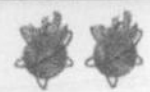

Category: Bone tumors and marrow abnormalities

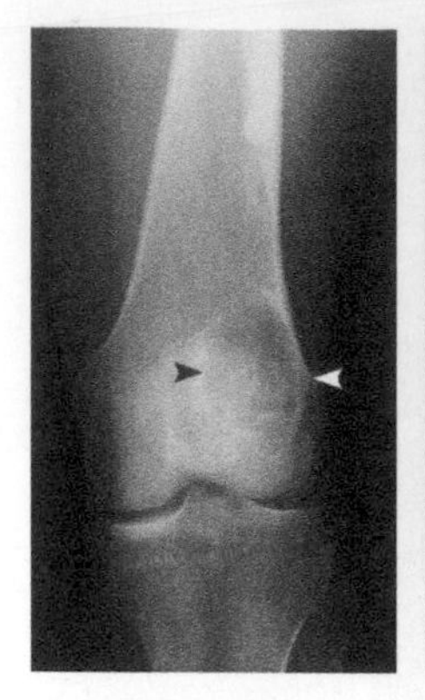

There is a lucent lesion in the distal lateral femoral condyle with a narrow zone of transition (*arrowheads*). Healed nonossifying fibroma is incidentally noted proximally.

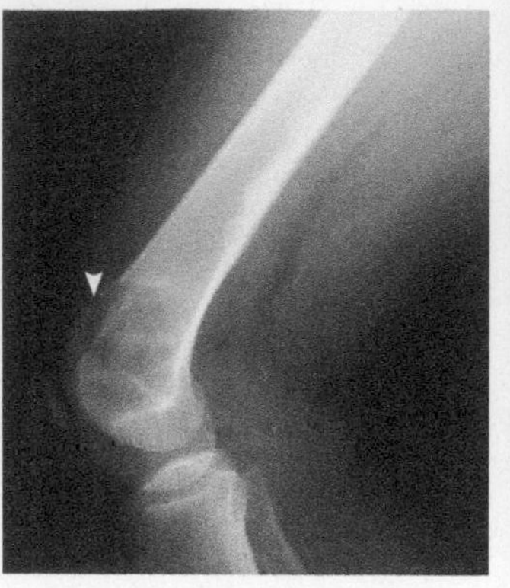

Mild cortical expansion and thinning are noted.

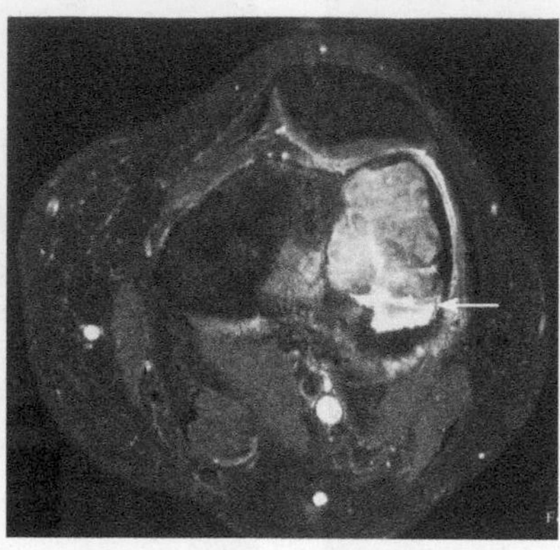

The lesion is T2 hyperintense with well-defined margins, and mild peripheral bone and soft-tissue edema. Mild bone expansion is noted. Fluid–fluid level is seen posteriorly (*arrow*).

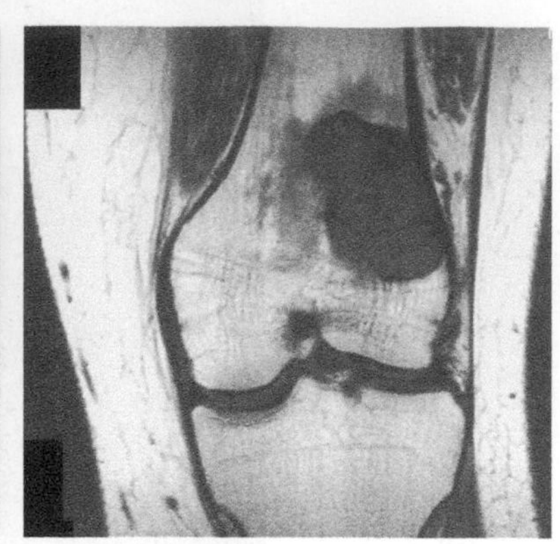

The lesion is T1 hypointense.

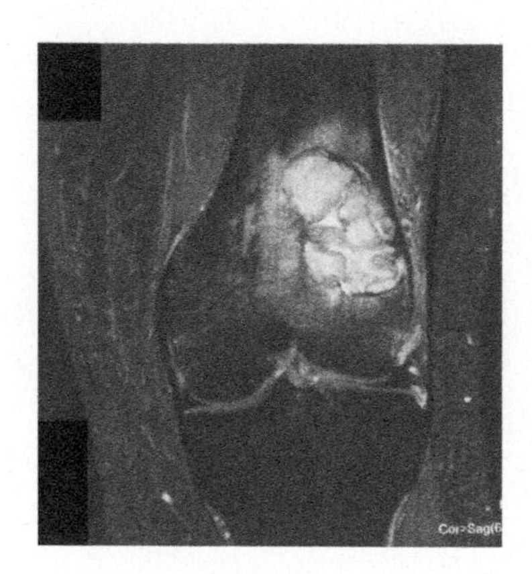

T2 hyperintensity with mild surrounding edema is seen.

Answers

1. There is a lytic mildly expansile subarticular lesion with coarse trabeculae and cortical thinning but no aggressive features. The location deep to the suprapatellar bursa is subarticular.
2. Aneurysmal bone cyst, giant cell tumor, desmoplastic fibroma, malignant fibrous histiocytoma (MFH) of bone and plasmacytoma.
3. A lytic expansile lesion in the subarticular region of the distal femur should always raise the concern for a giant cell tumor.
4. Giant cell tumor may occur as a rare complication of Paget disease. These typically occur in the skull and facial bones.
5. T1 hypointensity, T2 hyperintensity and signal heterogeneity. More than 60% of cases have hemosiderin from prior hemorrhage and will bloom on gradient-echo sequences.

Pearls

- Giant cell tumors typically occur at the end of long bones.
- The distal phalanges are also common, especially in cases of multiple giant cell tumors.
- Uncommon locations include the vertebrae, pelvic bones, and skull base.
- The lesions extend to the subarticular cortex, with expansion of bone and cortical thinning.
- Lesions are eccentric to the long axis of bone, and do not usually have a sclerotic rim.
- MRI may show fluid–fluid levels, and hemosiderin in more than 60% of cases.
- Recurrence is up to 50% if extended curettage is not performed, 10% if it is. Metastasis can occur in 10–25% of patients, usually to the lungs.

Suggested Readings

Aoki J, Tanikawa H, Ishii K, et al. MR findings indicative of hemosiderin in giant-cell tumor of bone: frequency, cause, and diagnostic significance. *AJR Am J Roentgenol.* 1996;166(1):145-148.

Swanger R, Maldjian C, Murali R, Tenner M. Three cases of benign giant cell tumor with unusual imaging features. *Clin Imaging*. 2008;32(5):407-410.

Increasing pain in the left thigh

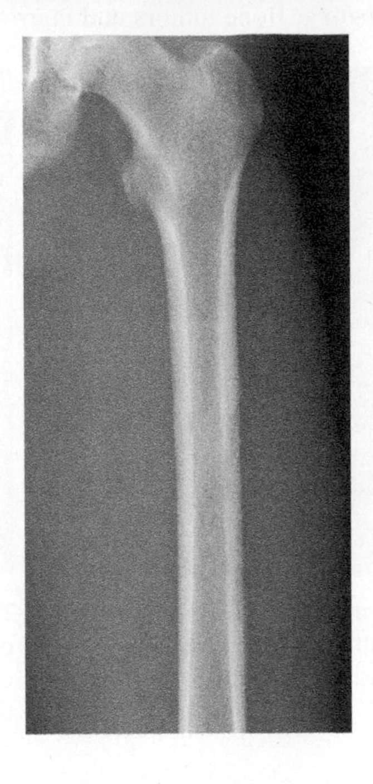

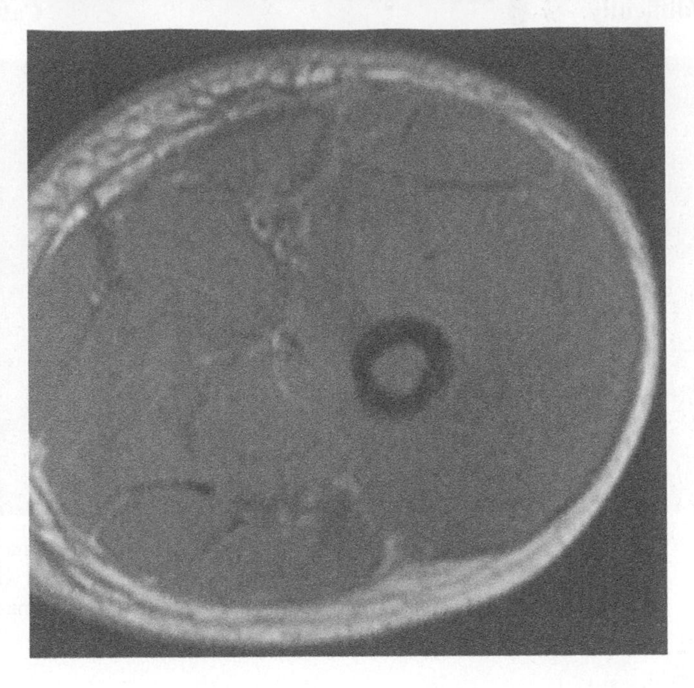

1. What are the radiographic findings?
2. What are the MRI findings?
3. What are included in the differential diagnosis?
4. What is the most likely diagnosis?
5. In this condition, what percentage of patients will demonstrate pure bone sclerosis?

Primary lymphoma of bone 1393

Case ranking/difficulty: 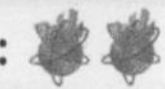

Category: Bone tumors and marrow abnormalities

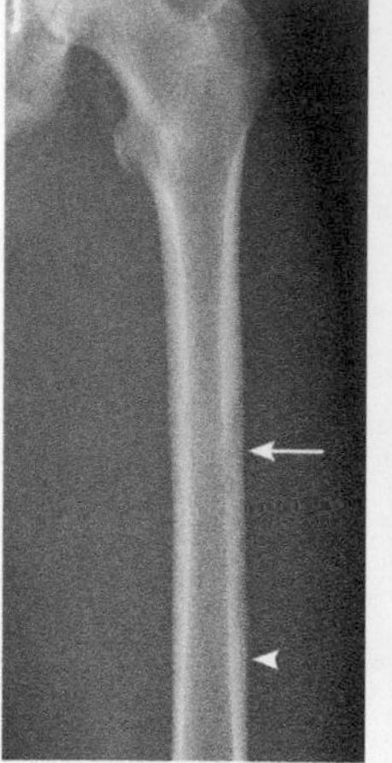

There is cortical erosion (*arrow*) and thinning with periosteal reaction (*arrowhead*), along the lateral femoral cortex.

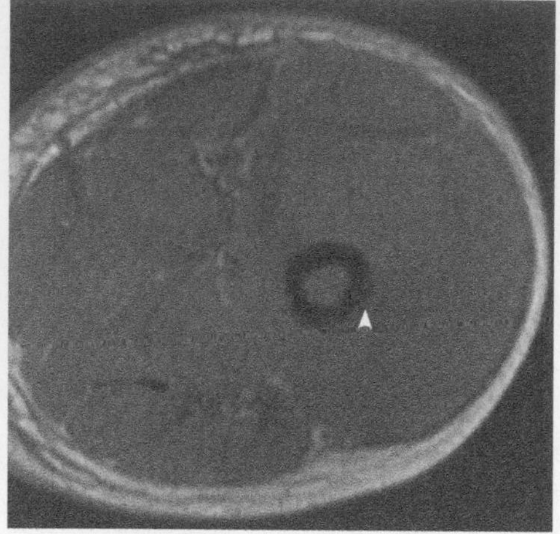

There is replacement of the marrow fat and lateral cortical erosion and thinning (*arrowhead*) with an isointense soft-tissue mass.

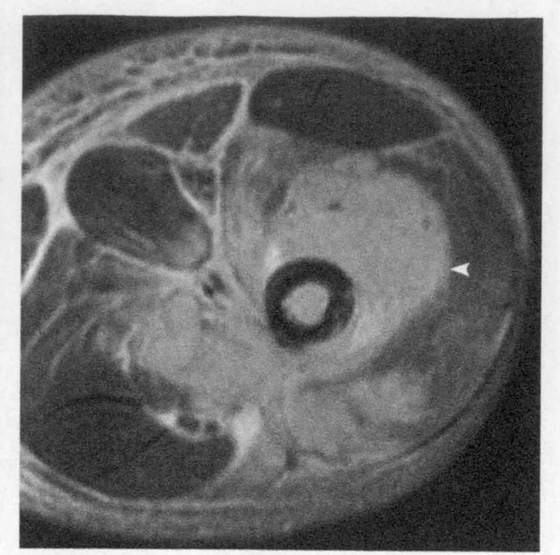

Tumor edema and soft-tissue mass are better appreciated with a disproportionately large soft-tissue mass.

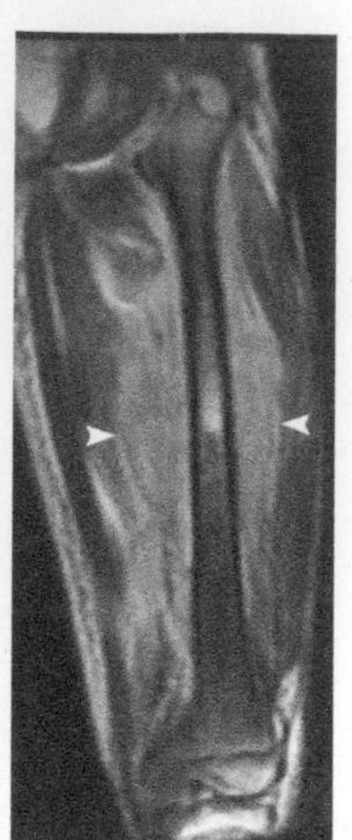

The large extraosseous component to this lesion is well appreciated. The soft-tissue mass is disproportionate to the cortical changes.

Answers

1. Osteolytic lesion in the lateral cortex, with periosteal reaction, soft-tissue mass, and no sclerosis.
2. There is T1 hypointensity, T2 hyperintensity, and a soft-tissue mass that is larger than the degree of bone destruction. Although sequestra can be seen in primary bone lymphomas, one is not demonstrated in this case.
3. Differential includes primary lymphoma of bone, Ewing sarcoma, multiple myeloma, osteosarcoma, and metastatic neuroblastoma (in younger patients).
4. Given the patient's age, large soft-tissue mass that is disproportionate to bone destruction, and the absence of sclerosis or generalized systemic disease, the most likely diagnosis is primary lymphoma of bone.
5. Only 5% of primary lymphoma of bone is purely sclerotic, although a mixed lytic/sclerotic picture is seen in up to 30% of patients.

Pearls

- Primary lymphoma of bone is uncommon.
- Bone involvement is primary, and there is no involvement of lymph nodes except perhaps regionally.
- Several criteria must be met for the lesion to be called primary lymphoma of bone:
  - Solitary bone lesion or multiple osseous lesions with no prior involvement of lymph nodes
  - Histological documentation of lymphoma
  - No lymph node involvement or only regional involvement
- Lesions are usually lytic or mixed lytic/sclerotic. Purely sclerotic lesions are seen in only 5% of patients.
- Sequestra may be seen in up to 11% of patients, differentiating this entity from other sarcomas.
- The soft-tissue mass is disproportionate to the degree of bone destruction. This finding is typically seen in lymphoma and other small, round, blue cell tumors.
- Periosteal reaction is uncommon, but may occur.

Suggested Readings

Kirsch J, Ilaslan H, Bauer TW, Sundaram M. The incidence of imaging findings, and the distribution of skeletal lymphoma in a consecutive patient population seen over 5 years. *Skeletal Radiol.* 2006;35(8):590-594.

Mulligan ME, McRae GA, Murphey MD. Imaging features of primary lymphoma of bone. *AJR Am J Roentgenol.* 1999;173(6):1691-1697.

Chronic knee pain

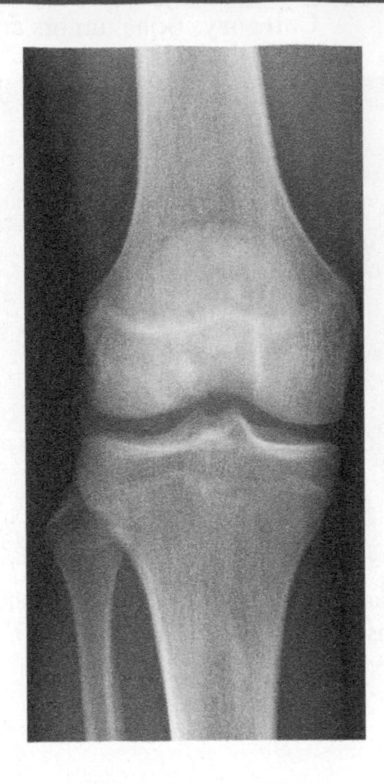

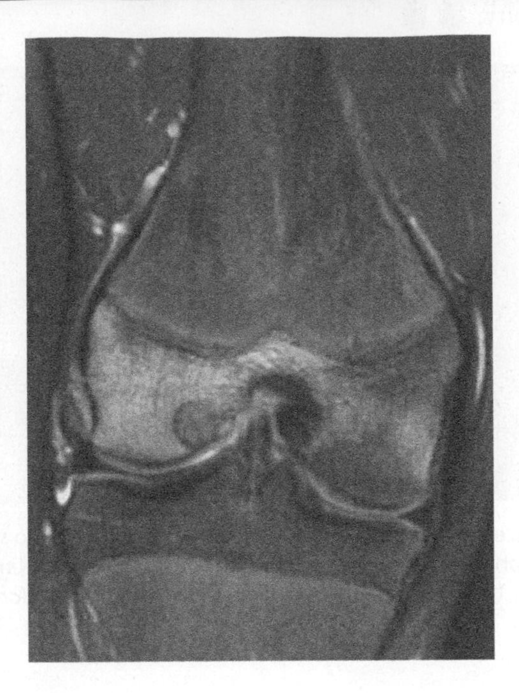

1. What are the radiograph findings?

2. What are the MRI findings?

3. What lesions are included in the differential, and what is the most likely diagnosis?

4. Why is the lesion typically heterogenous with foci of low signal on T2-weighted images?

5. What is the management for this lesion?

Chondroblastoma 1386

Case ranking/difficulty: 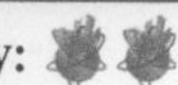

Category: Bone tumors and marrow abnormalities

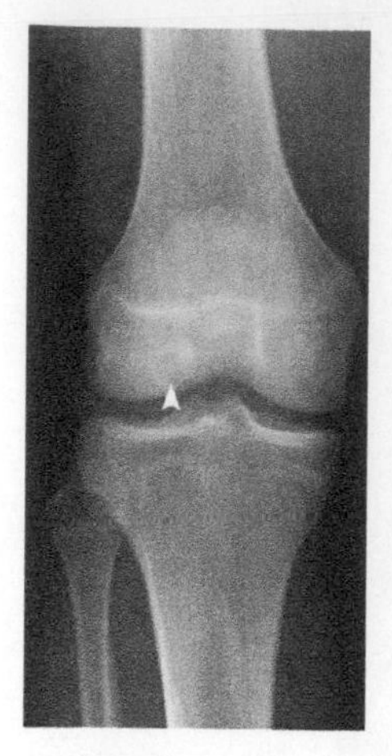

There is a well-defined lucent lesion in the lateral femoral epiphysis, with no matrix or cortical breach. The rim appears sclerotic.

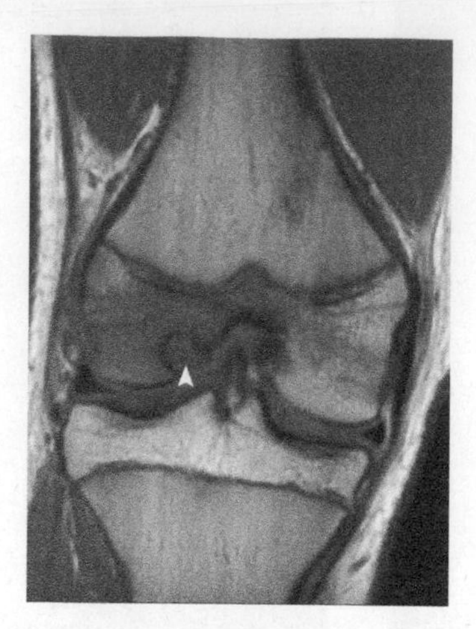

The lesion is isointense to skeletal muscle, with tiny hypointense foci suggesting calcification (*arrowhead*).

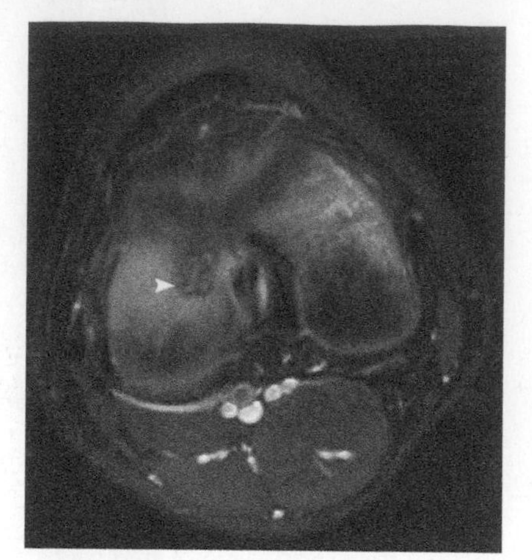

There is a mildly lobular configuration to the lesion.

Answers

1. There is a lucent nonexpansile lesion in the epiphysis of the lateral femoral condyle, with a sclerotic rim but no demonstrated matrix or periosteal reaction.
2. Well-defined lesion in the lateral femoral epiphysis with surrounding edema, but no cortical breakthrough or soft-tissue mass. The lesion is heterogenously isointense to hypointense on T2-weighted images with small foci of low T2 signal likely because of calcification. There are no fluid–fluid levels.
3. Based on the age of the patient, the location of the lesion, and the radiological features, the most likely diagnosis is a chondroblastoma. Clear cell chondrosarcomas occur in the epiphyses but usually after physeal closure, and the lesion is not expansile to suggest an aneurysmal bone cyst, which is also usually metaphyseal. Osteoblastomas are usually diaphyseal or metadiaphyseal.
4. Foci of low T2 signal can be seen in chondroblastomas, because of chondroblastic hypercellularity, calcifications, and hemosiderin.
5. The treatment for chondroblastomas is typically curettage and packing with methylmethacrylate. Care must be taken not to violate the joint articular surface, which can lead to joint seeding.

Pearls

- Chondroblastomas are tumors of chondroblasts that typically occur in young patients, before physeal closure.
- Lesions may extend into the metaphysis, or be located in the apophysis.
- Most lesions occur in the lower extremity and around the knee.
- Plain films will show a well-defined lucent lesion in the epiphysis with or without a thin sclerotic rim. Mild expansion or cortical scalloping can occur. A calcific matrix is seen in approximately 50% of cases.
- In rare cases, the tumor may arise in a nonepiphyseal site.
- MRI shows low T1 signal and variable T2 signal as a result of calcification, tumor hypercellularity, or hemosiderin. Enhancement is variable. Fluid–fluid levels may be seen.
- Recurrence is most common in purely epiphyseal lesions, and foot/ankle or proximal femur lesions.
- Pulmonary metastasis are uncommon, but when it does occur it is usually after tumor recurrence. Metastases may also rarely occur in benign disease.

Suggested Readings

Brien EW, Mirra JM, Kerr R. Benign and malignant cartilage tumors of bone and joint: their anatomic and theoretical basis with an emphasis on radiology, pathology and clinical biology. I. The intramedullary cartilage tumors. *Skeletal Radiol.* 1997;26(6):325-353.

Jambhekar NA, Desai PB, Chitale DA, Patil P, Arya S. Benign metastasizing chondroblastoma: a case report. *Cancer.* 1998;82(4):675-678.

Enlarging painful mass in clavicle

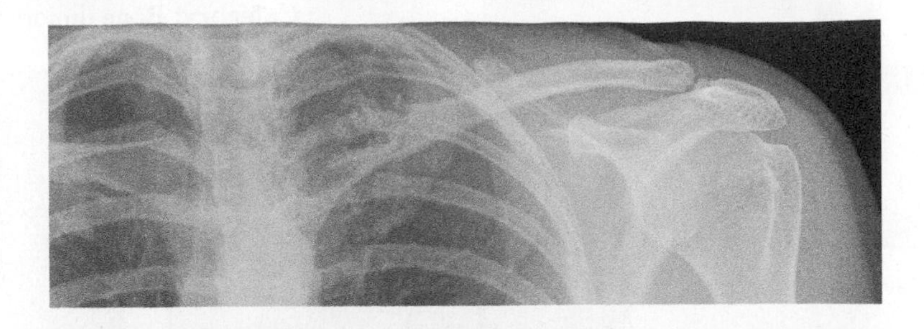

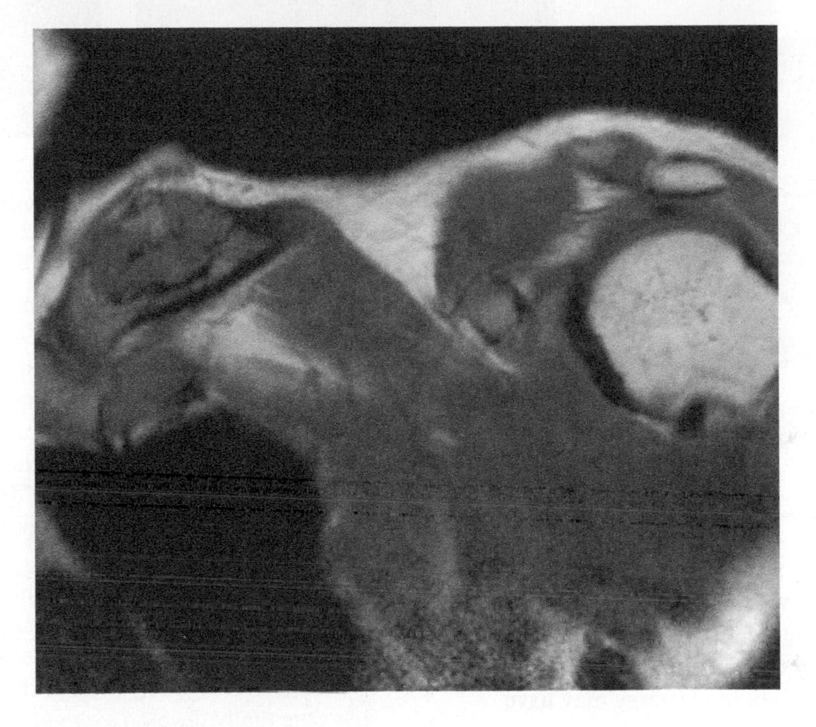

1. What is the differential diagnosis?

2. What is the most common age group for this entity?

3. What is the appropriate initial management for this entity?

4. What syndromes are associated with an increased risk of this condition?

5. What is the upper limit for cartilage cap thickness in benign chondroid lesions?

Chondrosarcoma 228

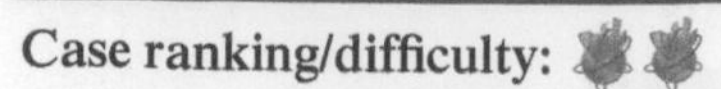

Case ranking/difficulty: **Category:** Bone tumors and marrow abnormalities

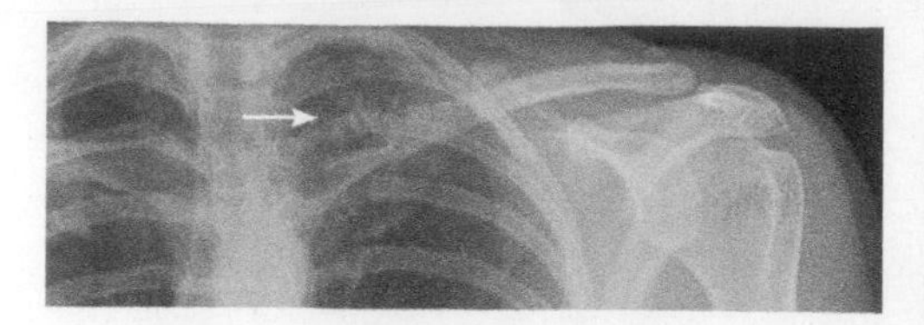

AP clavicle showing aggressive lytic lesion with matrix mineralization.

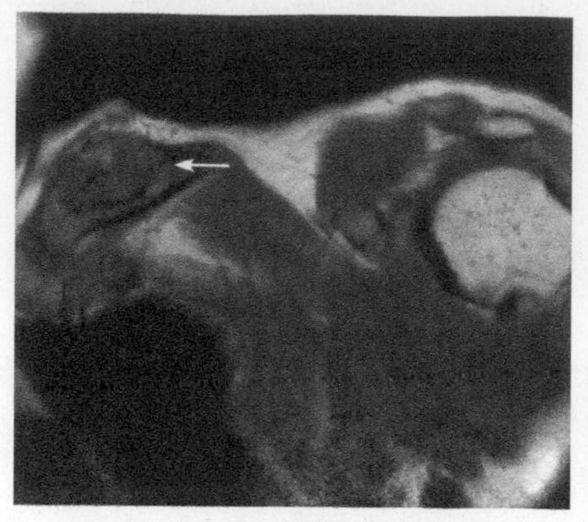

Aggressive lesion within proximal clavicle with low T1 signal (chondroid) elements.

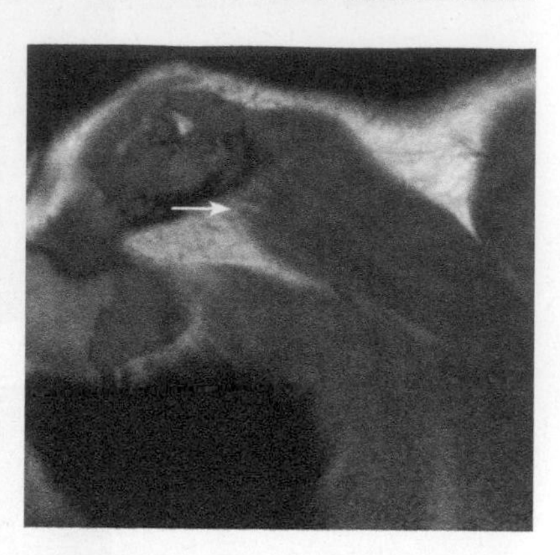

Chondrosarcoma is seen remote from the clavicular head of pectoralis major.

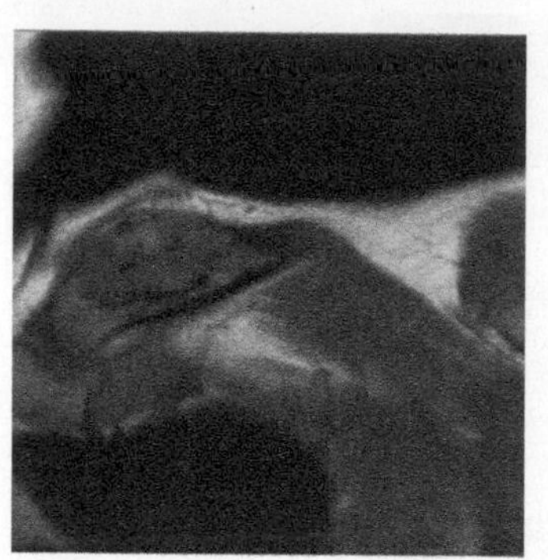

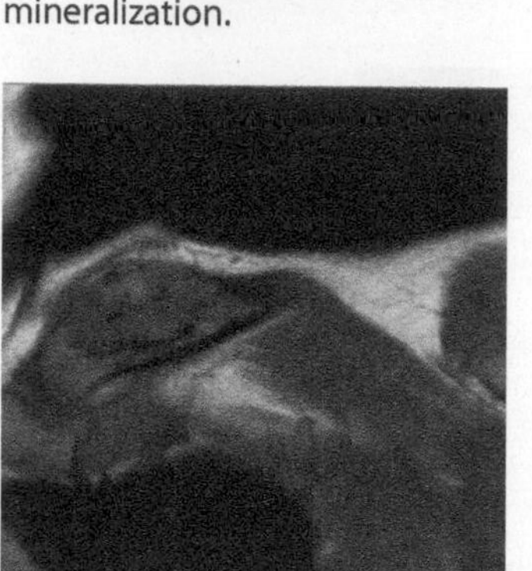

The lesion arises from the superior margin of the clavicle and has low T1 signal elements consistent with cartilage.

Answers

1. Chondrosarcoma typically occurs in the axial skeleton and is locally aggressive with typical chondroid ("rings-and-arcs") calcification, although loss of calcification by tumor destruction may be seen. Although infection or lytic metastases may have similar appearances, clinical correlation is important. Metastases are not usually solitary, however.
2. Most chondrosarcomas present after the sixth decade of life. They are very rare in adolescents, unlike osteogenic sarcomas.
3. Initial management of sarcomas must be via a multidisciplinary sarcoma service for optimal patient outcome. Injudicious biopsy may jeopardize future curative surgery. Discussion with a specialist surgeon is advised.
4. Maffucci and Ollier syndromes are associated with an increased risk of chondrosarcoma. The former is the association of multiple enchondromas with cutaneous hemangiomas, which increases the risk of chondrosarcoma by a factor of 20 from the normal population. Ollier disease is also associated with an increased risk of chondrosarcoma.
5. A cartilage cap thickness of up to 2 cm in an adult may be considered normal, although some authorities would recommend close follow-up of osteochondromas with 5- to 10-mm cartilage caps.

   MRI is the investigative modality of choice, although ultrasound may also be performed for this purpose.

Pearls

- Chondrosarcoma should be in the differential diagnosis of aggressive bone lesions in middle-aged and elderly patients. It is very rare before the fourth decade of life.
- The characteristic features of chondrosarcoma are matrix mineralization. Thorough evaluation of the nature of the calcification is essential to narrow the differential diagnosis from other primary bone tumors, for example, osteosarcoma.
- Chondrosarcoma is commonly found in typical locations, for example, pelvis, shoulder, diametaphyseal regions of long bones, and skull base, although any bone ossifying from cartilage can potentially develop a chondrosarcoma.
- It may occur by sarcomatous transformation of an enchondroma or osteochondroma. Increasing pain and an osteochondroma cartilage cap thickness greater than 2 cm warrant referral to a sarcoma center.
- A large soft-tissue mass is commonly associated with chondrosarcoma, although this is also a feature of small, round cell tumors and osteosarcoma.
- Syndromes are associated with an increased, risk of chondrosarcoma (eg, Ollier—enchondromatosis, and Maffucci syndrome—enchondromas plus hemangiomas).

Suggested Readings

Foran P, Colleran G, Madewell J, O'Sullivan PJ. Imaging of thoracic sarcomas of the chest wall, pleura, and lung. *Semin Ultrasound CT MR.* 2011;32(5):365-376.

Ozcanli H, Alimoglu E, Aydin AT. Malignant transformation of an enchondroma of the hand: a case report. *Hand Surg.* 2011;16(2):201-203.

Vanel D, Kreshak J, Larousserie F, et al. Enchondroma vs. chondrosarcoma: a simple, easy-to-use, new magnetic resonance sign. *Eur J Radiol.* 2012 Jan 5 [Epub ahead of print].

Vague pain and swelling in the left thigh for 1 year

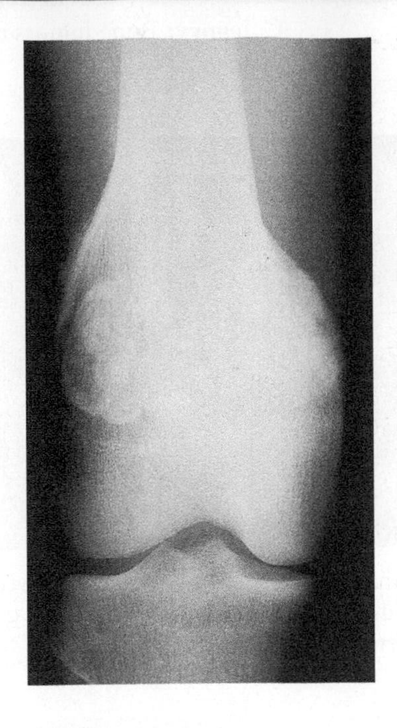

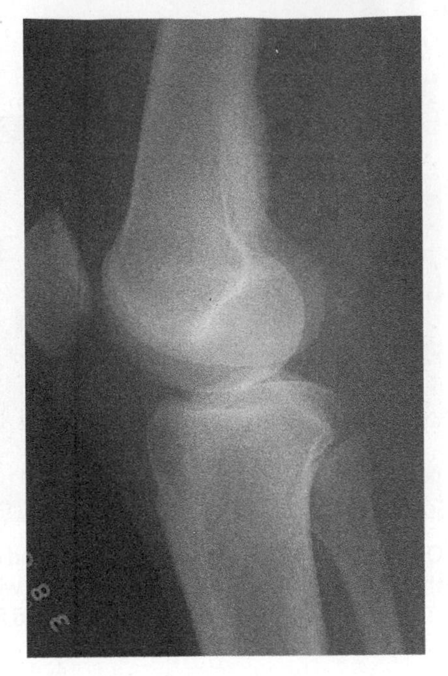

1. What are the radiograph findings?

2. What is the string sign?

3. This lesion has a poor prognosis. True or False?

4. What is the greatest risk of this lesion?

5. Dedifferentiation is usually to which tumors?

Parosteal osteosarcoma 1470

Case ranking/difficulty: 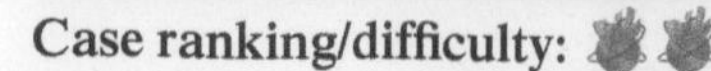

Category: Bone tumors and marrow abnormalities

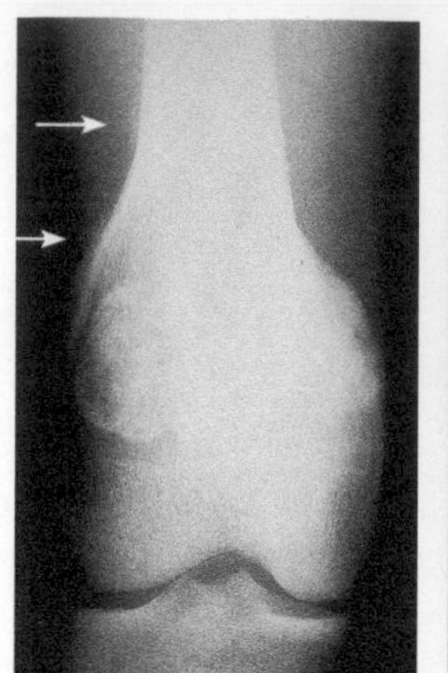

Dense distal femur with ossified mass laterally (*arrows*).

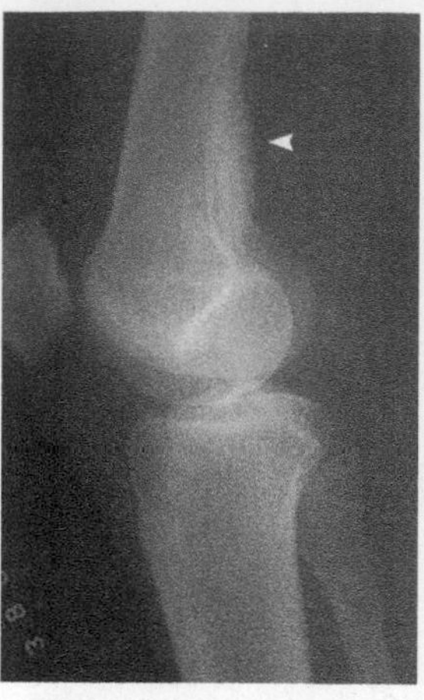

Ossified lesion with cortical thickening.

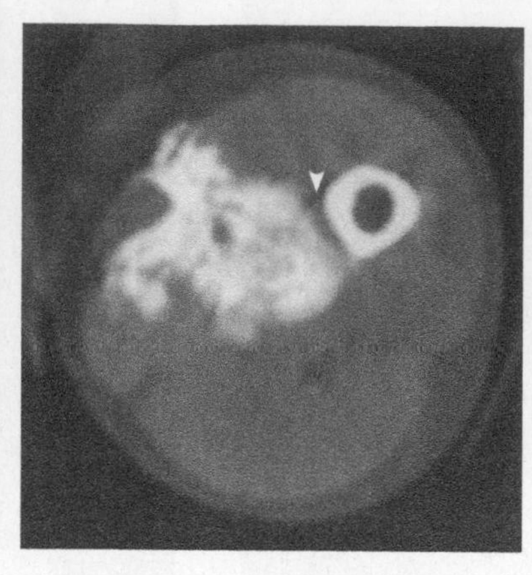

Large ossified mass adjacent to the distal femur with a lucent line between the mass and femur (*arrowhead*).

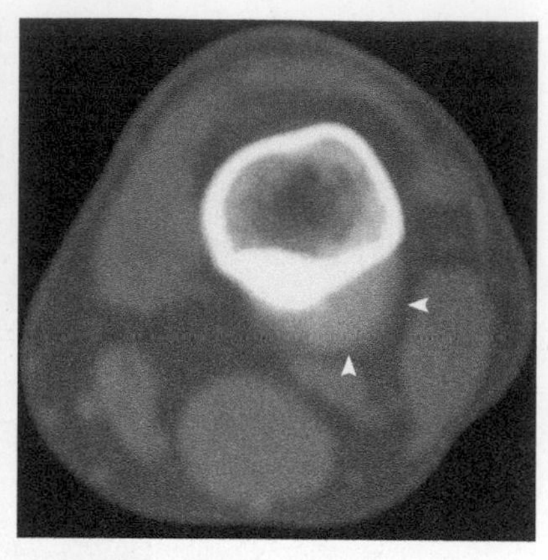

Soft-tissue component (*arrowheads*) in another patient.

Answers

1. There is s densely ossified mass posterior to the distal femur, with associated cortical thickening and no apparent corticomedullary continuity.
2. The string sign is a lucent line between the ossified mass and native bone caused by entrapped periosteum, and is seen in parosteal osteosarcomas.
3. Parosteal osteosarcomas have the best prognosis amongst osteosarcomas.
4. The greatest risk for parosteal osteosarcoma is dedifferentiation to a higher-grade tumor.
5. Dedifferentiation to a more aggressive tumor, when it occurs, is usually to a conventional osteosarcoma, fibrosarcoma, or malignant fibrous histiocytoma (MFH) of bone.

Pearls

- Parosteal osteosarcoma is the most common surface osteosarcoma.
- It has the best prognosis amongst osteosarcomas.
- A densely ossified lobulated mass abutting the cortex is typical, often with associated cortical thickening.
- Periosteal reaction is uncommon.
- The string sign may be present, which is a lucent line between the native bone and the mass.
- There is typically no cortical and medullary continuity, unlike an osteochondroma.
- The mass is less dense peripherally, with a larger unossified soft-tissue component and osteolysis corresponding with higher-grade tumor, or differentiation to a higher-grade tumor.
- Dedifferentiation usually occurs to a higher-grade conventional osteosarcoma, but also to MFH of bone or fibrosarcoma.

Suggested Readings

Jelinek JS, Murphey MD, Kransdorf MJ, Shmookler BM, Malawer MM, Hur RC. Parosteal osteosarcoma: value of MR imaging and CT in the prediction of histologic grade. *Radiology.* 1996;201(3):837-842.

Seeger LL, Yao L, Eckardt JJ. Surface lesions of bone. *Radiology.* 1998;206(1):17-33.

Yarmish G, Klein MJ, Landa J, Lefkowitz RA, Hwang S. Imaging characteristics of primary osteosarcoma: nonconventional subtypes. *Radiographics.* 2010;30(6):1653-1672.

Generalized bone pain

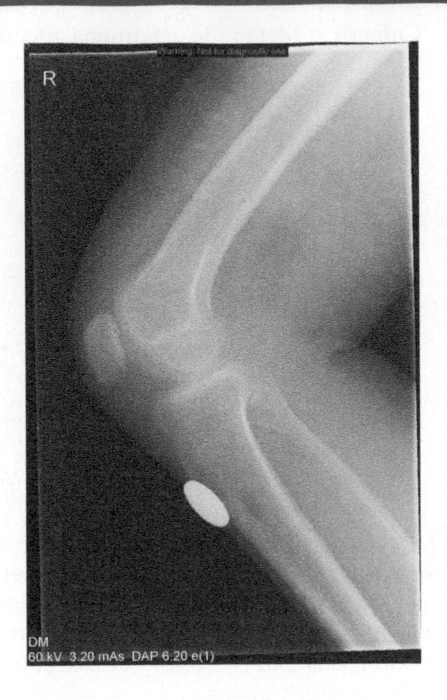

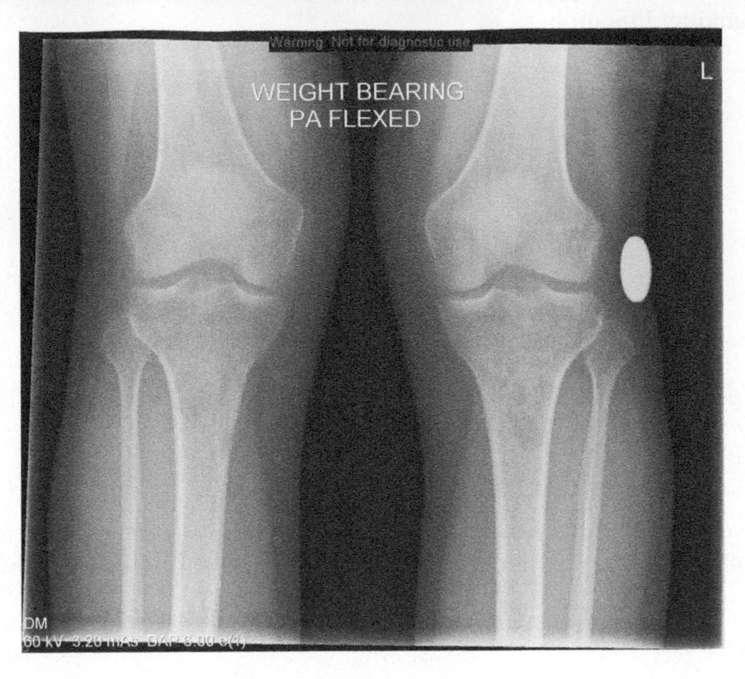

1. What is in the differential diagnosis of a lytic lesion?

2. Which endocrine abnormality is this entity most closely associated with?

3. What is the differential diagnosis of a sclerotic lesion?

4. Which cell type is responsible for the appearances of this condition?

5. What is the treatment of this bony abnormality?

Brown tumors (hyperparathyroidism) 488

Case ranking/difficulty: 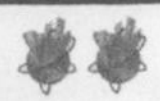

Category: Metabolic conditions affecting bone

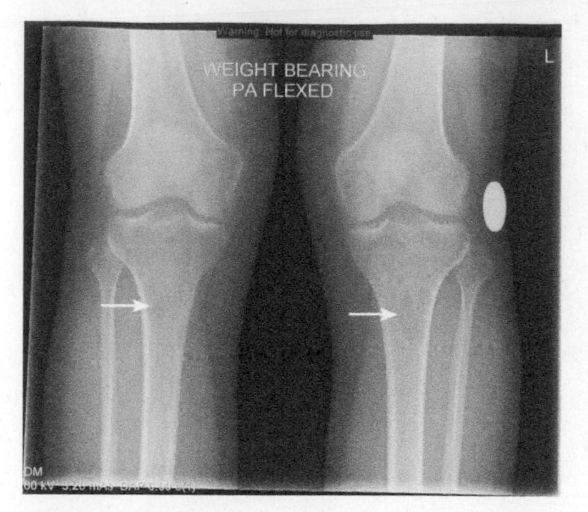

Bilateral well-defined lytic lesions with a narrow zone of transition.

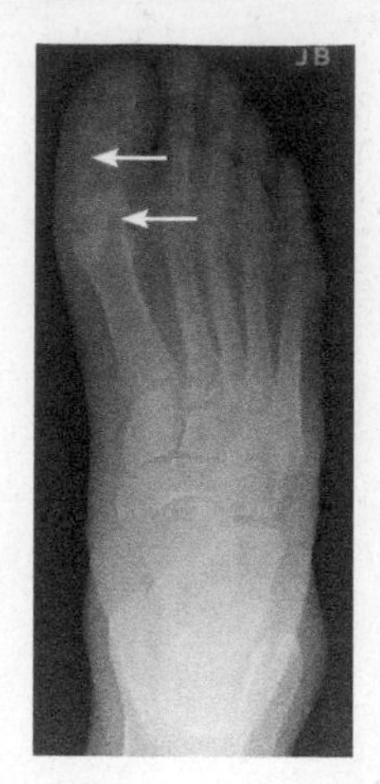

Multiple well-defined lytic lesions are seen.

⁹⁹Tc-MDP radionuclide scan demonstrates a superscan with generalized symmetric increase in skeletal activity and reduced renal and soft-tissue uptake. It is more common with secondary hyperparathyroidism.

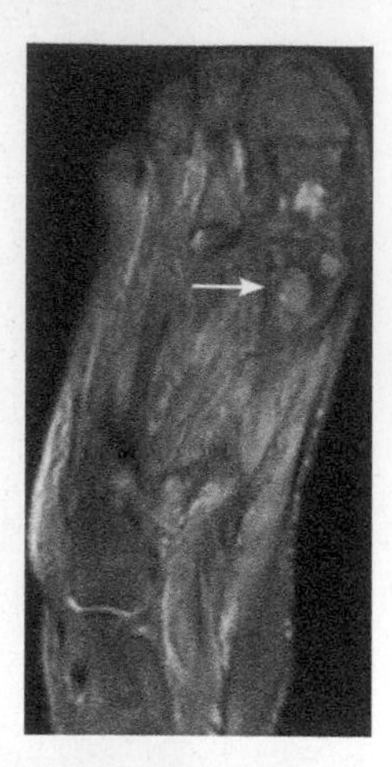

MRI demonstrates well-defined lesions of fluid signal with no cortical destruction.

Answers

1. Giant cell tumor, enchondroma and brown tumor are examples of lytic bone lesions. Other causes include fracture, fibrous dysplasia, eosinophilic granuloma, chondroblastoma, solitary bone cyst, nonossifying fibroma, infection, aneurysmal bone cyst, metastasis, and myeloma.

   It can be remembered with the pnemonic FEGNOMASHIC or FOGMACHINES.

2. Brown tumors have the greatest association with primary hyperparathyroidism. However, secondary hyperparathyroidism is more prevalent hence numerically there are more cases of brown tumor with this condition.

3. Any lytic lesion can become sclerotic when healed. Therefore possible causes include all causes of lytic lesions, in addition to typically sclerotic lesion, including enostosis, sclerotic metastasis, hemangioma, infarct, osteoid osteoma, chronic osteomyelitis, stress fracture, and osteopoikilosis.

4. Untreated hyperparathyroidism leads to osteoclast stimulation and bone lysis, resulting in osteoclastomas (brown tumors).

5. Correction of the underlying cause for hyperparathyroidism is all that is required to allow healing and sclerosis of the brown tumors and improvement in the bone pain.

Pearls

- The differential diagnosis of a well-defined lytic lesion in young patients includes brown tumors.
- Differentiation from other causes, for example, giant cell tumor is made by looking for associated features, for example, subperiosteal resorption, renal osteodystrophy, and the presence of multiple lesions.
- Imaging features may vary because of the presence of sclerosis, hemorrhage, or pathological fracture. Generalized features of hyperparathyroidism may be found on imaging for example, a superscan on ⁹⁹Tc-MDP bone scans.
- Treatment involves correction of the underlying hyperparathyroidism.

Suggested Readings

Hong WS, Sung MS, Chun KA, et al. Emphasis on the MR imaging findings of brown tumor: a report of five cases. *Skeletal Radiol.* 2011;40(2):205-213.

Noman Zaheer S, Byrne ST, Poonnoose SI, Vrodos NJ. Brown tumour of the spine in a renal transplant patient. *J Clin Neurosci.* 2009;16(9):1230-1232.

Hurt index finger while climbing several months ago

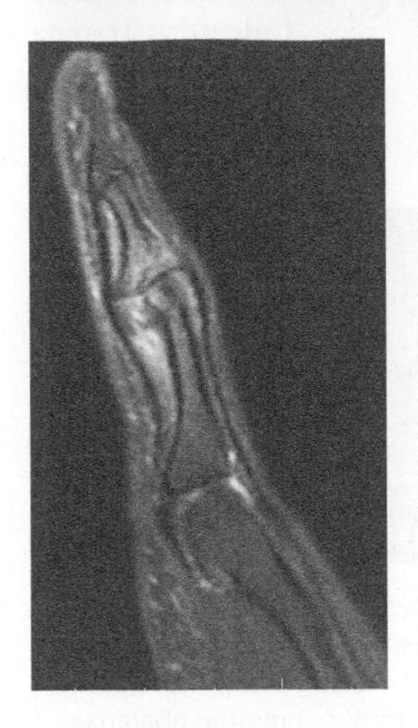 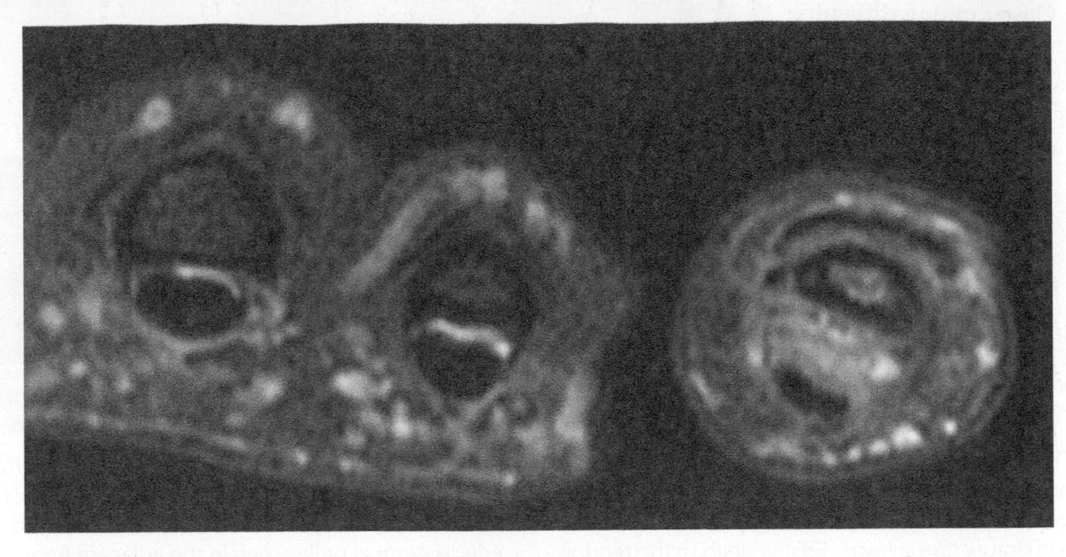

1. What are the MRI findings?
2. How many pulleys are in each finger?
3. Which pulley is most commonly injured?
4. Which pulley is most often affected in a trigger finger?
5. Bowstringing of the tendon is best appreciated on finger extension. True or False?

Pulley injury (climber's finger) 2308

Case ranking/difficulty: 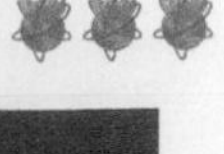 **Category:** Trauma

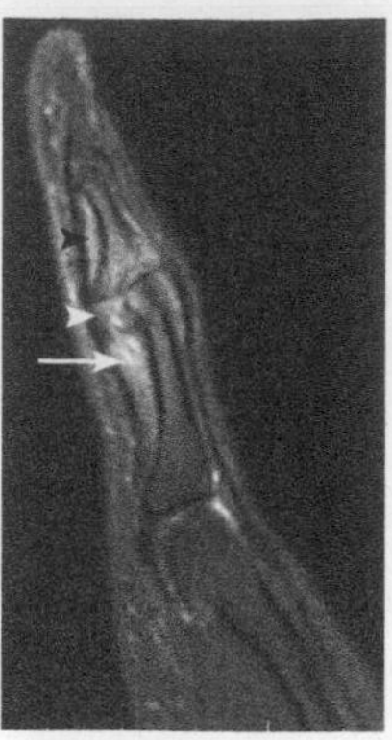

There is edema deep to the flexor tendon at the proximal phalanx, with "bowstringing" of the tendon (*arrow*). Heterogeneity of the volar plate consistent with injury (*arrowhead*). Edema deep to the tendon at the middle phalanx without bowstringing suggests low-grade A4 injury (*black arrowhead*).

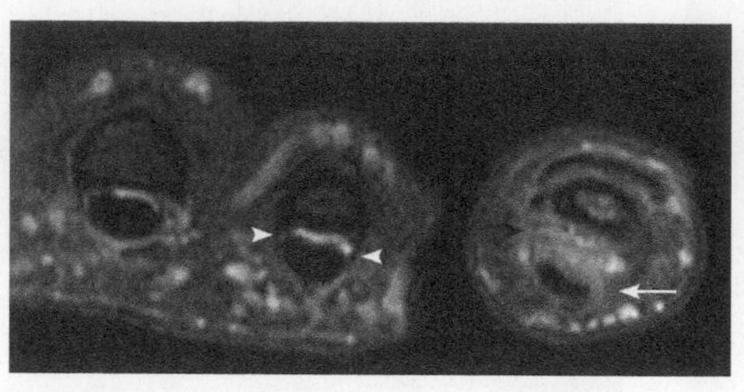

The A2 pulley shows high-grade tear medially (*arrow*) and intermediate-grade tear laterally (*black arrowhead*). There is separation of the tendon from bone with edema. Normal pulley seen in the adjacent finger (*white arrowheads*).

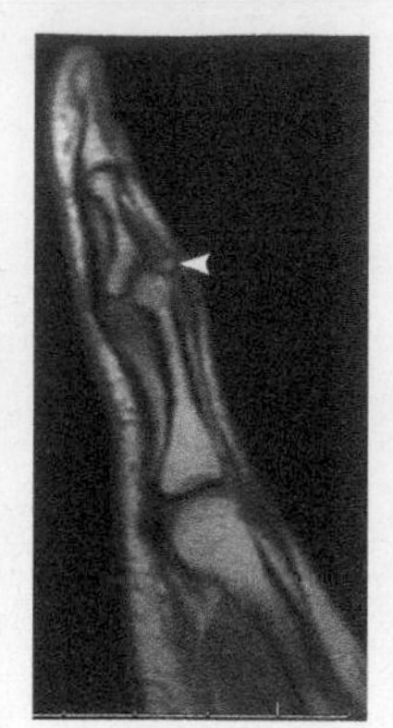

Avulsion fracture at the central slip attachment at the middle phalanx (*arrowhead*).

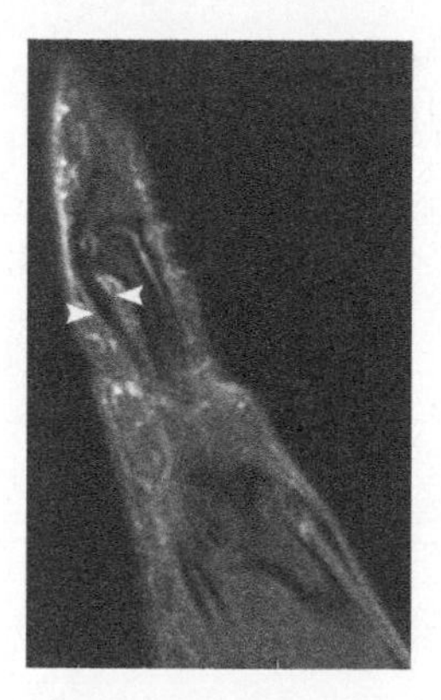

Another patient showing the mild thickening of the flexor tendon sheath consistent with the normal A2 pulley (*arrowhead*).

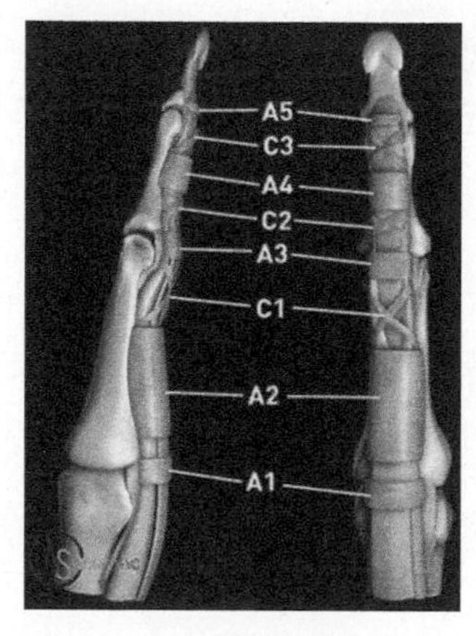

Illustration showing the finger pulleys. (Reprinted with permission from Radsource and Dr. Michael Stadnick.)

Answers

1. There is a high-grade injury to the A2 pulley with bowstringing and mild injury to the A4 pulley. There is also volar plate injury and avulsion fracture of the extensor tendon central slip insertion on the middle phalanx, with post-traumatic osteoarthritis and bone marrow edema.

2. There are 8 pulleys: 5 annular pulleys labelled A1 to A5, and 3 cruciate labelled C1 to C3.

3. The A2 pulley is the most important pulley, but also the most frequently injured. The A3 pulley is the second most injured, followed by A4.

4. The A1 pulley is most often affected in a trigger finger.

5. False. Finger flexion accentuates the bowstringing of the flexor tendon in a pulley injury, but is usually not performed because flexion may result in pain and subsequent motion artifact.

Pearls

- The flexor tendon pulleys help to keep the flexor tendon opposed to bone, facilitating normal finger biomechanics.
- There are 5 annular pulleys labelled A1 to A5, and 3 cruciate pulleys labelled C1 to C3.
- The annular pulleys contribute most to stability, especially A2 followed by the A4 pulley.
- The A2 pulley is most frequently injured, followed by A3 then A4.
- Mild pulley injury is manifested by edema deep to and surrounding the tendon, with possible associated tenosynovitis.
- More severe pulley injury will result in "bowstringing" with loss of apposition of the tendon to bone.
- Flexion of the finger on ultrasound or MRI will accentuate the finding of "bowstringing."

Suggested Readings

Awh MH. Pulley lesion of the fingers. *MRI Web Clinic*. 2005.

Hauger O, Chung CB, Lektrakul N, et al. Pulley system in the fingers: normal anatomy and simulated lesions in cadavers at MR imaging, CT, and US with and without contrast material distention of the tendon sheath. *Radiology*. 2000;217(1):201-212.

Klauser A, Frauscher F, Bodner G, et al. Finger pulley injuries in extreme rock climbers: depiction with dynamic US. *Radiology*. 2002;222(3):755-761.

Pain in the hip with snapping symptoms

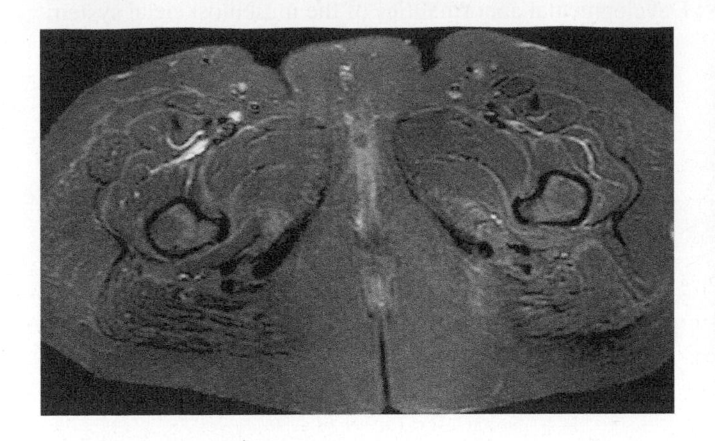

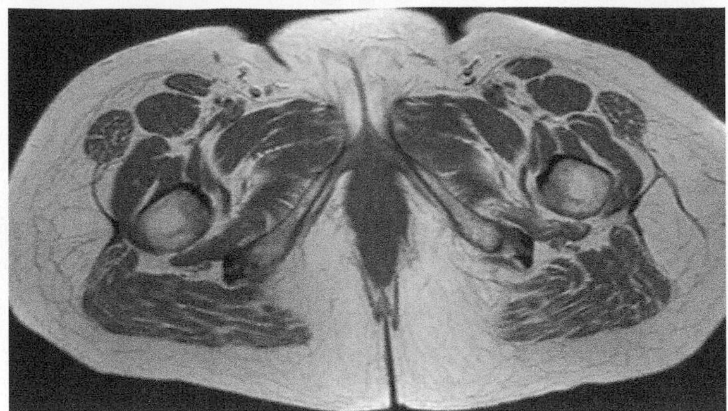

1. What are the MRI findings?

2. What is the differential diagnosis?

3. What is the most likely diagnosis?

4. What is the anatomy of the affected structure?

5. What leg movements exacerbates the symptoms of this entity?

Ischiofemoral impingement syndrome 1734

Case ranking/difficulty: 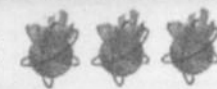 **Category:** Developmental abnormalities of the musculoskeletal system

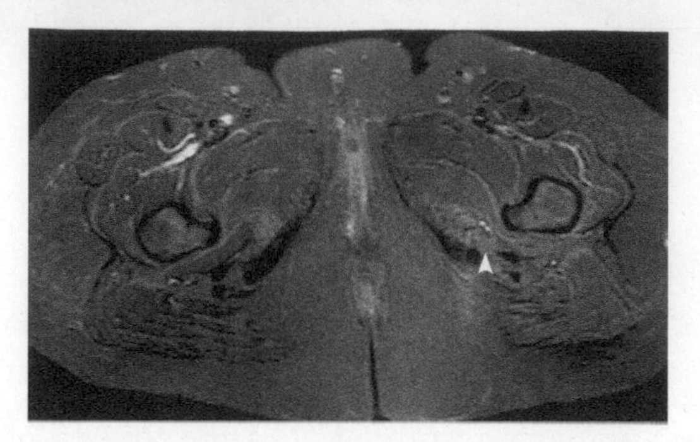

Edema in the left quadratus femoris muscle.

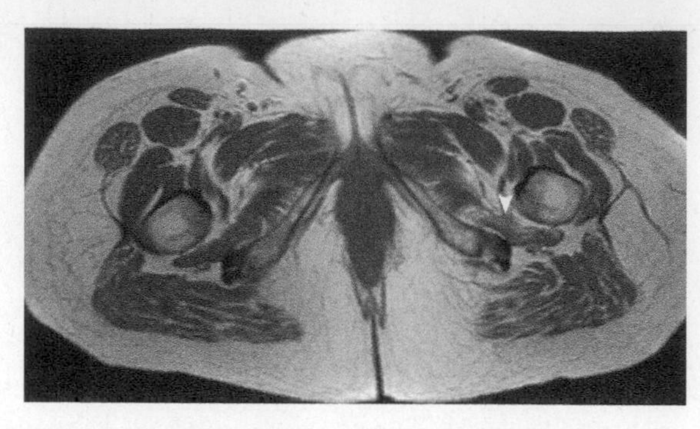

Fatty atrophy of the left quadratus femoris.

Answers

1. STIR image demonstrates edema, and high T1 signal indicates atrophy in the quadratus femoris. The ischiofemoral space is narrowed, and the quadratus femoris is atrophic in comparison to its counterparts.
2. The differential diagnoses include piriformis syndrome, iliopsoas bursitis, ischial bursitis, quadratus sprain, and acute quadratus tear.
3. Given the edema and atrophy of the quadratus femoris muscle, along with a narrowed ischiofemoral space, the diagnosis is ischiofemoral impingement.
4. Quadratus femoris is a quadrangular shape muscle that originates at the lateral margin of the obturator ring above the ischial tuberosity.

   It inserts on the posterior medial aspect of the proximal femur along the quadrate tubercle of the posterior intertrochanteric region.

   Superiorly the quadratus femoris is surrounded by fat and the inferior gemellus muscle, and inferiorly, it is close to the adductor magnus. The sciatic nerve is posterior and in close proximity.
5. Extension, adduction, and internal rotation are the main movements that lead to ischiofemoral impingement and subsequent pain.

Pearls

- In ischiofemoral impingement syndrome, there is an impingement of the quadratus femoris muscle in the ischiofemoral space.
- It is one of the cause of chronic buttock and hip pain.
- The syndrome is most commonly seen in middle-aged and older women, and may be bilateral in up to 25%. The anatomy of the female pelvis with its wider-spaced ischial tuberosities may be a predisposing factor. It may also be acquired, with hypertrophic changes at the ischial tuberosity being contributory.
- Ischiofemoral impingement should be differentiated from quadratus femoris muscle sprain or tear. In quadratus femoris strain, the edema is at the myotendinous junction, whereas in ischiofemoral impingement syndrome, the edema is at the level of ischiofemoral recess and may be associated with atrophy.
- Other differentials include lesser trochanteric, iliopsoas, and ischial tuberosity bursitis.
- Axial fat-saturated fluid-sensitive images are useful sequences as they demonstrate muscle edema and increased signal within the tendon. On axial T1-weighted images, atrophy of this muscle and narrowing of the ischiofemoral space is well appreciated.
- Conservative treatment includes analgesics and anti-inflammatory drugs.
- Surgical resection of the lesser trochanter has been described as an option for refractory cases.

Suggested Readings

Ali AM, Whitwell D, Ostlere SJ. Case report: imaging and surgical treatment of a snapping hip due to ischiofemoral impingement. *Skeletal Radiol.* 2011;40(5):653-656.

Kassarjian A, Tomas X, Cerezal L, Canga A, Llopis E. MRI of the quadratus femoris muscle: anatomic considerations and pathologic lesions. *AJR Am J Roentgenol.* 2011;197(1):170-174.

Torriani M, Souto SC, Thomas BJ, Ouellette H, Bredella MA. Ischiofemoral impingement syndrome: an entity with hip pain and abnormalities of the quadratus femoris muscle. *AJR Am J Roentgenol.* 2009;193(1):186-190.

Painful sternoclavicular joint with swelling and multiple skin pustules

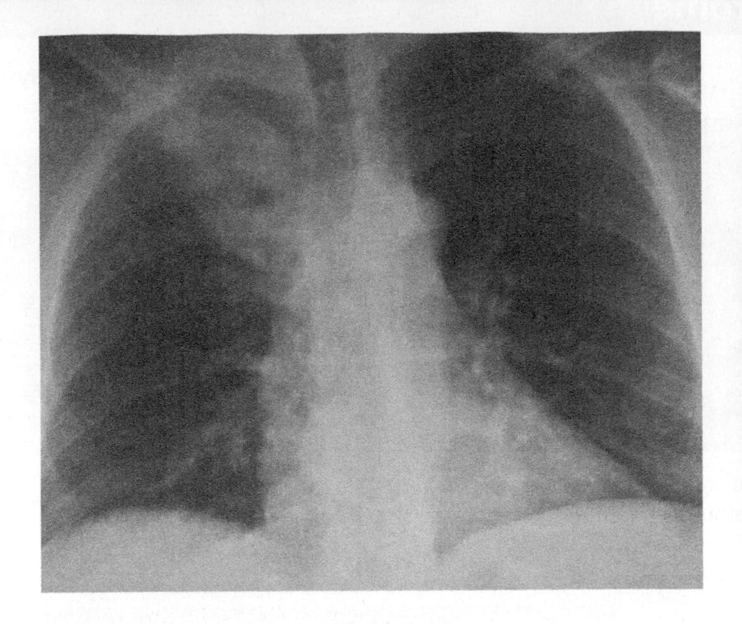

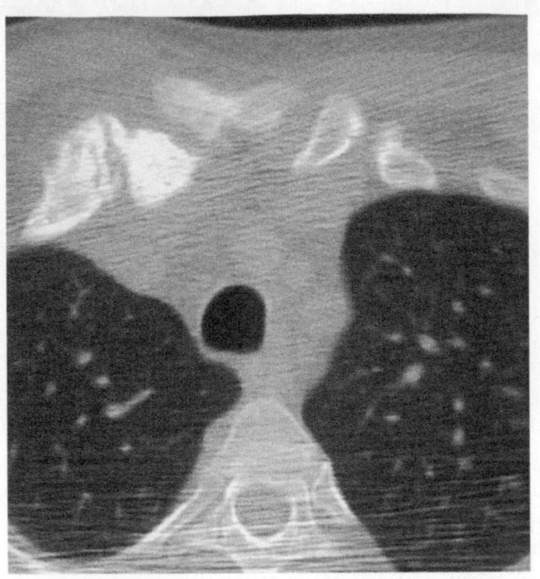

1. What are the radiograph findings?

2. What are the CT findings?

3. What is the differential diagnosis?

4. What is the likely diagnosis?

5. What are the treatment options?

SAPHO (synovitis, acne, palmoplantar pustulosis, hyperostosis and osteitis) syndrome 1545

Case ranking/difficulty: 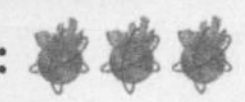

Category: Infections in the musculoskeletal system

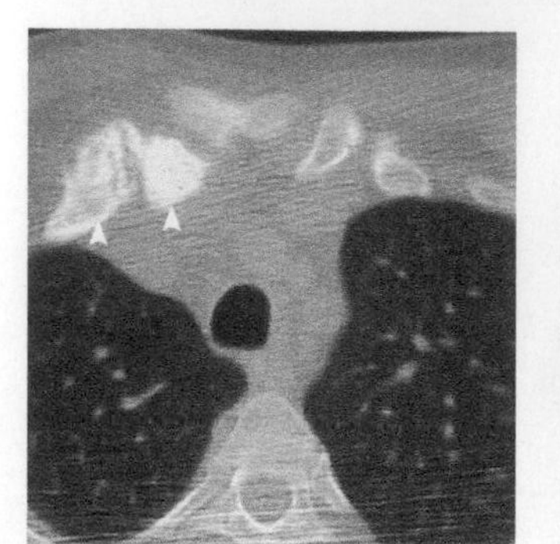

Hyperostosis, sclerosis and expansion of the medial clavicle and sternum.

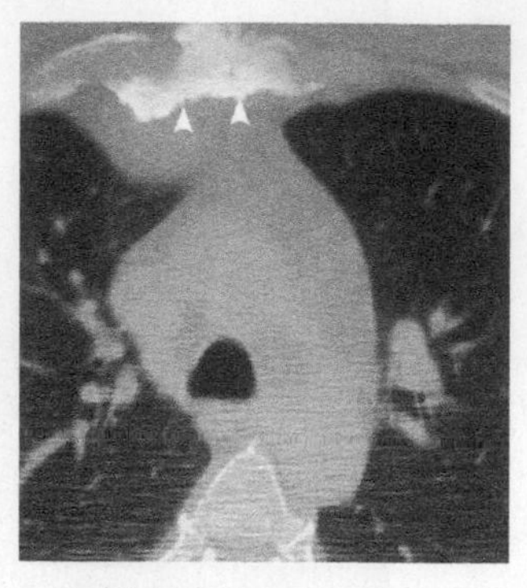

Erosion, sclerosis, hyperostosis, and expansion of the sternum.

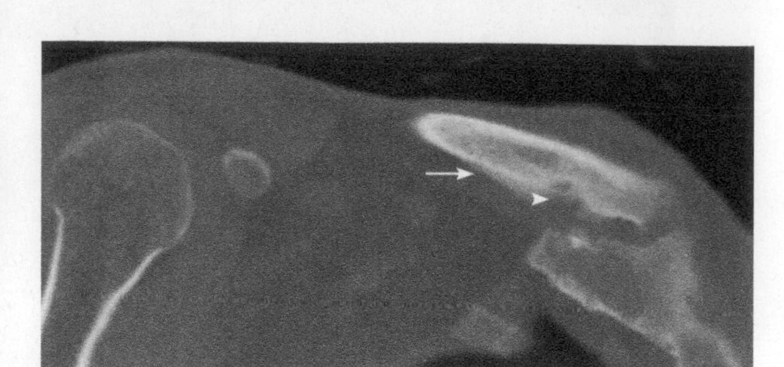

Different patient. Extensive sclerosis of the medial clavicle (*arrow*) and erosions (*arrowhead*).

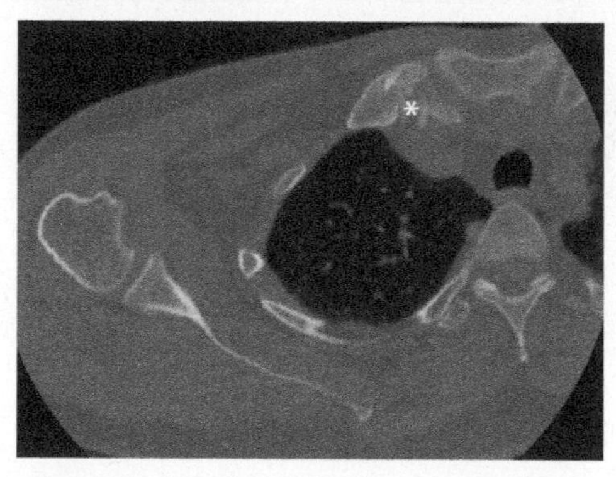

Different patient, less dramatic changes. Hyperostosis, sclerosis, and erosion (*asterisk*). Soft-tissue swelling is also seen.

Answers

1. Right sternoclavicular joint hyperostosis, sclerosis with erosion and soft-tissue swelling.
2. Hyperostosis, sclerosis, and erosions of the medial end of clavicle. There is also soft-tissue swelling.
3. The differential diagnosis involves bacterial, atypical or viral infection, autoimmune disease, metastasis, Ewing sarcoma, and osteonecrosis.
4. The diagnosis is SAPHO syndrome. SAPHO is an acronym for synovitis, acne, palmoplantar pustulosis, hyperostosis and osteitis.
5. The treatment options include analgesics, anti-inflammatory drugs, bisphosphonates, and immunomodulators.

Pearls

- SAPHO is a syndrome composed of synovitis, acne, palmoplantar pustulosis, hyperostosis and osteitis.
- The etiology is unknown, but may be infectious or an autoimmune response to infection.
- It most commonly involves the sternoclavicular joint demonstrating hyperostosis, osteosclerosis, and erosions with soft-tissue swelling. Long bones and axial skeleton can also be involved. There may be associated arthritis and ankylosis.
- SAPHO lesions can also uncommonly appear as an aggressive lesion within the long bones because of erosions, osteosclerosis, hyperostosis, and soft-tissue swelling.
- Plain film and CT scans are diagnostic and demonstrate variable hyperostosis, ankylosis, osteosclerosis, erosions, and soft-tissue swelling at the sternoclavicular joint.
- MRI can show marrow edema, soft-tissue abnormalities, and sternoclavicular joint effusion.
- The treatment involves NSAIDs, steroids, and analgesics, as well as immunomodulators.

Suggested Readings

Depasquale R, Kumar N, Lalam RK, et al. SAPHO: What radiologists should know. *Clin Radiol.* 2012;67(3):195-206.

Sweeney SA, Kumar VA, Tayar J, et al. Case 181: synovitis acne pustulosis hyperostosis osteitis (SAPHO) syndrome. *Radiology.* 2012;263(2):613-617.

Painful and swollen digit

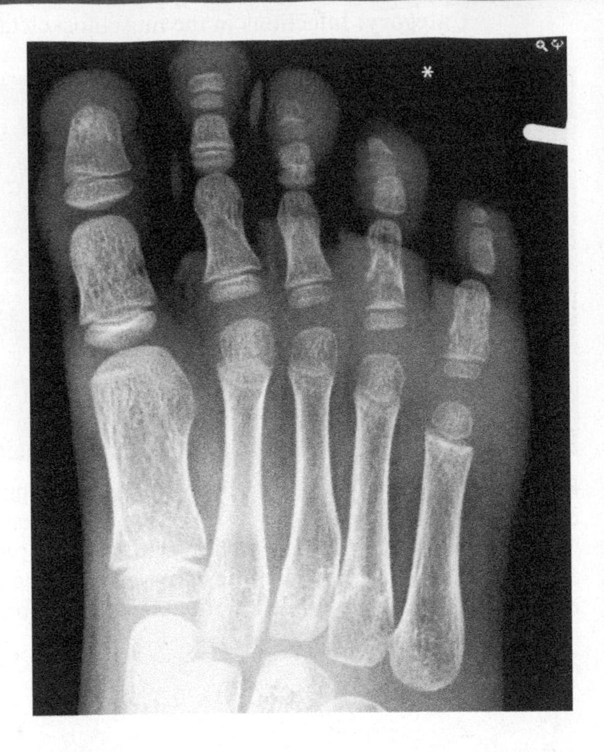

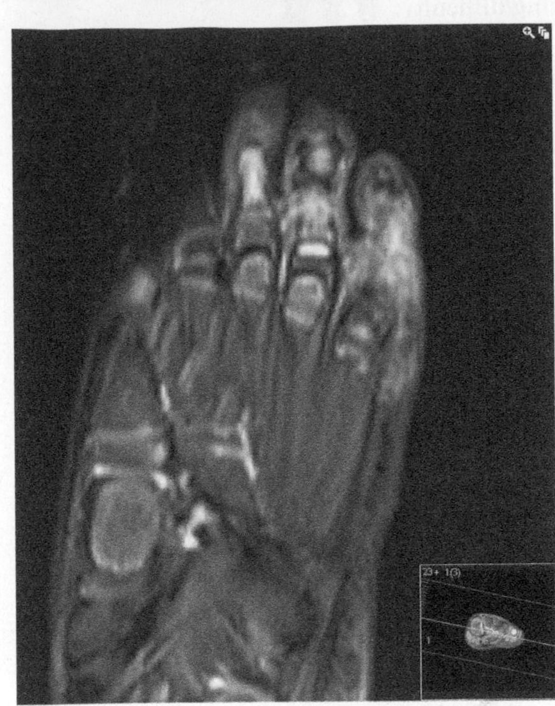

1. What is the descriptive term used for this entity?

2. In which age group is this condition most prevalent?

3. What is the differential diagnosis?

4. What are the possible treatments for this condition in other bones?

5. What are the most common digital bones to be involved with this condition?

Tuberculous dactylitis 1715

Case ranking/difficulty: 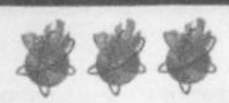 **Category:** Infections in the musculoskeletal system

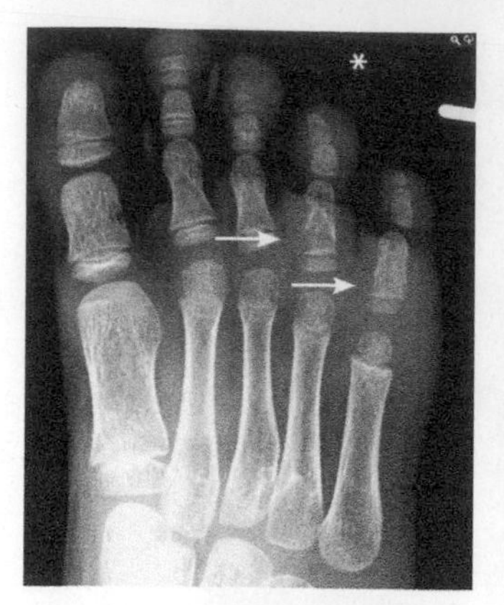

Soft-tissue swelling around fourth and fifth proximal phalanges. Expansion of digits with lucency and destruction of medial cortex.

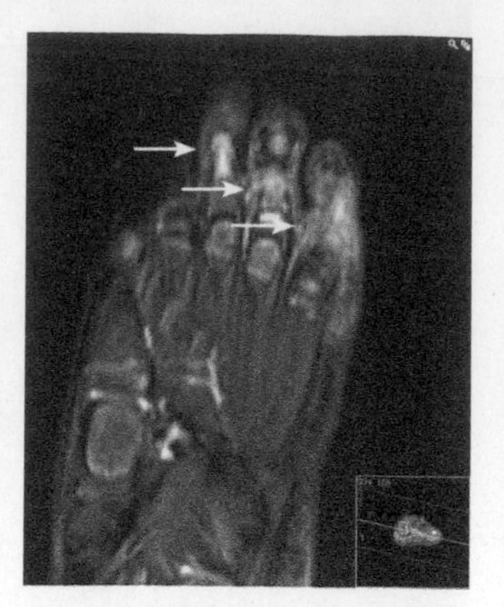

Corresponding fat-suppressed MRI image demonstrates high T2 weighted signal in the shaft of the third to fifth proximal phalanges with significant edema and cortical destruction.

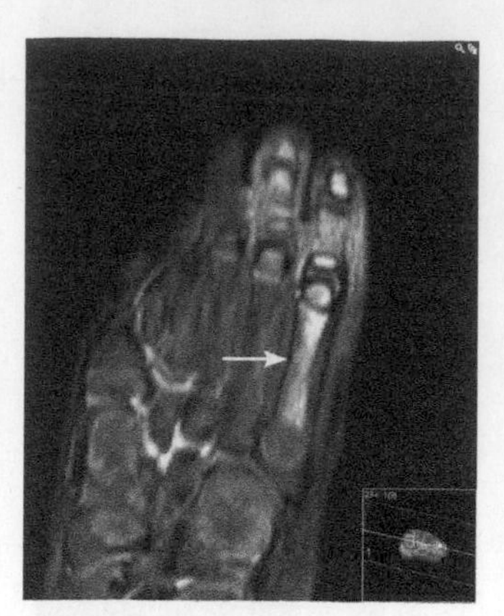

Fat-suppressed MRI demonstrates high signal within the fifth metatarsal in addition consistent with TB osteomyelitis.

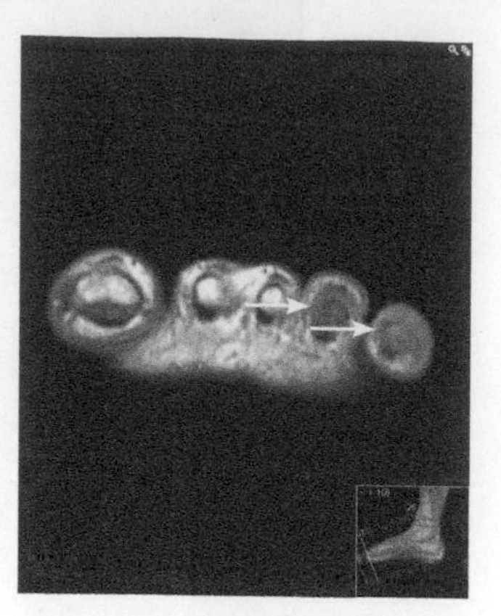

Marrow signal change (low T1) is seen in both fourth and fifth digits, which is typical of osteomyelitis. (Image courtesy of Dr. Denis Remedios.)

Answers

1. Spina "ventosa" means "wind-filled" and is a descriptive term used because of the appearance of expansion and multiple air-like lucencies. It is a typical feature of tuberculous digital osteomyelitis.

2. Eighty-five percent of patients with TB dactylitis are younger than the age of 6 years.

3. Lung cancer metastasis would not be found in the young age group. Sarcoidosis may look very similar, although again is found in a different age group (20 to 40 years of age). In a patient of this age group, however, TB and sarcoid would still both be in the differential. Leukemia may have similar appearances and has a large soft-tissue component.

4. Antituberculous chemotherapy is normally sufficient treatment for TB osteomyelitis. Occasionally, surgical curettage or fixation of a pathological fracture may be required.

5. The most common digits to be involved are the proximal phalanges of the index and middle fingers.

Pearls

- An expanded digit with lucencies and a large soft tissue mass is typical for TB dactylitis. The classical descriptive term on a radiograph for this entity is *spina ventosa*, a description of the appearance of the digits as "wind-filled" with numerous air-like lucencies.
- The diagnosis should be entertained in susceptible patient groups, for example, Asian, malnourished, immunosuppressed.
- Eighty-five percent of patients are younger than the age of 6 years.
- Most cases are treatable with antituberculous therapy alone; however, a bone biopsy may be required to make the diagnosis, and to guide appropriate treatment in cases of antibiotic resistance.

Suggested Readings

Malik S, Joshi S, Tank JS. Cystic bone tuberculosis in children—a case series. *Indian J Tuberc.* 2009;56(4):220-224.

Ritz N, Connell TG, Tebruegge M, Johnstone BR, Curtis N. Tuberculous dactylitis—an easily missed diagnosis. *Eur J Clin Microbiol Infect Dis.* 2011;30(11):1303-1310.

Sunderamoorthy D, Gupta V, Bleetman A. TB or not TB: an unusual sore finger. *Emerg Med J.* 2001;18(6):490-491.

1-day-old male with a history of deformity

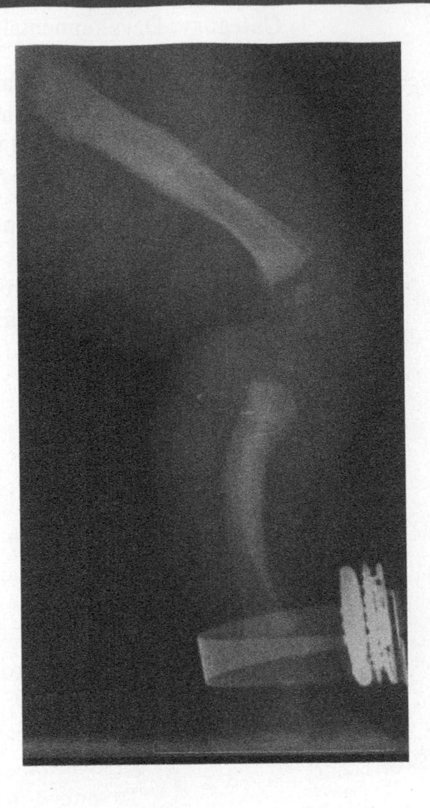

1. What are the radiographic findings?

2. What are the presumed etiologies?

3. What are included in the differential, and what is the most likely diagnosis?

4. What are the typical radiological features in this entity?

5. What is the management?

Congenital bowing of the tibia 1437

Case ranking/difficulty: ❋❋❋

Category: Developmental abnormalities of the musculoskeletal system

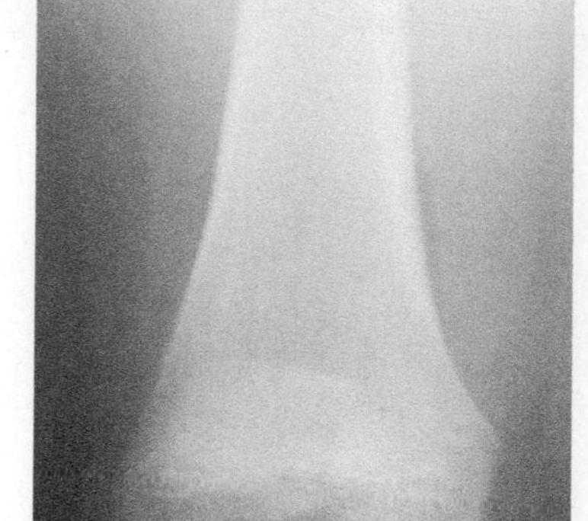

Comparison case of Blount disease, showing bowing in the medial–lateral plane.

Answers

1. There is posteromedial bowing of the tibia and fibula, with cortical thickening of the tibia. Mild cortical thickening of the femur is also seen.
2. An abnormal intrauterine position is the likely etiology, although fetal vascular insufficiency and localized skeletal dysplasia have also been implicated.
3. Tibial bowing can be seen in fibula hemimelia, neurofibromatosis, Blount disease, and physiological and congenital tibial bowing. The most likely diagnosis, based on age and direction of bowing, is congenital tibial bowing.
4. In congenital bowing, there is posteromedial bowing of the tibia and fibula with diaphyseal broadening and cortical thickening of the concave tibial cortex. Pseudoarthrosis occurs in neurofibromatosis.
5. Gradual remodelling occurs, so management is typically conservative or with bracing. If there is significant leg-length discrepancy, an osteotomy and leg lengthening may be performed, which may be combined with a contralateral epiphysiodesis.

Pearls

- Congenital tibial bowing affects the tibia and fibula in the newborn.
- An abnormal intrauterine position is the likely etiology.
- Bowing is posterior and medial in the vast majority of patients.
- In neurofibromatosis, bowing is anteriorly and laterally; in fibula hemimelia, it is anteriorly and medially.
- Physiological bowing and Blount disease result in varus angulation.
- Treatment is usually conservative with bracing, and gradual remodeling. Surgery is indicated in some cases.

Suggested Readings

Cheema JI, Grissom LE, Harcke HT. Radiographic characteristics of lower-extremity bowing in children. *Radiographics*. 2003;23(4):871-880.

Hofmann A, Wenger DR. Posteromedial bowing of the tibia. Progression of discrepancy in leg lengths. *J Bone Joint Surg Am.* 1981;63(3):384-388.

History of rheumatoid arthritis; wrist pain

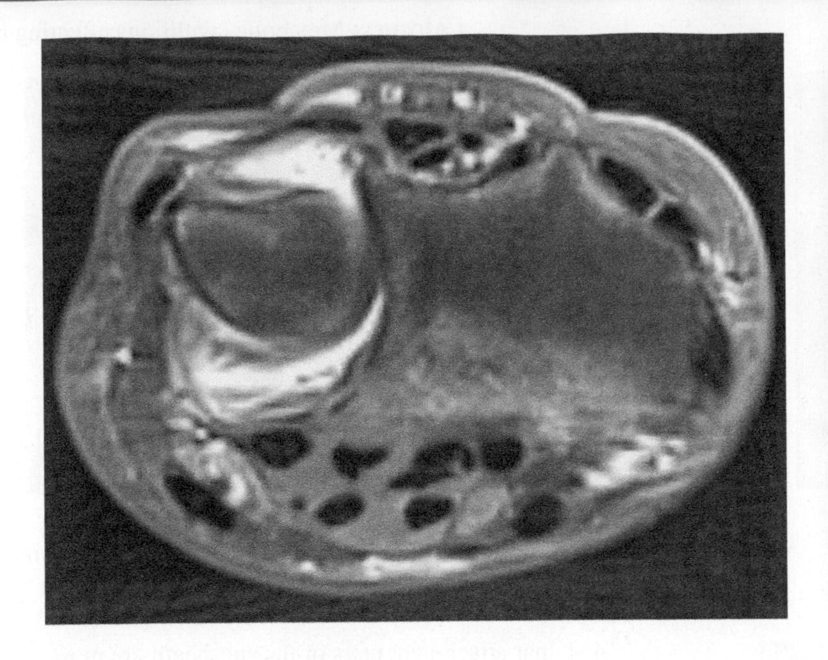
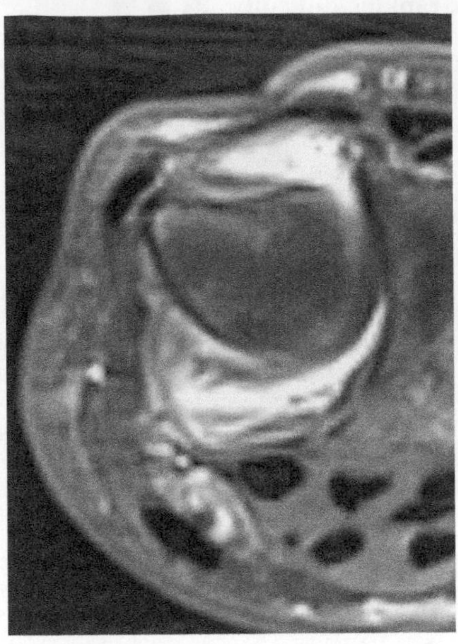

1. What are the MRI findings?
2. What is the typical mechanism of injury?
3. What are the restraints of the extensor carpi ulnaris (ECU) tendon?
4. Where does the ECU subsheath typically tear?
5. What tears has the worse prognosis, and what is the treatment for that tear?

Extensor carpi ulnaris (ECU) subluxation and subsheath tear 1425

Case ranking/difficulty: 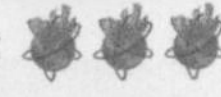

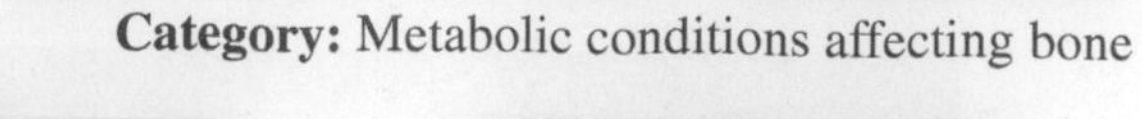

Category: Metabolic conditions affecting bone

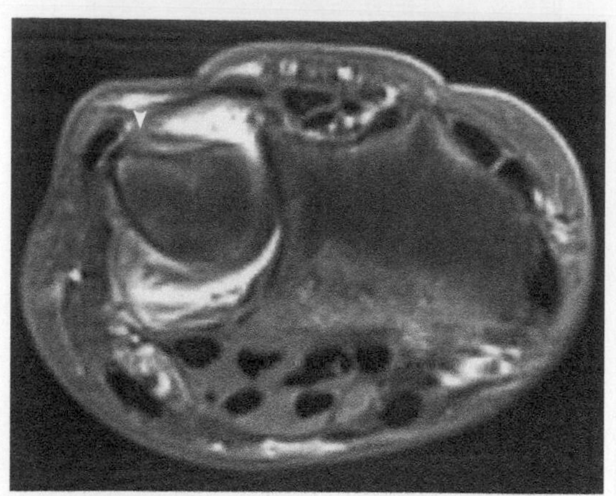

There is ulnar subluxation of the extensor carpi ulnaris (ECU) tendon. The ulnar aspect of the ECU subsheath is torn (*arrowhead*).

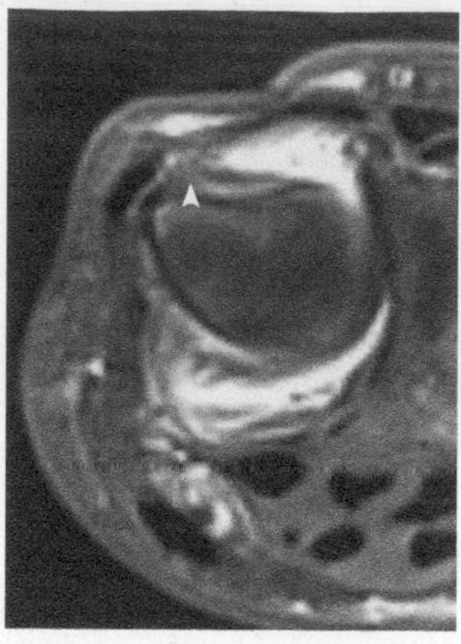

Magnified view shows ECU subluxation and subsheath tear (*arrowhead*).

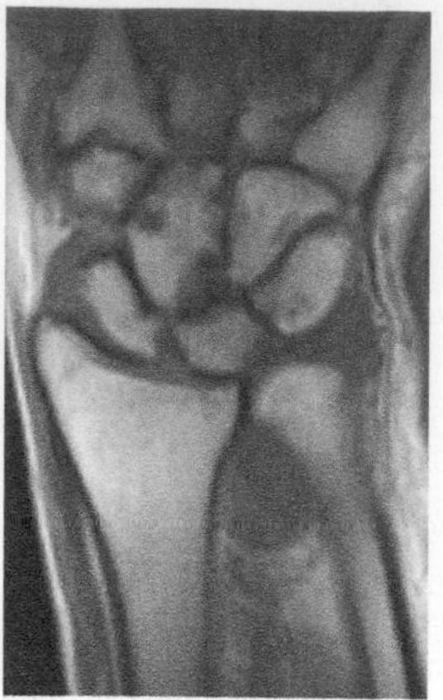

Cystic erosions from rheumatoid arthritis, and wrist and DRUJ effusions.

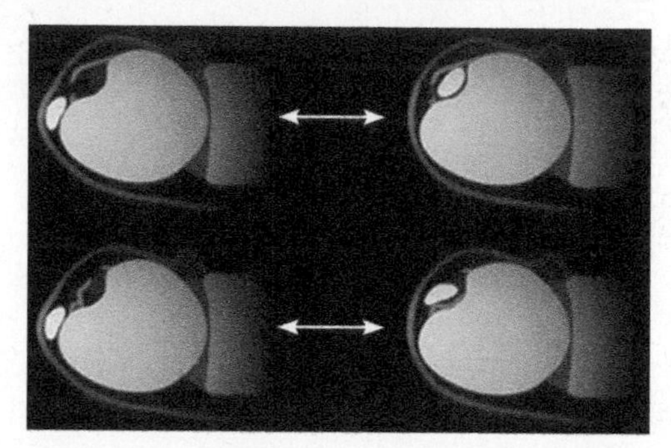

Ulnar-sided subsheath tears (*top row*) typically result in transient dislocation of the tendon followed by relocation upon pronation, with the tendon returning to a position beneath the subsheath. With radial-sided tears (*lower diagrams*), the tendon is more likely to lie on top of the torn subsheath following relocation. *Outer line* is the retinaculum, *inner line* is the subsheath. (Reprinted with permission from Radsource and Dr. Michael Stadnick.)

Answers

1. Tear of the ulnar attachment of the extensor carpi ulnaris (ECU) subsheath, with ulnar subluxation of the ECU tendon. There are also wrist and distal radioulnar joint effusions with synovitis.
2. Repetitive supination as in golf or tennis, distal radius and Galeazzi fractures, and rheumatoid arthritis have all been implicated in ECU subsheath tears and ECU subluxation.
3. The ECU subsheath is the major restraint of the ECU tendon. The subsheath also attaches near the base of the ulnar styloid process, and fractures of the styloid process result in instability of the ECU.
4. Ulnar attachment tears of the subsheath are most common, followed by radial attachment tears.
5. Radial tears have the worst prognosis. Management is typically conservative with casting in extension and radial deviation. Some authors advocate reconstructing the subsheath acutely.

Pearls

- The extensor carpi ulnaris (ECU) subsheath is attached to the distal ulna dorsally, and keeps the ECU from dislocating.
- Fractures of the distal radius may result in associated ulnar styloid process fractures and injury to the subsheath, as the latter attaches to the ulna styloid process.
- Rheumatoid arthritis and chronic repetitive supination, as in tennis and golf, can also lead to subsheath insufficiency.
- Radial-sided tears have a worse prognosis as the subluxing tendon will lie on top of the subsheath following pronation, preventing healing. These usually require surgical intervention.
- Ulnar-sided subsheath tears are treated conservatively.

Suggested Readings

Awh MH. Extensor carpi ulnaris subsheath injury. *MRI Web Clin.* February 2009.

Inoue G, Tamura Y. Recurrent dislocation of the extensor carpi ulnaris tendon. *Br J Sports Med.* 1998;32(2):172-174.

Pain following remote knee injury

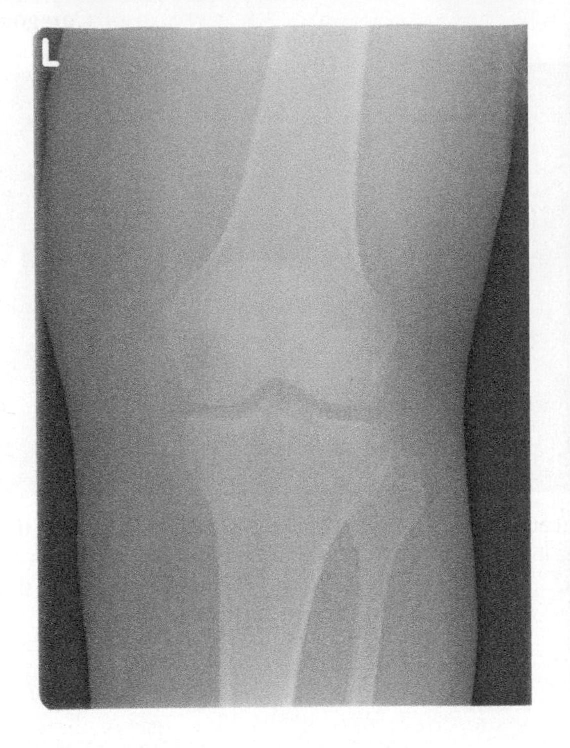

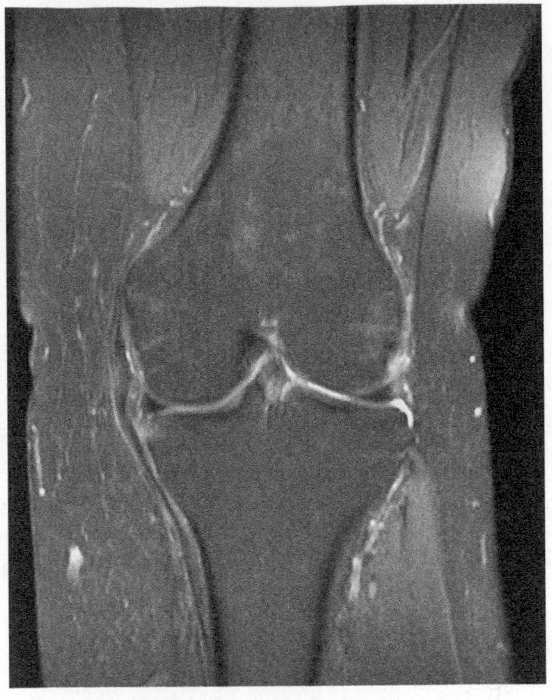

1. What is the abnormal structure in the radiograph?

2. What is the probable mechanism of injury?

3. What are the common associated soft-tissue injuries?

4. What is the imaging modality of choice for this entity?

5. What is the treatment for this entity?

Reverse segond fracture 1651

Case ranking/difficulty: 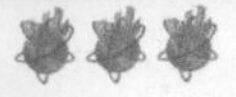

Category: Trauma

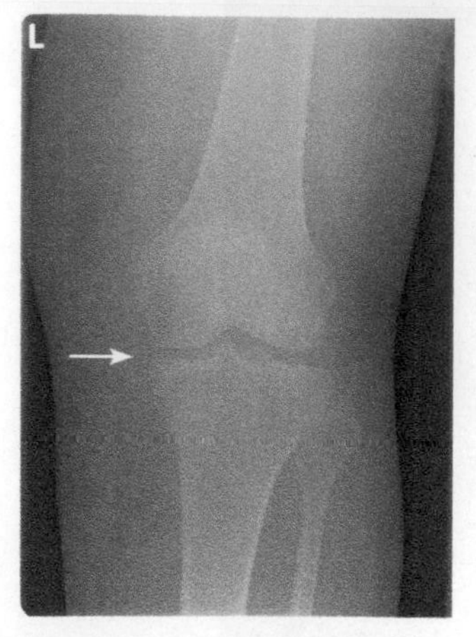

Avulsion fracture of medial tibial plateau consistent with a "reverse Segond" fracture.

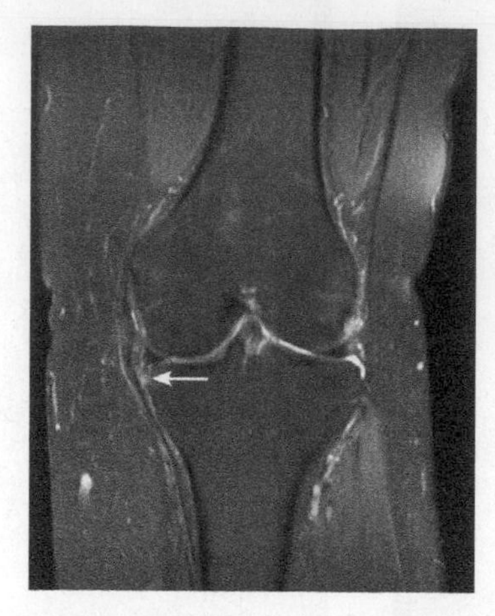

Avulsion of medial tibial plateau by deep fibers of MCL. There is edema in the MCL consistent with a partial tear.

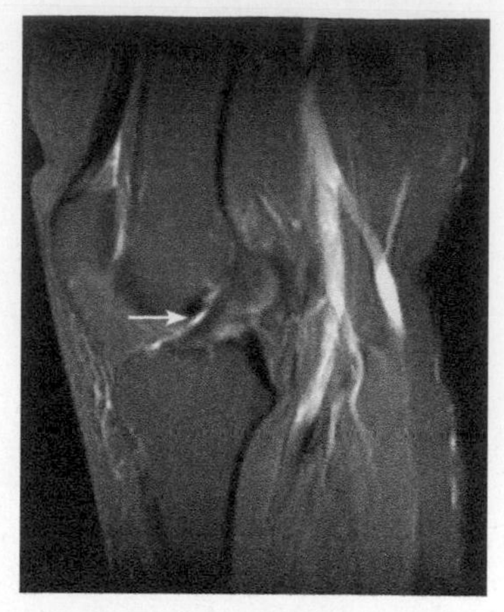

The ACL and PCL are intact in this patient, although they can be damaged with this mechanism of injury and should be carefully evaluated.

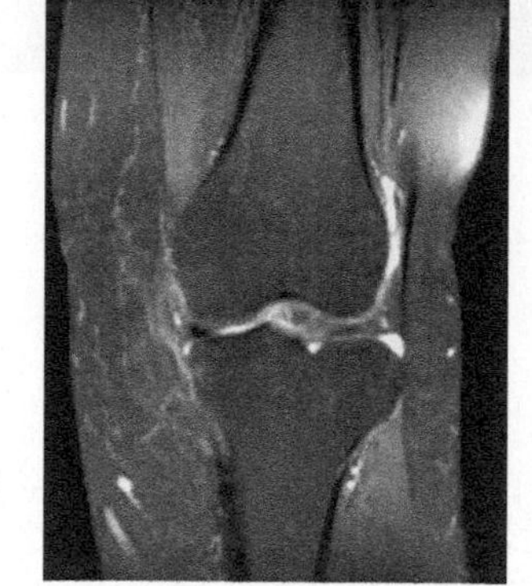

The lack of marrow edema, effusion, and other injuries are relatively unusual, although it is possible the injury occurred some time previously and the patient presented late.

Answers

1. The reverse Segond injury describes a medial capsular avulsion.
2. In common with pure MCL injuries, the presence of a medial capsular avulsion is strongly suggestive of a valgus strain injury mechanism. With this injury there is often a component of external rotation associated.
3. The reverse Segond fracture is strongly associated with tears of the deep fibers of the MCL, medial meniscus (especially root), and posterior cruciate ligament.
4. Although plain films are adequate initially to demonstrate the fracture, an MRI is mandatory to assess the extent of internal derangement, which is the more significant finding.
5. The fracture itself needs no treatment per se; however, the extent and grade of soft tissue injuries, in particular medial meniscal and MCL, determines the need for surgery. The PCL is usually not surgically repaired.

Pearls

- The presence of a tiny avulsion fracture adjacent to the medial tibial plateau should be treated with caution, as it is suggestive of more significant trauma and internal knee derangement.
- The fracture relates to avulsion of the deep fibers of the MCL or posterior oblique ligament at the proximal tibial insertion.
- The "reverse Segond" fracture involves valgus strain with external rotation.
- The most common associated injuries are the MCL, medial meniscus, and PCL.
- Treatment is determined by the presence of associated ligamentous injuries, which must be assessed by MRI.

Suggested Readings

Escobedo EM, Mills WJ, Hunter JC. The "reverse Segond" fracture: association with a tear of the posterior cruciate ligament and medial meniscus. *AJR Am J Roentgenol.* 2002;178(4):979-983.

Gottsegen CJ, Eyer BA, White EA, Learch TJ, Forrester D. Avulsion fractures of the knee: imaging findings and clinical significance. *Radiographics.* 2008;28(6): 1755-1770.

Hall FM, Hochman MG. Medial Segond-type fracture: cortical avulsion off the medial tibial plateau associated with tears of the posterior cruciate ligament and medial meniscus. *Skeletal Radiol.* 1997;26(9):553-555.

Patient with longstanding chronic condition who is on treatment

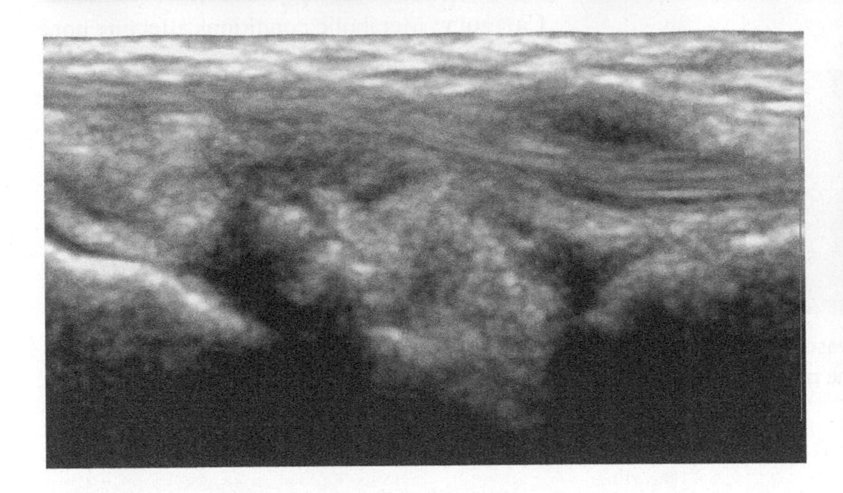

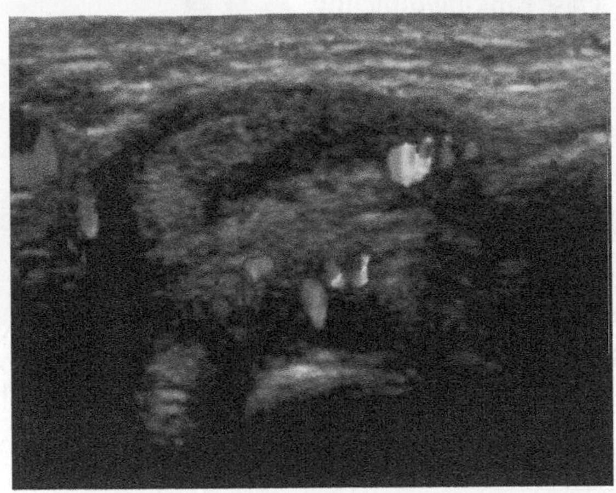

1. What are the ultrasound findings?
2. What is the differential diagnosis?
3. What is the role of ultrasound in monitoring the response to therapy?
4. What is the best scanning technique when evaluating the MCP joints?
5. What is the most reliable method of assessing disease activity?

Rheumatoid arthritis of hands (ultrasound) 1378

Case ranking/difficulty: 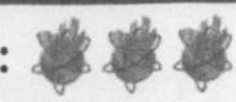

Category: Metabolic conditions affecting bone

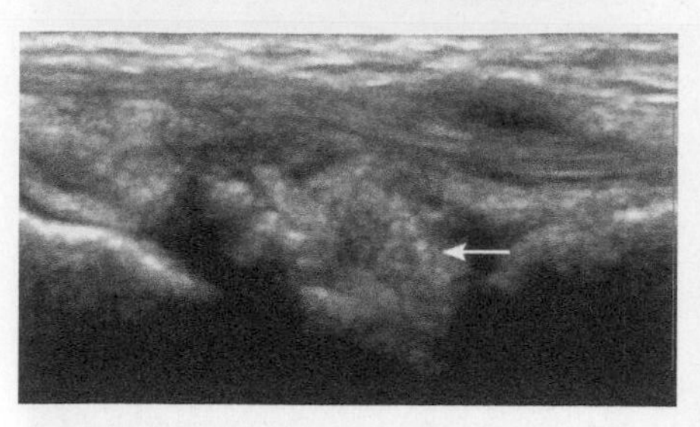

Echogenic pannus in the joint space.

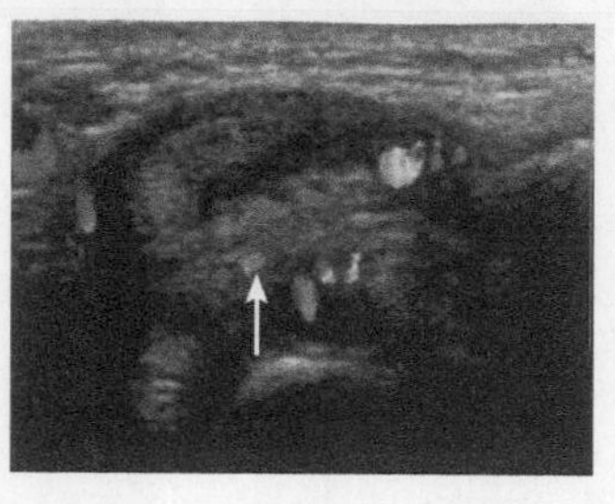

Minimal vascularity in and around the pannus.

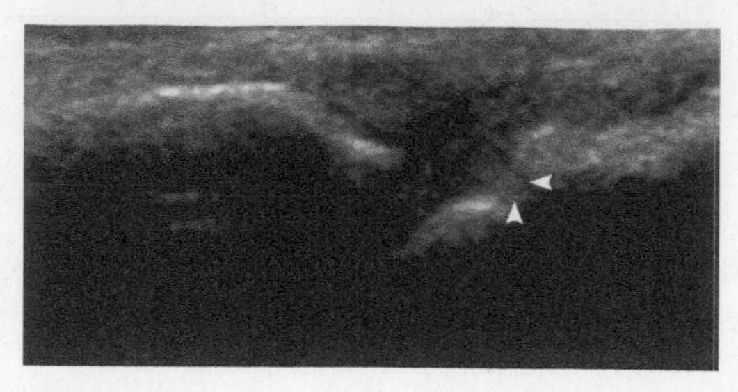

Small erosion is seen.

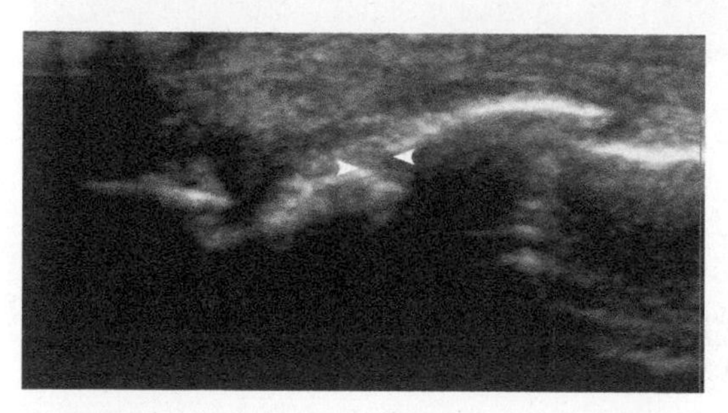

Small erosion is seen.

Answers

1. The ultrasound images show echogenic pannus in the MCP joint spaces with mildly increased vascularity. Minimal joint effusion and small erosions are seen. The increased vascularity is usually more intense, but this patient had been on Disease-Modifying antirheumatic Drugs.

2. Ultrasound is sensitive but nonspecific, so any inflammatory arthritis, including RA, gout, CPPD, and septic arthritis, would be included. The multiplicity of joints in this case excludes septic arthritis. Osteoarthritis would be expected to show osteophytes, but they are not demonstrated here.

3. Ultrasound will show changes in effusion, erosions, pannus size, and vascularity, and is an effective way of monitoring response to treatment.

4. A high-frequency probe (12 to 18 MHz), with power Doppler is used. A volar approach has been said to be superior to dorsal imaging.

5. Both MRI and quantitative power Doppler ultrasonography are effective in measuring the response of rheumatoid arthritis to therapy and to assess disease activity.

Pearls

- Ultrasound is useful in the early detection of changes of RA. It is sensitive, but not specific.
- High-frequency (12 to 18 MHz) imaging with a volar and dorsal approach in the hands is standard. The volar approach may be superior.
- Ultrasound can be used to follow the response to treatment.
- Synovial hypertrophy or pannus is echogenic, with increased vascularity on Doppler.
- The vascularity is dependent on disease activity and also on treatment.
- Joint effusion is hypoechoic or anechoic.
- Rheumatoid nodules can be seen as fluid filled cavities with round borders.
- Erosions are identified as irregularities in the echogenic cortex.

Suggested Readings

Lopez-Ben RR. Assessing rheumatoid arthritis with ultrasound of the hands. *AJR Am J Roentgenol.* 2011;197(3):W422.

Platzgummer H, Schueller-Weidekamm C. Radiological imaging in early diagnosis of rheumatoid arthritis: the role of ultrasound and magnetic resonance imaging [in German]. *Radiologe.* 2012;52(2):124-131.

History of chronic disease and pain in the bilateral shoulders

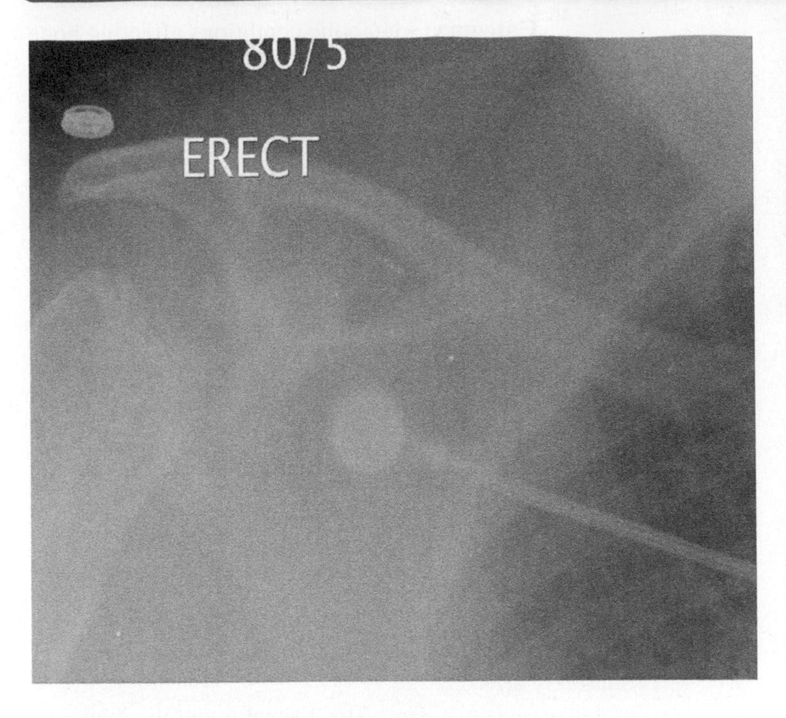

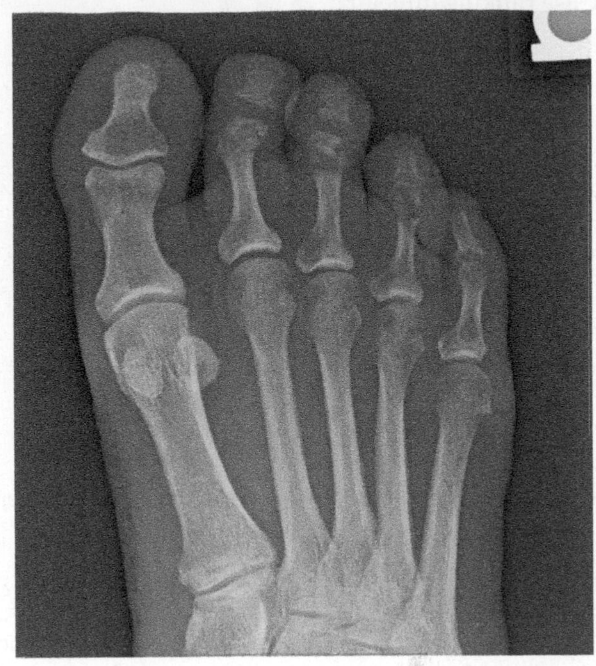

1. What are the radiograph findings?
2. What other entities are included in the differential diagnosis?
3. What is the most likely diagnosis?
4. What is the pathophysiology of this condition?
5. Which joints are typically affected in this condition?

Multicentric reticulohistiocytosis 1459

Case ranking/difficulty: 🐢🐢🐢

Category: Metabolic conditions affecting bone

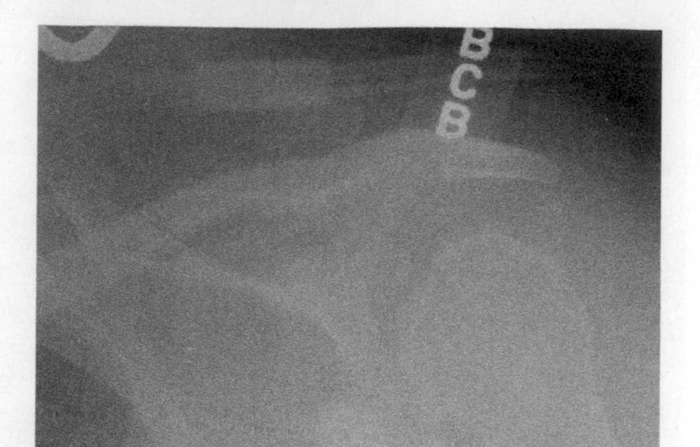

Joint space widening, erosions and cystic change. Changes are bilateral.

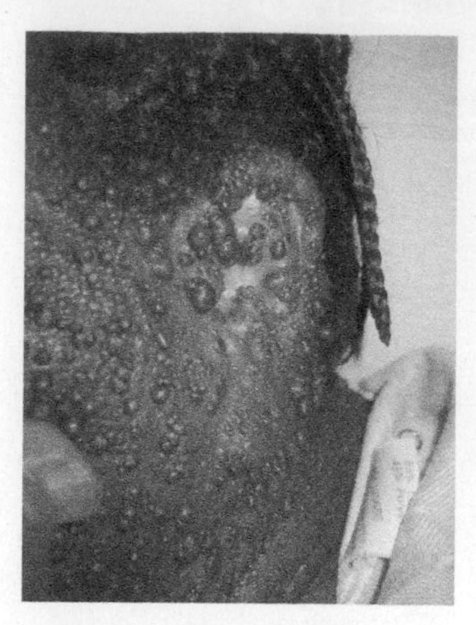

Multiple raised skin lesions.

Answers

1. Joint space widening, erosions, cystic change, and no periosteal reaction.
2. Gout, rheumatoid arthritis, psoriatic arthritis, neuropathic shoulder, sarcoid, and multicentric reticulohistiocytosis.
3. Given the presence of raised nodular skin lesions and a destructive arthritis with no periosteal reaction or sclerosis, the most likely diagnosis is multicentric reticulohistiocytosis.
4. Multicentric reticulohistiocytosis is characterized by the deposition of multinucleated giant cells in the skin, joints, and bones.
5. The PIP and DIP joints of the hands are most commonly involved, although any joint may be affected.

Pearls

- Multicentric reticulohistiocytosis (MRH) is a rare condition resulting in deposition of histiocytic multinucleated giant cells in the joints and skin. There is an association with tumors.
- The hands, especially the PIP and DIP joints, are most commonly affected.
- Joint disease is manifested by normal mineralization or mild osteopenia, with initially preserved or widened joint spaces due to intra-articular deposition of lipid laden histiocytes.
- Cysts and erosions are present. There is no periosteal reaction or bone sclerosis.
- Skin lesions are nontender nodules that are often raised, particularly around the PIP and DIP joints of the hands and especially the nail beds. However, deposition can occur anywhere, including the mucosa.

Suggested Readings

Scutellari PN, Orzincolo C, Trotta F. Case report 375: Multicentric reticulohistiocytosis. *Skeletal Radiol.* 1986;15(5):394-397.

Yap FB. Multicentric reticulohistiocytosis in a Malaysian Chinese lady: a case report and review of literature. *Dermatol Online J.* 2009;15(1):2.

Chronic neck pain with a history of mild dysphagia

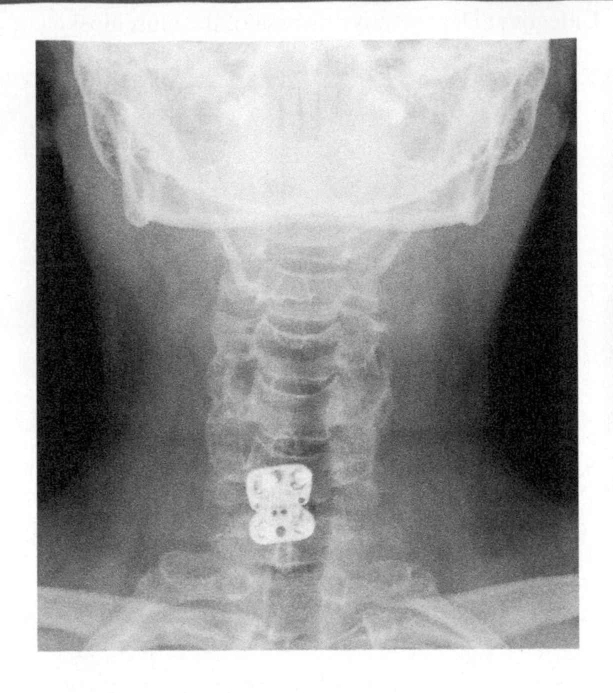

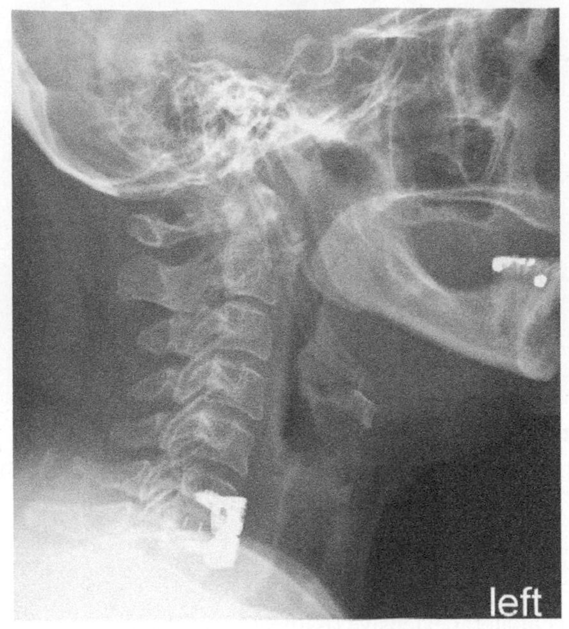

1. What are the radiograph findings?

2. What is the likely diagnosis?

3. How do these patients typically present?

4. What are some of the predisposing factors for this condition?

5. What is the treatment?

Eagle syndrome 1374

Case ranking/difficulty: 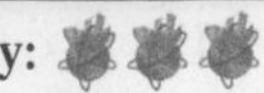 **Category:** Degenerative disease of the musculoskeletal system

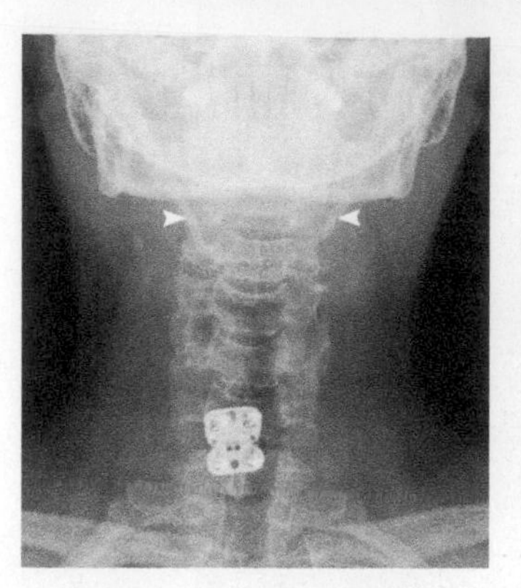

Extensive stylohyoid ligament ossification is seen.

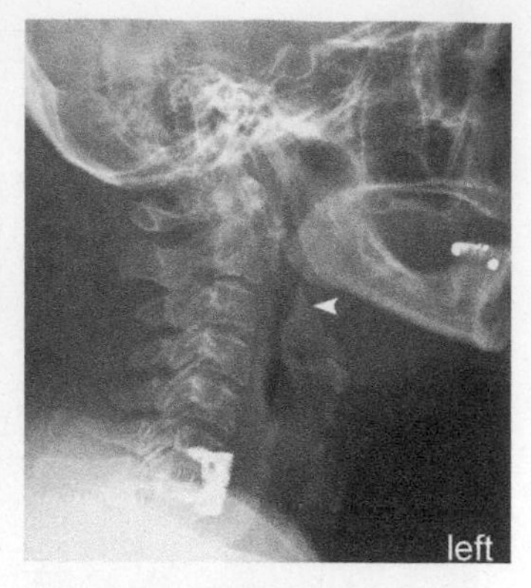

Extensive stylohyoid ligament ossification is well demonstrated on the lateral radiograph.

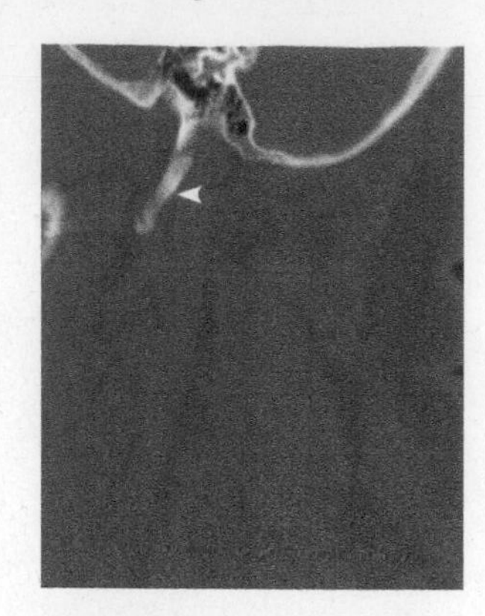

Extensive stylohyoid ligament calcification is well seen on the sagittal reformatted CT image.

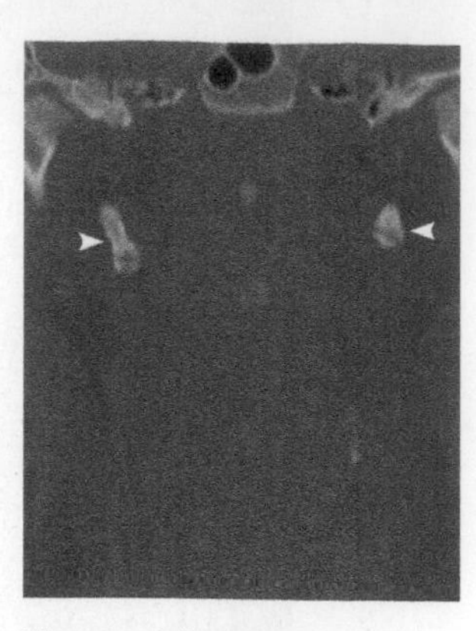

The partially interrupted stylohyoid ligament ossification is seen.

Answers

1. There is bilateral extensive ossification of the stylohyoid ligaments.
2. There is bilateral extensive stylohyoid ligament ossification consistent with Eagle syndrome.
3. Many patients with prominent styloid processes and/or stylohyoid ligament ossification are asymptomatic.

   Presenting symptoms include dysphagia, throat discomfort, symptoms related to carotid artery compression, and a foreign-body sensation.
4. Diffuse idiopathic skeletal hyperostosis (DISH) is an association. Previous tonsillectomy and trauma have been implicated as predisposing events. Patients with altered vitamin D metabolism in end-stage renal disease may also be predisposed.
5. In asymptomatic calcification/ossification, no treatment is required. In symptomatic patients, the initial management is analgesia with or without steroid injection. In refractory cases, surgical shortening or resection of the styloid process or stylohyoid ligament is performed.

Pearls

- Eagle syndrome is characterized by an elongated unilateral or bilateral styloid processes or stylohyoid ligament ossification greater than 3 cm.
- Etiology is unknown, but prior tonsillectomy and DISH have been described as associations. Trauma has also been implicated.
- Patients can often be asymptomatic, but throat discomfort and dysphagia may be presenting features.
- Compression of the carotid arteries may occur.
- Treatment is usually conservative with analgesia and/or steroid injections. In refractory cases, surgical shortening of the styloid process or ossified ligament, or removal, may be indicated.

Suggested Readings

Lorman JG, Biggs JR. The Eagle syndrome. *AJR Am J Roentgenol.* 1983;140(5):881-882.

Murtagh RD, Caracciolo JT, Fernandez G. CT findings associated with Eagle syndrome. *AJNR Am J Neuroradiol.* 2001;22(7):1401-1402.

History of long-term osteoporosis therapy, and now presents with a femoral fracture after minor trauma

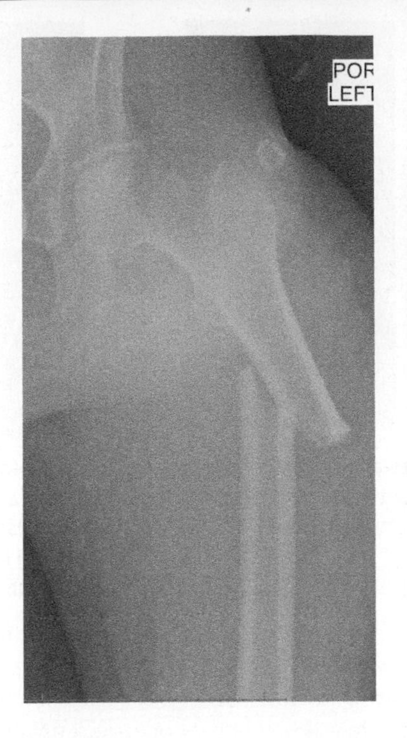

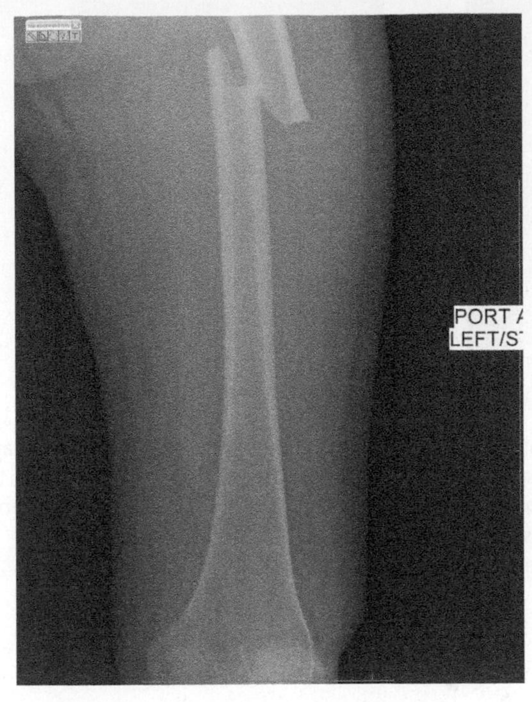

1. What are the pertinent radiographic findings?

2. What is the most likely etiology for this lesion?

3. How often is the lesion bilateral?

4. What is the incidence of this type of fracture?

5. What is the appropriate management for early stage disease?

Bisphosphonate-related femoral fracture 1341

Case ranking/difficulty: 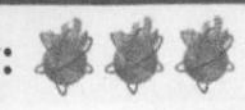 **Category:** Metabolic conditions affecting bone

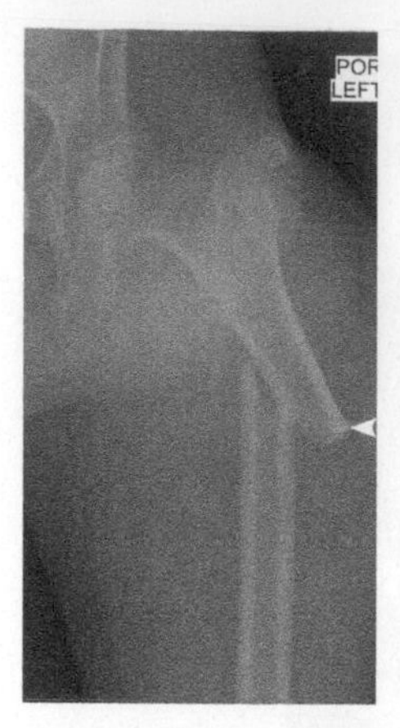

There is lateral cortical thickening (*arrowhead*) with a displaced angulated subtrochanteric fracture. The medial aspect of the fracture line is oblique.

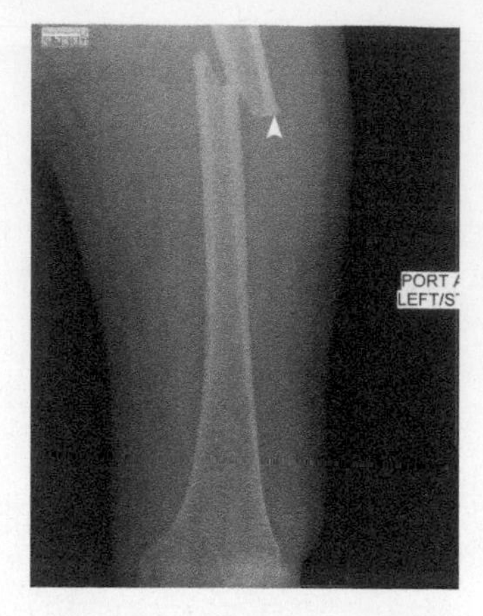

Lateral cortical thickening is noted.

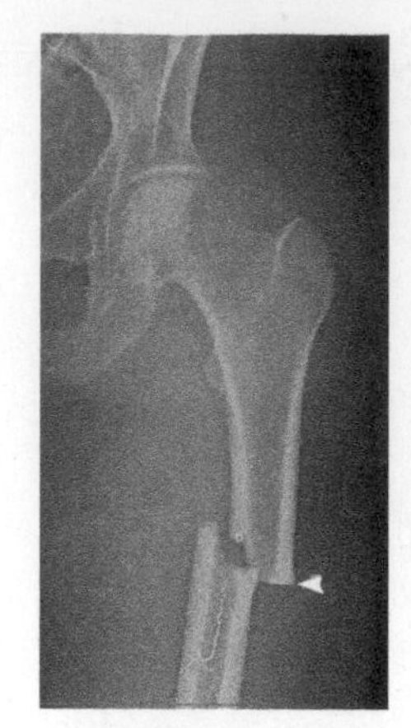

Lateral cortical thickening is better appreciated posttraction.

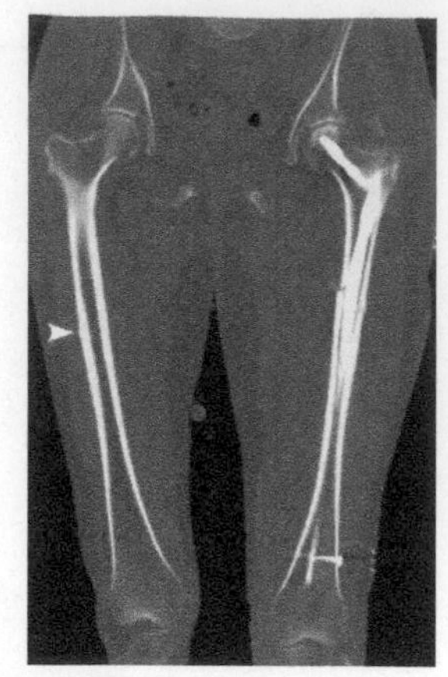

Coronal reformatted image postsurgical fixation of the left fracture, also shows mild cortical thickening in the subtrochanteric right femur, indicating bilateral disease.

Answers

1. There is a transverse displaced angulated subtrochanteric fracture. There is mild lateral cortical thickening which is typical in bisphosphonate related femoral insufficiency fractures.
2. A displaced subtrochanteric fracture in an older patient should raise the suspicion for bisphosphonate-related femoral fracture. Although the early stages of bisphosphonate-related insufficiency fractures can look like stress fractures or osteomalacia, the presence of a complete subtrochanteric fracture in a patient on long-term bisphosphonates is diagnostic.
3. Bisphosphonate fractures are bilateral in 53% of patients.
4. The incidence for bisphosphonate-related femoral fractures is 1 in 1000 annually.
5. Withdrawal of bisphosphonates alone has not proven effective in preventing the progression of early stage bisphosphonate-related insufficiency fractures to complete fractures. Prophylactic intramedullary rodding is indicated.

Pearls

- Long-term bisphosphonate therapy may result in an insufficiency-type femoral fracture in the lateral cortex that often progresses to a complete fracture.
- The fractures are subtrochanteric in location. A subtrochanteric fracture is an atypical location for femoral fractures in older patients, and should raise the concern for a pathological fracture.
- The fracture orientation is transverse or short oblique.
- Fractures may be bilateral in up to 53% of patients.
- Operative treatment is required, even in early incomplete fractures, as there is a propensity to progress to complete fractures with conservative treatment.

Suggested Readings

Banffy MB, Vrahas MS, Ready JE, Abraham JA. Nonoperative versus prophylactic treatment of bisphosphonate-associated femoral stress fractures. *Clin Orthop Relat Res*. 2011;469(7):2028-2034.

Porrino JA, Kohl CA, Taljanovic M, Rogers LF. Diagnosis of proximal femoral insufficiency fractures in patients receiving bisphosphonate therapy. *AJR Am J Roentgenol.* 2010;194(4):1061-1064.

Rogers LF, Taljanovic M. FDA statement on relationship between bisphosphonate use and atypical subtrochanteric and femoral shaft fractures: a considered opinion. *AJR Am J Roentgenol.* 2010;195(3):563-566.

History of chronic neck pain, with acute progressive quadriplegia

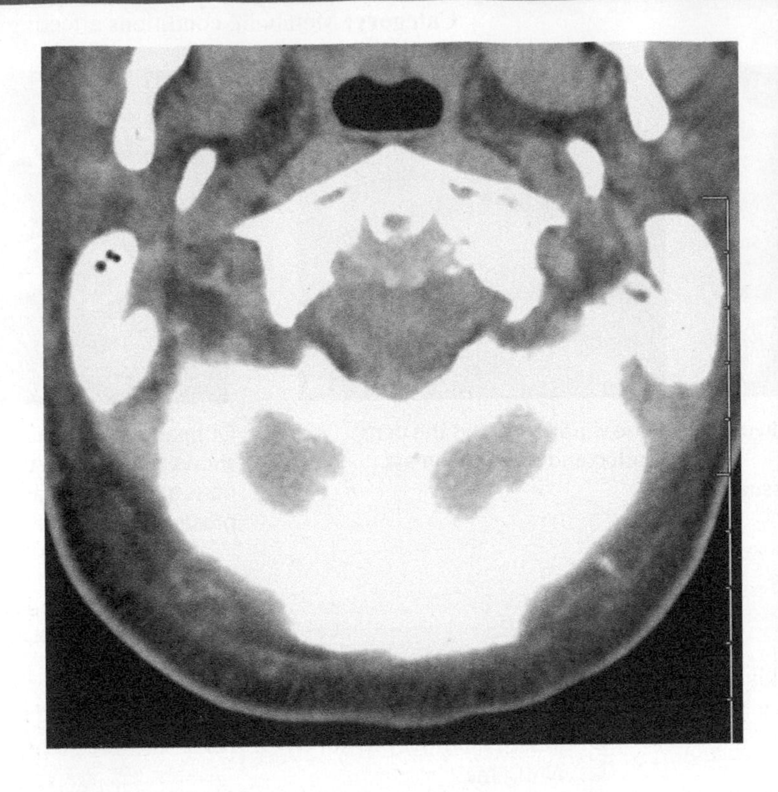

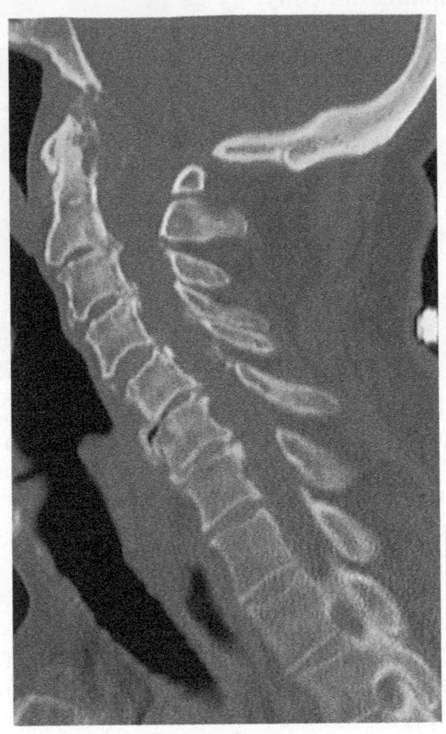

1. This entity typically occurs in which patient population?

2. What are the typical presenting symptoms?

3. In which part of the neck would calcification be considered an uncommon radiological feature in this condition?

4. What is the main predisposing factor for this entity?

5. What is included in the differential diagnosis?

CPPD crowned dens syndrome 1319

Case ranking/difficulty: 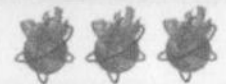

Category: Metabolic conditions affecting bone

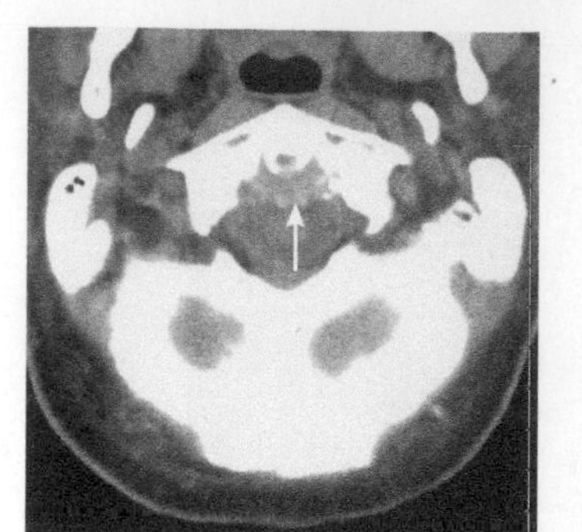

There is a calcified soft-tissue mass posterior to the dens, with erosion of the dens.

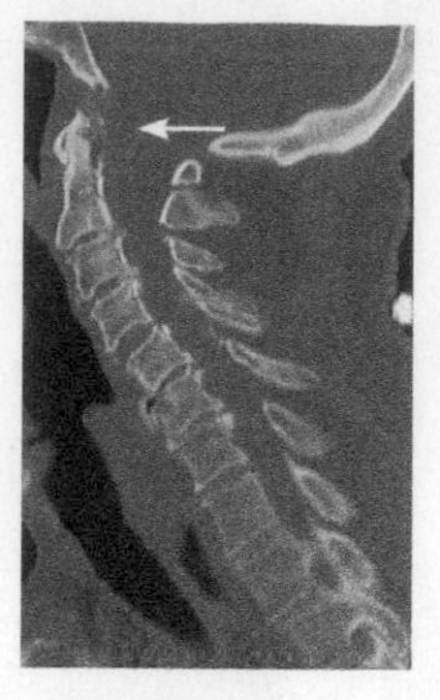

The dens and clivus erosion, with a calcified soft-tissue mass, is better delineated.

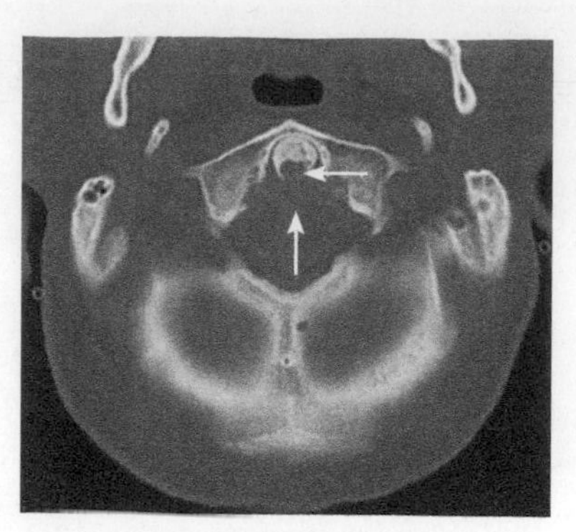

Bone windows shows the dens erosion and soft-tissue mass.

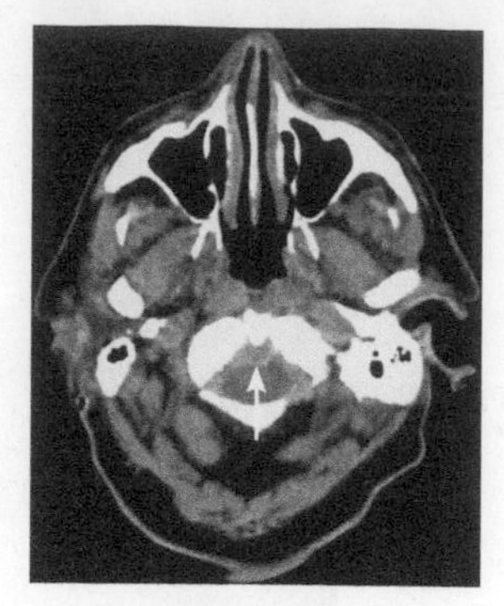

CT head scan 6 years prior shows that the soft-tissue mass at the dens was present, but smaller.

Answers

1. CPPD crowned dens syndrome has a reported higher incidence in older females and in patients with a history of CPPD.
2. The typical presentation is chronic neck pain that is progressive. Rarely, there is mass effect with cord compression and quadriplegia. Acute on chronic neck pain does occur.
3. Calcification in the longus coli muscle is more typical for calcium hydroxyapatite deposition disease, rather than CPPD. Vertebral artery calcification is not associated with CPPD.
4. A history of CPPD would strongly support the diagnosis of CPPD crowned dens syndrome.
5. A calcified extradural mass would raise the concern for a meningioma. HADD (hydroxyapatite deposition disease) is in the differential, but calcifications may be seen in the longus coli muscle in HADD. A tuberculous extradural abscess is disc centered.

Pearls

- A calcified soft-tissue mass centered around the dens should raise the possibility of CPPD Crowned dens syndrome.
- This entity occurs in older patients and in patients with a history of CPPD.
- Mass effect on the cord and adjacent osseous structures are uncommon, but does occur.
- CPPD crowned dens may be differentiated from calcium hydroxyapatite deposition by the presence of calcification in the longus coli muscle, which typically occurs in HADD (hydroxyapatite deposition disease) but not CPPD.
- In CPPD crowned dens, calcifications involve the alar and transverse ligaments.
- Unless there is mass effect, treatment is conservative.

Suggested Readings

Ali S, Hoch M, Dadhania V, Khurana JS. CPPD crowned dens syndrome with clivus destruction: a case report. *J Radiol Case Rep.* 2011;5(8):30-37.

Bouvet JP, le Parc JM, Michalski B, Benlahrache C, Auquier L. Acute neck pain due to calcifications surrounding the odontoid process: the crowned dens syndrome. *Arthritis Rheum.* 1985;28(12):1417-1420.

Chronic disease on treatment, with worsening right shoulder pain

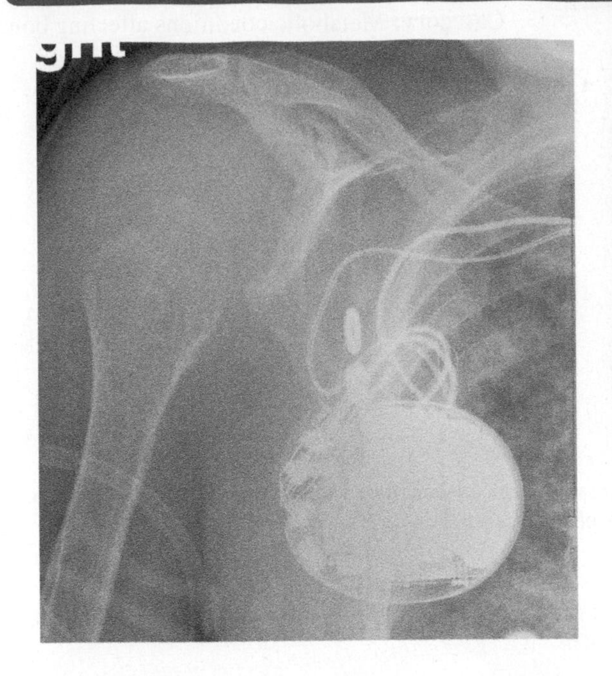

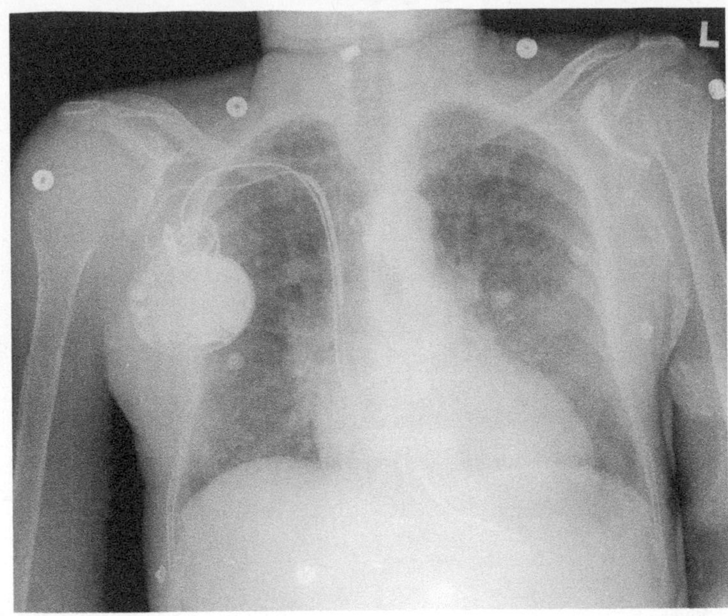

1. What are the findings in the shoulders?

2. What are included in the differential, and what is the most likely diagnosis?

3. What is the next most appropriate study?

4. Where are the common sites affected in this condition?

5. What are the findings to be expected on MRI?

Amyloid arthropathy 1379

Case ranking/difficulty:

Category: Metabolic conditions affecting bone

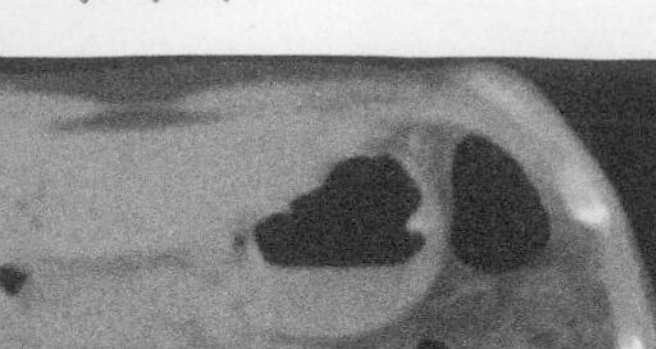

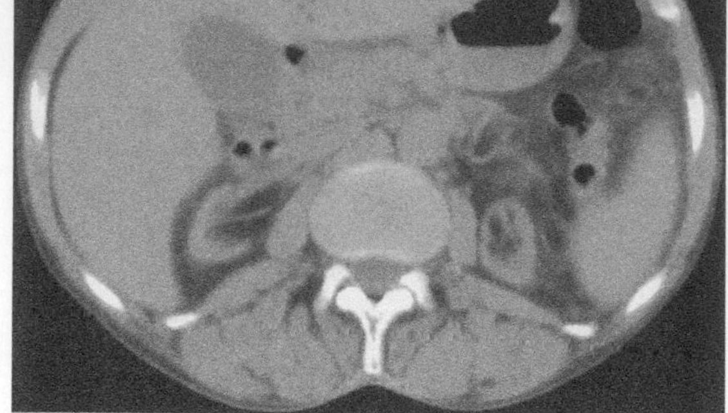

Axial CT image shows marked renal atrophy.

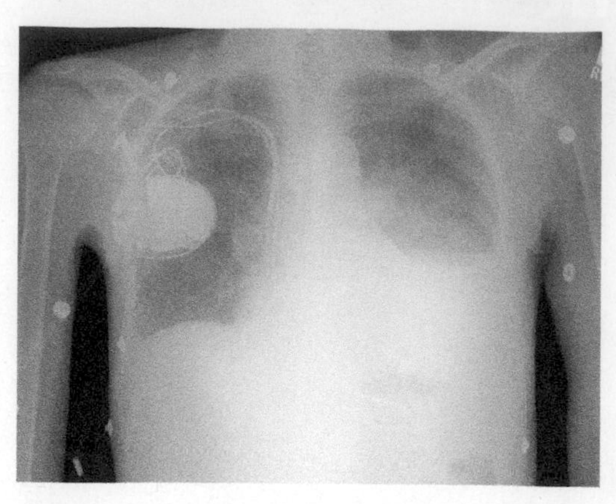

Chest radiograph 4 years prior showed normal shoulders and a large left pleural effusion.

Answers

1. There is joint space widening, cysts, erosions, and subluxation bilaterally, worse in the right shoulder.
2. Septic arthritis, amyloid arthropathy, rheumatoid arthritis, and PVNS are all included in the differential. Based on the history, nonfebrile state, and the bilaterality, the most likely differential is dialysis related amyloid arthropathy.
3. If septic arthritis needs to be excluded clinically, then joint aspiration is the next most appropriate study. If it does not need to be excluded, then MRI.
4. Amyloid spondyloarthropathy occurs predominantly, but not exclusively, in dialysis-related amyloid. The shoulders, spine, wrists, hips, knees, and carpal tunnels are most commonly affected.
5. Amyloid arthropathy is typically isointense to hypointense on all pulse sequences, with no paramagnetic effect as seen in PVNS. Contrast enhancement is variable.

Pearls

- Amyloid arthropathy results from the extracellular deposition of amyloid in the joint spaces and soft tissues.
- In dialysis patients, it is related to the inability of the dialysis membrane to remove amyloid protein.
- Cervical spine and shoulders are most commonly affected.
- Plain films show cysts, erosions and periarticular osteopenia. The joint space is preserved or widened until late in the disease.
- Soft-tissue masses may be seen.
- Amyloid is low signal on all MR sequences with no paramagnetic effect, differentiating it from PVNS. Contrast enhancement is variable.

Suggested Readings

Cobby MJ, Adler RS, Swartz R, Martel W. Dialysis-related amyloid arthropathy: MR findings in four patients. *AJR Am J Roentgenol.* 1991;157(5):1023-1027.

Sheldon PJ, Forrester DM, Learch TJ. Imaging of intra-articular masses. *Radiographics.* 2005;25(1):105-119.

Pain in the medial foot with a positive tinel sign; history of running and playing basketball

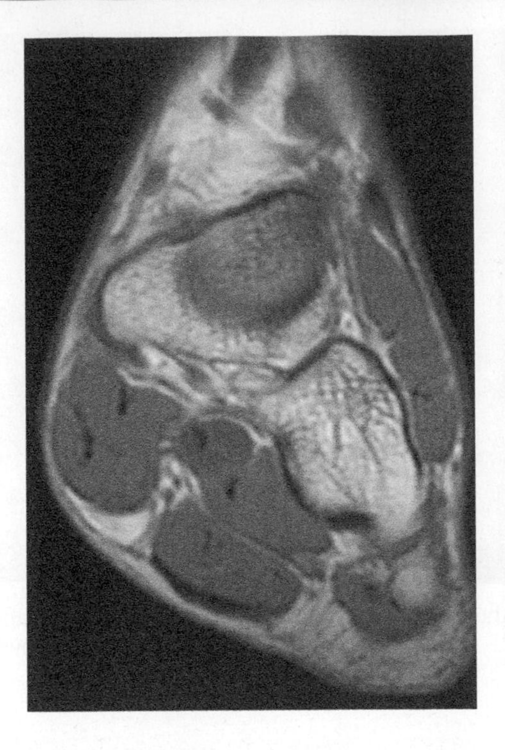

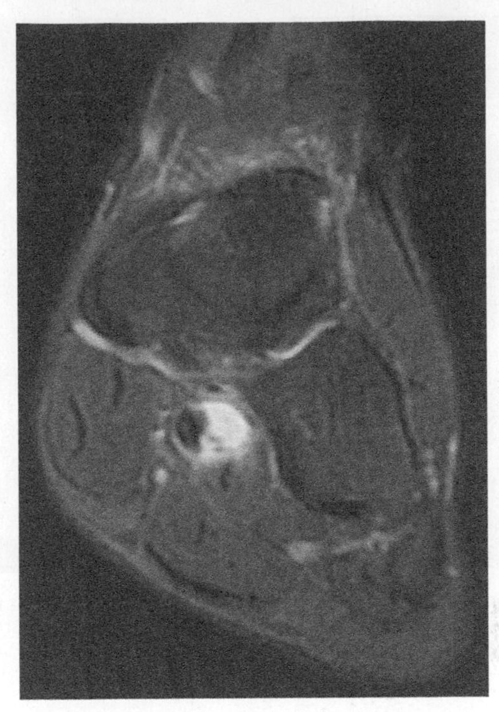

1. What are the MRI findings?

2. What additional MRI findings might you see?

3. Which nerve is affected in this condition?

4. More distal entrapment of the affected nerve may result in denervation of which muscles?

5. What factors may predispose patients to develop this condition?

Jogger's foot 1472

Case ranking/difficulty:

Category: Trauma

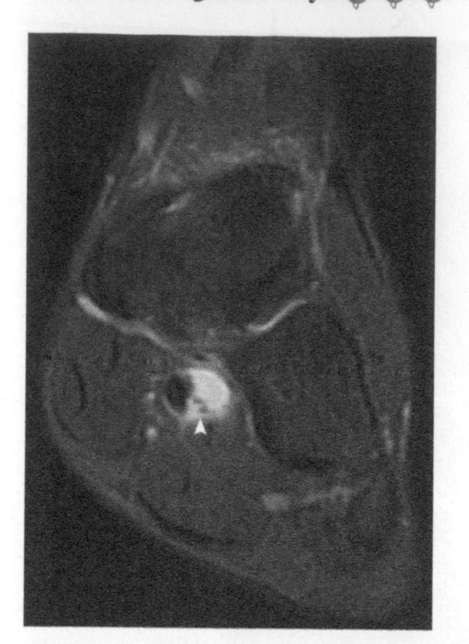

Marked tenosynovitis at the master knot of Henry is seen.

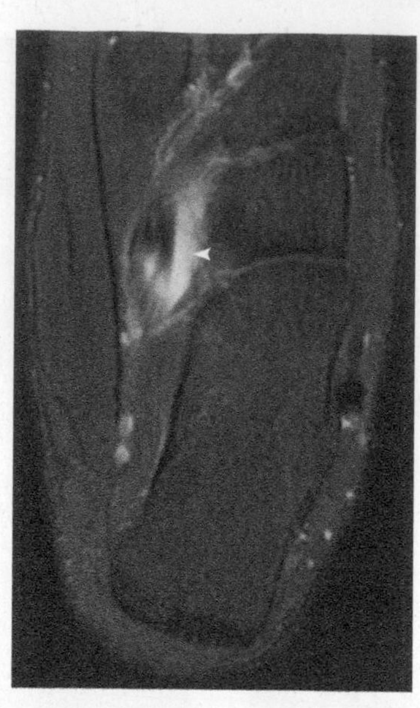

Tenosynovitis at the master knot.

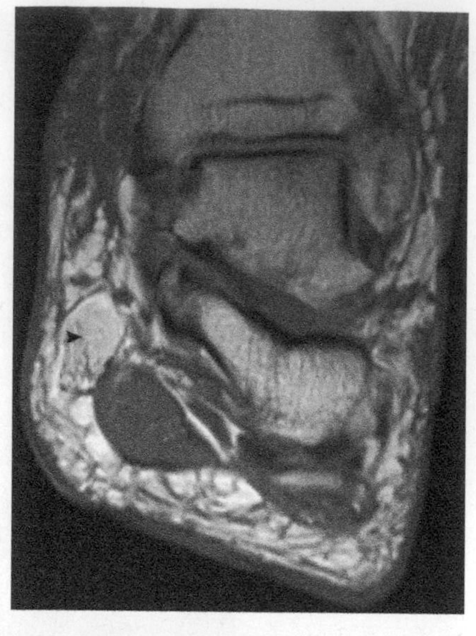

Fatty atrophy of the abductor hallucis in another patient (*arrowhead*).

Answers

1. There is extensive tenosynovitis of the flexor digitorum and flexor hallucis tendons at the master knot of Henry. No denervation changes are seen at this time.
2. Denervation atrophy of the abductor hallucis and flexor digitorum brevis muscles may eventually be seen in a jogger's foot. Pes planus and ganglion cysts may be predisposing factors.
3. Entrapment or irritation of the medial plantar nerve is the cause of a jogger's foot.
4. More distal entrapment of the medial plantar nerve may result in denervation of the flexor digitorum brevis and first lumbrical muscles.
5. Chronic repetitive stresses such as jogging, a ganglion cyst or other mass between the abductor hallucis and flexor digitorum brevis muscles, and pes planus are predisposing factors.

Pearls

- Jogger's foot is a result of irritation or entrapment of the medial plantar nerve.
- Patients present with medial foot pain and numbness.
- The nerve is entrapped at or just distal to the tarsal tunnel, or adjacent to the master knot of Henry.
- Pes planus may exacerbate the nerve compression.
- Chronic repetitive stress such as jogging or other sports results in tenosynovitis at the master knot and compression of the nerve.
- Denervation atrophy may eventually be seen in the abductor hallucis and flexor digitorum brevis muscles.

Suggested Readings

Delfaut EM, Demondion X, Bieganski A, Thiron MC, Mestdagh H, Cotten A. Imaging of foot and ankle nerve entrapment syndromes: from well-demonstrated to unfamiliar sites. *Radiographics*. 2003;23(3):613-623.

Donovan A, Rosenberg ZS, Cavalcanti CF. MR imaging of entrapment neuropathies of the lower extremity. Part 2. The knee, leg, ankle, and foot. *Radiographics*. 2010;30(4):1001-1019.

Chronic shoulder pain

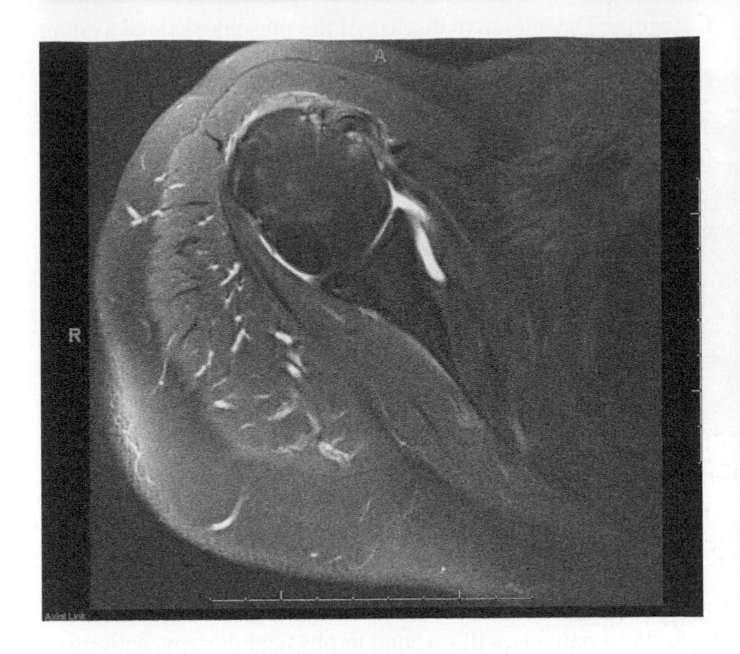

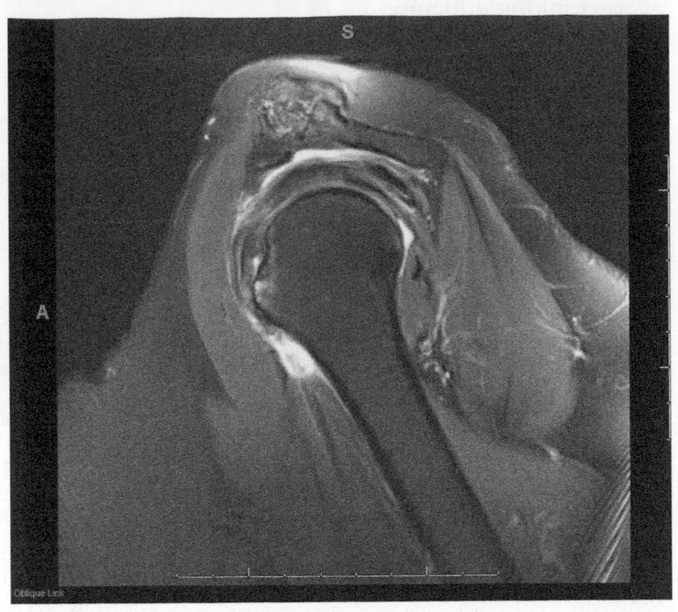

1. What are the pertinent imaging findings?

2. What are the typical radiologic findings in this entity?

3. What are the clinical features and associations of this form of impingement?

4. What is the best MRI protocol for evaluating this condition?

5. What are the treatment options?

Subcoracoid impingement 1351

Case ranking/difficulty: 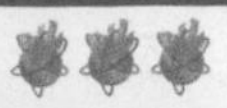

Category: Degenerative disease of the musculoskeletal system

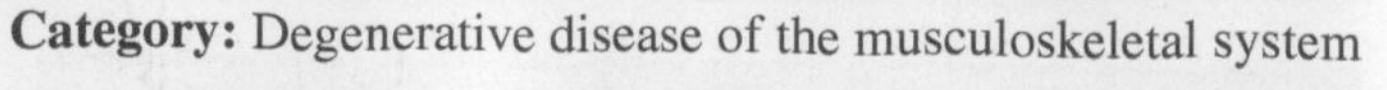

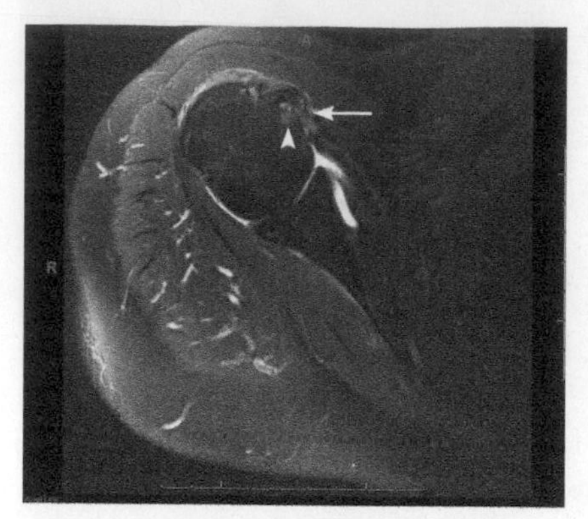

Narrowed subcoracoid distance with edema and cystic change in the lesser tuberosity (*arrowhead*). Subscapularis tendinosis (*arrow*) is seen.

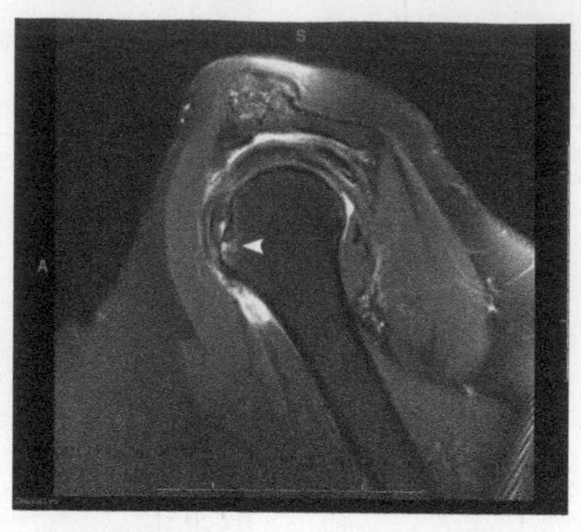

Edema and cystic change in the lesser tuberosity.

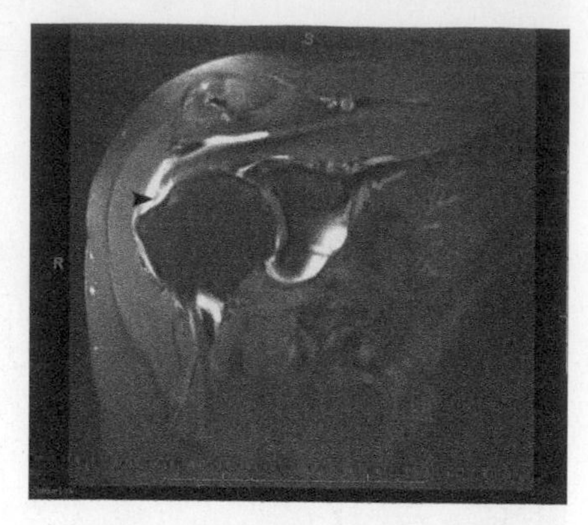

Acromioclavicular joint osteoarthritis with a full-thickness supraspinatus tear (*arrowhead*) are also demonstrated.

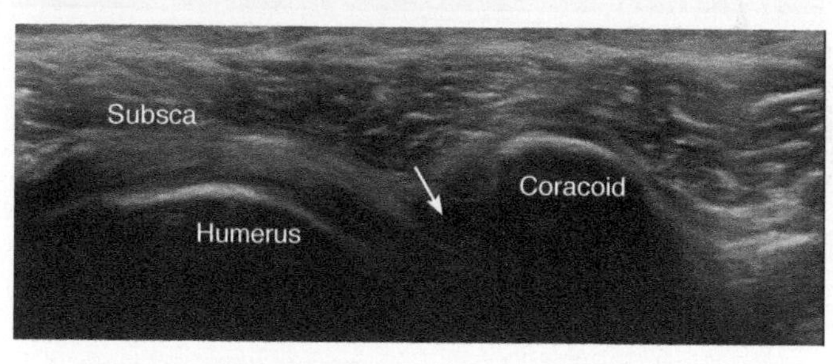

Another patient. Narrowing of the subcoracoid distance, with loss of the echogenic fibrillary pattern of the subscapularis tendon indicating tendinosis. The *arrow* shows a subcoracoid bursitis.

Answers

1. The coracohumeral distance is normally 8.4 to 11 mm; in this case it is 3 mm. There is associated edema and cystic change in the lesser tuberosity, and the subscapularis appears deformed and tendinotic, with a small tear.

2. Subcoracoid impingement occurs when there is a narrowed subcoracoid distance, typically less than 5.5 mm. There is often edema and cystic change in the lesser tuberosity, and tendinosis or tearing of the subscapularis.

   An association with a chevron(^)-shaped outlet has been described.

3. Subcoracoid impingement is often symptomatic with anterior shoulder pain, and greatest in internal rotation. Subacromial impingement is much more common, and that results in supraspinatus tears.

4. An axial fat-suppressed fast spin-echo T2-weighted sequence is the sequence of choice. An MRI arthrogram is not indicated.

5. Most patients will respond to physical therapy, activity modification and NSAIDs. Surgery is rarely indicated, but an open or arthroscopic coracoplasty can be performed in refractory cases.

Pearls

- A narrowed subcoracoid distance on ultrasound or MRI supports the clinical diagnosis of subcoracoid impingement.
- Ultrasound has the advantage of showing dynamic impingement, not just morphological detail.
- MRI shows a narrowed coracohumeral distance. Normal is 8.4 to 11 mm.
- A chevron (^) supraspinatus outlet is associated with subcoracoid impingement.
- Associated edema and cystic change in the lesser tuberosity and anterior humerus is often seen.
- Subscapularis tendinosis or tears may occur.

Suggested Readings

Giaroli EL, Major NM, Lemley DE, Lee J. Coracohumeral interval imaging in subcoracoid impingement syndrome on MRI. *AJR Am J Roentgenol.* 2006;186(1):242-246.

Okoro T, Reddy VR, Pimpelnarkar A. Coracoid impingement syndrome: a literature review. *Curr Rev Musculoskelet Med.* 2009;2(1):51-55.

History of trauma, presenting to the ER for abdominal pain and abdominal CT

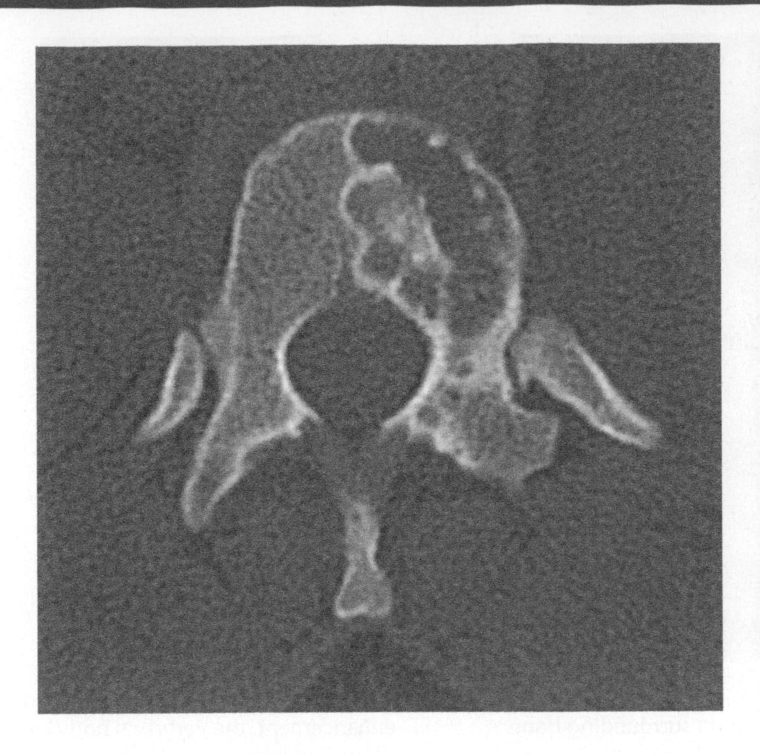

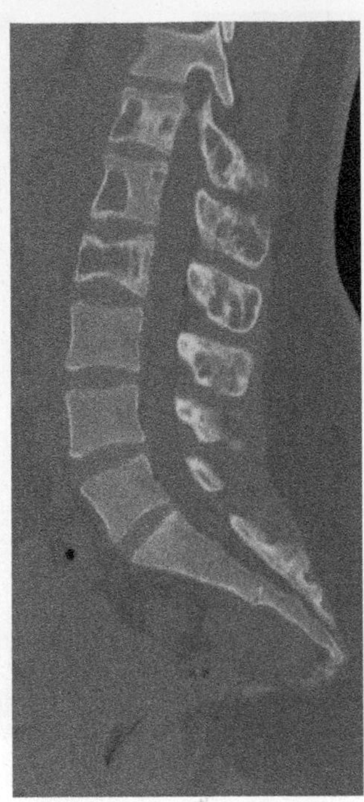

1. What are the relevant CT findings?

2. How would you expect these lesions to appear on MRI?

3. What is the differential diagnoses?

4. Based on the stated history and imaging features, what is the most likely diagnosis?

5. What condition is considered a part of the spectrum of this entity?

Lymphangiomatosis 1420

Case ranking/difficulty: 

Category: Developmental abnormalities of the musculoskeletal system

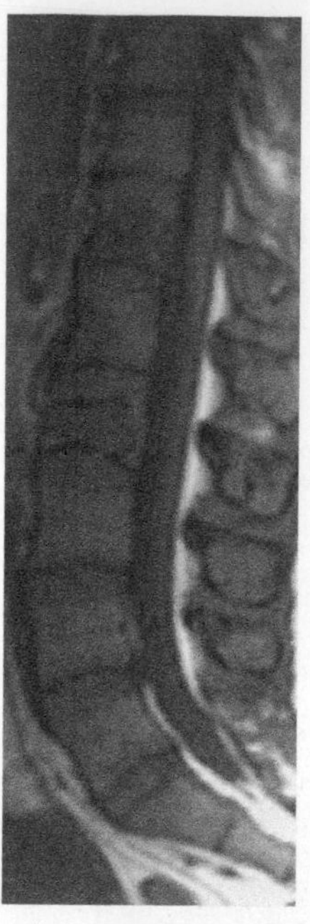

Lesions are mildly T1 hypointense centrally.

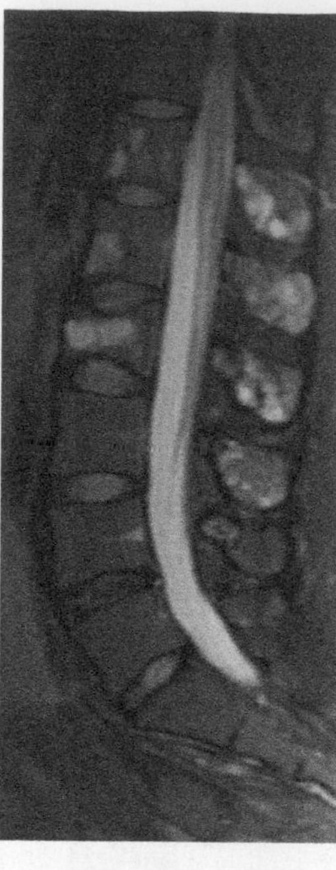

Lesions are T2 hyperintense. There is no surrounding bone marrow edema.

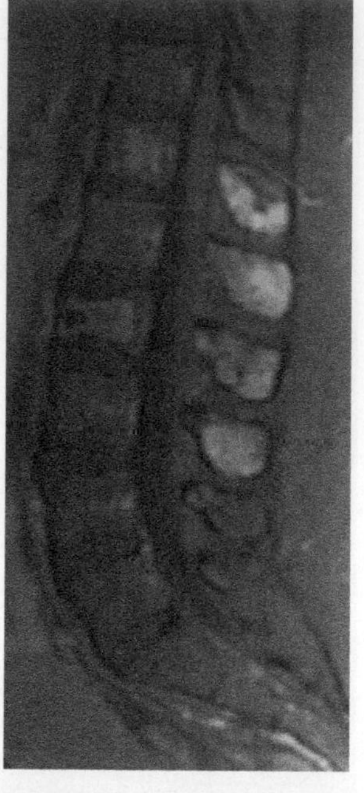

Posterior element lesions show diffuse enhancement, the vertebral body lesions show mainly peripheral enhancement.

Answers

1. Multiple vertebral lucent lesions involving the bodies and posterior elements, with mild expansion and no matrix. L3 is anteriorly wedged.
2. The lesions are cystic with no perilesional edema in uncomplicated cases. Edema may be seen after a pathological fracture.
3. Although metastasis and myeloma are quoted as differentials for this entity, the sclerotic rims and lack of soft-tissue components would make those unlikely differentials.
4. The most likely diagnosis is lymphangiomatosis.
5. Lymphangiomatosis and Gorham disease are considered as a spectrum of disease, rather than separate entities.

Pearls

- Lymphangiomatosis is part of the spectrum of "angiomatous" disorders that includes lymphangiomas, hemangiomas, and hybrids of the two.
- The pelvis, spine, skull, and long bones are commonly affected.
- Lesions may be solitary or multiple.
- Lesions are osteolytic, with a variable sclerotic rim and variable expansion. Cortical expansion may be marked and the cortex may appear destroyed.
- Some consider lymphangiomatosis and Gorham disease as part of a spectrum.
- MRI shows the cystic nature of the lesions.

Suggested Readings

Ozturk A, Yousem DM. Magnetic resonance imaging findings in diffuse lymphangiomatosis: neuroradiological manifestations. *Acta Radiol.* 2007;48(5):560-564.

Wong CS, Chu TY. Clinical and radiological features of generalised lymphangiomatosis. *Hong Kong Med J.* 2008;14(5):402-404.

Swelling of the great toe

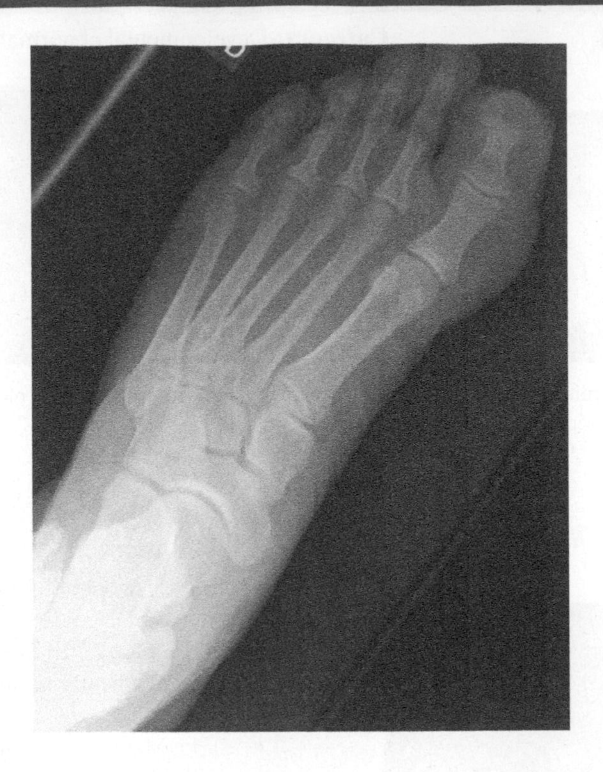

1. What are the radiograph findings?

2. What is the predominant component of the soft-tissue swelling?

3. What would be the next most appropriate study, and what might you expect to see?

4. What are included in the differential, and what is the most likely diagnosis?

5. What are some of the associations in this condition?

Macrodystrophia lipomatosa 1457

Case ranking/difficulty: 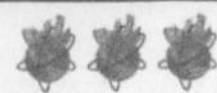 **Category:** Developmental abnormalities of the musculoskeletal system

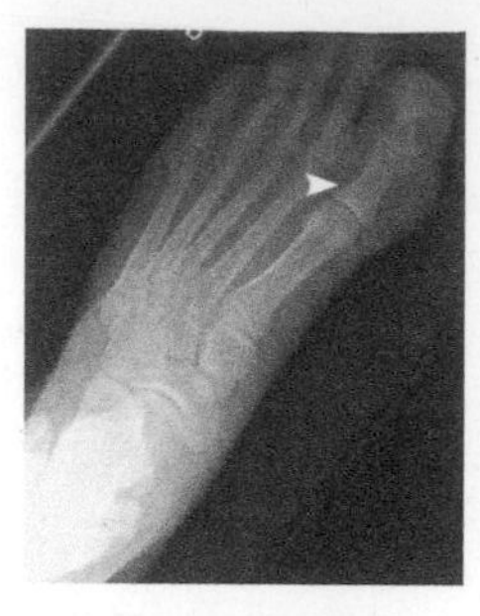

Soft-tissue swelling is seen in the great toe, with a fatty component. Mild periosteal reaction is seen (*arrowhead*).

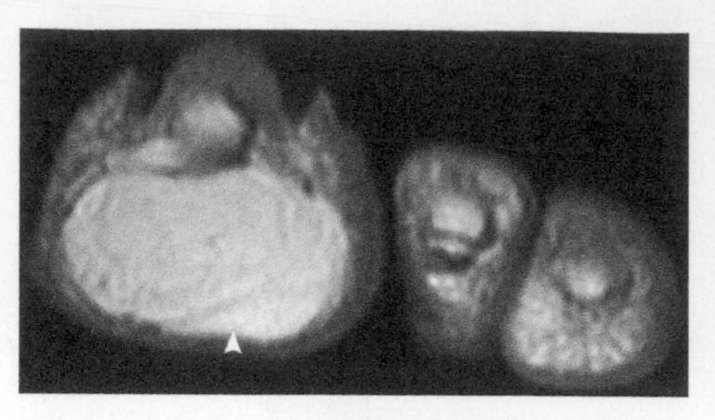

A large, predominantly fatty mass is seen in the plantar aspect of the great toe.

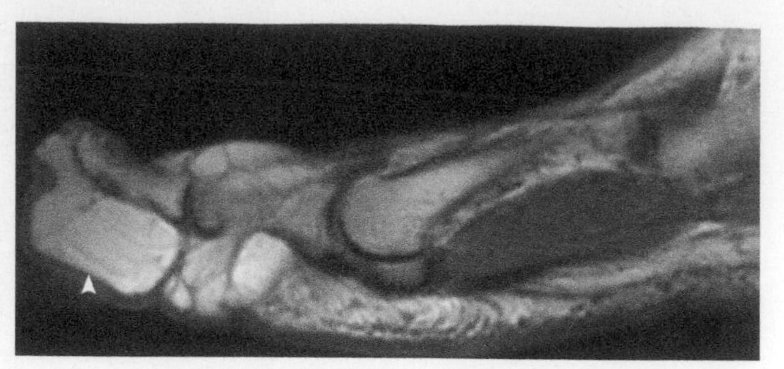

The fatty mass causes elevation of the digit.

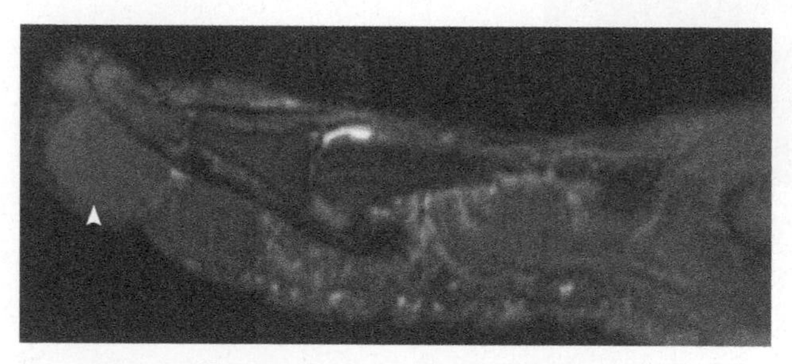

The mass completely saturates on fat-suppressed FSE T2-weighted images.

Answers

1. Extensive soft-tissue swelling of the first digit and mild periosteal reaction at the base of the first proximal phalanx.
2. The soft-tissue swelling is mainly fat.
3. MRI. Extensive fatty proliferation on the plantar aspect of the great toe would be expected. Periosteal new bone, enlarged tendons, cortical thickening, and fibrolipomatous hamartoma of the plantar nerve may be seen.
4. Neurofibromatosis, hemangiomatosis, lymphangiomatosis. The most likely diagnosis is macrodystrophia lipomatosa.
5. Fibrolipomatous hamartoma of the plantar or median nerves can be seen in macrodystrophia lipomatosa. Osseous and tendinous overgrowth may occur.

Pearls

- Macrodystrophia lipomatosa is a rare congenital nonhereditary disorder, characterized by the proliferation of all mesenchymal elements in the digit.
- Lesions typically are in the distribution of the plantar and median nerves.
- Marked fatty proliferation occurs with associated proliferation of periosteum and bone.
- The fatty lesion is usually in the plantar/palmar aspect of the digit and at the end.
- MRI shows a predominantly fatty lesion with minor fibrous elements that is unencapsulated but well defined, and with possible associated proliferation of the osseous and periosteal structures.

Suggested Readings

Chiang CL, Tsai MY, Chen CK. MRI diagnosis of fibrolipomatous hamartoma of the median nerve and associated macrodystrophia lipomatosa. *J Chin Med Assoc*. 2010;73(9):499-502.

Upadhyay D, Parashari UC, Khanduri S, Bhadury S. Macrodystrophia lipomatosa: radiologic-pathologic correlation. *J Clin Imaging Sci*. 2011;1(1):18.

Enlarging mass in dorsal soft tissues of the index finger

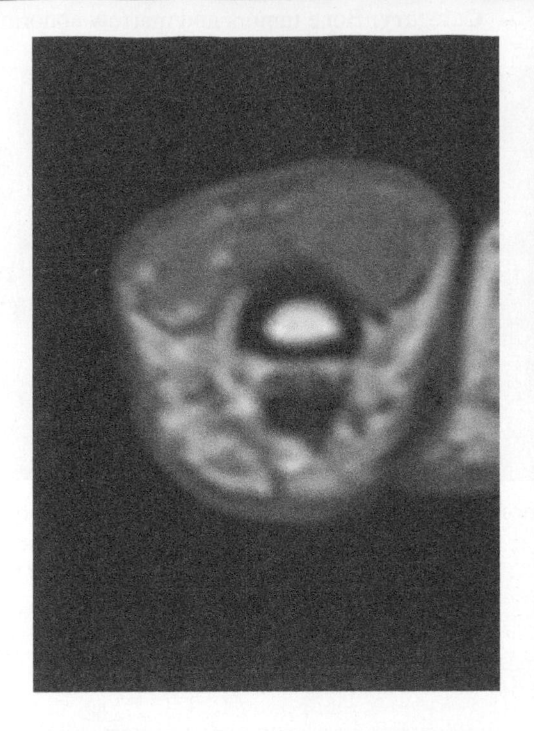

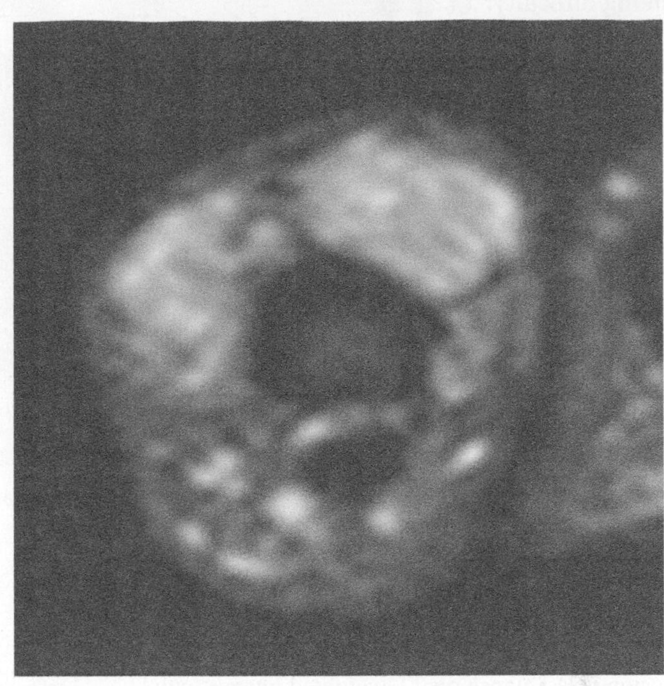

1. What are the signal characteristics shown in this lesion?

2. Based on signal characteristics, what are the most likely differential diagnoses?

3. What is the most common location for this lesion?

4. What is the recurrence and metastatic risk of this lesion?

5. What is the initial treatment?

Parachordoma 1316

Case ranking/difficulty: 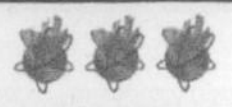

Category: Bone tumors and marrow abnormalities

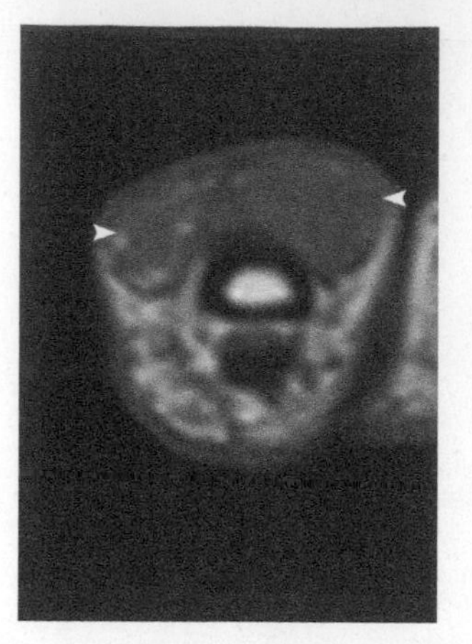

There is a well-defined soft-tissue lesion with peripheral interdigitated fat, surrounding the extensor digitorum tendon.

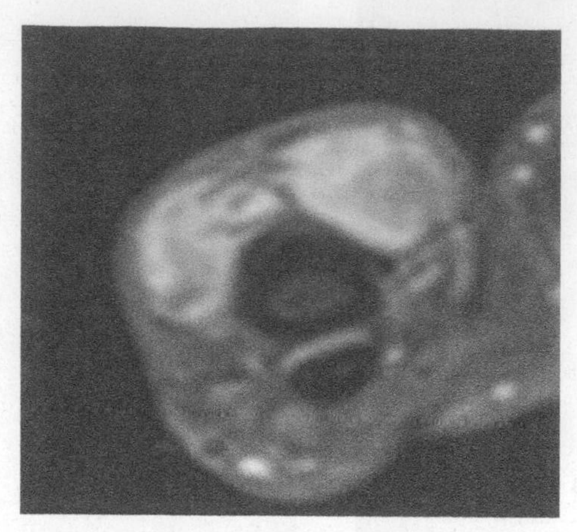

Mild heterogenous enhancement.

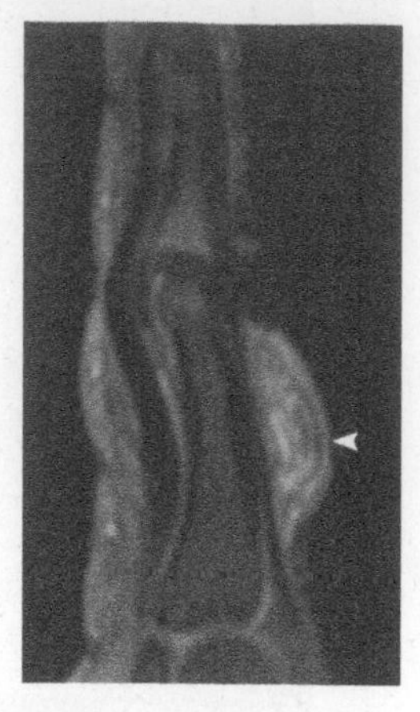

Well-defined mildly enhancing soft-tissue lesion intimately related to the extensor tendon.

Answers

1. This lesion is isointense on T1-weighted images with peripheral interdigitated fat, foci of increased T2 signal, and mild peripheral contrast enhancement.
2. The peripheral areas of fat could suggest a hemangioma, but the lack of significant contrast enhancement makes this less likely. Parachordomas are extremely rare, and have variable signal characteristics as in this lesion.
3. The most common location for parachordomas is in the extremities.
4. Parachordomas typically have an indolent course with slow growth, but late recurrence and metastasis do infrequently occur.
5. Initial treatment is by wide local excision.

Pearls

- Parachordomas are rare soft-tissue tumors, often occurring in the soft tissues of the digits.
- The extremities are most often affected, most often the lower extremities.
- There is a slight male predilection, most often in the fourth decade of life.
- Parachordomas were initially thought to be the soft-tissue equivalent of skeletal chordomas, but are now thought to be a distinct entity.
- Imaging characteristics are nonspecific, but are typically T2 hyperintense with variable contrast enhancement.
- Most demonstrate an indolent course, but late recurrence and metastasis have been reported.
- Treatment is by wide excision biopsy.

Suggested Readings

Ali S, Leng B, Reinus WR, Khilko N, Khurana JS. Parachordoma/myoepithelioma. *Skeletal Radiol.* 2013; 42(3):431, 457-458.

Clabeaux J, Hojnowski L, Valente A, Damron TA. Case report: parachordoma of soft tissues of the arm. *Clin Orthop Relat Res.* 2008;466(5):1251-1256.

De Comas AM, Deavers MT, Raymond AK, Madewell JE, Lewis VO. Intraneural parachordoma of the arm with regional metastases. *Skeletal Radiol.* 2011;40(7):943-946.

Swelling in the arm

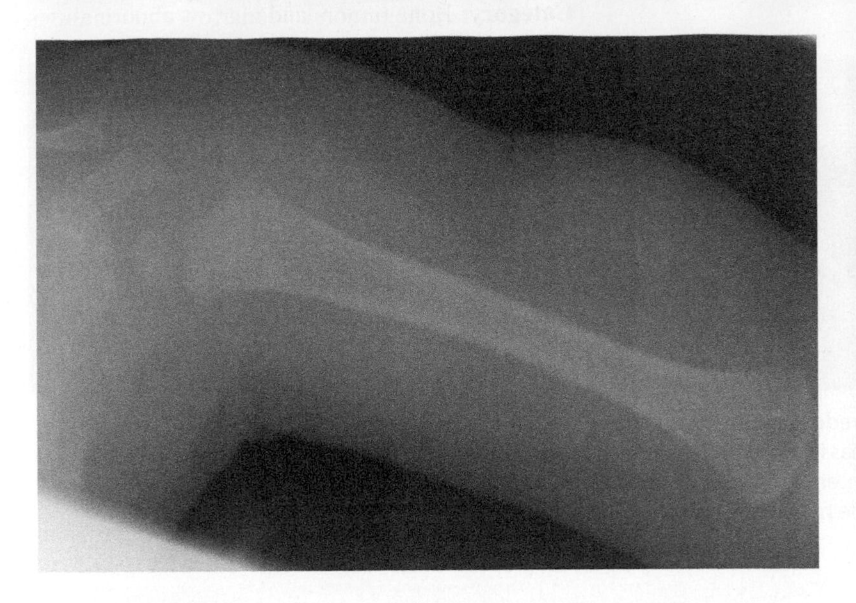

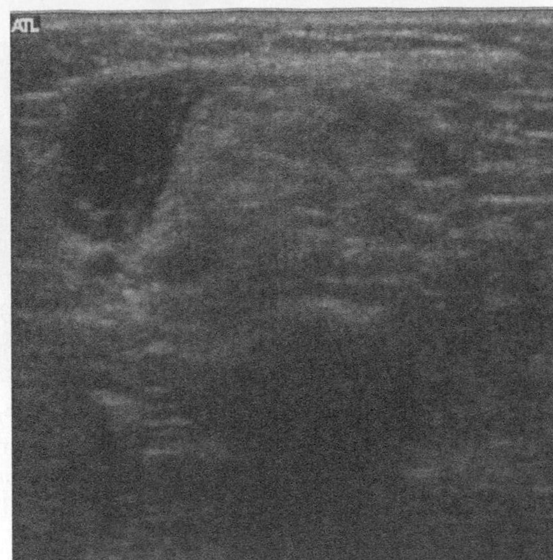

1. What are the radiograph findings?
2. What are the ultrasound findings?
3. What is the most likely diagnosis?
4. What is the natural history of these lesions?
5. What are the possible signal characteristics on MR images, and what is the significance?

Lipoblastoma 1571

Case ranking/difficulty: 

Category: Bone tumors and marrow abnormalities

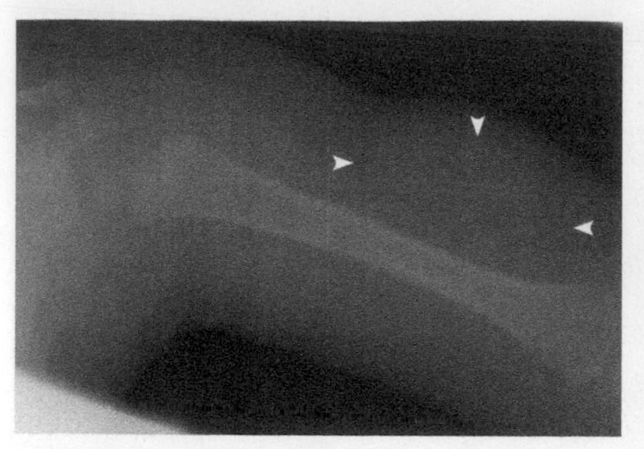

A predominantly fatty lesion with internal septations is seen in the arm.

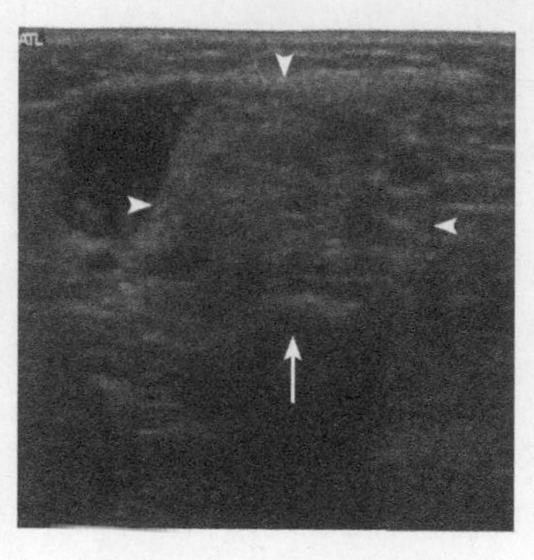

Predominantly hyperechoic mass (*arrowheads*) is seen in the anterior soft tissues adjacent to the humerus (*arrow*).

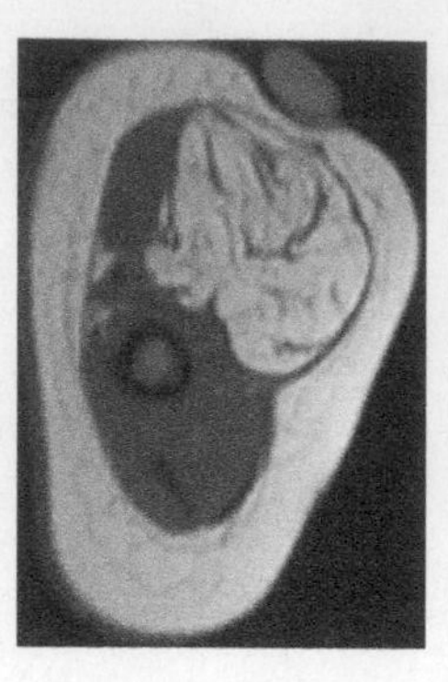

Fatty mass with internal septations.

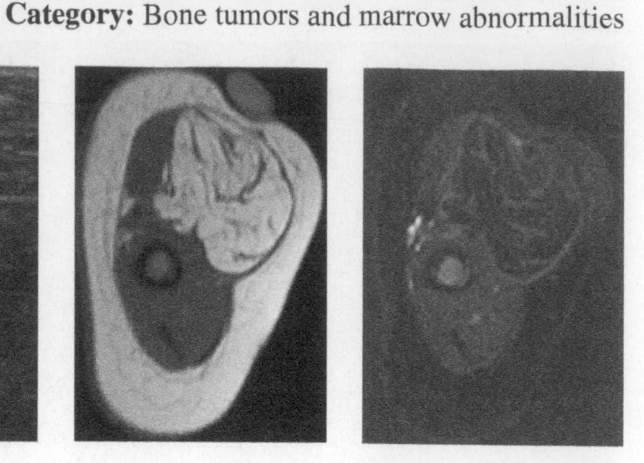

The mass saturates on fat-suppressed FSE T2-weighted images.

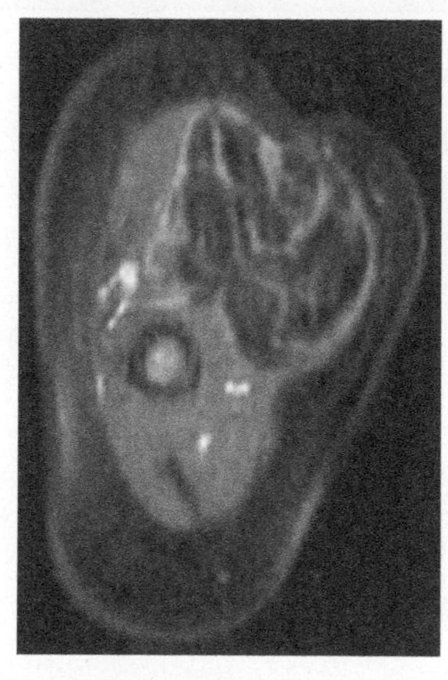

Heterogenous, predominantly septal, enhancement is seen.

Answers

1. There is a soft-tissue mass of fat density, with no bony attachment, destruction, or calcification.
2. Predominantly echogenic soft-tissue mass with internal septations and no internal vascularity.
3. Given the age of the patient and the fatty nature of the mass, the most likely diagnosis is lipoblastoma.
4. Lipoblastomas gradually increase in size and evolve into more mature lipomas.
5. T1 hyperintensity because of fat with fat suppression and internal septations. Focal areas of T2 hyperintensity reflect a myxoid component and can be seen in less mature lipoblastomas.

Pearls

- Lipoblastomas are rare benign mesenchymal tumors of embryonic white fat that occur in infancy and early childhood.
- They present as a painless slow growing soft-tissue mass in the extremities. Uncommonly, the trunk, mediastinum, neck, and retroperitoneum may be affected.
- Well-defined benign lipoblastoma accounts for 70% of cases. Diffuse lipoblastomatosis accounts for 30%.
- Lesions mature into typical lipomas over time.
- MRI is the best modality for investigating these lesions. The lesions are T1 hyperintense because of fat, and have internal septations and a variable margin. Diffuse lipoblastomas have a less-well-defined margin.
- A myxoid component is common in the early stage, which can be confused with a myxoid liposarcoma, but this component diminishes with time.
- Diffuse lipoblastomatosis can recur after excision.

Suggested Readings

Chung EB, Enzinger FM. Benign lipoblastomatosis. An analysis of 35 cases. *Cancer*. 1973;32(2):482-492.

Murphey MD, Carroll JF, Flemming DJ, Pope TL, Gannon FH, Kransdorf MJ. From the archives of the AFIP: benign musculoskeletal lipomatous lesions. *Radiographics*. 2004;24(5):1433-1466.

Painful mass on the dorsum of the foot

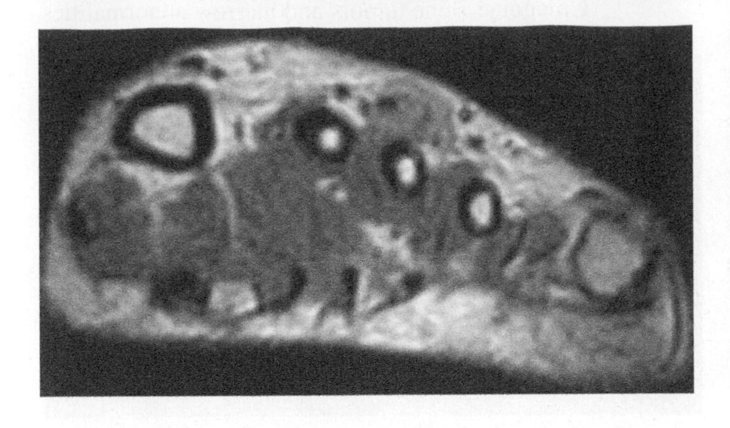

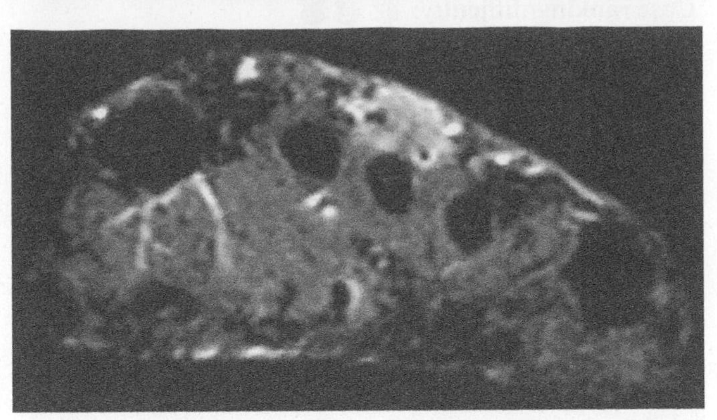

1. What are the MRI findings?

2. What are the most likely differentials?

3. What is the most common location for these tumors?

4. What are the most important predictors of outcome?

5. Where do metastases typically occur in these tumors?

Clear cell sarcoma of the foot 1558

Case ranking/difficulty: 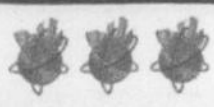

Category: Bone tumors and marrow abnormalities

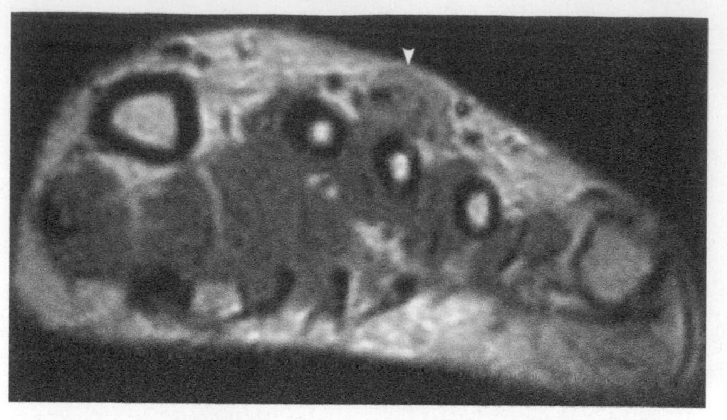

There is a T1 isointense to mildly hyperintense soft-tissue mass partially enveloping the extensor digitorum tendon.

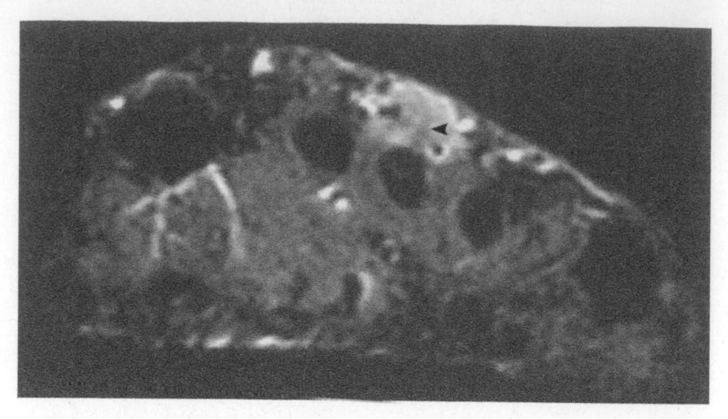

The lesion is mildly hyperintense with foci of low signal, suggesting melanin (*arrowhead*).

The soft-tissue mass is mildly T1 hyperintense to skeletal muscle.

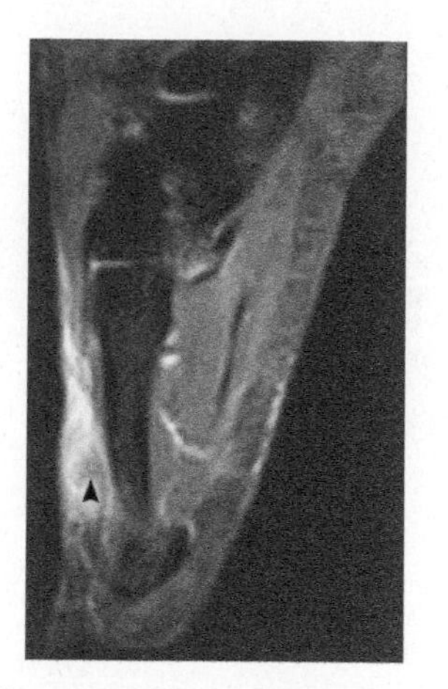

The lesion is T2 hyperintense with foci of low signal intensity consistent with melanin (*arrowhead*).

Answers

1. There is a well-defined soft-tissue mass with T1 and T2 hyperintensity and foci of T2 hypointensity.
2. T1 shortening with T1 hyperintensity is shown, indicating melanin content. Synovial sarcoma may show calcification (T1 and T2 hypointensity) and not melanin.
3. Although clear cell sarcomas can occur in many locations, the most common location is at the musculoaponeurotic structures of the foot and ankle.
4. Tumor size and necrosis are the best predictors of outcome.
5. Metastases typically are to regional lymph nodes and lungs.

Pearls

- Clear cell sarcomas of soft tissues are rare tumors accounting for less than 1% of soft-tissue sarcomas.
- They have a predilection for the extremities, particularly the musculoaponeurotic structures of the foot and ankle.
- Because of the melanin content of the lesion, they are often mistaken for malignant melanoma. They are, however, distinct entities.
- Melanin will cause T1 and T2 shortening on MRI, so T1 hyperintensity and T2 hypointensity can be expected. Marked variability in signal is seen, however.
- Tumor size and necrosis are the best predictors of outcome.
- Metastases are usually to regional lymph nodes and lungs.

Suggested Readings

Deenik W, Mooi WJ, Rutgers EJ, Peterse JL, Hart AA, Kroon BB. Clear cell sarcoma (malignant melanoma) of soft parts: A clinicopathologic study of 30 cases. *Cancer.* 1999;86(6):969-975.

Hourani M, Khoury N, Mourany B, Shabb NS. MR appearance of clear cell sarcoma of tendons and aponeuroses (malignant melanoma of soft parts): radiologic-pathologic correlation. *Skeletal Radiol.* 2005;34(9):543-546.

Leng B, Zhang X, Ali S, et al. Clear cell sarcoma: a case report with radiological and pathological features of an atypical case. *Case Rep Oncol.* 2012;5(2):449-454.

Chronic left shoulder pain

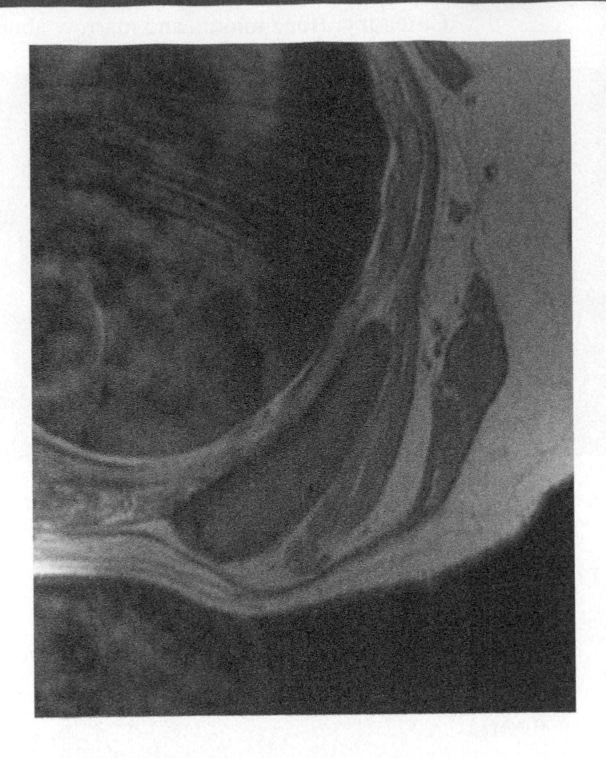

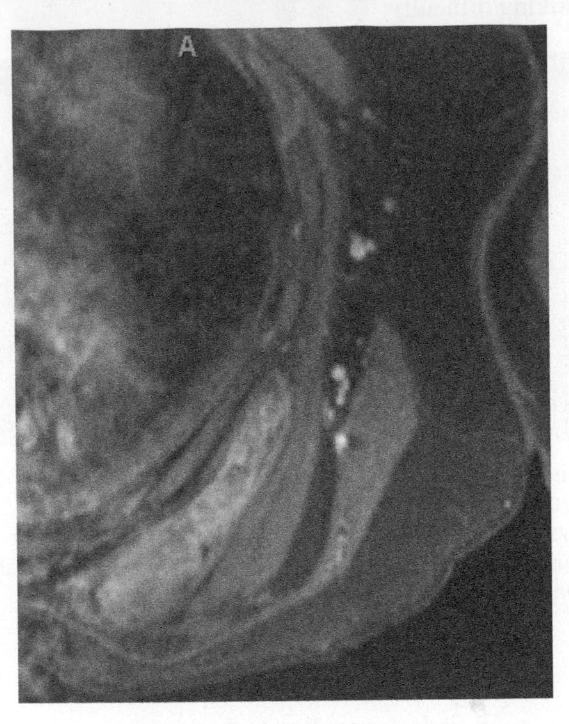

1. What are the demonstrated findings?

2. What are the demonstrated MRI characteristics?

3. What are included in the differential, and what is the most likely diagnosis?

4. What is the characteristic ultrasound appearance of this lesion?

5. What is the prevalence of this lesion on CT in patients older than age 60 years?

Elastofibroma dorsi 1369

Case ranking/difficulty: 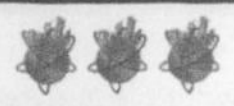

Category: Bone tumors and marrow abnormalities

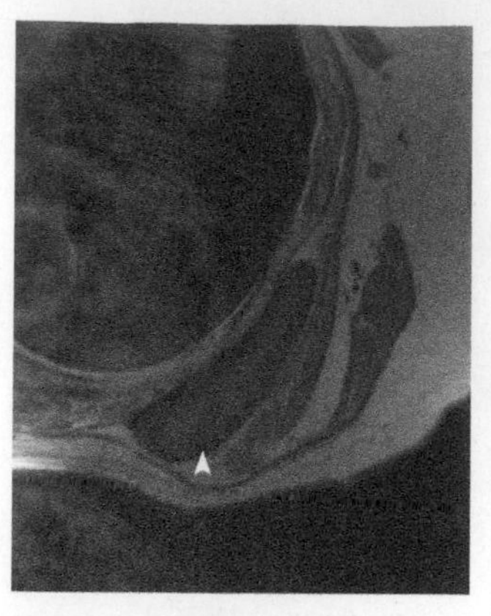

There is a well-defined subscapular mass that is peripherally T1 hypointense and centrally mildly hyperintense.

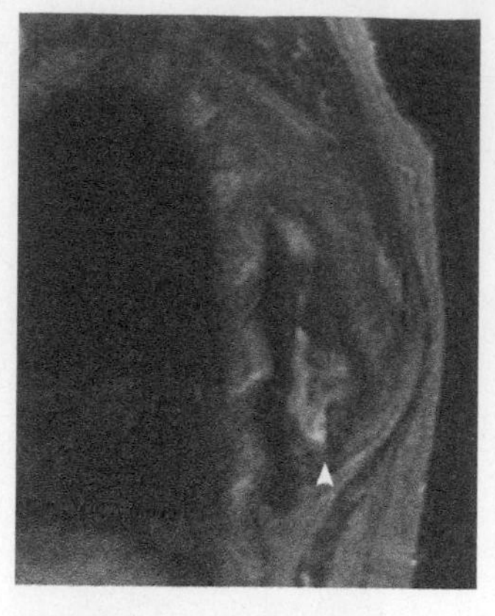

The subscapular location of the mass, between the inferior scapula and chest wall is appreciated. Central T2 hyperintensity is seen.

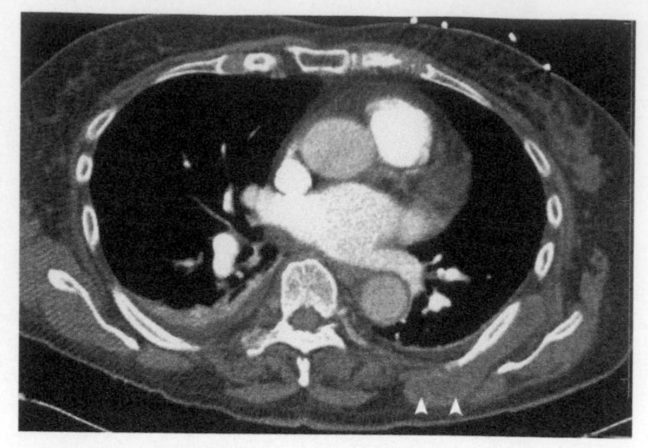

Well-defined subscapular mass with mild central hypodensity is seen.

Answers

1. There is a soft-tissue lesion deep to the serratus anterior muscle in an infrascapular location.
2. There is a well-defined but unencapsulated soft-tissue mass deep to the serratus anterior muscle, with T1 isointensity to hypointensity. There is heterogenous enhancement after contrast, and there is no local invasion or calcification.
3. The differential includes metastasis, liposarcoma, and desmoid tumor. However, the most likely diagnosis based on location and imaging characteristics is an elastofibroma dorsi.
4. Elastofibroma dorsi on ultrasound demonstrates a multilayered appearance with an echogenic fibroelastic stroma interspersed with hypoechoic fat.
5. The reported prevalence of this lesion on chest CT in patients older than age 60 years is 2%.

Pearls

- Elastofibroma dorsi are uncommon, benign, soft-tissue tumors with a classic infrascapular location deep to the serratus anterior and latissimus dorsi muscles.
- The tumor is more common in women, and has a slight right-sided predominance.
- The tumor is isoattenuating to muscle with interspersed areas of fat on CT.
- Ultrasound shows a characteristic multilayered pattern of hypoechoic fat and echogenic fibroelastic tissue.
- MRI shows a well-defined but unencapsulated lesion, with isointensity to skeletal muscle on T1- and T2-weighted images and foci of T1 hyperintense fat. There is variable enhancement.
- Wide surgical excision is curative.

Suggested Readings

Brandser EA, Goree JC, El-Khoury GY. Elastofibroma dorsi: prevalence in an elderly patient population as revealed by CT. *AJR Am J Roentgenol.* 1998;171(4):977-980.

Ochsner JE, Sewall SA, Brooks GN, Agni R. Best cases from the AFIP: elastofibroma dorsi. *Radiographics.* 2006;26(6):1873-1876.

Pain in the back for months

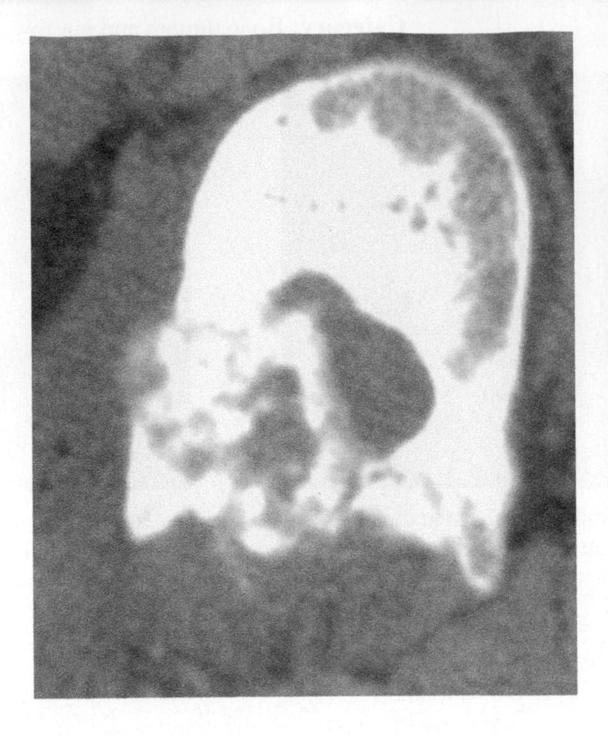

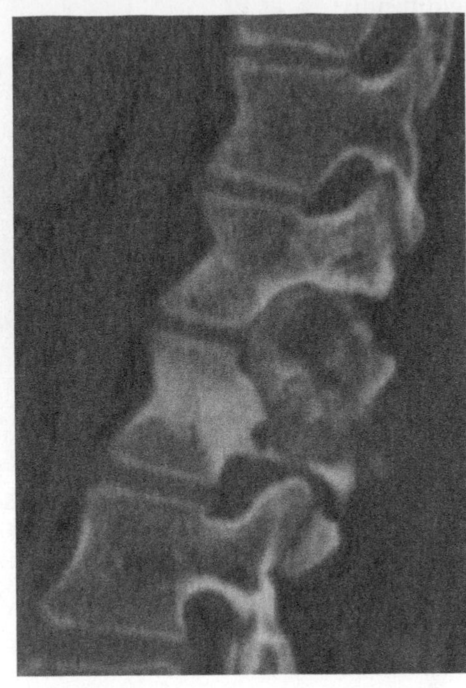

1. What are the CT findings?

2. What is the differential diagnosis, and what is the most likely etiology?

3. What are common locations for this lesion?

4. What differentiates the aggressive form of this lesion from the nonaggressive form?

5. What is the management for these lesions?

Aggressive osteoblastoma 1397

Case ranking/difficulty: 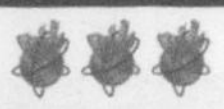

Category: Bone tumors and marrow abnormalities

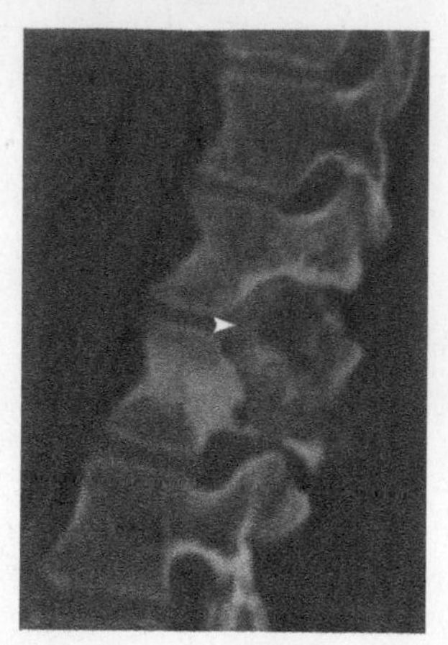

Sagittal reformatted images show an expansile posterior element lesion with a central mineralized matrix, cortical expansion, and breakthrough with adjacent vertebral sclerosis.

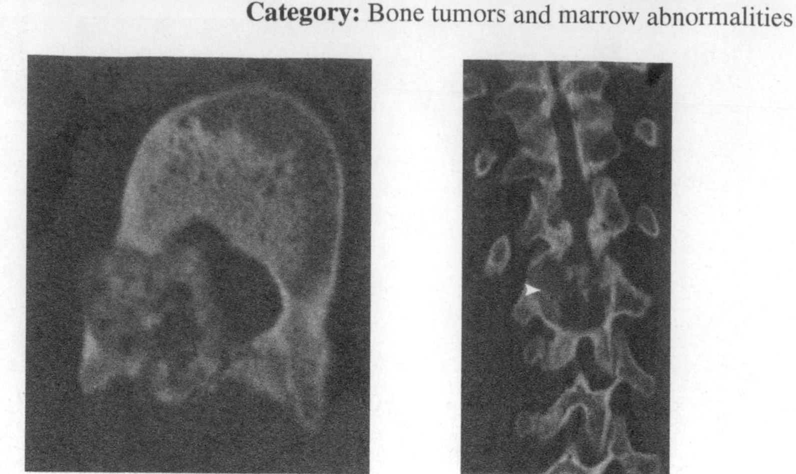

Similar findings as in the Figure on the extreme left.

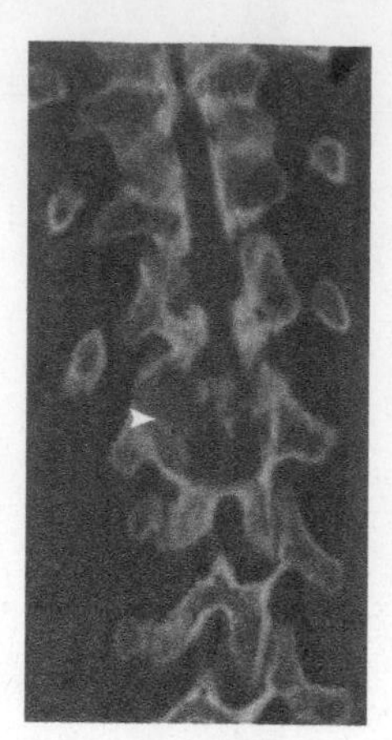

Coronal reformatted images show the highly mineralized matrix and bone expansion.

Answers

1. Lucent expansile lesion with central mineralization located in the posterior elements, and with cortical breakthrough. Sclerosis is seen in the vertebral body with bony remodelling.
2. Differential includes osteoblastoma, aneurysmal bone cyst, giant cell tumor, and a low-grade osteosarcoma. Given the age of the patient, size of lesion, and bony expansion, aggressive osteoblastoma is the favored diagnosis. Osteoid osteoma is not expansile.
3. Osteoblastomas typically occur in the posterior elements of the spine or the diaphysis of long bones. The metaphysis is less common.
4. An aggressive osteoblastoma is characterized by bony expansion, cortical breakthrough, and soft-tissue infiltration as shown in this case. Tumor recurrence is common. Metastasis is extremely uncommon and usually occurs if there is malignant transformation to an osteosarcoma, following radiation therapy.
5. Aggressive osteoblastomas usually require surgical excision, but unfortunately there is a high recurrence rate (up to 50%).

   In surgically unresectable tumors, radiation therapy and chemotherapy have been tried, but there is the risk of postradiation sarcoma.

Pearls

- Osteoblastomas are histologically similar to osteoid osteoma.
- They are, however, larger than 2 cm in size.
- Nocturnal pain and relief with aspirin, as seen in an osteoid osteoma, are not typical features.
- The lesion is commonly located in the posterior elements of the spine, and the diaphysis of long bones.
- Lesions are lucent and may have central mineralization. There can be mild expansion, especially in the spine, with surrounding sclerosis. Variable central mineralization is present.
- An aggressive osteoblastoma with cortical expansion and breakthrough and infiltration of the soft tissues has been described. These aggressive lesions can recur, but have no metastatic potential.
- Aggressive osteoblastomas are usually larger than 3 cm.
- MRI shows isointensity to hypointensity on T1-weighted images, with variable T2 signal.

Suggested Readings

Abramovici L, Kenan S, Hytiroglou P, Rafii M, Steiner GC. Osteoblastoma-like osteosarcoma of the distal tibia. *Skeletal Radiol.* 2002;31(3):179-182.

Ramirez JA, Sandoz JC, Kaakaji Y, Nietzschman HR. Case 3: aggressive osteoblastoma. *AJR Am J Roentgenol.* 1998;171(3):863, 867-868.

Pain in thigh; no history of trauma

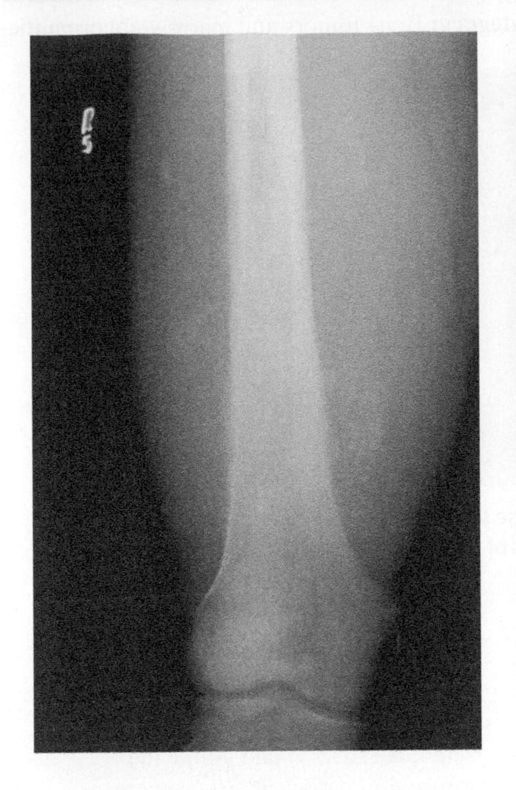

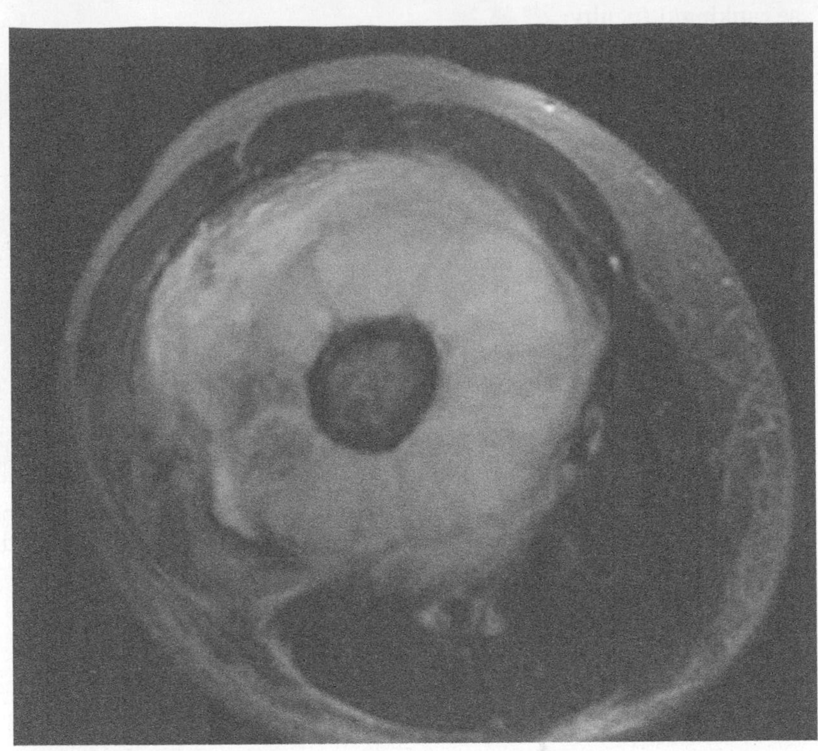

1. What are the radiographic features?

2. What is the differential diagnosis?

3. What is the most likely diagnosis?

4. What are the typical radiographic features?

5. What are the typical CT and MRI characteristics?

Periosteal osteosarcoma 1469

Case ranking/difficulty: 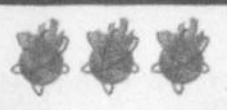 **Category:** Bone tumors and marrow abnormalities

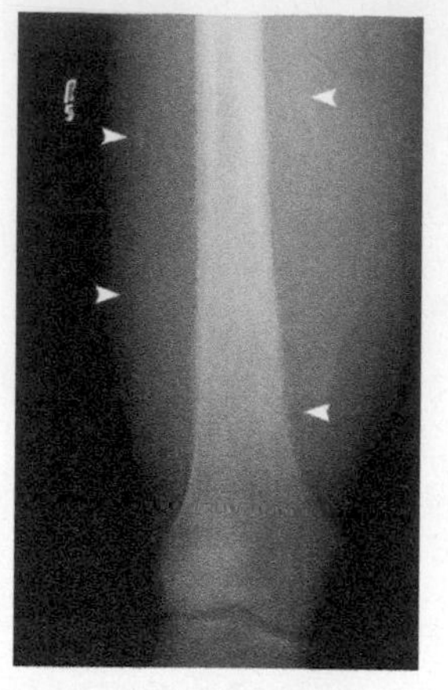

Diaphyseal soft-tissue mass, with aggressive periosteal reaction and mineralization (*arrowheads*).

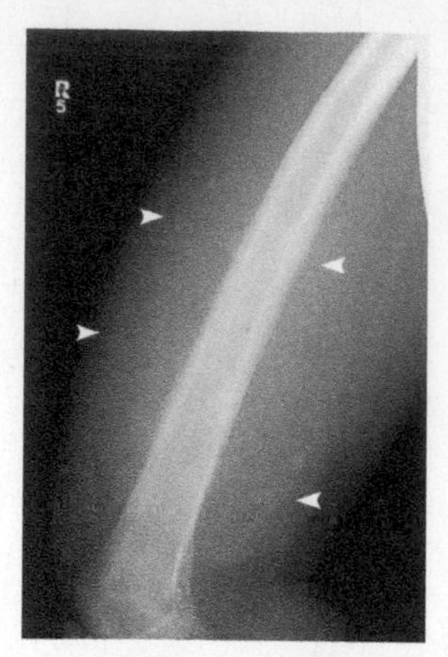

Diaphyseal soft-tissue mass, with aggressive periosteal reaction and mineralization (*arrowheads*).

T2 hyperintense soft-tissue mass with lack of medullary involvement.

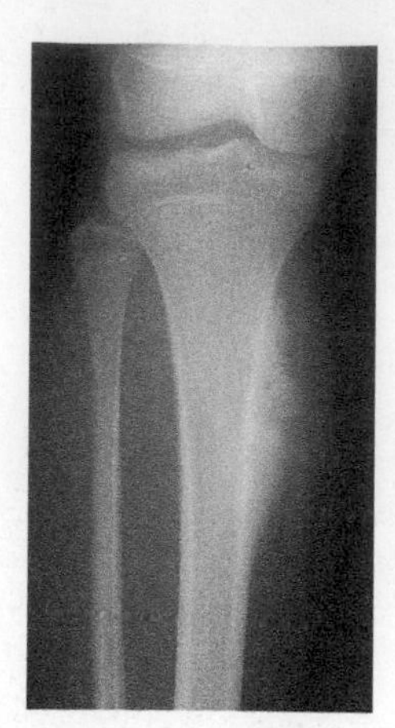

Another patient with more classic sunburst periosteal reaction and no cortical destruction.

Answers

1. There is a large soft-tissue mass and a lesion located in the diaphysis with aggressive periosteal reaction.
2. Differential includes high-grade surface osteosarcoma and periosteal, parosteal, and conventional osteosarcoma, as well as a juxtacortical chondrosarcoma.
3. Based on location and imaging characteristics, the most likely diagnosis is periosteal osteosarcoma.
4. Periosteal osteosarcomas are located in the diaphysis with more aggressive periosteal reaction, soft-tissue mass, cortical thickening, and scalloping than seen in parosteal lesions. However, medullary involvement is atypical.
5. Reflecting the cartilaginous nature of the tumor, the lesions are typically low density on CT and T2 hyperintense on MRI, with low signal foci as a result of periosteal reaction and new bone formation. The cortex is often thickened, but medullary involvement is uncommon.

Pearls

- Periosteal osteosarcoma is a surface osteosarcoma.
- Histological grade is intermediate between parosteal osteosarcoma and high-grade surface osteosarcoma (HGSO).
- Lesions are predominantly diaphyseal, like high-grade surface osteosarcoma (HGSO) and unlike the metaphyseal location of parosteal osteosarcoma.
- Medullary involvement is less common than parosteal osteosarcoma and HGSO, although it is a higher-grade lesion than parosteal osteosarcomas.
- Codman triangle and sunburst periosteal reaction is present.
- Cortical thickening and erosions with a soft-tissue mass are seen.
- Lesions are low density on CT and high signal on T2-weighted MR sequences.
- Prognosis is intermediate between HGSO and parosteal osteosarcoma.

Suggested Readings

Murphey MD, Jelinek JS, Temple HT, Flemming DJ, Gannon FH. Imaging of periosteal osteosarcoma: radiologic-pathologic comparison. *Radiology.* 2004;233(1):129-138.

Murphey MD, Robbin MR, McRae GA, Flemming DJ, Temple HT, Kransdorf MJ. The many faces of osteosarcoma. *Radiographics.* 2010;17(5):1205-1231.

Yarmish G, Klein MJ, Landa J, Lefkowitz RA, Hwang S. Imaging characteristics of primary osteosarcoma: nonconventional subtypes. *Radiographics.* 2010;30(6):1653-1672.

Pain in leg following a fall

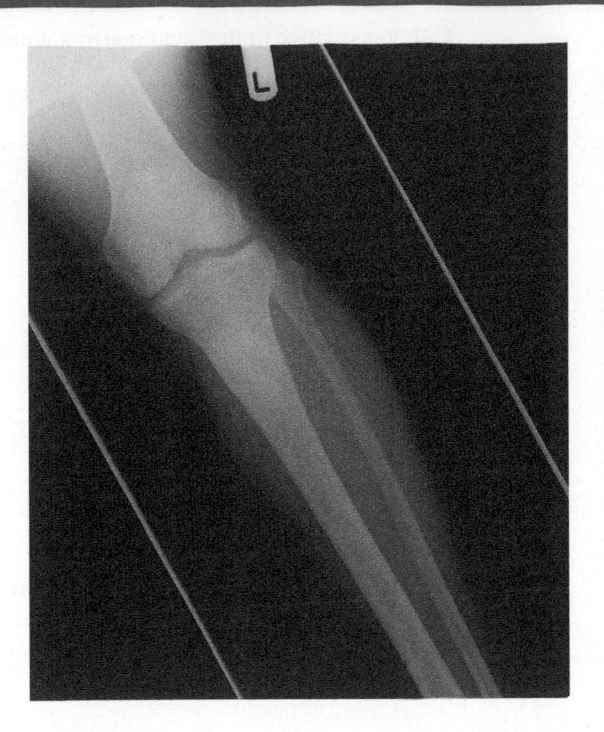

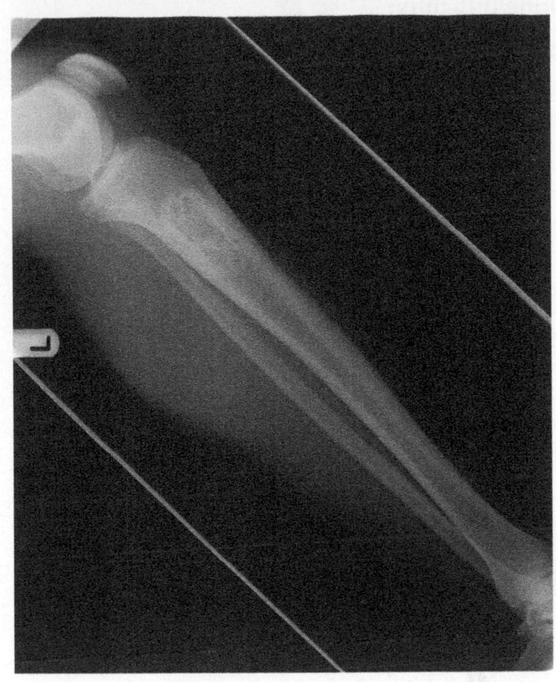

1. What is the differential diagnosis?

2. What is the incidence of this lesion among all cases of primary bone tumor?

3. Which features are not typical for this entity?

4. What is the correct treatment of this lesion?

5. What are the most common locations for this entity?

Chondromyxoid fibroma 1844

Case ranking/difficulty:

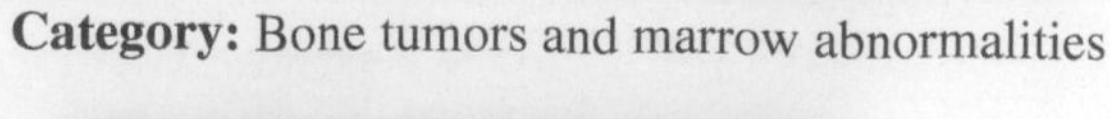

Category: Bone tumors and marrow abnormalities

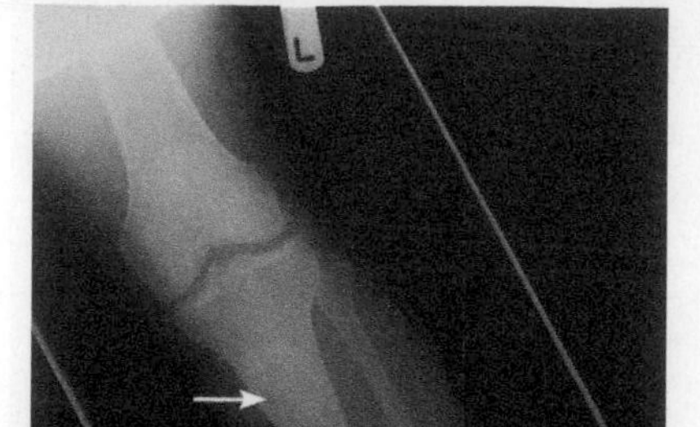

Expansile lesion with lytic and sclerotic elements at proximal tibial metaphysis. No periosteal reaction or cortical destruction.

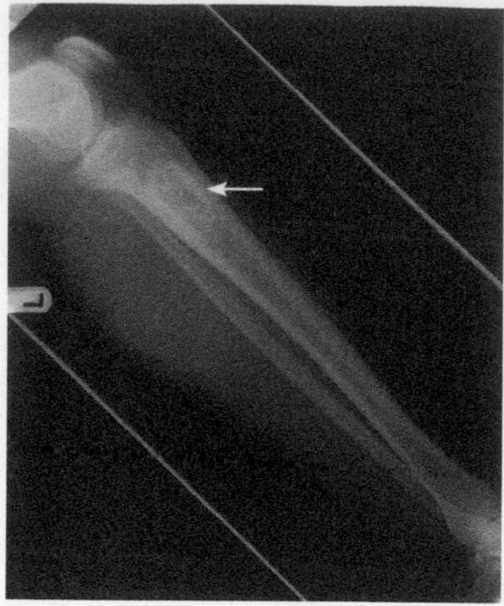

Lateral view demonstrates lesion with no associated soft-tissue swelling anteriorly and posteriorly, no periosteal destruction, nor cortical erosion. All these features are of a non-aggressive lesion.

Answers

1. The differential diagnosis of chondromyxoid fibroma (CMF) includes enchondroma, nonossifying fibroma, aneurysmal bone cyst, and chondrosarcoma (although features of CMF typically are non-aggressive).
2. CMF is a very rare tumor, which makes it difficult to diagnose confidently as a result. However, it has quite distinctive features: adolescent age group, usually lytic, often found about the knee, part of a fibrous/myxoid or chondroid matrix, but often appearing predominantly lytic.
3. CMF is always benign, although local recurrence is relatively common postcurettage. Aggressive features, such as cortical destruction, periosteal reaction, wide zone of transition, and soft-tissue component, are inconsistent with the diagnosis.

   They are eccentrically based in the cortex, and do not arise from the medulla.

   Most lytic lesions are susceptible to pathological fracture.
4. The correct treatment for chondromyxoid fibroma is curettage.

   The lesions are often painful, and can appear identical to a low-grade chondrosarcoma; consequently, histological confirmation of benignity is required.
5. The most common location for CMF is about the knee, with proximal tibial lesions the most frequent.

Pearls

- Chondromyxoid fibroma (CMF) is a very rare tumor so should not be at the top of a list of differential diagnoses for bone tumors of benign appearance about the knee.
- The lesion may consist of any combination of chondroid, myxoid, or fibrous elements.
- It may have predominantly lytic (most common), mixed lytic and sclerotic, or predominantly sclerotic appearances (rarely).
- The lesion most commonly presents in the second and third decades of life.
- The possibility of pathological fracture should be considered as a source of pain.
- The lesion often requires a biopsy to make a confident diagnosis.

Suggested Readings

Desai SS, Jambhekar NA, Samanthray S, Merchant NH, Puri A, Agarwal M. Chondromyxoid fibromas: a study of 10 cases. *J Surg Oncol.* 2005;89(1):28-31.

Kim HS, Jee WH, Ryu KN, et al. MRI of chondromyxoid fibroma. *Acta Radiol.* 2011;52(8):875-880.

Levine SM, Lambiase RE, Petchprapa CN. Cortical lesions of the tibia: characteristic appearances at conventional radiography. *Radiographics.* 2001;23(1):157-177.

Patient presents with a palpable mass in the posterior left thigh after falling down the stairs

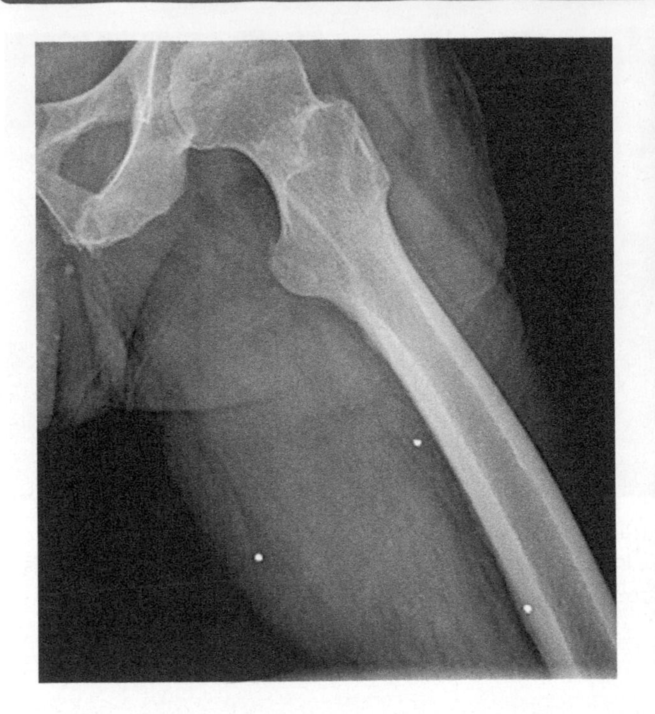

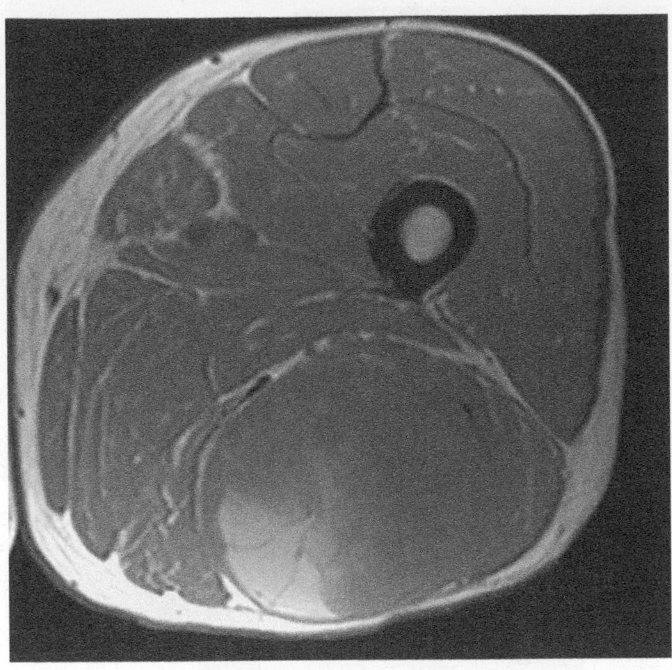

1. What is the typical presentation of this lesion?

2. What is the prognosis of this lesion?

3. What is the best predictor of outcome in this lesion?

4. What are the MRI characteristics of this lesion?

5. What characteristics do not exclude the diagnosis of this lesion?

Extraskeletal osteosarcoma 1317

Case ranking/difficulty: 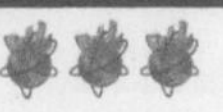

Category: Bone tumors and marrow abnormalities

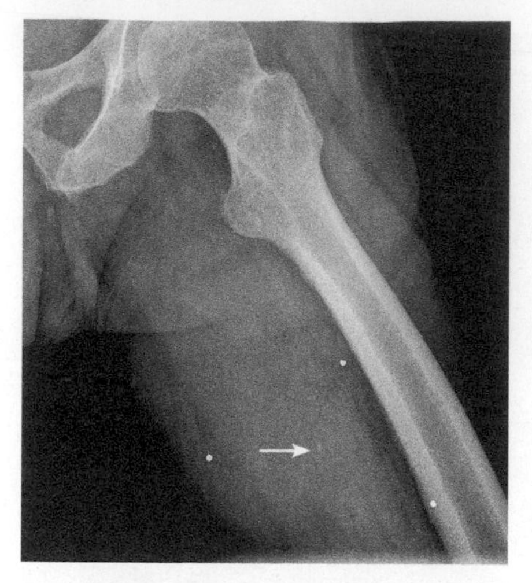

There is a small focus of ossification (*arrow*).

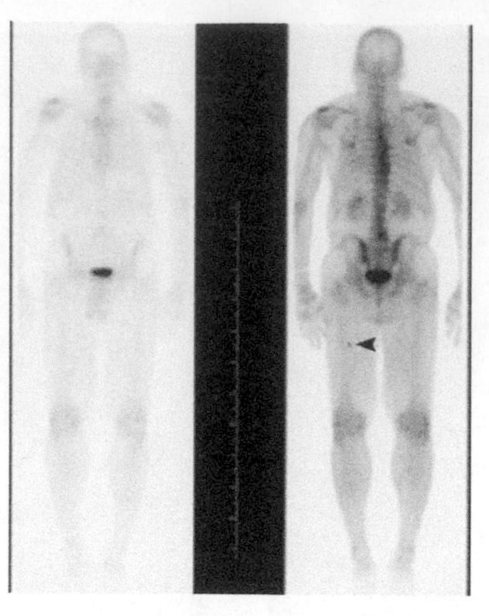

99mTc-MDP radionuclide bone scan shows focal uptake in the posterior thigh soft tissues.

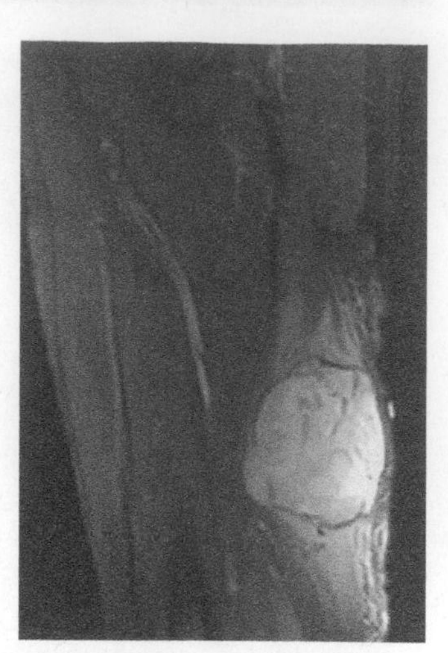

Marked necrosis and signal heterogeneity is seen. There is little peritumoral edema.

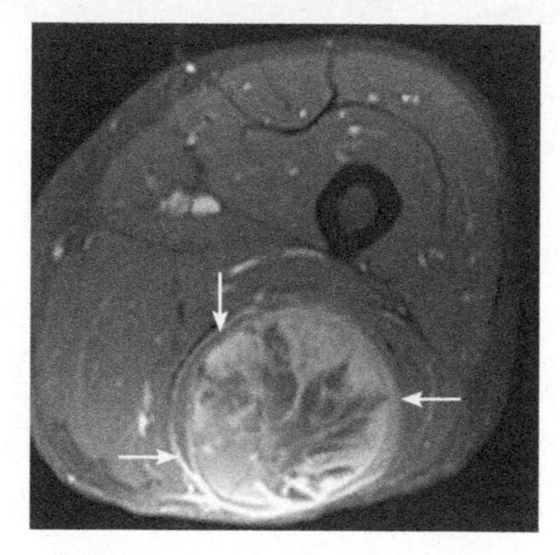

Heterogenous enhancement is seen. Pseudocapsule is demonstrated (*arrows*).

Answers

1. Extraskeletal osteosarcomas are typically discovered after trauma, with a palpable soft-tissue mass.
2. Local tumor recurrence and metastasis are frequent, with more than 50% of patients dying within 2 to 3 years of diagnosis.
3. Tumor size is the best predictor of outcome.
4. Lesions are typically pseudoencapsulated with areas of necrosis and hemorrhage. There is often attachment to the fascia.
5. A radiographically visible osteoid matrix is seen in only 50% of cases. Hemorrhage and necrosis are common.

Pearls

- Extraskeletal osteosarcoma is a rare form of osteosarcoma.
- Typically occurs in an older age group than conventional osteosarcoma.
- Typically large soft-tissue mass on presentation.
- A history of trauma often precedes discovery.
- The presence of a pseudocapsule can usually reduce the suspicion for a neoplastic lesion, but is often present in extraskeletal osteosarcomas.
- An osteoid matrix may or may not be demonstrated on imaging.
- An important imaging differential is myositis ossificans.
- The prognosis is poor, with frequent metastasis and local tumor recurrence.

Suggested Readings

Huvos AG. Osteogenic sarcoma. In: *Bone Tumor: Diagnosis, Treatment and Prognosis*. Philadelphia, PA: Saunders; 1991:85-156.

Varma DG, Ayala AG, Guo SQ, Moulopoulos LA, Kim EE, Charnsangavej C. MRI of extraskeletal osteosarcoma. *J Comput Assist Tomogr.* 1994;17(3):414-417.

Acute on chronic back pain with sudden loss of bladder and bowel function; history of prior spine surgery

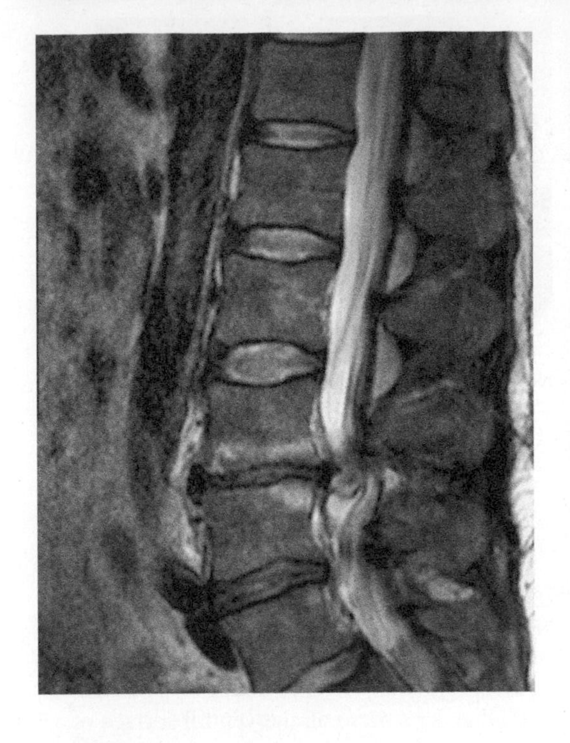

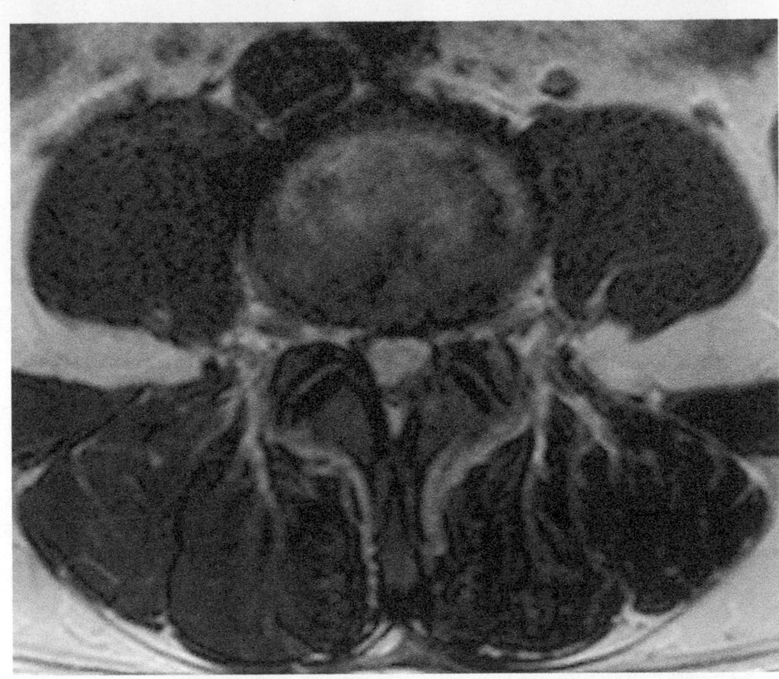

1. What are the MRI findings?

2. What are the differential diagnosis of intradural and extramedullary lesions?

3. What is the diagnosis?

4. What makes the diagnosis challenging?

5. How are these lesions classified?

Intradural disc prolapse 1004

Case ranking/difficulty: 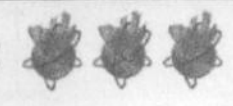

Category: Degenerative disease of the musculoskeletal system

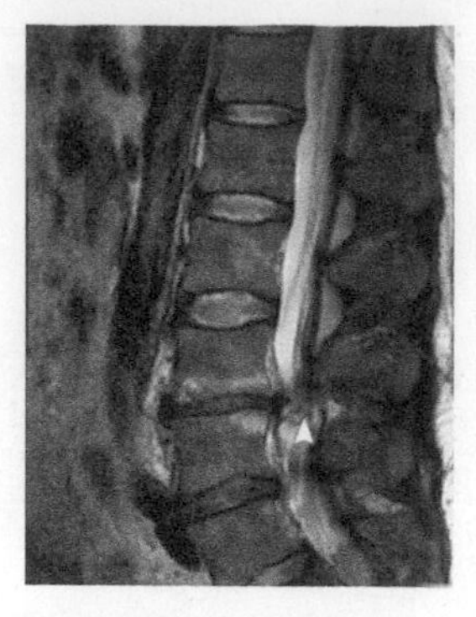

Intradural disc material causing cauda compression.

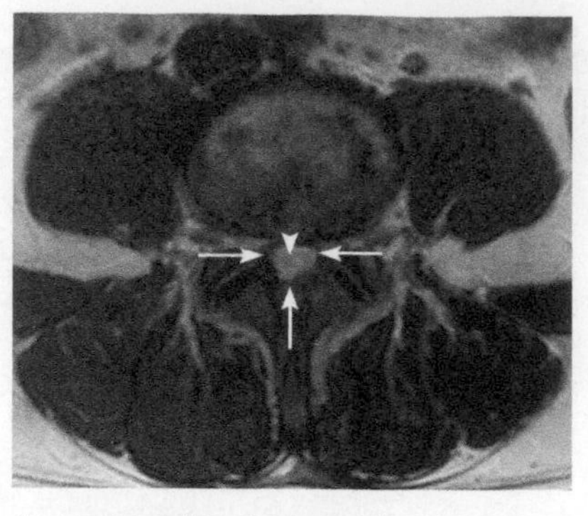

Central canal is obscured by cystic disc material and the normal nerve roots are displaced peripherally.

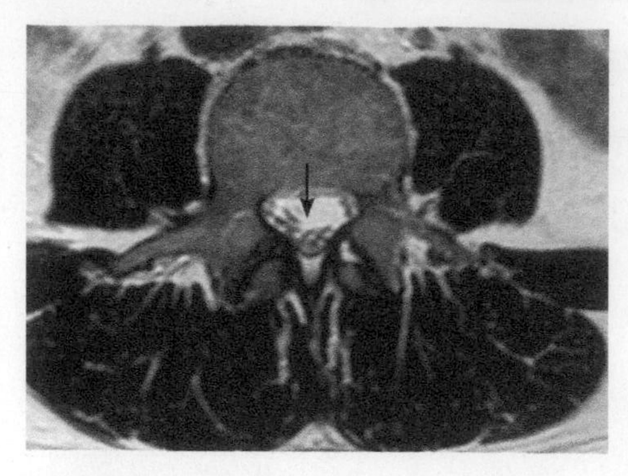

Normal nerve roots for comparison.

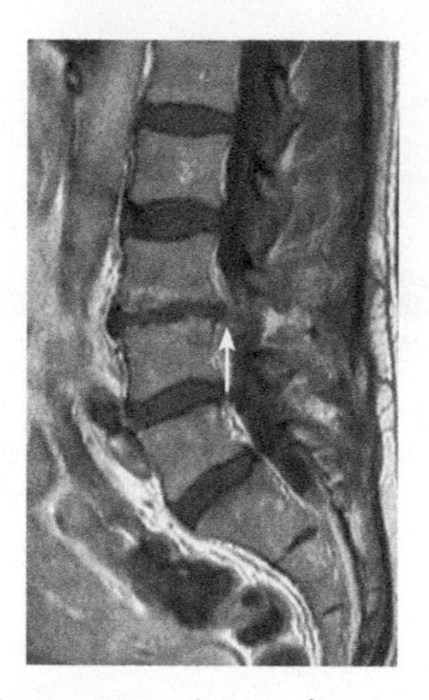

Post-contrast image showing entry of the disc material into the dural sac.

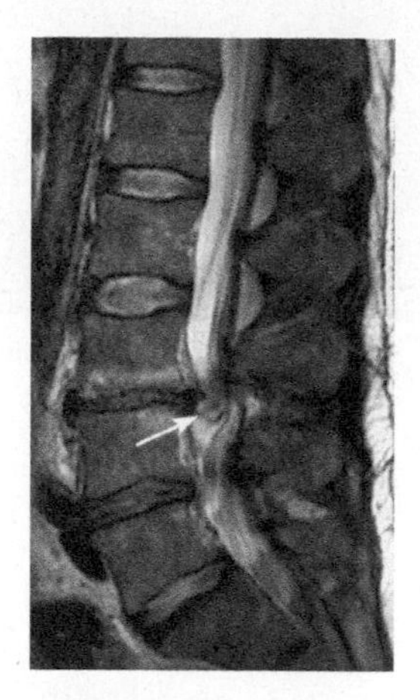

Intradural disc material.

Answers

1. Intradural and extramedullary lesion that is T2 hyperintense, peripherally displacing nerve roots.
2. The differential diagnosis includes herniated intradural disc material, meningioma, neurofibroma, and metastasis.
3. Cystic disc material is seen displacing the normal nerve roots peripherally, consistent with herniated intradural disc material.
4. The diagnosis can be made challenging by the presence of cystic changes and calcification of the disc suggesting other etiologies. In this case, the cystic disc material resembles CSF, and the nerve roots are displaced peripherally. The postoperative status of a patient, and the presence of congenital adhesions and a constitutionally narrow spinal canal, can also make the diagnosis difficult.
5. Type A: herniation of the disc into the dural sac; type B: herniated disc into the dural sheath in the preganglionic region.

Pearls

- Intradural herniated disc is a rare cause of cord or cauda equina compression.
- It accounts for 0.26% or 0.3% of all herniated disc cases, and is most common in lumbar region, usually at L4/5.
- Congenital adhesions between the ventral surface of the thecal sac and posterior longitudinal ligament acts as a predisposing factor.
- They can be difficult to diagnose, especially when they undergo cystic or calcified changes.
- According to Mut et al, they can be classified into 2 types.
  - Type A: herniation of a disc material into the dural sac
  - Type B: herniation into the dural sheath in the preganglionic region of the nerve root.
- MRI is the investigative modality of choice. Contrast-enhanced MRI is used to differentiate between intradural and extramedullary lesions such as neurofibroma, meningioma, and also between intradural lesions such as epidermoid and dermoid. Disc material does not enhance immediately after administration of contrast.
- Treatment usually involves urgent removal of the disc, especially when causing compressive symptoms.

Suggested Readings

Arnold PM, Wakwaya YT. Intradural disk herniation at L1-L2: report of two cases. *J Spinal Cord Med.* 2011;34(3):312-314.

Mut M, Berker M, Palaoğlu S. Intraradicular disc herniations in the lumbar spine and a new classification of intradural disc herniations. *Spinal Cord.* 2001;39(10):545-548.

Singh PK, Shrivastava S, Dulani R, Banode P, Gupta S. Dorsal herniation of cauda equina due to sequestrated intradural disc. *Asian Spine J.* 2012;6(2):145-147.

Bilateral lower back pain

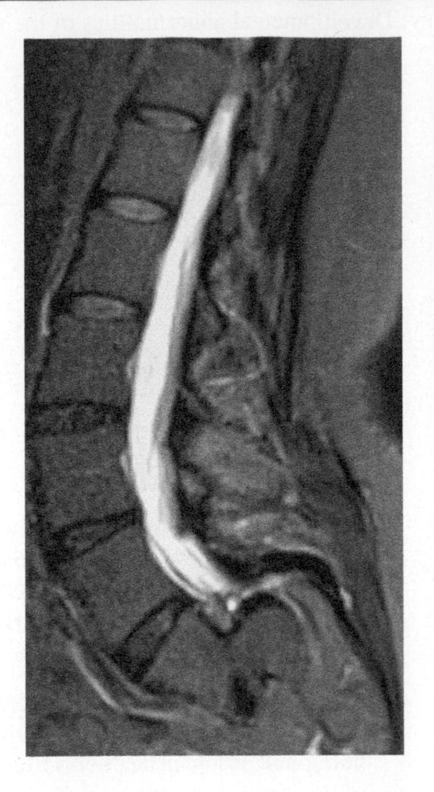

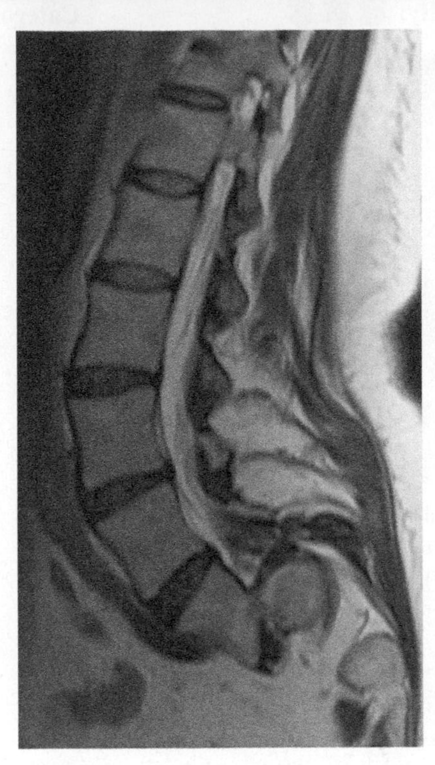

1. What is the diagnosis?

2. What are the common patient demographics for this condition?

3. Deficiency of which structure is usually responsible for this specific entity?

4. What are the usual complications of this condition?

5. What is the treatment of choice for progressive deformity/complications?

Dysplastic spondylolisthesis 41

Case ranking/difficulty: 

Category: Developmental abnormalities of the musculoskeletal system

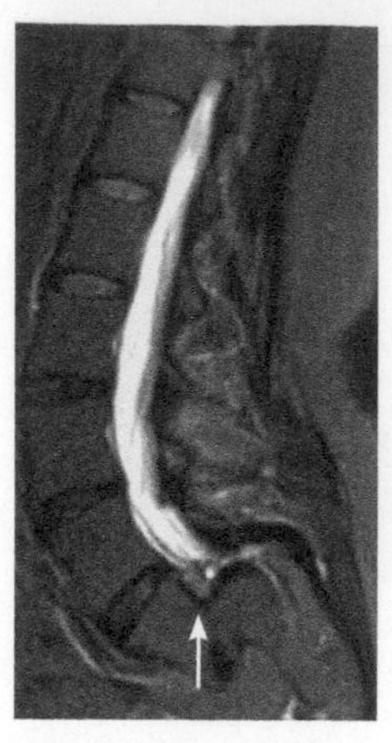

Dysplastic superior articular facet of S1 leads to 100% spondylolisthesis of L5 on S1. There are no pars defects.

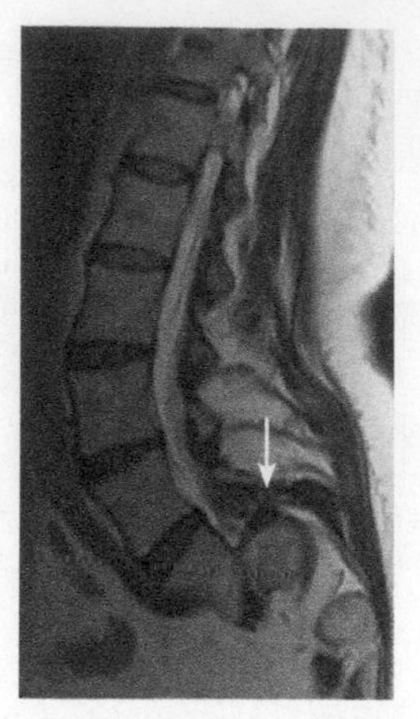

There is severe lateral recess and central canal stenosis at L5/S1 secondary to the spondylolisthesis.

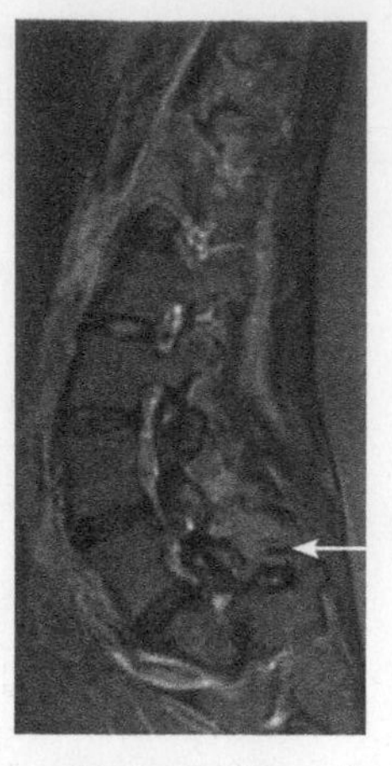

The dysplastic (horizontal) superior articular facets of S1 are well demonstrated on the sagittal images.

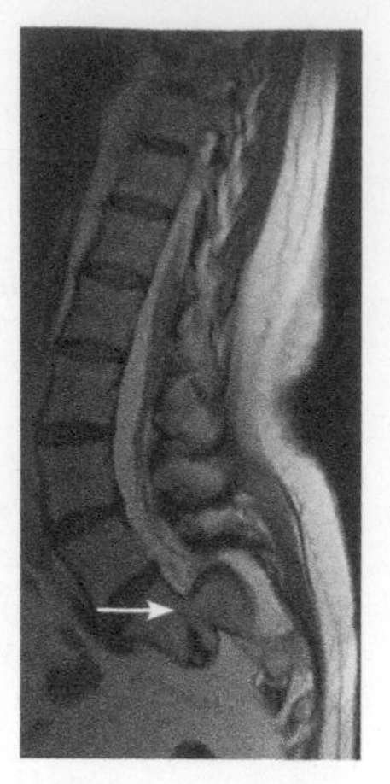

There is a diminutive fused L5/S1 articulation and compensatory lumbar hyperlordosis.

Answers

1. Dysplastic spondylolisthesis is a common but under recognized cause of slips identified in adolescents and young adults. It relates to congenital dysplasia of the posterior elements, usually superior articular facets of S1.
2. Dysplastic spondylolisthesis is congenital, more common in women and found more frequently in whites.
3. Dysplastic spondylolisthesis usually results from a congenitally malformed superior articular facet of S1.
4. Severe deformity leads to a hyperlordotic lumbar spine. There is usually L5/S1 disc degeneration. As the slip progresses, there may be severe central canal and lateral recess stenosis.
5. As slips progress they may require surgical intervention. A posterior decompression with fusion is the preferred approach as it allows the central canal to be decompressed and fixation prevents further progression of the slip and deformity.

Pearls

- Dysplastic spondylolisthesis is a common but under recognized cause of a slip in an adolescent or young adult at L5/S1.
- The key distinction between an isthmic and a dysplastic cause is the spinal canal, which is widened as a result of pars defects, and narrowed as a result of facet joint dysplasia and subluxation.
- The identification of a dysplastic (horizontal) superior horizontal articular facet of S1 is virtually pathognomic of this condition, although other dysplastic etiologies include abnormal vertically oriented facet joints.
- Spondyloptosis (100% slip) is probably only commonly seen in cases of dysplastic spondylolisthesis, hence if this degree of slip is noted, a congenital dysplastic etiology should be considered.
- The L5/S1 articulation is often partly fused and diminutive in this type of spondylolisthesis.
- Regular follow up is advised for consideration of surgery as high-grade dysplastic spondylolisthesis may have severe central canal stenosis and deformity.

Suggested Readings

Pucher A, Jankowski R, Szulc A, Stryczyński P, Strzyzewski W. Surgical treatment of dysplastic and isthmic spondylolisthesis. *Ortop Traumatol Rehabil.* 2005;7(6):639-645.

Vialle R, Dauzac C, Khouri N, Wicart P, Glorion C, Guigui P. Sacral and lumbar-pelvic morphology in high-grade spondylolisthesis. *Orthopedics.* 2007;30(8):642-649.

Subject Index

Accessory soleus muscle (1430)
Achilles paratenonitis (1698)
Achilles tendon tear (1598)
Achondroplasia (1460)
ACL reconstruction (114)
Acromioclavicular joint subluxation (480)
Aggressive osteoblastoma (1397)
Ameloblastoma (1551)
Amyloid arthropathy (1379)
Aneurysmal bone cyst (1438)
Ankylosing spondylitis (467)
Anterior impingement syndrome
of ankle (1199)
Anterior labroligamentous periosteal sleeve
avulsion (ALPSA lesion) (1398)
Anterolateral impingement (1318)
Arthrofibrosis of the knee (1429)
Athletic pubalgia (1455)
Avascular necrosis of hip (529)

Baxter neuropathy (1451)
Bisphosphonate-related femoral fracture (1341)
Bizarre parosteal osteochondromatous
proliferation: nora lesion (1536)
Blount disease (1439)
Brodie abscess (229)
Brown tumors (hyperparathyroidism) (488)
Bucket-handle tear of medial meniscus (1721)
Burst fracture of C1 (Jefferson) (527)

Caffey disease (infantile cortical
hyperostosis) (2311)
Calcaneal insufficiency avulsion fracture (1532)
Calcaneal lipoma (1404)
Calcaneus fracture: tongue type (2328)
Cam-type femoral acetabular impingement (1334)
Carpal tunnel syndrome (median neuritis) (1531)
Chondroblastoma (1386)
Chondromyxoid fibroma (1844)
Chondrosarcoma (228)
Chordoma (1412)
Chronic osteomyelitis of ischium (1722)
Clear cell sarcoma of the foot (1558)
Cleidocranial dysostosis (1436)
Congenital bowing of the tibia (1437)
Cortical desmoid (cortical avulsive injury) (1464)
CPPD crowned dens syndrome (1319)

De Quervain tenosynovitis (1649)
Diabetic osteomyelitis of foot (1701)
Diffuse idiopathic skeletal hyperostosis
(DISH) (1343)
Diffuse sclerotic metastases
(prostatic carcinoma) (104)
Discoid lateral meniscus (1410)
Distal biceps tendon rupture (1444)
Dorsal defect of the patella (1349)
Dysplastic spondylolisthesis (41)

Eagle syndrome (1374)
Elastofibroma dorsi (1369)
Enchondroma (1973)
Enteropathic sacroiliitis (1837)
Erosive Osteoarthritis (1729)
Essex-Lopresti fracture–dislocation (2318)
Ewing sarcoma (1839)
Extensor carpi ulnaris (ECU) subluxation and
subsheath tear (1425)
Extensor digitorum brevis manus (EDBM) (1449)
Extraskeletal osteosarcoma (1317)

Femoral neck stress fracture (1384)
Fibrolipoma of the median nerve (1446)
Fibromatosis: deep extra-abdominal (1454)
Fibrous dysplasia (339)

Galeazzi fracture–dislocation (1396)
Giant cell tumor (1413)
Giant cell tumor of the tendon sheath (1556)
Glenoid labral articular disruption (GLAD)
lesion (1547)
Gout (1330)

Haglund syndrome (1321)
Hamate-lunate impaction syndrome (1599)
Hamstring tear (1861)
Hemochromatosis-induced arthritis (1730)
Hibernoma (1596)
Hill-sachs defect (anterior dislocation
of the shoulder) (526)
Hoffa fracture (1315)
Hypertrophic osteoarthropathy (1323)

Iliotibial band friction syndrome (1367)
Infectious flexor tenosynovitis (1332)
Infectious sacroiliitis (1347)
Intradural disc prolapse (1004)
Intramuscular hemangioma (1458)
Ischiofemoral impingement syndrome (1734)
Isolated MCL sprain of knee (1703)

Jersey finger—flexor digitorum profundus
tendon rupture (1399)
Jogger's foot (1472)
Jumped facet (2357)
Jumper's knee (1557)
Juvenile idiopathic arthritis (1380)

Keloids (1550)
Kienböck disease (1555)

Lateral epicondylitis (209)
Lateral patellar dislocation (478)
Lateral ulnar collateral ligament (LUCL)
injury of elbow (2232)
Legg-calve-perthes disease (1735)
Lesser trochanter avulsion: metastatic
disease (1363)
Lipoblastoma (1571)
Lipoma arborescens of knee (1447)
Lisfranc fracture dislocation (1539)
Lung metastasis within the patella (1553)
Lyme arthritis (1340)
Lymphangiomatosis (1420)
Macrodystrophia lipomatosa (1457)
Madelung deformity (1339)
Maisonneuve fracture (1362)
Massive rotator cuff tear (1700)
Medial collateral ligament bursitis (1326)
Medial meniscal tear (335)
Melorheostosis (1860)
Meniscocapsular separation (1648)
Metastatic cauda equina compression (1006)
Milwaukee shoulder (1548)
Monteggia fracture–dislocation (1395)
Morel-Lavallee lesion (1005)
Morton neuroma (1419)
MRI geyser sign; os acromiale (1389)
Mucoid degeneration of the anterior cruciate
ligament (1324)
Multicentric reticulohistiocytosis (1459)
Multiple hereditary exostoses (1338)
Multiple lytic lesions of skull—pacchionian
granulations (1836)
Multiple myeloma (1725)
Myositis ossificans circumscripta (1542)

Necrotizing fasciitis (2368)
Neurofibroma (1442)
Non-accidental trauma (2209)
Nonosseous calcaneonavicular coalition (1320)

O'Donoghue triad (1541)
Occult scaphoid fracture (1387)
Os trigonum syndrome (1287)
Ossification of the posterior longitudinal
ligament (OPLL) (1342)
Osteochondral lesion of talar dome (1529)
Osteogenesis imperfecta (type III) (1463)
Osteoid osteoma (1391)
Osteopetrosis (2310)
Osteoporotic cauda equina compression (1007)
Osteosarcoma: conventional type (1414)

Paget disease (1825)
Parachordoma (1316)
Paralabral cyst with infraspinatus
denervation (1530)
Parosteal osteosarcoma (1470)
Particle disease (1376)
PASTA (partial articular supraspinatus tendon
avulsion) lesion (2250)
Patella sleeve avulsion fracture (1345)
Patellofemoral dysfunction (1720)
Pectoralis major tear (2305)
Perilunate dislocation (1394)
Periosteal osteosarcoma (1469)
Peroneal tendon subluxation (1377)
Pigmented villonodular synovitis
(PVNS) (1402)
Pincer-type femoroacetabular impingement
(FAI) (2355)
Pivot-shift injury of knee (1702)
Plantar fascia rupture (2262)
Plantar fasciitis (1331)
Plantar fibroma (1453)

Plantaris tear (1392)
Plexiform neurofibroma (1549)
Post-traumatic osteolysis of the clavicle (1552)
Posterior hip dislocation (1471)
Posterior sternoclavicular joint dislocation (1364)
Posterior tibial tendon subluxation (1473)
Posterolateral corner injury (1289)
Preaxial polydactyly (1461)
Primary lymphoma of bone (1393)
Proximal focal femoral deficiency (PFFD) (2309)
Pseudoaneurysm (1466)
Psoas abscess—tuberculosis (1716)
Psoriatic arthritis (1717)
Pulley injury (climber's finger) (2308)

Quadriceps tendon rupture (1400)

Radial ray anomaly (2344)
Reverse segond fracture (1651)
Rheumatoid arthritis (1381)
Rheumatoid arthritis of hands (ultrasound) (1378)
Rickets (1736)

Sacral insufficiency fracture (1537)
SAPHO (synovitis, acne, palmoplantar pustulosis, hyperostosis and osteitis) syndrome (1545)
Sarcoid (1534)
Scapholunate dissociation (1538)
Scheuermann disease (1452)
Scurvy (1737)
Segond fracture (1540)
Septic arthritis of the hip (1533)
Sickle cell anemia (1544)
SLE arthritis (1718)
Slipped capital femoral epiphysis (SCFE) (1445)
Stener lesion (1415)
Subacromial subdeltoid bursitis (1723)
Subcoracoid impingement (1351)
Superior labral anterior to posterior (SLAP) type III tear (1333)
Synovial osteochondromatosis (1450)
Synovial sarcoma (1562)

Talar neck fracture: Hawkins type 1 (1462)
Transient osteoporosis of hip (1435)
Triangular fibrocartilage tear (336)
Triceps tendon tear (1467)
Trigger finger (1719)
Trochanteric bursitis (1724)
Tuberculous abscess (493)
Tuberculous dactylitis (1715)
Tuberculous epidural abscess with cord compression (988)
Turf toe (1411)

Ulnar impaction syndrome (2367)
Ulnar impingement syndrome (1441)
Unicameral bone cyst (1325)

Wrisberg rip tear lateral meniscus (1344)

Difficulty Level Index

Easy Cases
1362, 526, 2328, 1384, 1537, 1445, 1387, 1538, 1394, 1471, 480, 1364, 1539, 335, 1703, 1541, 1540, 1721, 114, 1700, 1467, 1598, 1400, 1542, 1552, 1529, 1464, 2367, 1287, 1199, 1530, 209, 1321, 1723, 1724, 1698, 1531, 1331, 1725, 1553, 104, 1973, 1412, 1839, 1414, 1404, 1325, 339, 1338, 1453, 1447, 1533, 493, 1347, 1381, 1380, 1330, 1729, 1717, 1837, 1544, 1450, 1376, 1323, 1825, 2310, 1736, 1452, 1320, 1410, 1343, 1836, 1735, 529, 1007, 1006

Moderately Difficult Cases
2209, 2357, 1462, 2318, 1396, 1395, 1363, 1532, 1345, 1315, 527, 1702, 1289, 1344, 478, 2262, 2305, 1444, 1861, 1392, 1005, 1473, 1377, 1415, 1719, 336, 2250, 1648, 2232, 1399, 1411, 1649, 1557, 1455, 1326, 1367, 1429, 1324, 1720, 1599, 1441, 1555, 1318, 2355, 1334, 1451, 1389, 1547, 1398, 1333, 2344, 2309, 2311, 1463, 1460, 1461, 1436, 1439, 1860, 1339, 1430, 1349, 1449, 1737, 1548, 1730, 1718, 1534, 467, 1342, 1435, 2368, 1716, 1340, 229, 1701, 1722, 1332, 988, 1596, 1562, 1556, 1550, 1549, 1442, 1419, 1402, 1458, 1454, 1446, 1466, 1551, 1391, 1536, 1438, 1413, 1393, 1386, 228, 1470, 488

Most Difficult Cases
2308, 1734, 1545, 1715, 1437, 1425, 1651, 1378, 1459, 1374, 1341, 1319, 1379, 1472, 1351, 1420, 1457, 1316, 1571, 1558, 1369, 1397, 1469, 1844, 1317, 1004, 41

Author Index

Dhiren Shah
526, 480, 335, 1703, 1721, 114, 1700, 209, 1723, 1724, 1698, 1725, 104, 1973, 339, 493, 1717, 1837, 1836, 529, 527, 1702, 478, 1719, 336, 2250, 1648, 2232, 1649, 1720, 2355, 1718, 467, 1716, 229, 1701, 1722, 228, 488, 1715, 1651, 1844, 41

Sanjay Patel
1537, 1445, 1387, 1538, 1539, 1541, 1540, 1598, 1400, 1542, 1552, 1287, 1199, 1553, 1404, 1447, 1729, 1450, 1736, 1735, 1007, 1006, 1289, 2262, 1444, 1861, 1005, 1399, 1599, 1555, 1334, 1547, 1398, 1333, 1436, 1860, 1449, 1737, 1548, 1730, 1435, 1332, 988, 1596, 1402, 1446, 1536, 1734, 1545, 1004

Sayed Ali
1362, 2328, 1384, 1394, 1471, 1364, 1467, 1529, 1464, 2367, 1530, 1321, 1531, 1331, 1412, 1839, 1414, 1325, 1338, 1453, 1533, 1347, 1381, 1380, 1330, 1544, 1376, 1323, 1825, 2310, 1452, 1320, 1410, 1343, 2209, 2357, 1462, 2318, 1396, 1395, 1363, 1532, 1345, 1315, 1344, 2305, 1392, 1473, 1377, 1415, 1411, 1557, 1455, 1326, 1367, 1429, 1324, 1441, 1318, 1451, 1389, 2344, 2309, 2311, 1463, 1460, 1461, 1439, 1339, 1430, 1349, 1534, 1342, 2368, 1340, 1562, 1556, 1550, 1549, 1442, 1419, 1458, 1454, 1466, 1551, 1391, 1438, 1413, 1393, 1386, 1470, 2308, 1437, 1425, 1378, 1459, 1374, 1341, 1319, 1379, 1472, 1351, 1420, 1457, 1316, 1571, 1558, 1369, 1397, 1469, 1317

Acknowledgement Index

Stephen Huebner
1531, 1544, 1381, 1467, 1471, 1529, 1530, 1825, 1839, 1466, 1340, 1439, 1455, 1557, 2209

Christopher Fang
1542, 1446, 1596, 1599

Sayed Ali
1545